The
Biological
Aspects of
Normal Personality

The Biological Aspects of Normal Personality

Readings selected and comments written by

R.A.Prentky

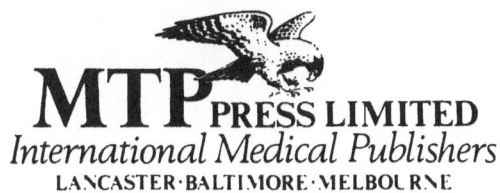

MTP PRESS LIMITED
International Medical Publishers
LANCASTER·BALTIMORE·MELBOURNE

Published by
MTP Press Limited
Falcon House
Lancaster, England

ISBN-13: 978-94-011-6216-6   e-ISBN-13: 978-94-011-6214-2
DOI: 10.1007/978-94-011-6214-2

British Library Cataloguing in Publication Data
Biological aspects of normal personality.
  1. Personality - Addresses, essays, lectures
  I. Prentky, R A
  155.2'34   BF698.9.B5

CONTENTS

PREFACE

It is the mission of this volume to accomplish two goals: (1) present a relatively *broad spectrum* or research focusing on biophysical aspects of personality, (2) select those studies examining *normal* personality. Both statements require brief clarification.

With regards to the first point, it will become evident why the qualifier 'relatively' is used. This area of inquiry is a recent one, only within the past several decades moving into the neighbourhood of scientific respectability. As such, investigation has been limited to a handful of laboratories in England and the Soviet Union. The pioneering work of Pavlov was succeeded by such dedicated disciples as Nebylitsyn, Teplov, Sokolov, Krasusky, Pushkin, Yermolaeva-Tomina, Rozhdestvenskaya, Ippolitov and Aleksandrova. The one reliable theme that has dominated Russian research is 'strength of nervous system'. A number of prolific British investigators, including Eysenck, Gray and Claridge, have also figured prominently. The race however has been run on pretty much the same track, an observation which is not intended to impune its worth. The result is that a disproportionate amount of the research presented here involves strength of nervous system and introversion/extraversion. Nevertheless, a feature of this collection is a selection of research from other areas of inquiry, such as behavioural genetics and a catchall category for neuroanatomical and neurochemical considerations.

As it stands, 'normal personality' is a straightforward enough idea. Most of us, I imagine, think that we have one. In fact, we rarely think about how 'normal' our personality is until we are confronted by a personality questionnaire, parlour game or parapsychological quiz. It is something like having a nurse or physician check our blood pressure. If it's about 130/70 we conclude we are

functioning normally. Similarly, if our MMPI profile falls entirely within the designated 'normal range' we conclude that our personality is functioning normally. Abnormal personality is thought of as so extreme (schizophrenia, manic-depression, neurosis and the like) that it bears no resemblance, surely nothing to do with 'normals'. Such reasoning is surely one of the factors contributing to the sparse research on normal personality (i.e. what is normal need not be investigated since, by definition, it is normal.). It is the thesis of this writer, and hopefully one of the messages derived from this book, that endogenous disturbances of personality represent extremes on a *continuum* of functioning, and not a biologically oblique dimension. Along the continuum are degrees of deviance. Too deviant, and we are labelled according to a DSM III category. Marginally deviant, and we are thought of as 'eccentric' or an 'oddball' but not crazy. Most of us do indeed fall under the major bulbous projection of the Gaussian curve, but none of us represent the 'mean' or epitomize the 'norm'. Our composit personality traits lie scattered along the abscissa somewhere under the umbrella. Obviously, the fine-tuned calibration of central tendency has no place at this puerile stage of investigation. However, the message is quite clear. The extraordinarily complex biochemical transmission of information in the human body is neither 'normal' or 'abnormal' but functions within tolerable ranges that vary within each individual. While at the moment we will be ignoring the tails of the distribution, it should be obvious that we cannot speak of the middle range of the distribution without casting shadows on the tails. Without such a conception of range in personality, it would be tantamount to impossible to speak of 'individual differences'. In analysis of variance terms we would be looking at a between group difference (normal vs abnormal), disregarding 'error' variance.

In modern parlance an "all-or-nothing' approach may be viewed as a synergistic theory of personality. If all biological switches are 'in series' all systems are 'go' for a normal personality. What distinguishes one personality from another is the manner in which the environment inscribes the blank slate. Abnormal personality occurs when one or more switches are out of series. The tabula rasa model suffers from parsimony. In particular, it leaves out endogenous inflences on personality which do not manifest themselves as clear aberrations. The notion of synergism, in this case, is also parsimonious as it suggests that when 'in phase' (all switches in sync) the slate will be normal. Were that the case, biology would account for no variation (or all variation) in personality.

It is not inconceivable that, as Nebylitsyn (1972) stated, one 'unified theory of neurophysiological factors of personality . . . (could) explain the innumerable dynamic variations in individual behaviour'. Nebylitsyn's complete thought on this matter is worth noting:

In the more remote perspective, we should focus attention on "deep" problems (such as that of the biological origins of individual differences in nervous system properties), since in the final analysis differences between strong and weak or between mobile and inert nervous systems should be determined by the nature of the processes occurring at the cellular level, at the level of microinformation. Each physiological individuality is basically a biochemical individuality. Sooner or later, in the agenda of scientific investigation, there will be questions about the individual microdynamics of the processes of cellular efficiency, of the spreading of the neural impulse, of threshold reactions, of adaptation and habituation, and of a whole series of neurophysiological phenomena which constitute the basis of individual differences in nervous system properties. Answers to these questions would reveal something of the essence of psychological individuality and would contribute greatly to our understanding of behaviorally significant aspects of such individuality, and possibly the extent to which these are regulated and altered by pharmacodynamic and biophysical means*.

I would like to extend a debt of gratitude to a former mentor and advisor, Dr William Revelle, for implanting and nourishing the germ that developed into my present infection. In the early stages of the development of this book I had the opportunity to exchange ideas with Professors Venables and Eysenck. I am most grateful for their encouragement and suggestions. I am also appreciative for the helpful remarks of Professors Rue Cromwell and Don Fowles. The need for a text such as this one arose during a graduate seminar I instructed on the biological bases of personality at the University of Massachusetts. To the students of that seminar I extend a warm thanks. Finally, I want to sincerely thank Shana Prentky, the one person who patiently provided three years of support for an often unmindful friend.

The preparation of this book was supported, in part, by Training Grant 00042 and Research Grant 25935, both from the National Institute of Mental Health.

RAP
Rochester, New York
October, 1978

*Nebylitsyn, V. D. *Fundamental Properties of the Human Nervous System*. p.293 London: Plenum Press, 1972.

Section One

Arousal Theory and Personality:
Methodological and Conceptual Issues

Editorial Commentary

on

Arousal Theory and Personality:
Methodological and Conceptual Issues

At the outset let me attempt to reduce the forthcoming maze of intricate and hopefully interrelated research to two basic themes. One theme takes place at the behavioural level, where it is a common observation that a primary symptom in abnormal personality involves attention and information processing. Classic notions to this effect were first advanced by Cameron (1951) and Chapman (1956a, b; 1958) in the fifties and McGhie and Chapman (1961) and Shakow (1962) in the early sixties. During the acute phase of illness, schizophrenics attend to a wide range of stimuli, 'overincluding' or 'orienting' to irrelevant stimuli in the process. Furthermore, they appear very slow to 'habituate'. Both the barrage of excess input and the failure to habituate to it cause a marked impairment in performance. It was also observed that chronic or more regressed schizophrenics seemed to process information with blinders on, tunnel vision so-to-speak. They 'underincluded' and habituated rapidly to whatever they did process. It should be pointed out that disorders involving processing of and habituation to sensory input are many and varied. Additionally, the habituation process seems integrally tied to stress (Levin, 1971). Since stress is a cardinal precipitant of many disorders, it appears that the whole system of input regulation and processing was fundamental to mental health.

The second theme lies at the neurophysiological level. Numerous attempts have been made to explain behavioural deficit in terms of 'arousal level'. Pavlov (1941) first argued that subcortical excitation of the cortex could result in low behavioural arousal due to reactive cortical inhibition *or* high behavioural arousal as a response to the excitation. Pavlov's theory will receive considerable elaboration in the next chapter. Malmo (1957, 1959) maintained that the reticular formation in the midbrain was responsible for generating excessive levels of excitation. Mednick (1958) attributed the acute phase of schizophrenia to over-responsivity to stimuli from heightened drive (arousal) level and the chronic phase to under-responsivity and a dampened drive level. Fish (1961) also argued that schizophrenia was attributable to over-activity of the reticular formation. Venables (1964, 1966) postulated that chronic schizophrenics were over-aroused, and that this condition indicated a failure of the reticular formation to selectively filter incoming stimuli. Venables concluded that the reticular formation functioned to select stimuli in modulating arousal levels in normal individuals. Broen and Storms (1966) theorized that 'latent' inappropriate responses 'surface' during periods of high arousal. High arousal produces 'response competition' by elevating the strength of formerly subdominant and inappropriate responses. Response competition then gives rise to the disorganization apparent in much schizophrenic behaviour. Epstein (1967) has argued that schizophrenia results from an 'inadequately modulated inhibitory system for controlling excitation'. In the normal case, the inhibitory system is 'fine-tuned', increments in inhibition and excitation being effectively balanced. In the abnormal case, an 'all-or-none' situation exists; excitation is blocked completely or experienced intensely. Tecce and Cole (1972) hypothesized that schizophrenic behaviour is a non-monotonic (inverted-U) function of arousal and a positive, monotonic function of attention. Tecce and Cole conceptualized 'attention' as a hypothetical organismic process which facilitates selection of relevant stimuli from the environment. Arousal was defined as a hypothetical energizing process, unselective and affecting only intensity of response. The net result is a tidy theoretical package that integrates the concepts of attention and arousal. The inverted-U-shaped function mentioned by Tecce and Cole is a ubiquitous one in personality research. It is a simple relationship stating that the *maximum* values of the dependent variable (performance usually) are found at the intermediate range of the independent variable (arousal or attention). Increases or decreases in the independent variable *diminish* the dependent variable (note the graphical illustrations in Section 2 commentary). (Of course, in the simple U-shaped function, *minimum* values of the DV are located at the intermediate range of the IV.) We have then a relatively vague conception of a possible physiological mechanism underlying the major behavioural deficit in severe psychopathology — regulation and processing of stimulus input. One strategy that has been adopted to further elucidate the physiological mechanisms responsible for pathological symptom formation is to examine peripheral measures of nervous system activity, such as electrodermal or cardiac activity. This research is represented by the extensive work of Venables (1963, 1966, 1969, 1974) and Gruzelier (1973, 1975, 1976, with Venables, 1972, 1974a, 1974b, 1975a, 1975b). Psychopathology is not the focus of this volume. Consequently, discussion of the development of research on arousal and schizophrenia will not be pursued. However, as will become evident, just as extreme deviations in nervous system activity may prompt highly pathological behaviour, moderate deviations may signal idiosyncratic behaviours within the normal range characteristically labelled as traits of personality.

This section is devoted to general problems arising in the study of personality from a neurophysiological or psychophysiological perspective. To begin with, the psychophysiological approach has its primary *raison d'etre* in establishing *electrical* correlates of behaviour. The neurophysiological approach seeks to establish *neurological* or neuroanatomical correlates of behaviour. In both cases a one-to-one correspondence is assumed. When behaviour varies, physiology varies accordingly. Physiological mechanisms serve as indicators of behavioural states. However, it is *not* appropriate to conclude that the appearance of a particular behaviour reflects the underlying physiological mechanism. If no behaviour is observed to occur, no physiological parameter can be recorded. Thus, the concurrence of behaviour and physiology is an important methodological problem, somewhat reminiscent of the James-Lange vs. Cannon debate over the temporal relationship between cognition and behaviour.

Some basic statistical considerations include alpha error resulting from multiple comparisons and significant main and interaction effects that fail to include the means comprising the main effect or the simple effects comprising the interaction. These are obviously general statistical issues, though they crop up with 'reliable' frequency in psychophysiological research. L.I.V. contamination is a more specific statistical problem that demands attention. The Law of Initial Values refers to the effect of differences in initial levels of psychophysiological activity on post-manipulation changes. For example, in a typical drug study comparing schizophrenics and normals, it is imperative that pre-drug measurement be taken and subtracted from post-drug effects. Such precaution is obviously called for when one considers the pre-manipulation assumptions about the psychophysiological differences between the contrasted groups. As an example, schizoprenics are often observed to have a higher resting heart rate than normals, regardless of drugs. In this particular situation, a covariance technique that removes variance due to individual differences in basal level should prove more satisfactory than algebraic difference scores. Another statistical problem, quite specific to this research, is the non-linearity of most psychophysiological processes. Nonlinear properties derive from the transformation of electrical signals at the receptor or synaptic junction into recordable information, as well as the presence of feedback mechanisms throughout the nervous system that produce artifactual noise which must be filtered out (Vaughn, 1975). For these and other biophysical reasons, potentials recorded from the skin and scalp may not accurately reflect the physiological activity being monitored.

Rather than introducing the research on endogenous factors in normal personality on an overly sanguine note, it was decided to confront the reality of the insuperable riddles of the brain. While we have only begun our trek into the near-to-unchartered domain of the cranium, there is no reason for not believing that a modicum of inspiration and a profusion of perspiration will ultimately yield a precise stereotaxic map of the brain and, with it, definitive answers to the question of the influence of the brain on personality.

References

Broen, W. E. and Storms, L. H. (1966). Lawful disorganization: The process underlying a schizophrenic syndrome. *Psychological Rev.* 73, 265–279

Cameron, N. and Magaret, A. (1951) *Behaviour Pathology*. (Boston: Houghton Mifflin)

Chapman, L. J. (1956a). Distractibility in the conceptual performance of schizophrenia. *J. Abnorm. Social Psychol.*, 53, 286–291

Chapman, L. J. (1956b). The role of type of distracter in the "concrete" conceptual performance of schizophrenics. *J. Personality*, 25, 130–141

Chapman, L. J. (1958) Intrusion of associative responses into schizophrenic conceptual performance. *J. Abnorm. Social Psychol.*, 56, 374–379

Epstein, S. (1967). Toward a unified theory of anxiety. In B. A. Maher (ed.) *Progress in Experimental Personality Research*, (New York: Academic Press)

Fish, F. (1961). A neurophysiological theory of schizophrenia. *J. Mental Sci.*, 107, 828–838

Gruzelier, J. H. (1973). Bilateral asymmetry of skin conductance orienting activity and levels in schizophrenics. *Biol. Psychol.*, 1973, 1, 21–41

Gruzeller, J. H. (1975). The cardiac responses of schizophrenics to orienting, signal and non-signal tones. *Biol. Psychol.*, 3, 143–155

Gruzelier, J. H. (1976). Clinical attributes of schizophrenic skin conductance responders and non-responders. *Psychol. Med.*, 6, 245–249

Gruzelier, J. H. and Venables, P. H. (1972). Skin conductance orienting activity in a heterogeneous sample of schizophrenics. *J. Nerv. Ment. Dis.*, 155, 277–286

Gruzelier, J. H. and Venables, P. H. (1974a). Bimodality and lateral asymmetry of skin conductance orienting activity in schizophrenics: Replication and evidence of lateral asymmetry in patients with depression and disorders of personality. *Biol. Psychiatry*, 8, 55–73

Gruzelier, J. H. and Venables, P. H. (1974b). Two-flash threshold, sensitivity and B in normal subjects and schizophrenics. *Q. J. Exp. Psychol.*, 26, 594 (b)

Gruzelier, J. H. and Venables, P. H. (1975a). Relations betwen two-flash discrimination and electrodermal activity, re-examined in schizophrenics and normals. *J. Psychiatri. Res.*, 12, 73–85

Gruzelier, J. H. and Venables, P. H. (1975b). Evidence of high and low levels of physiological arousal in schizophrenics. *Psychophysiology*, 12, 66–73

Levine, S. (1971). Stress and behavior. *Sci. Am.*, 224, 26–31

Malmo, R. B. (1959). Activation: A neurophysiological dimension. *Psychol. Rev.*, 66, 367–386

Malmo, R. B. (1957). Anxiety and behavioral arousal. *Psychol. Rev.*, 64, 276–287

McGhie, A. and Chapman, J. S. (1961). Disorders of attention and perception in early schizophrenia. *Br. J. Med. Psychol.*, 34, 103–116

Mednick, S. A. (1958). A learning theory approach to research in schizophrenia. *Psychol. Bull.*, 55, 316–327

Pavlov, I. P. (1941). *Conditioned Reflexes and Psychiatry*. (trans. W. H. Gantt) (New York: International University Press)

Shakow, D. (1962). Segmental set: A theory of the formal deficit in schizophrenia. *Arch. Gen. Psychiatry*, 6, 1–17

Tecce, J. J. and Cole, J. O. (1972). Psychophysiological responses of schizophrenics to drugs. *Psychopharmacologia*, 24, 159–200

Vaughn, H. (1975) Physiological approaches to psychopathology. In M. L. Kietzman, S. Sutton, and J. Zubin (eds.), *Experimental Approaches to Psychpathology*. (New York: Academic Press)

Venables, P. H. (1963). The relationship between level of skin potential and fusion of paired light flashes in schizophrenics and normals. *J. Psychiatr. Res.*, 1, 279–287

Venables, P. H. (1964). Input dysfunction in schizophrenia. In B. A. Maher (ed.), *Progress in Experimental Personality Research*. (New York: Academic Press)

Venables, P. H. (1966). A comparison of two flash and two click thresholds in schizophrenic and normal subjects. *Q. J. Exp. Psychol.*, 18, 371–373

Venables, P. H. (1969). Sensory aspects of psychopathology. In J. Zubin & C. Shagass (eds.), *Neurobiological Aspects of Psychopathology*. (New York: Grune & Stratton)

Venables, P. H. (1974). The recovery limb of the skin conductance response in "high risk" research. In S. A. Mednick, F. Schulsinger, J. Higgins, & B. Bell (eds.), *Genetics, Environment and Psychopathology*. (Amsterdam: North–Holland Publishing Company)

From M. A. Wenger, B. T. Engel and T. L. Clemens (1957). Behavioral Science, 2, 216-221, *by kind permission of the authors and Behavioral Science.*

STUDIES OF AUTONOMIC RESPONSE PATTERNS: RATIONALE AND METHODS[1]

by M. A. Wenger, B. T. Engel, and T. L. Clemens

University of California at Los Angeles

This report briefly summarizes the results of eighteen years of research on the measurement of autonomic functions in human subjects during rest, and presents a discussion of hypotheses and methodology for the study of autonomic response patterns.

Most of the report is devoted to a discussion of instrumentation and methods of measurement employed in current investigations. The following variables are measured: electrical resistance of palmar skin; respiration rate; finger, face, and axillary temperatures; heart rate, potentials and rhythms; changes in finger and leg blood volume; systolic and diastolic blood pressures; stroke volume of the heart; pupillary diameter; stomach and lower bowel motility; salivary output; and selected muscle action potentials. Most responses are amplified and recorded continuously and simultaneously by means of chopper type Offner amplifiers. Pupillary diameter and systolic and diastolic blood pressure are time sampled; the former by means of a Bolex motion picture camera, the latter by means of a Gilson automatic blood pressure recorder. Stomach motility is recorded continuously by means of a new method—a magnetometer which remotely detects the movements of a small ingested magnet. Lower bowel motility is recorded by a bipolar electrode.

IN 1939 the senior author and his associates initiated work designed to test the following restatement of the Eppinger and Hess hypothesis (3):

The differential chemical reactivity and the physiological antagonism of the adrenergic and cholinergic branches of the autonomic nervous system permit of a situation in which the action of one branch may predominate over that of the other. This predominance, or autonomic imbalance, may be phasic or chronic, and may obtain for either the adrenergic or the cholinergic system. Autonomic imbalance, when measured in an unselected population, will be distributed continuously about a central tendency which shall be defined as autonomic balance (5).

[1] This investigation was supported (in part) by research grant M-788 from the Institute of Mental Health, National Institutes of Health, Public Health Service.

The work involved the measurement of a number of autonomically innervated functions in a population of children, the intercorrelation and factorial analysis of the data, and the estimation of the obtained autonomic factor for the individual children. Such factor estimates were called "Scores of Autonomic Balance," and their distribution was found to be approximately normal. It was concluded that the original Eppinger and Hess hypothesis was supported, and that it fitted the obtained results better than did the restatement; i.e., the obtained factor could more logically be interpreted as a sympathetic-parasympathetic continuum than as representing relative dominance of adrenergic or cholinergic divisions.

Further studies with children (6, 7, 10)

and with adults (8) led to the following conclusions:

1. Individual differences in autonomic functioning during controlled rest exist in both children and adults.

2. These differences, measured in terms of an autonomic factor, are continuously distributed and are presumed to be normally distributed in an unselected population. Vagotonia and sympathicotonia, as described by Eppinger and Hess, are regarded as representing extremes on such a continuum.

3. The autonomic factor for a given individual tends to remain constant from year to year, but it may be altered phasically or chronically by changes in external or internal stimulation.

4. Autonomic factor scores are related to certain personality patterns and to certain diagnostic categories, such as anxiety psychoneurosis, battle fatigue, and asthma.

5. Autonomic factor scores do not necessarily reflect a consistent pattern of autonomic balance or imbalance. That is, some individuals demonstrate autonomic patterns wherein some functions suggest an apparent dominance of the sympathetic branch and others indicate an apparent dominance of the parasympathetic branch. Individual differences in patterns of action, therefore, are considered to be significant.

6. Autonomic factor scores from resting data are not necessarily related to autonomic reactivity under stimulation.

The last conclusion is based on a study, not yet published, which found that frequencies of symptoms reported under nine autonomomimetic drugs were related to scores of autonomic balance, but that autonomic reactivity under the drugs was related more closely to autonomic reactivity to a placebo. This study and many other observations convinced us that measures of autonomic balance in a resting state must be supplemented by measures of response patterns to stimuli for which the normative response is established, if ANS data are to prove of more than limited usefulness in the prediction of behavior.

Although many investigators have studied reactivity of discrete ANS functions, and a few have used several variables in their studies,[2] the validity of one, or a few, ANS variables as a measure of total ANS response has never been investigated. A comprehensive and systematic research seemed indicated. Accordingly, our present program on "Studies of Autonomic Response Patterns" was undertaken.

This program, which got under way in 1954, has the following specific objectives:

1. To develop practicable techniques of measurement and statistical analysis of autonomic response patterns in man.

2. To investigate resting, primary, recovery, and secondary autonomic response patterns in man to a variety of physical and psychological stimuli in order to determine (a) group central tendencies to specific stimuli, (b) the nature of individual response pattern differences, and (c) the possibility of classifying stimuli according to group response patterns.

3. To investigate the value of autonomic response patterns in standard test situations for the prediction of psychosomatic and other abnormal reactions to subsequent stressors.

4. To investigate the relationship of autonomic response patterns to personality.

5. To test the hypothesis that emotional behavior in man is characterized by at least eight fundamentally different autonomic response patterns.

6. To determine the most significant variables in autonomic response patterns, so that the number of variables in future research may be reduced.

Certain general hypotheses also may be mentioned:

I. Patterns of autonomic response in man demonstrate consistent variation according to the stimuli which elicit them.

II. Differential autonomic response patterns in man provide a basis for an objective classification of stimulus effect.

III. Consistent individual differences in autonomic response patterns to a given stimulus occur in both primary and secondary responses.

IV. Individual differences in autonomic response patterns, supplemented by differences in autonomic balance, furnish a basis

---

[2] This work is reviewed in connection with other publications from this project.

M. A. WENGER, B. T. ENGEL, AND T. L. CLEMENS

for the prediction of men who cannot well withstand physical and psychological stress and men who may develop specific psychosomatic and other psychological disorders.

V. Such predictions will afford a background for preventive therapy which will serve to decrease the frequency of psychological disorders.

The long-term objectives of the program are to test the above-stated hypotheses by simultaneous measurement of as many ANS responses as prove practicable, as elicited by a wide range of physical, physiological, and psychological stimuli, with a follow-up study of subjects with respect to life-stress reactions and disorders.

The remainder of this report describes our methods of measurement.

(A) *General Apparatus:* Twelve channels of recording include an 8-channel Offner[3] type D3 Electroencephalograph, three type 133 Offner DC amplifiers, and one special channel. The console accommodates a 24-inch Offner Dynograph (polygraph) which employs 11 standard pen-motors with 6 ohm coils and one special 600 ohm pen-motor. Six paper speeds are available: .125, .25, .625, 1.25, 2.5 and 6.25 cm./sec. Our typical recording speed is .125 cm. per sec., or about 3″ per minute. A special filter switching panel provides for independent variable time constants when recording through the pre-amplifiers of the D3; and the chopper-type amplifiers employed in this apparatus permit drift-free DC recording when the pre-amplifiers are by-passed. Impedance matching in the latter case is accomplished by means of coupling transformers to which a balancing circuit is added to allow manual recentering of the pens. Such couplers are comparable to the Offner Input Coupler, type 9138. The 12th amplifier is specially constructed for the recording of stomach motility. It drives the 600 ohm pen and is described elsewhere (11).

Two other channels of information are used: (a) A Gilson[4] Automatic Blood Pressure Recorder (4) provides automatic inflation and deflation of a standard area cuff at any of four time intervals (1″, 5″, 30″, 60″), or by manual control. The pulse sound from the brachial artery is detected by a Brush pressure microphone, amplified, and recorded on chart paper which moves only as the cuff deflates. A second pen records the inflation pressure, which is pre-set, and the curve of deflation. The chart is calibrated in mm. Hg., and the points of *appearance* and *marked muffling* (1st and 4th blood pressure phases) can be read on the deflation curve as systolic and diastolic blood pressure respectively. (b) A Bolex, 16 mm. motion picture camera loaded with Eastman cine-kodak high speed infrared film, emulsion #2183, is used to record changes in the pupils of the eyes and/or facial expression. Two Sylvania infrared self-contained reflector type heat lamps are placed three feet from the subject and directed at his face. The increase in temperature on the face is negligible[5] since the lamps are operated at 55 rather than 110 volts AC. A type 200 C, 5 amp. General Radio Company variac is used to reduce voltage input to the lamps. The camera may be operated manually by remote cable control or by a motor-driven trigger. For most work the latter is employed with one exposure every three seconds. Calibration is accomplished with a black grease pencil mark of known length drawn directly below the subject's left eye.

All of the above apparatus except the camera and its automatic trigger are contained in one room. In an adjoining semi-soundproofed room is a shielded cage (size 9 x 6 x 6 ft.) which houses the cot for the subject and the pick-up units which are described in the following sections. The cot consists of a foam-rubber mattress on a firm wooden base so that no movements of metal structures occur. The head of the cot is adjustable, with hinges at 21 inches from the top. The typical elevation is 6½ inches. (Initial work employed a chaise-lounge with rope support for the pad, which is shown in published pictures of our laboratory [12, p. 268]. It has been supplanted by a structure which is longer, wider, and higher.)

[3] Offner Electronics, Inc., Chicago 25, Illinois.
[4] Gilson Medical Electronics, Madison, Wisconsin.

[5] The temperature at the concentration point of the two lights was found to rise 1° C within ten minutes and to maintain this level for 40 minutes.

A window between the rooms permits observation of the subject, and furnishes reflected light to the subject's room—the only lighting typically employed. An intercommunication system permits constant monitoring of sounds from the subject's room, and communication with the subject when desired. Any or all of the communication may be recorded on a long-playing tape recorder. An air conditioner provides constant room temperature in all seasons.

(B) *Recordable Variables:* Three of the recordable physiologic variables already have been mentioned: Pupillary diameter and systolic and diastolic blood pressure. Others are described in the following paragraphs. All utilize the Offner AC/DC equipment, and are selected according to the experiment.

1. *Electrical Skin Resistance:* For recording skin resistance, a constant current of 40 microamperes is impressed through electrodes made of zinc plates 2 cm. in diameter, encased in a plastic cup. Contact with the skin is made with an agar zinc sulfate electrode paste.[6] A Darrow-type bridge (2) with a range of 500,000 ohms is utilized, and the output is DC amplified. Calibration is determined by bridge regulation.

2. *Respiration:* The pick-up for respiration consists of an aluminum plate .035 inches thick, $5\frac{1}{2}$ inches long and $1\frac{1}{2}$ inches wide. The center is bent into an arch within which a Baldwin SR4 type C-14 strain gauge[7] (nominal resistance 2000 ohms) is cemented. The ends of the aluminum plate are attached to a cloth strip which fastens around S's chest. As respiratory movements bend the plate, the strain gauge is stretched and its electrical resistance changes concomitantly. This variable resistor is one arm of a Wheatstone bridge which is powered by

a $22\frac{1}{2}$ volt battery. The output is DC amplified. Amplitude is not calibrated.

3. *Skin Temperature:* Temperatures of the face, finger, and axilla (and room temperature) are recorded through a DC amplifier by means of Western Electric type 14B thermistors. Resistances of the thermistors vary from approximately 2000 ohms at 23° C to approximately 975 ohms at 41° C. Each thermistor functions as one arm of a Wheatstone bridge which is powered by a $1\frac{1}{2}$ volt battery. All temperatures are recorded on one channel by means of a constant speed, motor-driven, selector switch which samples face and axillary temperatures once and finger temperature twice every 10 seconds. Room temperature is selectively recorded by means of a separate, manually operated switch. Calibration is accomplished by substituting known resistances for the thermistors, whose resistances at given temperatures have been predetermined. The sensitivity of each thermistor is controlled by means of a voltage divider from the bridge power supply. Thermistors are attached with adhesive tape which also covers the sensing element, to the right cheek and tip of the second finger of the right or left hand depending upon experimental requirements. A third thermistor, mounted on a sponge rubber pad and placed in the axilla, is held in position by the pressure of the subject's arm. Room temperature is recorded from a free thermistor.

4. *Heart Rate and Variability:* Heart rate appears on several channels. The most dependable measure is the typical EKG obtained from AC recording with standard electrodes. Lead II usually is employed. In some experiments a cardiotachometer[8] is used with DC amplification to measure the period of each heart cycle. The pick-up electrodes are the same as those for the EKG except that lead IV is used to obtain maximum QRS potentials. Condensor discharge time reflects individual heart periods, and determines the deflection of the recording pen. Calibration involves a constant speed motor with a series of contacts designed to establish records equivalent to 30, 90, 120 and 180 heart cycles per minute.

---

[6] Forty grams of Penick's USP No. 1 powdered agar-agar, 3 grams zinc sulfate ($ZnSO_4$), in 257 ml. of distilled H_2O. The solution, premixed cold in a 600 ml. Pyrex beaker, is placed into a 1″ bath of boiling water and cooked with constant stirring for 1 minute and 45 seconds. After cooling it is placed in air-tight jars.

[7] Baldwin-Lima-Hamilton Corp., Philadelphia 42, Pa.; or the entire pick-up unit is available from Electro-Medical Engineering Co., Burbank, Calif.

[8] Constructed by Electro-Medical Engineering Co., Burbank, Calif.

5. *Finger Plethysmograph:* A small plastic cup is placed over the index finger so that 4 cc. of the finger are enclosed. The system is made air-tight with caulking compound. Tygon plastic tubing (size $\frac{3}{8}''$ diameter) connects the cup to a P97-0.05D-350 Statham pressure transducer[9] used as a gauge transducer. Blood volume changes in the finger then activate the unit which is powered by a 10 volt battery. Amplification is either DC, as is typical, or AC. The latter has certain advantages and is being investigated (1). A balancing and calibrating circuit described by Statham is utilized. Calibration is accomplished by switching a resistor in parallel with one arm of the transducer bridge. The resulting pen displacement equals that produced by a digital volume change of .01 cc.

6. *Leg Plethysmograph:* A standard blood pressure cuff is placed around the calf of the left leg, and inflated to 20 mm. Hg. Pressure changes from the cuff produced by changes in blood volume of the leg activate a Statham P5-0.2D-1800 differential pressure transducer powered by a 28 volt battery. The output typically receives DC amplification, but AC recording is being investigated.

7. *Stomach Motility:* Only a brief description will be given here since the technique for recording this function is discussed elsewhere (9, 11). The subject swallows a $\frac{3}{16}'' \times \frac{1}{2}''$ plastic-coated cast Alnico #5 magnetic rod,[10] the movements of which are remotely detected by a modified Waugh Magnetometer.[11] A magnetic phase detector generates a variable current which is proportional to the lines of magnetic force cut by the magnet. The signal is increased by means of an AC amplifier and then is filtered to give a DC signal. Recording is either by standard Offner DC equipment or with our special amplifier (11).

8. *Muscle Potentials:* Muscle activity of frontalis or of the flexors and extensors of the left forearm is measured in some experiments with silver electrodes, 8 mm. in diameter and 10 cm. apart. Cambridge electrode jelly is used to maximize conductance; and the electrodes are secured to the skin by means of collodion. The Offner D-3 has a built-in calibrator which covers a range of 10 to 1000 microvolts in seven steps. This is utilized to calibrate muscle potentials and other AC signals.

9. *Salivation:* We have made many attempts to record salivation continuously, either by weight or volume displacement. Such measurement requires a wide range of operation with great stability and sensitivity. The most promising technique at present consists of a lever system comprising a steel plate, $8\frac{1}{2}$ inches in length, 3 inches wide, and .08 inches thick, attached solidly to a plastic block on one end and engaging a Statham G1-1-1000 force transducer on the other end. A graduated 100 ml. cylinder is fastened to this plate. One tube from the double-hole stopper closing the cylinder goes to a rubber-tipped saliva ejector which is placed in the subject's mouth, and another goes to a negative pressure pump. As saliva is collected in the cylinder the added weight bends the plate slightly and activates the transducer which is very sensitive, having a maximum range of 2 oz. and a maximum displacement of .003 inches. 20 volts is impressed across the transducer bridge and the output receives DC amplification. A 1000 MFD, 25V Cornell-Dubilier dielectric capacitor is placed across the output to filter out disturbances caused by the negative pressure pump and movements of the subject. The calibrating resistor is chosen to give a pen displacement equivalent to a weight of 2 ml. of H_2O introduced into the collecting bottle. Increases in rate of salivary flow are reflected by a steeper slope of the recorded line.

10. *Ballistic Index of Cardiac Output:* The pick-up for this measure is an Astatic L-12-U crystal phonograph cartridge with a maximal signal output of 4 volts. A 4.3 megohm load resistor is placed across the output terminals. The cartridge is encased in sponge rubber without a phonograph needle and is strapped to the subject's leg six inches above the ankle. The signal receives AC amplification and calibration is in microvolts. The

---

[9] Statham Laboratories, Inc., Los Angeles 64, Calif.

[10] Terry Sales Corporation, 2910 South La Cienega Blvd., Culver City, Calif.

[11] Now manufactured by E. M. Irwin, 1238 S. Gerhart Avenue, Los Angeles 22, Calif.

record provides a crude measure of cardiac output.

11. *Radial Pulse:* Exploratory work has been done employing a Statham P81-5G-350 transducer placed over the radial artery in an effort to obtain a continuous measure of systolic and diastolic blood pressure. Attachment has been made with rubber sponges and straps, or with a plastic band shaped to curve around the wrist and hold the transducer in place. Initial results with this technique appear promising but a number of improvements are necessary. In particular the system is too sensitive to movements by the subject. A more appropriately shaped transducer and a better method of attachment are indicated.

12. *Motility of the Lower Bowel:* A bipolar electrode of our own design is inserted into the lower bowel through the anus and is held in place by the internal sphincter. Both AC and DC records of changes in potentials have been obtained from a few subjects. If further work indicates that significant data are obtainable by this method the electrode will be described elsewhere.

REFERENCES

1. Clemens, T. L., & Wenger, M. A. A comparison of DC and AC recording of finger blood volume. (In preparation; to be submitted, *J. appl. Physiol.*)

2. Darrow, C. W. Uniform current for continuous standard unit resistance records. *J. gen. Psychol.*, 1932, 6, 471–493.

3. Eppinger, H., & Hess, L. *Die Vagotonie*, Berlin, 1910. (Trans. *Vagotonia*; Mental and Nervous Disease Monograph, No. 20; New York: Nerv. and Ment. Dis. Publ. Co., 1915).

4. Gilson, W. E. An automatic blood pressure recorder. *Electronics*, May 1942.

5. Wenger, M. A. The measurement of individual differences in autonomic balance. *Psychosom. Med.*, 1941, 3, 427–434.

6. Wenger, M. A. The stability of measurement of autonomic balance. *Psychosom. Med.*, 1942, 4, 94–95.

7. Wenger, M. A. Seasonal variations in some physiologic variables. *J. lab. clin. Med.*, 1943, 28, 1101–1108.

8. Wenger, M. A. Studies of autonomic balance in Army Air Forces personnel. *Comp. Psychol. Monog.*, Vol. 19, No. 4; Berkeley: University of California Press, 1948.

9. Wenger, M. A., Engel, B. T., & Clemens, T. L. Stomach motility as recorded by the magnetometer method. (To be submitted, *Gastroenterol.*)

10. Wenger, M. A., & Ellington, M. The measurement of autonomic balance in children: Method and normative data. *Psychosom. Med.*, 1943, 5, 241–253.

11. Wenger, M. A., Henderson, E. B., & Dinning, J. S. A magnetometer method for recording gastric motility. (Submitted, *Science.*)

12. Wenger, M. A., Jones, N. F., & Jones, M. H. *Physiological psychology.* New York: Holt, 1956.

(Manuscript received December 3, 1956.)

The scientist has his guesses as to how the finished picture will work out; he depends largely on these in his search for other pieces to fit; but his guesses are modified from time to time by unexpected developments as the fitting proceeds. These revolutions of thought as to the final picture do not cause the scientist to lose faith in his handiwork, for he is aware that the completed portion is growing steadily. Those who look over his shoulder and use the present partially developed picture for purposes outside science, do so at their own risk.

—A. S. EDDINGTON in *The Nature of the Physical World*

From E. Duffy (1957). Psychological Review, *64*, 265-275, *by kind permission of the American Psychological Association.*

THE PSYCHOLOGICAL SIGNIFICANCE OF THE CONCEPT OF "AROUSAL" OR "ACTIVATION"

ELIZABETH DUFFY

The Woman's College of the University of North Carolina

The concept of "arousal," "activation," or "energy mobilization," as developed by the writer over a period of many years (7, 9, 10, 11, 13), and employed by others in various contexts (15, 18, 25, 40), has wide applicability in psychology.[1] A fuller discussion of the topic will be presented elsewhere. Pending its appearance, however, it may be of interest to point out some of the areas which this concept should serve to illuminate.

It has been argued in previous papers (10, 12) that all variations in behavior may be described as variations in either the direction[2] of behavior or the intensity of behavior. Only one part of this argument is essential for the present purpose. Whatever may be the reaction to the attempt to reduce the descriptive categories of psychology to two basic types of concept, we can proceed without dispute provided only it is agreed that intensity is a characteristic of behavior which can be abstracted and studied separately. It is the intensity aspect of behavior which has been variously referred to as the degree of excitation, arousal, activation, or energy mobilization.

I have argued that such abstraction from the totality of behavior is a necessary procedure if the psychologist is to be enabled to manipulate variables in a way likely to provide solutions to some of his problems. Confusion of the direction of behavior with the intensity of behavior, resulting in their fortuitous combination in certain psychological concepts (10) and in the "trait" names used to describe personality (12), was suggested as a possible basis for some of the unrewarding findings in many psychological investigations. Since the intensity of response can vary independently of the direction of response, it was proposed that it should be measured independently and its correlates investigated.

Perhaps a parallel may be seen in the analysis of sensory function.[3] Before

[1] The terms "activation" and "arousal," as used here, do not refer specifically to the activation pattern in the EEG. On the contrary, they refer to variations in the arousal or excitation of the individual as a whole, as indicated roughly by any one of a number of physiological measures (*e.g.*, skin resistance, muscle tension, EEG, cardiovascular measures, and others). The degree of arousal appears to be best indicated by a combination of measures.

[2] "Direction" in behavior refers merely to the fact that the individual does "this" rather than "that," or responds positively to certain cues and negatively to others.

[3] For this suggestion of a parallel, I am indebted to Dr. R. B. Malmo, who, in the fall of 1955, was kind enough to read the major portion of my manuscript for a forthcoming book, and to discuss it with his staff.

ELIZABETH DUFFY

progress could be made in the study of sensation and its physical correlates, it was necessary to separate the dimension of intensity from that of other sensory characteristics. In audition, for example, loudness was distinguished from pitch, and was related to a different type of variation in the physical stimulus. In vision, brightness was separated from hue, and each of these aspects of vision was related to the appropriate type of variation in the stimulus. Little progress in the understanding of sensation could have been made until suitable abstractions from the total sensory experience had been achieved, and these identifiable aspects of the totality had been investigated separately.

Measurement of the intensity of response (i.e., the degree of excitation, arousal, activation, or energy mobilization), it has been pointed out, may be achieved, at least in rough fashion, through various means (9, 10, 13, 15). Among the physiological measures which may be employed are skin conductance, muscle tension, the electroencephalogram (EEG), pulse rate, respiration, and others. These measures show intercorrelations, although the correlation coefficients are not always high since there is patterning in the excitation of the individual, the nature of which appears to depend upon the specific stimulus situation and upon organic factors within the individual.[4] Nevertheless, there is evidence also of "generality" of the excitation. Hence a concept of arousal, or energy mobilization, appears to be justified.

It should be noted that the physiological measures which serve as indicants of arousal, and which correlate at least to some degree with each other, include

[4] The patterning of excitation is discussed more fully in the manuscript referred to in Footnote 3. It is believed that a more adequate concept of excitation, or activation, is thereby developed.

measures of autonomic functions, of skeletal-muscle functioning, and of the functioning of the higher nerve centers. It is clear that it is the *organism*, and not a single system, or a single aspect of response, which shows arousal or activation.

The historical roots of the concept of activation lie in Cannon's concept of "energy mobilization" during "emotion" (3). Unlike Cannon's concept, however, the present concept of activation or arousal is designed to describe the intensity aspect of *all* behavior (10, 12). Referred to as the "degree of excitation," it was, in 1934, defined as "the extent to which the organism as a whole is activated or aroused" (9, p. 194). Both its definition and its proposed mode of measurement have in more recent publications followed the line suggested at that time (10, 13). When, however, studies of the electroencephalogram provided data on the behavioral correlates of changes in the EEG, it was sugggested that this measure also provided an indication of the degree of arousal (13).

To those unfamiliar with the concept of activation, confusion frequently arises between the degree of internal arousal (referred to by the concept) and the vigor and extent of overt responses. While the degree of internal arousal usually correlates fairly closely with the intensity of overt response, a discrepancy between the two may be introduced by the intervention of inhibitory processes, a phenomenon which has not received the degree of attention to which it is entitled. An additional source of confusion is the tendency on the part of some to confuse activation or excitability with vitality. Actually, it is suggested that these two characteristics are more likely to be negatively related than to be positively related. The tendency to be frequently and intensely aroused leads no doubt to fatigue and to a consequent reduction in vitality.

The chief point in regard to arousal, which I have repeatedly made (10, 11, 12, 13), is that arousal occurs in a *continuum*, from a low point during deep sleep to a high point during extreme effort or great excitement, with no distinguishable break for such conditions as sleep or "emotion." Evidence supporting this contention has been presented specifically for skin conductance, muscle tension, and the EEG (13). Recently Lindsley has elaborated upon the conception as it applies to the EEG (25), although earlier, in his "activation theory of emotion" (24, pp. 504–509), he had been of the opinion that "emotion" and sleep were conditions which were correlated with certain changes in the EEG, while conditions intermediate between the two were held to be as yet unexplained.

The factors which produce variations in the degree of arousal are various. They include, apparently, drugs, hormones, variations in physical exertion, and variations in what is commonly referred to as the degree of motivation. It appears that differences in the degree of arousal in different individuals may have a genetic or an environmental basis, or both. This conclusion is suggested from animal studies and from the relatively few studies of human beings in which the problem has been considered.

One of the potential contributions to psychology of the concept of arousal is that of breaking down the distinction between "drives" or "motives" and "emotion" (10, 11). The same kinds of physiological changes may be observed to occur in these variously designated conditions, and, depending upon the degree of arousal, to produce the same sorts of effect upon behavior. It has been contended that "emotion" is in no sense a unique condition, and that our

investigations should not be directed toward the study of "emotion" as such (9).

In the study of "motivation," the concept of arousal is of distinct service. By means of the physiological measures which serve as indicants of arousal, we may secure a direct measure of the degree (intensity) of "motivation." [5] Any other measure must of necessity be less direct. When all factors affecting the level of arousal except the degree of incentive value or threat value are held constant, measurement of the degree of arousal affords a measure of the "motivating" value of a given situation. It also affords, incidentally, an objective measure of what is called the "stress" imposed by a situation.

Physiological measurements made in a wide variety of situations have shown the expected correspondence between the degree of arousal and the apparent degree of significance of the situation— i.e., its incentive value or its threat value (13). For example, men undergoing flight training were found to show more tension of the muscles during the solo stage of training than during other stages, and during the maneuvers of take-off and landing than during other maneuvers (39). Galvanic skin responses obtained during replies to questions about provocative social problems were found to be smaller if the replies were in harmony with group opinion than if they were not, and "Yes" responses were found in general to be associated with smaller galvanic reactions than "No" responses (34).

The concept of activation holds fur-

[5] The concept of "motivation," as currently employed, is a "compound" concept which incorporates a description of both the "drive level," or arousal aspect, of behavior and also the direction taken by behavior, i.e., the selectivity of response. These two aspects of behavior may vary independently, though both are characteristically affected by a certain stimulus-condition such as hunger.

ther significance for psychology by virtue of the fact that variations in the degree of activation are, on the average, accompanied by certain variations in overt response.[6] The degree of activation appears to affect the speed, the intensity, and the coordination of responses. In general, the optimal degree of activation appears to be a moderate one, the curve which expresses the relationship between activation and quality of performance taking the form of an inverted U. This conclusion, as it relates to muscular tension and performance, was suggested by me in 1932 (8, pp. 544–546), by Freeman in several papers published around that time (15), and later by Courts (4). That it holds also for other indicators of the degree of activation is suggested by Freeman's finding that skin resistance and reaction time, measured simultaneously on a single subject for 105 trials over a number of days, gave an inverted U-shaped curve when plotted on a graph (14). More recently the EEG has been found to show the same sort of relationship to reaction time (22).

The effect of any given degree of activation upon performance appears to vary, however, with a number of factors, including the nature of the task to be performed and certain characteristics of the individual—such as, perhaps, the ability to inhibit and coordinate responses under a high degree of excitation (8). Organismic interaction is the basic explanatory principle suggested to account for the particular effects upon performance of various degrees of activation. Such organismic interaction may also, it appears, have some effect upon sensory thresholds. Again the possibility presents itself that the relationship may take the form of an inverted U-shaped curve.

[6] These studies are reviewed in the manuscript referred to in Footnote 3.

When performance has been observed to vary under certain conditions, such as those of drowsiness, of fatigue, or of "emotion," it is suggested that the variation may be due, at least in part, to the effect of varying degrees of arousal. The disorganization of responses frequently reported during "overmotivation" or "emotion," for example, may be conceived of as resulting in part from too high a degree of arousal. Such a condition would be represented at one end of the U-shaped curve. A similar disorganization of responses, found sometimes during drowsiness or fatigue, would be represented at the other end of the curve showing the relationship between arousal and performance. In any case, it seems clear that prediction of overt response to a given set of stimulating conditions can be increased in accuracy when there is knowledge of the degree of internal arousal.

It appears also that, under similar stimulation, individuals differ in the degree of their arousal and in the speed with which they return to their former level of functioning. Moreover, there is evidence of consistency in this individual variation. Apparently the individual who responds with intensity in one situation will, on the average, respond with intensity in other situations also, as compared with other individuals. While the degree of arousal varies with the situation, the rank in arousal tends to be preserved. Different individuals appear to vary around different central tendencies —i.e., to differ in responsiveness. The easily aroused, or more responsive, individual has been found to show this responsiveness in many different forms, some of which will be described below.

For instance, subjects who showed a large number of galvanic skin responses when there was no observable stimulation also showed less adaptation of the galvanic skin response (GSR) to repeated stimulation (33).

Similarly, the frequency of the alpha rhythm in normal adults has been reported to show a significant relationship to ratings on the behavioral continuum called "primary-secondary function" (32). Individuals in whom the alpha rhythm was more rapid tended to show more "primary functioning," or to be "quick, impulsive, variable, and highly stimulable." Those with relatively low frequencies of the alpha rhythm tended to show more "secondary functioning," or to be "slow, cautious, steady, with an even mood and psychic tempo. . . ." Mundy-Castle hypothetically ascribed these behavioral differences to differences in excitability within the central nervous system, the "primary functioning" individuals showing the greater excitability. A difference in neural excitability was also suggested as the explanation of his finding that there was a significant difference in the EEG activity evoked by rhythmic photic stimulation between subjects with a mean alpha frequency above 10.3 cycles per second and those with a mean alpha frequency below that rate.[7] He offered the same explanation of the greater incidence of "following"[8] in the beta range by those subjects showing little alpha rhythm, even when the eyes were closed, as compared with those subjects showing persistent alpha rhythms (32).

Gastaut and his collaborators have also reported individual differences in cortical excitability (17). While their major purpose was not the investigation of individual differences, they made the incidental observation that calm individuals had a slow, high-voltage alpha rhythm (8–10 c./s.), with little "driving" of occipital rhythms by photic stimulation. Neurons showed a long recuperation time, synchrony of response was said to be noticeable, and recruitment poor. "Nervous" individuals, on the other hand, were said to have a high-frequency, low-voltage alpha rhythm (10–13 c./s.), which at times was not perceptible. They were described as having a short neuronal recuperation time, little synchrony of response, good recruitment, and considerable driving by photic stimulation. In other words, "calm" as compared with "nervous" individuals showed less cortical excitability.

Differences in the EEG's of different individuals under similar stimulating conditions appear to be correlated also with differences in another form of responsiveness—i.e., differences in the threshold of deep reflexes. It has been reported that normal subjects with deep reflexes which are difficult to elicit showed a high percentage of alpha activity and little or no fast activity, while those with deep reflexes which were hyperactive had little alpha activity and a high percentage of fast activity (21). However, while groups at the two extremes of reflex responsiveness differed significantly in the percentage of alpha activity, there was wide variation in the extent of such activity within any one of the groups formed on the basis of reflex status. Amplitude of rhythm was observed to be greatest in EEG records showing pronounced alpha activity.

Proneness to develop anxiety under stress, which may perhaps be regarded as a form of hyperresponsiveness, has been found, in both normal subjects and psychiatric patients, to be associated with a significantly smaller percentage

[7] It is believed, he says, that "electrical rhythms in the brain can be initiated or augmented by a process similar to resonance; in other words, if an area of the brain is subjected to rhythmic impulses corresponding to its own latent or actual frequency, it may itself oscillate for as long as stimulation is maintained" (33, p. 319). It is thought that the area may also be activated by stimulation harmonically related to its own.

[8] "Following" refers to electrical responses in the cortex occurring at the stimulus frequency.

ELIZABETH DUFFY

of resting brain-wave activity in the alpha region when this activity is determined by automatic frequency analysis (35). The anxiety-prone groups showed more fast activity (16–24 c./s.), or more slow activity (3–7 c./s.), below the alpha range. The significance of the slow activity is not as clear as that of the fast activity. Fast activity may be presumed to be indicative of a high level of excitation. It has been observed, for example, at the beginning of EEG recording in normal subjects who are unusually apprehensive about the procedure, and it has been found to disappear with reassurance and the attainment of relaxation (24). It appears at least possible that the slow activity may be due to fatigue from previous states of intense arousal.

In an investigation employing prison farm inmates, schizophrenics, and control subjects, to whom a group of psychological tests were given. it was reported that EEG activity above 16–20 c./s. appeared in significant amounts only in the records of those who, as rated by the psychological tests, showed anxiety to a marked degree (20). Slow activity was said not to be very prevalent, but when it did occur, to be found most often among the patients.

These and other studies suggest that anxiety-proneness may be conceived of as a form of overarousal or hyperresponsiveness. The EEG's of the anxiety-prone seem very similar in most instances to the EEG's of other subjects whose exceptional responsiveness to the environment is indicated by active reflexes, or by ratings on "primary function."

Degree of tension of the skeletal muscles is another indicator of responsiveness, or ease and extent of arousal, in which differences between individuals have been found. In almost every investigation in which tension of the skeletal musculature has been measured,

wide differences between individuals in the degree of tension have been noted.[9] In the same stimulus situation, one individual would respond with a relatively low degree of. tension, another with a moderate degree, and a third with a high degree of tension. Moreover, when observed in a *different* stimulus situation, the subjects. while varying in their absolute level of tension, would tend to preserve their ranks with respect to tension of the muscles. It was thus shown that different individuals vary around different central tendencies, so that one individual might be characterized as being in general tense, and another as being in general relaxed.

In early studies of muscular tension. the writer found, in two separate investigations, that nursery school children showed marked individual differences in grip pressure while engaged in various tasks, and that there was a significant correlation between the grip pressure on one occasion and that on another, and during one task and during another (6. 7). Grip pressure scores were found to be independent of the strength of grip as indicated by dynamometer scores, but to be related to ratings on excitability and on adjustment to the nursery school, the tense children being rated as more excitable and, on the average. less well adjusted.

Arnold also found that individuals tended to preserve their rank in the group with respect to pressure from the hand during repetition of the same task and during the performance of different tasks (2).

A study of airplane pilots in training revealed that some showed excessive muscle tension (pressure on stick and on rudder pedal) in both take-offs and

[9] Differences in muscle tension will, for the purposes of this discussion, refer to differences in pressure exerted by some group of muscles or to .differences in electric potentials from muscles.

landings, while others showed little tension on either maneuver (39). No individuals were found who in general tended to be tense during take-offs alone or during landings alone.

Further evidence that individuals who are more highly activated than others in one stimulus situation, as indicated by tension of the skeletal muscles, are more responsive to a wide variety of stimuli, is presented in studies by Lundervold (26). "Tense" subjects, as compared with "relaxed" subjects, were found to show more activity in the muscles when external conditions were changed, as by an increase in noise, the lowering of the room temperature, or the introduction of certain stimuli which caused irritation or anger. In these persons, there was not only more activity in the single muscle, but also electrical activity in more muscles, including muscles which did not participate directly in the movement. At the end of thirty minutes of noise, fifty per cent of the tense subjects, as compared with none of the relaxed subjects, showed more action potentials than they had shown before the noise began.

A similar relationship between muscular tension and another form of responsiveness was earlier shown by Freeman and Katzoff, who found a significant correlation between grip-pressure scores and scores on the Cason Common Annoyance Test (16). Subjects with higher pressure scores tended to be more frequently or intensely annoyed—i.e., to show greater responsiveness of the sort referred to as "irritability."

It appears that, on the whole, skeletal-muscle tension in one part of the body tends to be positively related to that in other parts of the body, though the relationship between the tension in any two areas may not be very close. Parts of the body more remote from each other, or more widely differentiated in function, yield tension measures which

are less closely related than those which are closer together or functionally more similar. When tension measures taken from different parts of the body, recorded during different tasks, or made at widely separated intervals of time, nevertheless show a significant positive correlation with each other, it must, however, be concluded that there is at least some degree of "generality" in skeletal-muscle tension. Moreover, from measuring the responsiveness of the skeletal-muscle system, we may apparently predict to some extent the response of highly integrated systems of reaction described as "personality traits." Indeed, in a study in which no direct measure of muscular tension was employed, but in which ratings on muscular tension and measures of sixteen physiological variables were intercorrelated and submitted to factor analysis, a factor defined as muscular tension showed correlation with certain personality characteristics (36).

Since conditions of high activation may perhaps increase the likelihood of disorganization of motor responses, it is not surprising that measures of tremor and other forms of motor disorganization have been found to be related to the severity of conflicts (31) and to neuroticism (1, 19, 23, 28, 29, 30). Measures of irregularity in pressure appear to be among the measures which discriminate best between a normal and a psychiatric population, a finding which might be expected if, as suggested by the writer (8) and by Luria (27), irregular pressure tracings are indicative of poor coordination or lack of control of responses.

Other indicants of arousal have also been shown to be related to more complex forms of response. For example, it has been said that a reasonably accurate prediction of a person's respiratory rate at a given time during a flight could be made on the basis of knowl-

ELIZABETH DUFFY

edge of his "normal" respiratory rate and the name of the maneuver to be performed (39).

Similarly, when an "autonomic factor" was obtained from twenty physiological measures related to the functioning of the autonomic nervous system, it was found that individuals differed greatly in scores on this factor, but that the correlation coefficient between early and later factor scores did not drop below .64 over a two-year period (38). Children at one extreme of the autonomic-factor scores were reported to differ significantly from those at the other extreme in certain personality traits (37).

Individuals differ, not only in the degree of excitation produced by stimulation, but also in the speed with which the processes affected return to their prior level of functioning. Moreover, differences in recovery time cannot be accounted for solely by differences in the degree of arousal, for they are found when recovery is measured *in relation to the degree of arousal*. Darrow and Heath, who first made use of this measure, computed a "recovery-reaction quotient" by dividing the extent of recovery in skin resistance by the extent of decrease in resistance which had occurred as a result of stimulation (5). The recovery-reaction quotient was reported to be related to many different measures of " 'neurotic' and emotionally unstable tendencies." The investigators concluded that it was one of their best indicators of the absence of neurotic trend, but that the coefficients of correlation were not high enough to justify the use of the measure for prediction in individual cases. It would appear that the speed of recovery from arousal is an extremely significant aspect of response, and one which deserves further investigation.

Individuals who are exceptionally responsive to the environment may show their responsivity in behavior which,

from a directional point of view, may be described in diverse ways. A tendency toward a high degree of arousal does not determine which aspects of the environment an individual will approach or will have a tendency to approach (i.e., have a favorable attitude toward); nor does it determine which aspects of the environment he will withdraw from or have a tendency to withdraw from (i.e., have an unfavorable attitude toward). On the contrary, the orientation of the individual in his environment is determined largely by other factors. These are, of course, the factors, both genetic and environmental, which have given to various aspects of his environment the nature of their significance, or their "cue-function:" There are, nevertheless, differences in the way in which approach or withdrawal occurs which may conceivably be derived from differences in the level of activation. Among these appear to be differences in such aspects of behavior as alertness, impulsiveness, irritability, distractibility, and the degree of organization of responses. Moreover, greater responsiveness may, it is suggested, facilitate the development of aggression or withdrawal, enthusiasm, or anxiety. The more responsive individual in a certain kind of environment is no doubt more susceptible to the effects of that environment. Presumably he may become, depending upon circumstances, more anxiety-prone, more conscientious, more sympathetic, more devoted, or more irascible than a less responsive person would become under similar circumstances. We should therefore expect to find some association between a high degree of activation and easily aroused or intense responses of various kinds (e.g., anxieties, resentments, enthusiasms, or attachments). From knowledge of the individual's tendencies with respect to activation we should not, however, be able to predict the direction which his behavior would take. A more dependable association might be expected between individual differences in excitability and differences in the "dynamic" characteristics of behavior such as those mentioned above.

The effect of a high degree of arousal upon overt behavior varies, no doubt, with variations in the degree of inhibitory ability (9), or, as Luria has described it, with variations in the strength of the "functional barrier" between excitation and response (27).[10] Depending upon this factor, a high degree of activation may, I suggest, lead to impulsive, disorganized behavior or to sensitive, alert, vigorous, and coordinated responses to the environment. Evidence in support of these statements is at present so meager, however, as to leave them in the category of speculations. It is to be hoped that further investigation will provide the basis for a more confident statement of the relationship between "personality" characteristics and individual differences in the level of activation.

SUMMARY

The concept of arousal or activation appears to be a significant one for the ordering of psychological data. Differences in activation, as shown in a wide variety of physiological measures, appear to be associated with many other differences in response.

In different stimulus-situations, the same individual differs in the degree of arousal. Measurement of the physiological indicants of arousal affords, when

10 Luria reports that children show weakness of the functional barrier between excitation and motor response, as indicated by poor performance on a test requiring that a key be pressed down as slowly as possible (28). The writer noted that, during a discrimination performance, younger nursery school children, with irregular grip-pressure tracings, had a higher proportion of their errors in the category of "impulsive" errors, or errors of over-reaction (8).

other factors are constant, a direct measure of the "motivating" or "emotional" value of the situation to the individual. The concept serves to break down the distinction between the arousal aspect of "drives" or "motives" and that of "emotion," and to suggest instead a continuum in the degree of activation of the individual.

Differences in activation in the same individual are, it is suggested, accompanied by differences in the quality of performance; the relationship may be graphically represented by an inverted U-shaped curve. Further data are needed, however, to establish the validity of this hypothesis.

In the same stimulus situation there are differences between individuals in the degree of arousal. These differences tend to persist, and thus to characterize the individual. Moreover, the easily aroused, or responsive, person shows this responsiveness in many forms. It has been observed in the ease with which deep reflexes are elicited, and in the extent, frequency, and duration of reactions to stimulation, both of the skeletal musculature and of various functions controlled by the autonomic nervous system. It has been shown also in differences in cortical potentials, which are presumably indicative of differences in the excitability of higher nerve centers. These various forms of responsiveness show, in general, positive intercorrelations, though the coefficients of correlation are apparently not high enough for a measure of any one mode of responsiveness to serve as an adequate measure of the general responsivity of the individual. They appear, however, to give justification to the conception of a responsive or an unresponsive individual, not merely responsive or unresponsive skeletal musculature, skin resistance, or cortical potentials.

Differences in arousal are shown also in responses of greater inclusiveness and

Elizabeth Duffy

of higher integration—i.e., in responses frequently classified as personality traits. Combining with one or another directional aspect of behavior, a persistent high degree of arousal may, it appears, be observed in many complex characteristics, such as anxiety-proneness or aggressiveness.

Facts such as those presented above suggest that the concept of activation may prove useful in many different areas of psychology.

REFERENCES

1. Albino, R. C. The stable and labile personality types of Luria in clinically normal individuals. Brit. J. Psychol., 1948, 39, 54–60.
2. Arnold, M. B. A study of tension in relation to breakdown. J. gen. Psychol., 1942, 26, 315–346.
3. Cannon, W. B. Bodily changes in pain, hunger, fear and rage. New York: Appleton, 1915, 1929.
4. Courts, F. A. Relations between muscular tension and performance. Psychol. Bull., 1942, 39. 347–367.
5. Darrow, C. W., & Heath, L. L. Reaction tendencies related to personality. In K. S. Lashley (Ed.), Studies in the dynamics of behavior. Chicago: Univer. of Chicago Press, 1932. Pp. 59–261.
6. Duffy, E. Tensions and emotional factors in reaction. Genet. Psychol. Monogr., 1930, 7, 1–79.
7. Duffy, E. The measurement of muscular tension as a technique for the study of emotional tendencies. Amer. J. Psychol., 1932, 44, 146–162.
8. Duffy, E. The relationship between muscular tension and quality of performance. Amer. J. Psychol., 1932, 44, 535–546.
9. Duffy, E. Emotion: an example of the need for reorientation in psychology. Psychol. Rev., 1934, 41, 184–198.
10. Duffy, E. The conceptual categories of psychology: a suggestion for revision. Psychol. Rev., 1941, 48, 177–203.
11. Duffy, E. An explanation of "emotional" phenomena without the use of the concept "emotion." J. gen. Psychol., 1941, 25, 283–293.
12. Duffy, E. A systematic framework for the description of personality. J. abnorm. soc. Psychol., 1949, 44, 175–190.
13. Duffy, E. The concept of energy mobilization. Psychol. Rev., 1951, 58, 30–40.
14. Freeman, G. L. The relationship between performance level and bodily activity level. J. exp. Psychol., 1940, 26, 602–608.
15. Freeman, G. L. The energetics of human behavior. Ithaca: Cornell Univer. Press, 1948.
16. Freeman, G. L., & Katzoff, E. T. Muscular tension and irritability. Amer. J. Psychol., 1932, 44, 789–792.
17. Gastaut, H. et Y., Roger, A., Corriol, J., & Naquet, R. Étude électrographique du cycle d'excitabilité cortical. EEG clin. Neurophysiol., 1951, 3, 401–428.
18. Hebb, D. O. Drives and the C.N.S. (conceptual nervous system). Psychol. Rev., 1955, 62, 243–254.
19. Jost, H. Some physiological changes during frustration. Child Develpm., 1941, 12, 9–15.
20. Kennard, M. A., Rabinovitch, M. S., & Fister, W. P. The use of frequency analysis in the interpretation of the EEG's of patients with psychological disorders. EEG clin. Neurophysiol., 1955, 7, 29–38.
21. Kennard, M. A., & Willner, M. D. Correlation between electroencephalograms and deep reflexes in normal adults. Dis. nerv. System, 1943, 6, 337–347.
22. Lansing, R. W., Schwartz, E., & Lindsley, D. B. Reaction time and EEG activation. Amer. Psychologist, 1956, 11, 433.
23. Lee, M. A. M. The relation of the knee jerk and standing steadiness to nervous instability. J. abnorm. soc. Psychol., 1931, 26, 212–228.
24. Lindsley, D. B. Emotion. In S. S. Stevens (Ed.), Handbook of experimental psychology. New York: Wiley, 1951. Pp. 473–516.
25. Lindsley, D. B. Psychological phenomena and the electroencephalogram. EEG clin. Neurophysiol., 1952, 4, 443–456.
26. Lundervold, A. An electromyographic investigation of tense and relaxed subjects. J. nerv. ment. Dis., 1952, 115, 512–525.
27. Luria, A. R. The nature of human conflict (Transl. and ed. by W. H. Gantt). New York: Liveright, 1932.
28. Malmo, R. B., Shagass, C., Bélanger, D. J., & Smith, A. A. Motor control in psychiatric patients under experimen-

tal stress. *J. abnorm. soc. Psychol.,* 1951, **46**, 539–547.

29. MALMO, R. B., SHAGASS, C., & DAVIS, J. F. Electromyographic studies of muscular tension in psychiatric patients under stress. *J. clin. exp. Psychopath.,* 1951, **12**, 45–66.

30. MALMO, R. B., & SMITH, A. A. Forehead tension and motor irregularities in psychoneurotic patients under stress. *J. Pers.,* 1955, **23**, 391–406.

31. MORGAN, M. I., & OJEMANN, R. H. A study of the Luria method. *J. appl. Psychol.,* 1942, **26**, 168–179.

32. MUNDY-CASTLE, A. C. Electrical responses of the brain in relation to behavior. *Brit. J. Psychol.,* 1953, **44**, 318–329.

33. MUNDY-CASTLE, A. C., & McKIEVER, B. L. The psychophysiological significance of the galvanic skin response. *J. exp. Psychol.,* 1953, **46**, 15–24.

34. MURRAY, H. A. *Explorations in personality.* New York: Oxford Univer. Press, 1938.

35. ULETT, G. A., GLESER, G., WINOKUR, G., & LAWLER, A. The EEG and reaction to photic stimulation as an index of anxiety-proneness. *EEG clin. Neurophysiol.,* 1953, **5**, 23–32.

36. WENGER, M. A. An attempt to appraise individual differences in level of muscular tension. *J. exp. Psychol.,* 1943, **32**, 213–225.

37. WENGER, M. A. Preliminary study of the significance of measures of autonomic balance. *Psychosom. Med.,* 1947, **9**, 301–309.

38. WENGER, M. A., & ELLINGTON, M. The measurement of autonomic balance in children: method and normative data. *Psychosom. Med.,* 1943, **5**, 241–253.

39. WILLIAMS, A. C., JR., MACMILLAN, J. W., & JENKINS, J. G. *Preliminary experimental investigations of "tension" as a determinant of performance in flight training.* Civil Aeronautics Admin., Div. of Res., Rep. No. 54, Washington, D. C. January, 1946.

40. WOODWORTH, R. S., & SCHLOSBERG, H. *Experimental psychology.* (Rev. ed.) New York: Holt, 1954.

(Received October 22, 1956)

From R. B. Malmo (1959). Psychological Review, *66*, 367-386, *by kind permission of the author and the American Psychological Association.*

ACTIVATION: A NEUROPSYCHOLOGICAL DIMENSION [1]

ROBERT B. MALMO

Allan Memorial Institute, McGill University

There have been three main lines of approach to the problem of activation: (*a*) through electroencephalography and neurophysiology, (*b*) through physiological studies of "behavioral energetics," and (*c*) through the learning theorists' search for a satisfactory measure of drive. Before attempting a formal definition of activation, I shall briefly describe these three different approaches to the concept.

Neurophysiological approach: Lindsley's Activation Theory. [2] The neuro-

physiological approach to activation had its origin in electroencephalography (EEG). Early workers in the EEG field soon discovered that there were distinctive wave patterns characterizing the main levels of psychological functioning in the progression from deep sleep to highly alerted states of activity (Jasper, 1941). In deep sleep large low-frequency waves predominate. In light sleep and drowsy states the frequencies are not as low as in deep sleep, but there are more low-frequency waves than in the wakeful states. In relaxed wakefulness there is a predominance of waves in the alpha (8–12 c.p.s.) range that gives way to beta frequencies (approximately 18–30 c.p.s.) when the *S* is moderately alert. Under highly alerting and exciting conditions beta waves predominate. In addition to the increased frequency of the waves under these conditions of heightened alertness there is also a change from a regular synchronized appearance of the tracing to an irregular desynchronized tracing, usually of reduced amplitude.

[1] Support for some of the research reported herein has come from the following sources: National Institute of Mental Health, National Institutes of Health, United States Public Health Service: Grant Number M-1475; Medical Research and Development Division, Office of the Surgeon General, Department of the United States Army: Contract Number DA-49-007-MD-626; Defence Research Board, Department of National Defence, Canada: Grant Number 9425-04; and National Research Council of Canada: Grant Number A. P. 29.

Grateful acknowledgment is made to A. Amsel, R. C. Davis, S. M. Feldman, P. Milner, M. M. Schnore, R. G. Stennett, D. J. Ehrlich and L. R. Pinneo for constructive criticism of the manuscript.

The main parts of this paper were presented in a Symposium entitled, "Experimental Foundations of Clinical Psychology," under the chairmanship of Arthur J. Bachrach, at the University of Virginia, April 1–2, 1959. To Ian P. Stevenson, who was the discussant of my paper on that Sympsoium, I owe a debt of gratitude for his very helpful comments.

[2] I am using neuropsychology in a rather broad sense, meaning to include the work often referred to by the term "psychophysiology." This usage implies that the chief problems being studied are psychological ones, and it also stresses the importance of neurophysiological techniques. It is true

that, strictly speaking, many of the physiological techniques in use are not neurophysiological ones; yet our main interest lies in the central neural control of the physiological functions under study rather than in the peripheral events themselves.

Later on in the paper I shall attempt a formal definition of activation. For the first section of the paper, I believe that it will be sufficient to say that in using the term "activation" I am referring to the intensive dimension of behavior. "Arousal" is often used interchangeably with activation; and level of drive is a very similar concept. For instance, a drowsy *S* is low, an alert *S* is high in activation.

For Lindsley's theory, desynchronization (called "activation pattern") became the single most important EEG phenomenon. My use of the term "desynchronization" is purely descriptive. Desynchronization or "flattening" in the EEG tracing was consistently found associated with increased alertness in a large variety of experiments with animal and human Ss. The consistency and generality of this phenomenon suggested the existence of mechanisms in the brain mediating behavioral functions having to do with levels of alertness, although at the time that the original observations were made it was not at all clear what these neural mechanisms were.

With the discovery of the ascending reticular activating system (ARAS), however, there was rapid and very significant advance in theory and experimentation. Some of the most important general findings have been as follows: (*a*) Lesions in the ARAS abolished "activation" of the EEG and produced a behavioral picture of lethargy and somnolence (Lindsley, 1957). (*b*) The "activation pattern" in the EEG was reproduced by electrical stimulation of the ARAS. Furthermore, in the monkey, Fuster (1958) recently found that concurrent ARAS stimulation of moderate intensity improved accuracy and speed of visual discrimination reaction. He also found that higher intensities had the opposite effect, producing diminution of correct responses and increase of reaction times. Interpretation of these latter findings is complicated by the fact that they were obtained with stimulation intensities higher than the threshold for the elicitation of observable motor effects such as generalized muscular jerks. It is not stated whether intensity of stimulation was systematically studied. In any event, these observations of deleterious effect from high intensity stimulation are of considerable interest because they are what might be expected according to the activation theory.

The activation theory as first stated by Lindsley (1951)—although introduced in the handbook chapter on emotion—was, from the outset, conceived by him to be broader than an explanatory concept for emotional behavior. The theory was elaborated by Hebb (1955) in an attempt to solve the problem of drives. With the continuous flow of new experimental data on the ARAS (Lindsley, 1957), this area of neuropsychological investigation appears to be heading toward an important breakthrough. I shall attempt to state very briefly the main points of the current theory, drawing upon the ideas of several authors. According to this theory, the continuum extending from deep sleep at the low activation end to "excited states" [3] at the high activation end is very largely a function of cortical bombardment by the ARAS, such that the greater the cortical bombardment the higher the activation. Further, the relation between activation and behavioral efficiency (cue function or level of performance) is described by an inverted **U** curve. That is, from low activation up to a point that is optimal for a given function, level of performance rises monotonically with increasing activation level, but beyond this optimal point the relation becomes nonmonotonic: further increase in activation beyond this point produces a fall in performance level, this fall being

[3] The expression "excited states" is frequently used to refer to the upper end of the activation continuum. In using this term I do not wish to imply increased overt activity. In fact, overt activity may be reduced to a very low level at the high end of the continuum, when—for example—a person is immobolized by terror.

directly related to the amount of the increase in level of activation.

Principles of neural action that could account for the reversal in the effects of nonspecific neural bombardment of the cortex by the ARAS have long been known (Lorente de Nó, 1939, p. 428). Circulation of neural impulses in a closed chain of neurons (or "cell assembly" to use Hebb's [1949] term) may be facilitated by impulses arriving outside the chain (e.g. from the ARAS). According to Lorente de Nó's schema, such extraneous impulses have the effect of stimulating certain neurons subliminally thus making it possible for an impulse from within the chain to finish the job, that is make it fire at the appropriate time in the sequence, when alone, without the prior hit, it would have failed to fire it.

Again, according to the same account by Lorente de Nó (1939, p. 428), the deleterious effects of overstimulation from impulses outside the chain can be explained. A neuron in the chain may fail to respond to stimulation if owing to repeated activity it acquires a high threshold, and this failure to transmit the circulating impulses would mean cessation of activity in a cell assembly. I proposed this kind of explanation previously (1958) to account for the downturn in the inverted U curve as an alternative to Hebb's suggestion that "the greater bombardment may interfere with the delicate adjustments involved in cue function, perhaps by facilitating irrelevant responses (a high D arouses conflicting $_sH_R$'s?)" (Hebb, 1955, p. 250).

It seems reasonable to suppose that as diffuse bombardment from the ARAS greatly exceeds an amount that is optimal for some simple psychological function being mediated by a particular cell assembly, the operation of that cell assembly will be impaired, and that the performance being mediated by it will suffer accordingly. This line of reasoning suggests that the inverted U relation should be found in quite simple psychological functions. Present evidence appears to support this suggestion. A recent (unpublished) experiment by Bélanger and Feldman, that I shall describe later in this paper, indicates that in rats the inverted U relation is found with simple bar pressing performance, and an experiment by Finch (1938) suggests that even such a simple response as the unconditioned salivary response yields the inverted U curve when plotted against activation level.

It may be noted that according to a response competition hypothesis, the inverted U relation should appear most prominently in complex functions where opportunities for habit interference are greater than they are in the case of simple functions. According to the response competition hypothesis, in the limiting case where response is so simple that habit interference is negligible, the relation between response strength and activation level should be monotonic. Therefore, finding the nonmonotonic relation in such simple responses as bar pressing and salivation raises strong doubts that the habit interference explanation can account for the seemingly pervasive phenomenon of the inverted U curve.

Principle of activation growing out of work on behavioral intensity. Even before the EEG work on desynchronization, the behavioral evidence had suggested the existence of some brain mechanism like the ARAS. The writings of Duffy (1951, 1957), Freeman (1948), and others of the "energetics" group have long stressed the importance of an intensity dimension in behavior.

In an attempt to obtain a measure

of this intensity variable, Duffy relied mainly on records of muscular tension (1932) while Freeman's favorite indicator was palmar conductance (1948). These workers concluded from their experiments that there was a lawful relationship between a state of the organism, called "arousal," "energy mobilization," "activation," or simply "intensity" and level of performance. Moreover they suggested that the relationship might be described by an inverted U curve(Duffy, 1957). This suggestion has proved heuristic as indicated by the current experimental attack on the inverted U hypothesis (Stennett, 1957a; Bindra, 1959; Cofer, 1959; Kendler, 1959).

The inverted U shaped curve has been shown to hold in numerous learning and performance situations where the amount of induced muscle tension was varied systematically (Courts, 1942). It is tempting to conclude that tension induction is simply one of the many ways to increase activation level, but as Courts' (1942) discussion suggests this conclusion would be premature. It is possible that squeezing on a dynamometer, a typical means of inducing tension in these experiments, may produce generalized activation effects as some data from Freeman indicate (1948, p. 71). But Freeman's data are insufficient to establish this point, and there are alternative explanations for the relationship between the performance data and induced tension (Courts, 1942). By repeating the induced-tension experiments with simultaneous recordings of EEG and other physiological functions it would be possible to determine how general the effects of inducing tension actually are. Such direct tests of the activation hypothesis are very much needed.

Drive and activation. A third approach to the activation principle was made by learning theorists, especially those of the Hull school. I have argued elsewhere (Malmo, 1958) that general drive (D), without the steering component, became identical in principle with activation or arousal. Set aside for the moment the attractive possibility of using ARAS as a neural model for mediation of D, and consider only the methodological advantages of physiological measures in the quantification of D. It seems that none of the other attempts to measure D have been really satisfactory, and that physiological indicants where applied have been surprisingly effective. Learning theorists up to the present time have made only very occasional use of physiological measures. For instance, in arguing that a previously painful stimulus had lost its drive properties, Brown (1955) cited the absence of physiological reaction when the stimulus was applied. More recently, Spence (1958) has reported some success with physiological measures in his studies of "emotionally-based" drive.

In keeping with traditional views concerning the place of physiological measures in psychology, on those few occasions that they were employed at all they were applied to aversive or emotionally based drive. According to the activation principle, however, it should be possible to use physiological measures to gauge appetitionally based as well as aversively based drive. This means, for instance, that in a water deprivation experiment there should be close correspondence between number of hours of deprivation and physiological level. That is, heart rate, for example, should be higher in an animal performing in a Skinner box after 36 hours of deprivation than after 24, higher still after 48 hours of deprivation and so on. In my Nebraska Symposium paper I stated that, as far as I was aware, this kind of experiment had not been reported (Malmo. 1958, p. 236).

Bélanger and Feldman in Montreal have recently completed such an experiment, and, as can be seen by inspecting Fig. 1, the results were as predicted by the activation hypothesis. Heart rate in rats showed progressive change corresponding with increasing hours of water deprivation. Although there were only seven rats in the group. this change in heart rate was highly significant. Deprivations were carried out serially on the same group of animals, commencing at 12 hours and proceeding to 24, 48 hours and so on with sufficient hydration (four to seven days) between deprivation periods to prevent any cumulative effects from affecting the experiments. Heart rate was picked up by means of wire electrodes inserted in the skin of the animals and was amplified and registered graphically by means of a Sanborn electrocardiograph. Particular care was

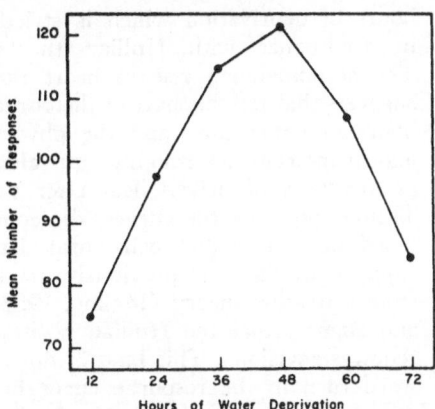

FIG. 2. Data from Bélanger and Feldman showing relation between water deprivation and Skinner box performance in rats ($N = 7$). See text for explanation.

taken to record heart rate under nearly the same conditions of stimulation each time, that is, when the animal was pressing on the lever in the Skinner box or during drinking from the dispenser immediately after pressing. Under these conditions it was not possible to obtain sufficient heart-rate data at the 12-hour deprivation interval. Testing the animal under constant stimulating conditions is a very important methodological consideration. Some exploratory observations indicated that heart-rate measurements taken in a restraining compartment did not agree with those taken under the carefully controlled stimulus conditions provided by the Skinner box. I shall return to this finding later on because, aside from its methodological importance, I believe that it has considerable theoretical significance as well.

Figure 2 presents the behavioral data which are again in remarkably good agreement with prediction from the activation hypothesis. Up to the 48-hour deprivation interval there is an increasing monotonic relationship between number of bar presses and

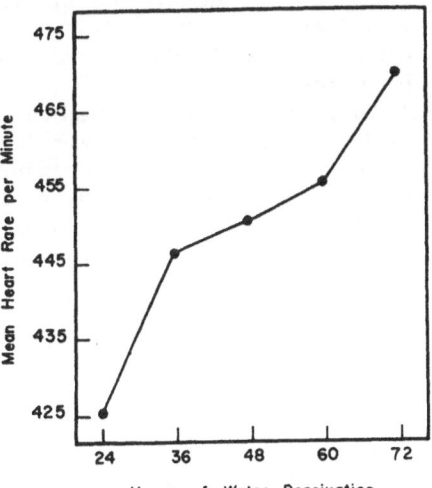

FIG. 1. Data from Bélanger and Feldman showing relation between water deprivation and heart rate in rats ($N = 7$). See text for explanation.

hours of deprivation which is strictly in accordance with Hullian theory. The accompanying rise in heart rate suggests that for this part of the curve, hours of deprivation and the physiological indicant are roughly equivalent as measures of drive. But after the 48-hour point on the curves, the combined heart rate and behavioral data support predictions previously made from activation theory (Malmo, 1958) and suggest that the Hullian position requires revision. This kind of downward turn in the response curve has usually been attributed to a physical weakening of the animal due to the deprivation of food or water. In the absence of physiological data such an assumption appeared reasonable in many cases, although it did not account for response decrement in certain experiments where physical weakening seemed to be ruled out (Finan, 1940; Freeman, 1940; Fuster, 1958; Kaplan, 1952; Stennett, 1957a). Attack on this problem with physiological methods should soon provide a definitive answer concerning the main determinants of this response decrement. The present experiment represents an important first step in a program of animal studies that should go a long way towards solving this problem. It is not claimed that this one experiment demolishes the inanition hypothesis, but it does seem that the results are opposed to it. Heart rate in the Minnesota starvation experiments was found lowered in the weakened individuals (Malmo, 1958, p. 252) whereas heart rate in the present experiment was markedly increased during the period when number of responses was declining. Moreover, Bélanger was careful to record the weights of the animals all through the experiments, and he observed only very slight changes in weight, even at the 72-hour deprivation interval. Again, it should be stressed that all through the experiment the animals received four to seven days of hydration between conditions. Furthermore, it is interesting to note that the animals continued to press the bar at fairly regular intervals in the high deprivation conditions (with response decrement). That is, their behavior did not appear as though they had "given up." The acts of pressing continued to occur regularly, only they were separated by longer temporal intervals than under more optimal conditions of deprivation.

The increasing monotonic curve for heart rate did not seem to be simply due to the physical conditions of exertion associated with the act of bar pressing. It is true that up to the peak of the performance curve increasing heart rate was accompanied by increasing frequency of bar pressing, but past this point, heart rate continued to show rise despite the decline in exertion due to bar pressing. One might conjecture that exercise may have had greater effect on heart rate under extreme deprivation, but this would be counterbalanced—to some extent, at least—by the reduced number of presses.

To control for possible serial effects in this experiment there were two checks. First, he obtained similar findings from a second group of rats in which the order of deprivation conditions was reversed, commencing with the 72-hour deprivation condition, and finishing with the 12-hour condition. Second, the group of rats that had the ascending order of deprivation intervals were tested one week after the end of the experiment under the 60-hour deprivation condition. Mean number of responses was 96.7 and mean heart rate was 458.9 beats per minute, thus providing good agreement with the results that were obtained in the main experiment.

Finally, it is possible to speculate along various lines about how the heart rate data could be accounted for without involving the concept of activation. Obviously, further experimentation is needed, but it is encouraging nonetheless that the first animal experimentation specifically designed to explore the relation between appetitional drive and activation turned out according to prediction.

CHARACTERISTICS OF ACTIVATION

The three approaches described in the previous section appear to lead to the same fundamental concept of activation. It will, of course, be difficult to state a precise definition of activation that will satisfy everyone. Neurophysiologically oriented workers will maintain a healthy scepticism concerning the so-called "peripheral" indicants of activation. The "energetics" group while welcoming the extended use of what is essentially their own methodology will in company with some learning theorists look askance at theoretical models that verge on neurologizing. Despite differences in point of view, however, it seems worthwhile to attempt to deal with certain major characteristics of activation on which we may expect a large measure of agreement.

Activation level a product of multiple factors. When a man is deprived of sleep for some 60 hours his activation level appears higher than it was before he had suffered sleep loss. Physiological indicants reveal an upward shift in activation level that is gradual and progressive throughout the vigil (Malmo, 1958). Having once demonstrated these physiological changes it is tempting to dispense with physiological recording in further work, assuming that 60 hours of deprivation will invariably produce a heightened state of activation. Such an assumption, however, cannot be made. An example will make clear why this assumption is untenable. A sleep-deprived S requires constant stimulation to prevent him from going to sleep. It is a general finding in such studies that despite the best intentions of the S to remain awake he will "catnap" if left alone. When he is working at a task trying to keep his efficiency from falling, the effect of major sleep loss is to produce a large increase in activation level. The important point to see here, however, is that the higher activation level is a combined product of the stimuli and their demands on him plus the condition of sleep loss. Without such stimulation, the S would surely fall asleep and we know from our studies of sleep that physiological levels drop very rapidly as one drifts into sleep. It is obvious, therefore, that in the absence of the task, physiological indicants at 60 hours' deprivation would show lower, not higher, activation in comparison with the rested condition.

That the "drive state" is in large part determined by environmental stimulating factors is indicated also by the observations of Bélanger and Feldman in their water deprivation experiments. Incidental observations suggested that, in addition to being more variable, heart rates recorded from the animal in a restraining compartment seemed to be consistently lower than those that were recorded when the animal was pressing the lever or drinking. In the restraining compartment the animal could view the lever through glass so that apparently mere sight of the lever was insufficient stimulation to produce the full effect upon heart rate that was produced by the acts of pressing on the lever and drinking. It thus appeared that, with deprivation time approximately the same, activation level differed appreciably depending upon the conditions of external stimulation. These observations were merely incidental ones in this experiment, and they should be repeated; but they encourage the point of view that activation level is in large part a function of environmental stimulating conditions. The experiments of Campbell and Sheffield (1953) seem to point in the same direction. In the absence of sufficient environmental stimulation, food deprived rats are no more active than satiated ones, but with stimulation they are much more active than the satiated controls.

Returning to the example of the water deprived rat in the Skinner box, the two major factors determining the level of activation in that situation are (a) the internal conditions produced by deprivation and (b) the environmental stimulating conditions. To restate a point previously made, level of activation does not seem to be simply determined by the condition of deprivation alone. This would mean that depriving an animal of water per se could not produce some direct effect on motor mechanisms such as a simple discharge into the cardiac accelerating mechanism, leading to increased heart rate. Instead of some direct effect of this kind leading immediately over to some observable effector action, deprivation appears to have a sensitizing effect that is undetectable (or latent). According to this view, when appropriate stimulation does occur, the previously latent effect of deprivation will show itself in the heart rate: within limits, the longer the period of deprivation the higher the heart rate. Furthermore, according to activation theory, the same central mechanism that increases heart rate also acts to increase bombardment of the cerebral cortex.

As previously stated, this central mechanism is presumed to be the ARAS.[4]

What could be the means of sensitizing cells in the ARAS by a condition such as deprivation of water or food? If some hormone like epinephrine were released by deprivation, it is conceivable that this hormone could act to sensitize the ARAS cells in degree proportional to the amount of time that the animal had been deprived. As a matter of fact, hormonal sensitization of neural mechanisms is a currently active area of research (Saffran, Schally, & Benfey, 1955; Dell, 1958).

There are some real difficulties in defending the position that the ARAS is a unitary intensity-mediating mechanism, because the ARAS does not appear to be a homogeneous anatomical system. Indeed, as Olszewski (1954) has shown, these central brain stem structures appear very complex and highly differentiated. This unreassuring fact must not be forgotten, but neither should it be accepted as precluding the unitary function. As Lashley points out in the discussion of Olszewski's paper, structural differences are not reliable indices of function when unsupported by other evidence.

As a matter of fact, there is some important functional evidence which encourages the unitary view despite the structural complexity of the ARAS. Dell (1958) has found that: "Epinephrine does not activate selectively mammillothalamocingular systems, . . . but instead activates the ascending reticular system *en masse*, thus leading to a generalized cortical arousal" (p. 370). Control experiments showed

[4] It is very likely that the descending reticular activating system is involved here too, but, at the present stage of knowledge in this field, it does not seem wise to introduce further complications into the neuropsychological model.

that the activation effect was due to a direct action of the epinephrine at the reticular level and not to an effect on the cerebral cortex. Similar results have been obtained by Rothballer (1956).

Another kind of difficulty for the quantitative view would be posed by showing that patterned discharge from the ARAS to the cortex (not merely total quantity of discharge) was the crucial factor in supporting some behavioral action. Don't the effector patterns of standing, walking, and righting pose just such a difficulty? The relation of midbrain mechanisms to posture seems to be clearly one in which patterns of discharge from the midbrain are important. But the decorticate mammal (guinea pig, rabbit, cat, dog) in which the cortex of both hemispheres has been removed shows approximately normal postural and progressional activities (Dusser de Barenne, 1934, p. 229). Since the activation concept under review deals with bombardment of the cerebral cortex, it appears that these non-cortically mediated response patterns fall outside of phenomena under present consideration.

I should add, finally, that my admittedly speculative suggestion concerning hormonal sensitization is by no means essential to the main point which is that the behavioral evidence clearly shows the effects of deprivation to be latent (i.e. unobservable) under certain conditions. Moreover, this stress placed on the latent effects of deprivation is not mere hairsplitting. In addition to being required for an explanation of the Montreal experiments, this concept of latent deprivation effects appears to account in large measure for the findings of Campbell and Sheffield (1953), and more generally for the failure of random activity

to adequately serve as a measure of drive or activation (Malmo, 1958).

Activation and the S–R framework. As the product of interaction between internal (perhaps hormonal) conditions and external stimulating ones, activation cannot be very reasonably classified as either stimulus or response. This means that the physiological measurements that are used to gauge level of activation do not fit very well into the S–R formula. It is perhaps useful to think of these physiological conditions as part of O in the S–O–R formula (Woodworth & Schlosberg, 1954, p. 2).

The momentary physiological reaction to a discrete stimulus like the sudden rise in palmar conductance accompanying pin-prick is not of primary concern to us in our study of activation. This kind of S–R reaction, important as it undoubtedly is for investigating other problems, is of little relevance for the study of activation, compared with the longer lasting changes. As Schlosberg has put it to me in personal communication, in employing skin conductance to gauge level of activation, one observes the "tides" and not the "ripples." I do not mean to disparage studies that use physiological reactions as R terms in the strict S–R sense. It is just that in this paper I am concerned with physiological functions only insofar as they are related to activation.

It may be queried whether we are dealing with a needless and hairsplitting distinction by saying that activation is not a response. However, the kind of difference I have in mind appears quite distinct and useful to keep in mind, though it should not be stressed unduly. Basically, it is the same distinction which Woodworth and Schlosberg (1956) make when they draw particular attention to the difference between slow and rapid changes in skin conductance. As examples of rapid changes in skin conductance, there are the "GSRs" as R terms in conditioned responses, and in free association tests. Examples of slow skin-conductance changes, on the other hand, are the gradual downward drifts that occur over hours during sleep (see Fig. 4), the slow downward changes in skin conductance in Ss as they become gradually habituated to an experimental situation (Davis, 1934; Duffy & Lacey, 1946), and (going up the activation scale) the progressive upward changes in conductance during a vigil (Malmo, 1958).

I would not deny that there are stimuli and responses going on in the physiological systems, but at the present time I see no way of identifying and handling them. It should be added, however, that this does not give one license to completely disregard the antecedents of physiological changes. For instance, if the hand of a sleeping S becomes hot by being covered with heavy bedclothing the local thermal sweating induced thereby will bring about a sudden rise in palmar conductance which has nothing to do with activation. Or sleep may by induced by certain drugs which have a specific stimulating effect on respiration, such that respiration rate will not fall during sleep as it usually does (see Fig. 5 for curve obtained under nondrug conditions). Furthermore, artifacts due to movement and postural shifts may prevent muscle potentials from serving as reliable indicants of activation level.

Limitations of the activation concept. I am not attempting to solve the problem of selection, i.e., the problem of finding the neurophysiological mechanisms that determine which cues in the animal's environment are prepotent in the sense of winning out over other cues in triggering off a pattern of ef-

fector action. This point seems clear enough, especially when it is stressed that activation has no steering function; and yet there is still the risk that some critics may misunderstand and state as one shortcoming of this theory that it does not adequately handle the problem of selection. The theory may be open to criticism on the grounds that it is limited, but it should not be criticized for failing to do something which it was not intended to do.

It will be noted that in general an attempt is made to raise theoretical questions that stand a good chance of being answered by available experimental techniques. Schematically, the experimental paradigm is as follows:

Activation
    level : Low Moderate High
Expected perform-
    ance level : Low Optimal Low

It is important to stress that the measure denoted by "moderate activation level" has meaning only in relative (not in absolute) terms. That is, the level is "moderate" because it is higher than that of the low activation condition, and lower than the level of the high activation condition. Comparisons are invariably of the within-individual, within-task kind, which means that the level of activation which is found to be optimal for one task is not directly compared with the level of activation which is found to be optimal for a different task. Thus, at the present stage of theorizing, no attempt is made to deal with the question of whether tasks which differ in complexity, for example, also differ with respect to the precise level of activation which is optimal for each one. However, I have dealt elsewhere (Malmo, 1958) with the related question of response competition, suggesting an alternative to the response competition explanation for decrement in performance with increased activation (or D).

Again, the theoretical formulations may be criticized for being too narrow. But it must be kept in mind that their narrowness is due to the close nexus between theory and experiment in this program. These formulations may also be criticized for an unjustifiable assumption in the postulation of a communal drive mechanism. One may well ask where the evidence is that proves the existence of a state of general drive. In dealing with this kind of question, it is essential to refer back to the outline of the experimental paradigm. The experimental induction of the three discriminable activation levels referred to in the outline depends upon the controlled variation of certain conditions in the S's environment. The fact that by varying conditions as dissimilar as appetitional deprivations and verbal incentives it is possible to produce similar shifts in physiological indicants provides a sound basis for introducing the operationally defined concept of activation level that cuts across traditional demarcation lines of specific drives. All this, of course, does not constitute final proof for a communal drive mechanism. Certainly further data are required before it is even safe to conclude equivalence of drive conditions in the alteration of physiological levels, to say nothing of proving the existence of a communal drive mechanism.

INTERRELATIONS BETWEEN PHYSIOLOGICAL INDICANTS OF ACTIVATION

Criticism directed against physiological measures as indicants of activation usually involves one or both of the following points. The first objection is that intercorrelations between physiological measures are so low that it is unreasonable to consider their use

for gauging a single dimension of behavior. A second objection is that activation properly refers to events in the brain and that the correspondence between these central events and what may be observed in such peripheral functions as heart rate, respiration, muscle tension and the like is not close enough to permit valid inferences from the peripheral events to the central ones. In the following section, I shall attempt to answer these criticisms.

Intra- and interindividual correlations among physiological indicants of activation. In an unpublished paper, Schnore and I have discussed certain misconceptions that have confused some critics of physiological methods. The most serious misunderstanding concerns correlations among physiological measures. It is true that *inter*individual correlations are low, but this fact is actually irrelevant insofar as using these measures to gauge activation is concerned. The important question is whether significant *intra*individual correlations are found in a sufficiently high proportion of individuals, and the answer appears to be yes (Schnore, 1959).

What the low *inter*individual correlations mean, of course, is that an individual in any given situation may have a heart rate that is high relative to the mean heart rate for the group, and at the same time have a respiration rate or a blood pressure that is low relative to the group mean. These findings are in line with the principle of physiological specificity that is now supported by several lines of evidence.[5]

[5] The general principle of physiological specificity states that under significantly different conditions of stimulation individuals exhibit idiosyncratic but highly stereotyped patterns of autonomic and somatic activation. I use the term *physiological specificity* as a generic reference to autonomic-response stereotypy (Lacey & Lacey, 1958) to symptom specificity (Malmo & Shagass,

Physiological specificity is a separate problem that is in no way crucial for the activation hypothesis. An illustration will make this clear. Take a rather extreme example of an individual with very *high* heart rate (say 95 when the mean for his group under specified conditions is 75) and very *low* palmar conductance (50 micromhos when the group mean is 100). In an experiment with varied incentive, in going from a low incentive to a high incentive condition this *S* will likely show an increase in heart rate from 95 to say 110 and an increase in palmar conductance from 50 to say 60 micromhos. The main point is that even though the *S*'s heart rate is already high compared with the mean for his group, it goes still higher (concordantly with palmar conductance) when the stimulating situation increases the level of activation. This is the kind of intraindividual correlation between physiological measures [6] that is required for gauging the dimension of activation and, to repeat, the evidence strongly indicates that the intraindividual correlations are sufficiently high for this purpose.

RELATIONS BETWEEN CENTRAL AND PERIPHERAL INDICANTS OF ACTIVATION

As previously noted, the pioneer EEG workers observed definite changes in EEG pattern accompanying major shifts in the conscious state of the *S*. Moreover, they recognized a continuum

of increasing activation usually referred to as the sleep-waking-excitement continuum, just as other workers like Freeman (1948) and Duffy (1957) employing peripheral measures of palmar sweating and muscular tension recognized it. Among the early workers in this field, Darrow (1947) studied EEG and other measures simultaneously, but only very recently have techniques been made available that can provide the kind of quantitative EEG measurements required for critical comparisons along the activation continuum. That is, from simple inspection of the raw EEG tracing it is possible to see gross differences between sleeping and waking, or between a drowsy, relaxed state and one of extreme alertness. But for experiments on activation it is necessary to have an instrument that will reveal measureable differences for "points" lying closer to each other on the activation continuum. For example, it is essential to have a measure that will discriminate reliably between a moderately alert and a highly alert state. For such discriminations the method of inspection will not do, and a device for objective quantification of the wave forms is required.

Because of its complexity the EEG tracing has been difficult to quantify, and although gross differences in activation level could be detected by simple inspection of the tracing, this method was too crude for more detailed work. However, with the advent of EEG frequency analysers, quantification of the EEG looked promising because these analysers were designed to provide quantified EEG data for each of many different narrow frequency bands. Unfortunately, these instruments have not proved useful because of insufficient stability. In our laboratory we have been trying band-pass filters to provide stable quantification of various selected

---

1949), and to stereotypy of somatic and autonomic activation patterns (Schnore, 1959).

[6] It is not claimed, however, that all physiological measures are equally useful for the purpose of gauging activation level On the contrary, as Schnore's experiments have suggested, some measures appear superior to others, and eventually we may be able to select the most discriminating ones and thus improve our measurement (Schnore, 1959).

frequency bands in which we are primarily interested (Ross & Davis, 1958). Results thus far appear highly encouraging.

Data indicating relationships between EEG and other physiological functions. In a recent sleep deprivation experiment, we found that palmar conductance and respiration showed progressive rise during the vigil, indicating increasing activation with deprivation of sleep. In the same experiment we recorded EEG and, by means of a band-pass filter, obtained a quantified write-out of frequencies from 8–12 per second, in the alpha range. It will be recalled that the classical picture of activation is reduction in the amount of alpha activity. Therefore, what we might expect to find in this experiment is progressive decrease in the amount of alpha activity. As a matter of fact, this is exactly what was found (Malmo, 1958, p. 237).

As Stennett (1957b) has shown, however, the relationship between EEG alpha activity and other physiological variables is sometimes curvilinear. In the sleep deprivation experiments physiological measurements were taken under highly activating conditions and at this high end of the continuum further increase in activation seems invariably to decrease the amount of alpha activity. But at the lower end of the continuum with the S in a drowsy state, increased activation has the opposite effect on alpha activity. An alerting stimulus, instead of producing a flattening of the EEG tracing, will actually produce an augmentation of the alpha activity. This has sometimes been referred to as a "paradoxical" reaction, although it seems paradoxical only when it is assumed that the relation between activation level and alpha amplitude is a decreasing monotonic one throughout the entire activation continuum. But Sten-

nett (1957b) has shown that the relationship is not monotonic. From his data he plotted a curve which has the shape of an inverted **U**. From this curve it would be predicted that with a drowsy S, stimulation should *increase* alpha amplitude. From the same inverted **U** curve it would also be predicted that an S whose activation level was sufficiently high (past the peak of the curve) before stimulation would show a *decrease* in alpha amplitude. Actually, some unpublished experiments on startle by Bartoshuk fit these predictions very well.

Recent data indicate the usefulness of a 2–4 c.p.s. band-pass filter in experiments on sleep. The data in the figures that follow represent mean values from three men who slept all night in our laboratory after serving as Ss in our sleep deprivation experiments.

Bipolar sponge electrodes, soaked in electrode jelly and attached to the S by Lastonet bands, were used for the parietal EEG placement (two thirds of the distance from nasion to inion, and 3 cm. from the midline on each side). The primary tracing was recorded by an Edin Electroencephalograph, and the two secondary tracings were integrations of the EEG potentials that were passed through band-pass filters for selective amplification of signals in the 2–4 and 8–12 c.p.s. frequency bands. Measurements on the secondary tracings were carried out with special rulers, and these measurements were converted to microvolt values by reference to calibration standards.

Method of recording and measuring palmar conductance was similar to that described by Stennett (1957a).

Electrocardiograms were picked up from electrodes placed on contralateral limbs, and heart rates were determined from measurements of electrocardiota-

Robert B. Malmo

chometric tracings. Respiration rates were obtained by means of a Phipps and Bird pneumograph.

All three Ss slept well throughout the night (approximately from 10 P.M. to 9 A.M. after some 60 hours without sleep). Physiological recordings were carried out continuously during the whole period of sleep in each case, and except for occasional attention to electrodes (e.g. application of electrode jelly and saline to electrodes) the Ss were undisturbed.

Four pairs of cellulose sponge electrodes were attached to the four limbs (to the pronator teres muscles of the arms and the peroneal muscles of the legs) for the purpose of recording muscle potentials. Primary muscle-potential tracings were recorded on the chart of a custom built Edin electromyograph (EMG). Electronic integrators (employing the condensor charge–discharge principle, like those used for the secondary EEG tracings), attached in parallel across the galvanometers of this EMG unit, integrated

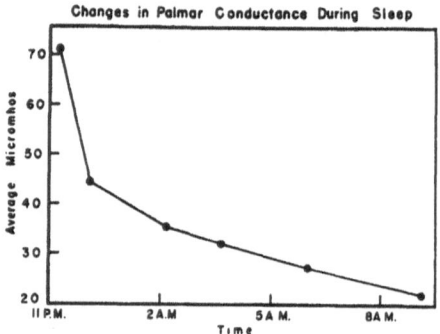

Fig. 4. Mean palmar conductance values from the same Ss, at the same times during sleep as in Fig. 3.

the muscle potentials over successive 4-second periods.

These muscle-potential tracings were used to record movements and periods of restlessness during sleep. Five-minute periods free from muscle-potential activity and preceded by at least 5 minutes of movement-free tracings were chosen for measurement in order to provide the values plotted in Fig. 3–5. The actual times plotted on the baseline represent the medians for the three Ss. In each instance the three times were close to one another.

In Fig. 3 observe that following a brief rise early in sleep the upper curve for 2–4 c.p.s. falls continuously during the entire period of sleep. This curve is consistent with published accounts of changes in EEG during sleep noted by inspection of the raw tracings (Lindsley, 1957, p. 68). Early in sleep there is an increase in slow waves around 2–4 cycles per second, but as sleep continues these waves are replaced by even slower ones. As far as I am aware, the data in Fig. 3 represent the first use of a 2–4 band-pass filter to quantify the EEG. The curve for 8–12 c.p.s. EEG also shows some fall, and the voltage is low in accordance with the well-known dis-

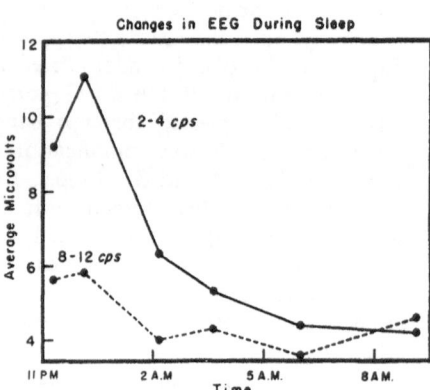

Fig. 3. Mean EEG values from three healthy young male Ss during a night's sleep. Subjects had been sleep-deprived. Band-pass filters were used in connection with electronic integrators to provide quantitative data in the two different frequency bands.

appearance of alpha waves from the raw tracings during sleep.

Figures 4 and 5 show data for palmar conductance, heart rate, and respiration, that were recorded at the same time as the EEG data. From the second plotted point on, there is rather close resemblance between these curves and the one for 2–4 c.p.s. EEG. It seems likely that a band-pass filter for fast frequencies in the beta range might yield a continuously falling curve commencing with drowsiness and continuing through the onset and early stages of sleep. There are serious technical difficulties in quantifying the next step of frequencies above the alpha band, but we are hopeful that a band-pass filter that has recently been constructed in our laboratory will overcome these difficulties.

Direct alteration of ARAS activity by means of electrical stimulation and related animal experimentation. The most relevant experiment on direct stimulation of the ARAS is, as far as I know, the one by Fuster (1958) that was mentioned earlier. By stimulating in the same part of the ARAS that produces the EEG picture of activation, Fuster was able to produce improved discrimination performance in the monkey. Presumably, this effect

was achieved by causing a larger number of impulses from the ARAS to bombard the cortex. The assumption would be that before the onset of electrical stimulation the cortex was not receiving sufficient bombardment for optimal performance (Hebb, 1955) and that ARAS stimulation brought total bombardment in the cortex closer to the optimal value. The situation may not be as simple as this, but the success of the Fuster experiment encourages further experimentation along these same lines. Finding that level of performance can be altered by electrical stimulation of the ARAS opens up the exciting possibility that if amount of neural activity in the ARAS can be measured, we might find a direct correlation between a central measure of activation and level of performance. For instance, the Bélanger and Feldman experiment described earlier might be repeated with the addition of recordings from the ARAS. The aim of such an experiment would be to determine whether the continuous rise in the heart rate curve with increasing deprivation times could be matched by a similar rise in amplitude of deflections from recording in the ARAS with implanted electrodes. Recent neurophysiological experiments appear encouraging with respect to the feasibility of such an approach (Li & Jasper, 1953, pp. 124–125; Magoun, 1958, p. 68).

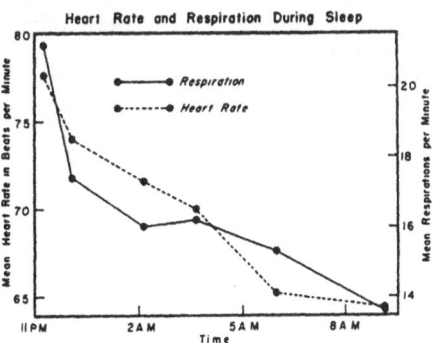

FIG. 5. Mean values for heart rate and respiration from the same *S*s at the same times during sleep as in Fig. 3 and 4.

EFFECTS OF INCREASED ACTIVATION ON LOCALIZED SKELETAL-MUSCLE TENSION IN PSYCHIATRIC PATIENTS

The implication of activation theory for various clinical phenomena might very well be the topic of a separate paper. Certainly there is not space to deal at length with the topic here. I have chosen, therefore, to present a

ROBERT B. MALMO

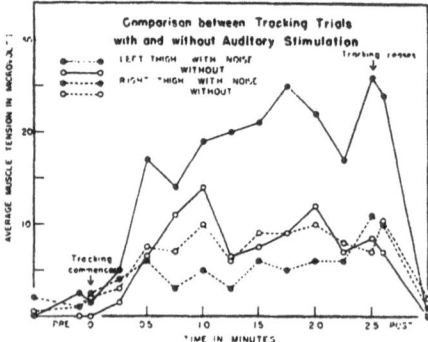

FIG. 6. Mean muscle tension from left thigh and right thigh from patient with complaint of tensional discomfort in the left thigh. Note that when patient was performing the tracking task under distraction (loud noise), tension rose in the left thigh but not in the right. See text for explanation.

few recent observations, chiefly in order to suggest how level of activation may be studied in relation to a clinical phenomenon.

The graph in Fig. 6 illustrates what appears to be a general finding in patients complaining of tensional discomfort in a localized muscular site. The data for the curves plotted in the figure were obtained from a psychiatric patient, a 42-year old woman who complained of muscular discomfort localized in the left thigh. In the session when these data were taken electromyograms (EMGs) were recorded from various muscles over the body; those from the left and right thighs are shown in the figure. The patient was engaged in pursuit tracking using an apparatus similar to the one employed by Surwillo (1955, 1956). Figure 6 shows that when a loud distracting noise, of the kind described by Schnore (1959), was presented during tracking, the tension in the left thigh was very much higher than that of the right thigh. When tracking was carried out under distraction free con-

ditions this tensional difference between thighs was not observed.

Interpretation of these data seems quite straightforward. When level of activation was increased by presenting a loud distracting noise the effect was shown entirely in one muscle group, the left thigh, which was the symptom area in this patient. Simultaneous recordings of tension from other parts of the body showed that the tension was specific to the left thigh and was not merely increased on the whole left side of the body.

The specificity of the left thigh in indicating the higher activation is quite clear. Observe that tension in the thigh muscles on the opposite side of the body actually fell slightly under the activating condition.

The same procedure was carried out with a second patient, a young girl of 28, who complained of a distressing feeling of tightness in the neck on the right side. Results were similar to the ones obtained in the previous case, with activation again showing its effect specifically in the symptom area. When the loud distracting noise was turned on during tracking, tension in this area showed marked increase whereas tension in the muscles on the left side of the neck showed no rise whatever.

Very similar results were obtained from two additional patients whose areas of tensional discomfort were localized in still different parts of the body. One woman with complaint of tension on the left side of her neck served as a useful control for the patient previously described with tension localized in the opposite side of the neck. No tracking experiment was carried out with this patient. Apparently the sight of the EMG recording room for the first time was itself sufficient to increase the amplitude of muscle potentials from the symptom area so that they become appreciably higher than those on the opposite side of her neck. The other woman (fourth patient in this series) complained of tensional discomfort that appeared to originate in the left shoulder. EMGs were recorded from the left and right shoulders of this patient while she lay in bed listening to the playback of a recorded interview. During the first part of the playback, tension was about the same on the two sides of the body. But when the topic concerning her dead sister commenced to come over the speaker, tension in the left shoulder became much greater than that in the right.

As far as could be determined, the EMG data from all these patients were consistent in suggesting that for skeletal-muscle tension in patients with well-developed tensional symptoms, increasing the activation level up to a certain point has the effect of raising muscle tension in one localized muscle group, the one in which the patient complained of tensional discomfort. It was not necessary for the patient to actually feel the discomfort during the experimental session for this differential result to appear. I have been using the term "symptom area" to refer to the muscle group where the discomfort was localized when present.

Interesting findings that appear to parallel those from the patients were obtained from three young male nonpatient Ss in our recent investigation of sleep deprivation. As previously mentioned, evidence from EEG, palmar conductance, and respiration indicated that activation during tracking increased progressively with hours of sleep deprivation. In addition to these other physiological tracings, EMGs from various areas over the body were also recorded. One muscle area, a different one for each S, showed significant rise in tension over the vigil. It

was the neck muscles in one S, the forehead in another, and the biceps muscle of the right arm in the third. In each case the one muscle showed statistically significant rise in tension, and in none of the Ss was there significant tensional rise in any other muscle. In fact, there was regularly progressive and very significant fall in the tension of the left forearm in all three Ss. As far as I know, none of the men actually complained of tensional discomfort in the areas showing rise in tension during the vigil.

Where high level activation is long continued as in a vigil or in certain psychoneurotic patients, it appears that skeletal tension may become localized to a single muscle group. The discomfort associated with this tension in some patients can become extremely severe. It should be noted that in one-session experiments, where rise in activation was for relatively short intervals of time, tensional rise occurred in more than one muscle group (Surwillo, 1956; Stennett, 1957a).

Methodologically, these results are important because they reveal a difference between EMGs and some other physiological measures with respect to gauging activation. Unlike heart rate or respiration rate that invariably yields one measure no matter how it is recorded, there are as many measures of muscle tension as there are muscles that can be recorded from. It appears that when sufficient care is taken, EMGs may be very valuable in helping to gauge activation, but that considerable caution is required in the interpretation of results, and especially in the interpretation of negative results.

From the clinical point of view it seems an interesting speculation that the patient's localized muscle tension may itself actually increase the general activation level. (I do not mean the level of muscle tension all over the body.) Two main assumptions are involved in this suggestion. The first one is that the area of localized muscle tension in the patient acts like tension that is induced, for example, by having an *S* squeeze on a dynamometer. From the generalized effects of tension induction on learning and performance it is clear that the effects of increased muscle tension are quite general ones. Though crucial physiological data are missing in these experiments, as previously mentioned, one very likely explanation of these results is that the local increase in muscle tension somehow produces an increase in the general level of activation, with rise in heart rate and blood pressure, with fall in level of EEG alpha, and so on. This is the second assumption. The results of two recent experiments are in line with this assumption. Meyer and Noble (1958) found that induced tension interacted with "anxiety" in verbal-maze learning ("anxiety" measured by means of the MAS [Taylor, 1953]), while Kuethe and Eriksen (1957) in a study of stereotypy likewise reported a significant interaction between these two variables when "anxiety" was experimentally produced by means of electric shocks. The MAS appears to select individuals who are significantly above the mean in activation, and from the results of Schnore (1959) and Feldman (1958) it seems safe to conclude that anticipation of shock also leads to increased levels of physiological activity. In short, generalizing from the induced tension experiments, it seems reasonable to suppose that a patient's muscular tension in a small focal area might have the general effect of increasing activation. If such is the case symptomatic treatment might have significant general as well as specific effects. Although based on only one patient, Yates' (1958)

results from symptomatic treatment of tics seems encouraging with respect to the feasibility of research in this general area.

Summary

The neuropsychological dimension of activation may be briefly described as follows. The continuum extending from deep sleep at the low activation end to "excited" states at the high activation end is a function of the amount of cortical bombardment by the ARAS, such that the greater the cortical bombardment the higher the activation. The shape of the curve relating level of performance to level of activation is that of an inverted U: from low activation up to a point that is optimal for a given performance or function, level of performance rises monotonically with increasing activation level; but past this optimal point the relation becomes nonmonotonic: further increase in activation beyond this point produces fall in performance level, this fall being directly related to the amount of the increase in level of activation.

Long before the discovery of the ARAS the behavioral evidence of Duffy, Freeman, and others of the "energetics" group had suggested the existence of some such brain mechanism. Moreover, learning theorists of the Hull school have in their concept of the general drive state come very close to the activation principle. Up to the present time they have employed physiological measures only sparingly and have restricted their use to the aversive aspects of drive. But with evidence that such measures may also be applied to nonaversive (appetitional) drive, it seems likely that the present rather unsatisfactory measures of drive may eventually be replaced by physiological indicants.

Activation has a number of main

characteristics that may be listed as follows: (*a*) Activation has no steering function in behavior. (*b*) It is considerably broader than emotion. (*c*) Activation is not a state that can be inferred from knowledge of antecedent conditions alone, because it is the product of an interaction between internal conditions such as hunger or thirst, and external cues. (*d*) Activation does not fit very well into the S-R formula. It is a phenomenon of slow changes, of drifts in level with a time order of minutes (even hours) not of seconds or fractions thereof. (*e*) Activation is a quantifiable dimension and the evidence indicates that physiological measures show a sufficiently high intraindividual concordance for quantifying this dimension.

It is suggested that activation is mediated chiefly through the ARAS which seems, in the main, to be an intensity system. Neurophysiological findings strongly suggest that it may be possible to achieve more precise measurement of activation through a direct recording of discharge by the ARAS into the cerebral cortex. Research on this problem is urgently needed.

The concept of activation appears to have wide application to phenomena in the field of clinical psychology. As one illustration, in this paper, activation was applied to clinical phenomena of tensional symptoms.

REFERENCES

BINDRA, D. *Motivation. A systematic reinterpretation.* New York: Ronald, 1959.

BROWN, J. S. Pleasure-seeking behavior and the drive-reduction hypothesis. *Psychol. Rev.*, 1955, **62**, 169–179.

CAMPBELL, B. A., & SHEFFIELD, F. D. Relation of random activity to food deprivation. *J. comp. physiol. Psychol.*, 1953, **46**, 320–326.

COFER, C. N. Motivation. *Annu. Rev. Psychol.*, 1959, **10**, 173–202.

COURTS, F. A. Relations between muscular tension and performance. *Psychol. Bull.*, 1942, **39**, 347–367.

DARROW, C. W. Psychological and psychophysiological significance of the electroencephalogram. *Psychol. Rev.*, 1947, **54**, 157–168.

DAVIS, R. C. Modification of the galvanic reflex by daily repetition of a stimulus. *J. exp. Psychol.*, 1934, **17**, 504–535.

DELL, P. C. Humoral effects on the brain stem reticular formations. In H. H. Jasper, L. D. Proctor, R. S. Knighton, W. C. Noshay, & R. T. Costello (Eds.), *Reticular formation of the brain.* Toronto: Little, Brown, 1958. Pp. 365–379.

DUFFY, ELIZABETH. The measurement of muscular tension as a technique for the study of emotional tendencies. *Amer. J. Psychol.*, 1932, **44**, 146–162.

DUFFY, ELIZABETH. The concept of energy mobilization. *Psychol. Rev.*, 1951, **58**, 30–40.

DUFFY, ELIZABETH. The psychological significance of the concept of "arousal" or "activation." *Psychol. Rev.*, 1957, **64**, 265–275.

DUFFY, ELIZABETH, & LACEY, O. L. Adaptation in energy mobilization: changes in general level of palmar skin conductance. *J. exp. Psychol.*, 1946, **36**, 437–452.

DUSSER DE BARENNE, J. G. The labyrinthine and postural mechanisms. In C. Murchison (Ed.), *A handbook of general experimental psychology.* Worcester, Mass.: Clark Univer. Press, 1934. Pp. 204–246.

FELDMAN, S. M. Differential effect of shock as a function of intensity and cue factors in maze learning. Unpublished doctoral dissertation, McGill Univer., 1958.

FINAN, J. L. Quantitative studies of motivation. I. Strength of conditioning in rats under varying degrees of hunger. *J. comp. Psychol.*, 1940, **29**, 119–134.

FINCH, G. Hunger as a determinant of conditional and unconditional salivary response magnitude. *Amer. J. Physiol.*, 1938, **123**, 379–382.

FREEMAN, G. L. The relationship between performance level and bodily activity level. *J. exp. Psychol.*, 1940, **26**, 602–608.

FREEMAN, G. L. *The energetics of human behavior.* Ithaca, N. Y.: Cornell Univer. Press, 1948.

FUSTER, J. M. Effects of stimulation of brain stem on tachistoscopic perception. *Science*, 1958, **127**, 150.

HEBB, D. O. *The organization of behavior.* New York: Wiley, 1949.

ROBERT B. MALMO

HEBB, D. O. Drives and the C.N.S. (conceptual nervous system). *Psychol. Rev.,* 1955, **62**, 243–254.

JASPER, H. H. Electroencephalography. In W. Penfield & T. C. Erickson (Eds.), *Epilepsy and cerebral localization.* Springfield, Ill.: Charles C Thomas, 1941, 380–454.

KAPLAN, M. The effects of noxious stimulus intensity and duration during intermittent reinforcement of escape behavior. *J. comp. physiol. Psychol.,* 1952, **45**, 538–549.

KENDLER, H. H. Learning. *Annu. Rev. Psychol.,* 1959, **10**, 43–88.

KUETHE, J. L., & ERIKSEN, C. W. Personality, anxiety, and muscle tension as determinants of response stereotypy. *J. abnorm. soc. Psychol.,* 1957, **54**, 400–404.

LACEY, J. I., & LACEY, BEATRICE C. Verification and extension of the principle of autonomic response-stereotypy. *Amer. J. Psychol.,* 1958, **71**, 50–73.

LI, C. L., & JASPER, H. H. Microelectrode studies of the electrical activity of the cerebral cortex in the cat. *J. Physiol.,* 1953, **121**, 117–140.

LINDSLEY, D. B. Emotion. In S. S. Stevens (Ed.), *Handbook of experimental psychology.* New York: Wiley, 1951. Pp. 473–516.

LINDSLEY, D. B. Psychophysiology and motivation. In M. R. Jones (Ed.), *Nebraska symposium on motivation 1957.* Lincoln: Univer. Nebr. Press, 1957. Pp. 44–105.

LORENTE DE NÓ, R. Transmission of impulses through cranial motor nuclei. *J. Neurophysiol.,* 1939, **2**, 402–464.

MAGOUN, H. W. *The waking brain.* Springfield, Ill.: Charles C Thomas, 1958.

MALMO, R. B. Measurement of drive: An unsolved problem in psychology. In M. R. Jones (Ed.), *Nebraska symposium on motivation 1958.* Lincoln: Univer. Nebr. Press, 1958, 229–265.

MALMO, R. B., & SHAGASS, C. Physiologic study of symptom mechanisms in psychiatric patients under stress. *Psychosom. Med.,* 1949, **11**, 25–29.

MEYER, D. R., & NOBLE, M. E. Summation of manifest anxiety and muscular tension. *J. exp. Psychol.,* 1958, **55**, 599–602.

OLSZEWSKI, J. The cytoarchitecture of the human reticular formation. In J. F. Delafresnaye (Ed.), *Brain mechanisms and consciousness.* Springfield, Ill.: Charles C Thomas, 1954. Pp. 54–76.

ROSS, W. R. D., & DAVIS, J. F. Stable bandpass filters for electroencephalography. *IRE Canad. Convention Rec. 1958,* Paper No. 860, 202–206.

ROTHBALLER, A. B. Studies on the adrenaline-sensitive component of the reticular activating system. *EEG Clin. Neurophysiol.,* 1956, **8**, 603–621.

SAFFRAN, M., SCHALLY, A. V., & BENFEY, B. G. Stimulation of the release of corticotropin from the adenohypophysis by a neurohypophysial factor. *Endocrinology,* 1955, **57**, 439–444.

SCHNORE, M. M. Individual patterns of physiological activity as a function of task differences and degree of arousal. *J. exp. Psychol.,* 1959, **58**, 117–128.

SPENCE, K. W. Theory of emotionally based drive (D) and its relation to performance in simple learning situations. *Amer. Psychologist,* 1958, **13**, 131–141.

STENNETT, R. G. The relationship of performance level to level of arousal. *J. exp. Psychol.,* 1957, **54**, 54–61. (a)

STENNETT, R. G. The relationship of alpha amplitude to the level of palmar conductance. *EEG Clin. Neurophysiol.,* 1957, **9**, 131–138. (b)

SURWILLO, W. W. A device for recording variations in pressure of grip during tracking. *Amer. J. Psychol.,* 1955, **68**, 669–670.

SURWILLO, W. W. Psychological factors in muscle-action potentials: EMG gradients. *J. exp. Psychol.,* 1956, **52**, 263–272.

TAYLOR, JANET A. A personality scale of manifest anxiety. *J. abnorm. soc. Psychol.,* 1953, **48**, 285–290.

WOODWORTH, R. S., & SCHLOSBERG, H. *Experimental psychology.* New York: Holt, 1954.

YATES, A. J. The application of learning theory to the treatment of tics. *J. abnorm. soc. Psychol.,* 1958, **56**, 175–182.

(Received May 4, 1959)

From W. I. Hume and G. S. Claridge (1965). Life Sciences, *4,* 545-553, *by kind permission of the authors and Pergamon Press.*

A COMPARISON OF TWO MEASURES OF "AROUSAL" IN NORMAL SUBJECTS

W. I. Hume, B.Sc.

G. S. Claridge, Ph.D.[*]

Department of Psychological Medicine,
University of Glasgow,
Southern General Hospital,
Glasgow, S.W.1.

The purpose of this study was to investigate the relationship, in a normal sample, between the subjective report of the fusion threshold of paired light flashes and the ongoing level of skin potential.

Leiderman & Shapiro[1] showed that sleeping Ss had a lower potential level than when they were awake and resting, and that this in turn was lower than the level under stimulating conditions. Thus as S became more "aroused"[2] his potential level increased. (It should be mentioned here that the actual potentials are negative in sign, but this is a methodological artifact and we shall refer to the absolute sign only). In an unpublished study in the authors' laboratory it was found that the two-flash threshold (TFT) was significantly lowered when S had his hand immersed in a bath of water at 10°C. This stimulus is subjectively highly arousing and one would thus expect that the more aroused S is, the lower will be his two-flash threshold. It would then be predicted that the TFT will

―――――――
[*]This study was supported in part by the Mental Health Research Fund; G.D. Searle & Co., Ltd.; Parke Davis & Co., Ltd. and A. Wander, Ltd.

"AROUSAL" IN NORMAL SUBJECTS

correlate negatively with skin potential; high potentials being associated with good discrimination (i.e. a low threshold measure). However Venables[3] reported a significant <u>positive</u> correlation between the two measures in normals, those Ss with a high skin potential being relatively poorer at discriminating between the flashes.

In view of the unexpected natures of Venables' findings, it was thought desirable to replicate his study as far as possible.

SUBJECTS

20 non-patient Ss took part in the experiment. Most of them were nurses. The age range was 18-40 years. It has been shown that age does not affect the TFT within these limits[3]. 17 of the Ss were female.

TWO-FLASH THRESHOLD

The apparatus was the same as that described by Venables[3] except for a slight alteration in the flash interval circuit. The flash duration was varied in steps between 1 and 40 msecs. The interval between the members of each pair of flashes could be varied from 5-500 msecs in 10 msecs steps. Pairs of flashes were presented at 5 second intervals. The threshold was determined by the method of limits: the inter-flash interval was increased until S indicated he could see two flashes, then it was decreased until he could see only one. Each interval was presented at least twice and it was not changed until S had given two consecutive identical judgements. The threshold was taken as the interval where S changed his judgement from 1 to 2 and vice versa. Two values were thus obtained, for increasing and decreasing intervals respectively; the final

"AROUSAL" IN NORMAL SUBJECTS

value being the mean of these two.   S indicated his judgement
by pressing a button with his left hand.   This is a typical
example of the procedure:-

   80-2,2; 70-2,2; 60-2,1[*],1.   Decreasing threshold=60 msecs.

   50-1,1; 60-1,1; 70-2[*],2.   Increasing threshold=70 msecs.

    The mean value is 65 msecs, and this was taken as the two-
flash threshold.   The asterisks denote the point where the
potential was measured.   Where the discrepancy between
increasing and decreasing thresholds was greater than 20 msecs,
the data were rejected.   The flash durations used were 1,5,10,
20,30 and 40 msecs.   They were presented in a random order for
each S.

SKIN POTENTIAL

    The electrodes were silver-silver chloride prepared
according to Venables and Sayer[4].   KCl was the electrolyte, in
a concentration of 0.5 gm/100 mls.   The electrode disc was
stuck in the end of a $\frac{1}{4}$" long plastic cylinder, forming a cup.
A small piece of sponge was soaked in the electrolyte and put in
the electrode cup which was then stuck onto the prepared skin
site with adhesive tape.   The skin had been washed with methylated spirit, and the site under the inactive electrode carefully
sanded to rupture the stratum lucidum and thus destroy any
potential generated at the site[5].   The active electrode was
placed on the palmar surface of the proximal segment of the
middle finger of the right hand;   the inactive electrode was on
the ventral aspect of the wrist.   Amplification was by a Grass
5P-1 DC amplifier, input impedence 1 megohm.   A balance
potential was put in series with the subject so that the zero

"AROUSAL" IN NORMAL SUBJECTS

point on the write-out chart corresponded to this potential.
Deviation from this zero was never more than 5 mV. This
procedure is virtually identical to that of Venables, as far as
the important variables are concerned.

PROCEDURE

S sat in a semi-sound proof room kept at a constant
temperature of $70^{\circ}C$, and illuminated by a 40W orange bulb placed
under the table supporting the two-flash unit. This enabled S
to be observed through a one-way screen. S was instructed to
keep his head in contact with a shaped head-rest to ensure that
the image of the flashes fell on roughly the same area of the
retina all the time. After placement of the electrodes S was
told to sit quietly for 2 minutes, then to respond to the flashes
when they appeared, by pressing the button. E then left the
room and began recording. When S's potential had steadied,
the flashes were switched on and extreme values of the intervals
were presented initially to ensure that S had understood the
instructions and was responding correctly, and to allow for
habituation of the potential response to the flashes.

RESULTS

Initially the potential level decreased steadily, but once
S was responding to the flashes, the level stabilised and
remained almost constant throughout the experiment. It can
thus be assumed that S's arousal level did not change during
the experiment. The potential measure used was the mean of the
two values when S changed his judgement for increasing and
decreasing intervals. These points are indicated by asterisks
in the example given earlier. The potential was measured to the

TABLE 1

Means, Standard Deviations and Ranges of Two-Flash Threshold (TFT), and Skin Potential for Various Flash Durations.

	Flash Duration (msecs.)					
	1	5	10	20	30	40
TFT (msecs.)	68.25	60.50	58.95	53.06	47.35	41.18
s.d.	10.40	8.65	8.97	8.35	6.21	10.50
Range	40-95	40-75	35-75	30-70	35-60	10-60
Pot.(-mV)	34.53	34.89	35.65	34.89	33.75	35.56
s.d.	15.41	15.66	16.10	17.01	15.54	16.65
Range	8.1-68.0	8.8-67.4	7.5-70.3	6.6-69.4	6.4-64.7	8.3-66.5
N	20	20	19	18	17	17

"AROUSAL" IN NORMAL SUBJECTS

TABLE 2.

Product-Moment Correlations between Two-Flash Threshold and
Skin Potential at Various Flash Durations*

	Flash Duration (msecs.)					
	1	5	10	20	30	40
r	-0.51	-0.27	-0.30	-0.39	-0.06	-0.31
Sig. Level	5%	n.s.	n.s.	n.s.	n.s.	n.s.
N	20	20	19	18	17	17

* The actual potential values are negative, but the sign was
ignored in calculating the correlations.

nearest 0.1 mV.

The results of statistical analysis of the data are presented in Tables 1 and 2.

DISCUSSION

It has previously been shown that the threshold for the discrimination of flashes is a function of the total sensory input, i.e. a combination of intensity and duration of flashes, and the background intensity[6]. Since the mean threshold for 1 msec. flashes was not different from Venables' it can be assumed that, as far as the discriminating mechanism in the nervous system is concerned, the physical determinent of the threshold, (i.e. the total sensory input) was identical in the two cases. The mean and range of our potential values are slightly greater than Venables', but the difference is not significant. We thus have two virtually identical experiments giving diametrically opposite results. Rose (personal communication) has also compared the TFT with an electrodermal measure (skin conductance) and obtained results which agree with those reported here for the 1 msec. flashes; i.e. high conductance (high arousal) being associated with good discrimination. On the other hand, Eysenck and Warwick[7] found no relation between these two variables. The confusion is worsened by the fact that Venables replicated his own findings on a second group of normals.

It will be noted that, of the 6 correlations computed, only one was significant, and that only at the 5% level. It is likely that this is a chance result because, if the relation between potential and threshold is a valid one, it should be

"AROUSAL" IN NORMAL SUBJECTS

revealed irrespective of the flash duration, since there is a linear relation between threshold and duration. However, the other non-significant correlations are all negative, and show a trend towards a value of about -0.3, indicating the possibility of a slight negative relation between the two measures.

The most obvious explanation of the discrepancies between the various results discussed above is in terms of sampling differences. If the correlation between two measures in a large group is zero, it is possible to extract sub-groups for which the correlation can be either significantly positive or negative. As the number in the sub-group increases, the correlation tends towards that for the total group. This is particularly relevant if the two measures used are related to personality. It is possible to choose a sub-group which appears to be randomly selected, but which, in fact, is homogeneous with respect to some personality factor which affects one or both of the measures. This is especially true if the Ss are volunteers - they do not constitute a random sample as far as personality is concerned.

On the available evidence it is not possible to say which of the reported correlations between skin potential and TFT is the most valid. As mentioned earlier one would expect a negative correlation, i.e. high arousal reflected by large potential levels being associated with high arousal (good discrimination, i.e. low values) on the TFT. But several studies comparing measures of sensory and autonomic "arousal" have shown a prominent lack of correlation between different measures in normal groups[8,9]. With psychiatric groups on the other hand, significant correlations have been found between the same

"AROUSAL" IN NORMAL SUBJECTS

measures[8,10]. Venables[3] also found a negative correlation between TFT and skin potential in a group of chronic schizophrenics. The relation between any two measures of arousal will depend on the group of subjects used, and on the particular measures themselves.

SUMMARY

The relation between the two-flash threshold and level of skin potential was investigated in a group of non-patient subjects, for 6 flash durations. Only at the 1 msec. duration was the correlation significant (-0.51) and only then at the 5% level. The discrepancy between these results and those reported by Venables for a virtually identical experiment is thought to be due to sampling differences.

REFERENCES

1. P.H. LEIDERMAN & D. SHAPIRO, J. Psychosom. Res. 7, 277,(1964)

2. R.B. MALMO, Psychol. Rev. 64, 265 (1959).

3. P.H. VENABLES, J. Psychiat. Res. 1. 279 (1963).

4. P.H. VENABLES & E. SAYER, Brit. J. Psychol. 54, 251 (1963).

5. S. ROTHMAN, Physiology and Biochemistry of the Skin, University of Chicago Press. (1954).

6. P.J. FOLEY, J. Opt. Soc. Amer. 51, 737 (1961).

7. H.J. EYSENCK & K.M. WARWICK, Experiments in Motivation, (ed. H.J. Eysenck), Pergamon Press, London. P.152. (1964).

8. G.S. CLARIDGE & R.N. HERRINGTON, J. ment. Sci. 106, 1568 (1960).

9. R.A. STERNBACH, EEG clin. Neurophysiol. 12, 609 (1960).

10. S.R. KRISHNAMOORTI & C. SHAGASS, Recent Advances in Biological Psychaitry, Vol. VI. (ed. J. WORTIS), Plenum Press, New York. P. 256 (1964).

From S. P. Taylor and S. Epstein (1967). Psychosomatic Medicine, *29*, 514-525, *by kind permission of the authors and Elsevier North-Holland.*

The Measurement of Autonomic Arousal

Some Basic Issues Illustrated by the Covariation of Heart Rate and Skin Conductance

STUART P. TAYLOR, Ph.D.,* and SEYMOUR EPSTEIN, Ph.D.

Empirical evidence is presented to demonstrate that there is no *true* relationship between such physiological measures as heart rate and skin conductance, but that (depending on circumstances) heart rate and skin conductance covary directly, inversely, or not at all. It is contended that a solution to the general measurement of arousal will not be found by transforming single measures, by innovations in data reduction, or by combining measures. Instead, the solution lies in learning more about the unique properties of different physiological systems by establishing how they vary as a function of the parameters of stimulus input—such as intensity, rate of stimulation, and time since stimulus onset.

THE FINDING of low intercorrelations among physiological measures (cf. Ax[1] and Lacey and Lacey[10]) has been a source of disturbance to a number of psychologists seeking an index of general arousal. Lazarus and colleagues[11] state that low correlations are "embarrassing to those who propose a general activation or arousal syndrome."

To deal with this problem, two general solutions have been proposed, one of which is to use multiple measures. Duffy[2] states: "it is probable that a combination of measures is more satisfactory than any measures taken singly." Proponents of the second approach have attempted to prove that low correlations are an artifact produced by inappropriate procedures or improper units of measurement. This has led to a search for procedures, transformations, and methods of data reduction to improve the correlations. It is further argued, from the same viewpoint, that intrasubject correlations, which have generally been found to be higher than intersubject correlations, are more germane to the concept of general arousal. In this respect, Schnore[15] notes that "it is possible . . . to obtain a zero correlation between any two variables when the correlation is computed among Ss, while the correlation between the same two variables can be perfect if computed within an S." Lazarus *et al.*[11] conclude

From the Psychology Department, University of Massachusetts, Amherst, Mass.

Supported by Research Grant MH 01293 from the National Institute of Mental Health, U. S. Public Health Service (S. Epstein).

*Present Address: Department of Psychology, Kent State University, Kent, Ohio.

Received for publication Aug. 11, 1966.

that the traditional "inter-individual correlation . . . obtained across subjects does not properly reflect the organization of autonomic activity in any given person, or in subjects in general."

In a study comparing reactions of heart rate and skin conductance during observation of a stressful film, Lazarus *et al.* reported a mean intrasubject correlation of .54 and concluded that while the correlation was not perfect, "nevertheless, we need not abandon the conviction of many decades that there is a substantial generality to autonomic nervous system reactions and that it is not altogether inappropriate to employ single measures of autonomic reactivity." Based on the assumption that "persistent efforts to improve methods of scoring the autonomic variables might reveal much closer relationships between such variables," Malmstrom *et al.*[12] attempted to improve the correspondence between heart rate and skin conductance levels of Ss observing a stressful movie by utilizing "the method of mean cyclic maxima," which controls for short-term cyclic changes in heart rate by averaging the peaks on a cardiotachometer record over brief intervals. It is noteworthy that while the method of mean cyclic maxima improved the over-all correspondence between skin conductance and heart rate, some of the findings on heart rate as related to stress points in the movie continued to be anomalous. The authors concluded: "A close inspection of the curves . . . suggests that many questions are raised by the results, although in general the summary statement that heart rate and skin conductance tend to rise and fall together over times is accurate."

The problem inherent in the two positions discussed above is that they both rest upon the assumption that the basic relationship between two autonomic measures, such as heart rate and skin conductance (to each other and to a general concept of arousal), is essentially positive and linear, and that the failure to obtain high correlations can be attributed to error of measurement in some form or other. The first position leads to an attempt to compensate for the error in a single measure by pooling across many measures, all of which are presumed to contribute to total arousal, much as the different scales in an intelligence test contribute to an over-all IQ. The second position leads to an attempt to improve individual measures. It is the contention of this paper that the basic assumption underlying both positions is incorrect. It should be noted that the author's position is not that the concept of general arousal is necessarily invalid, but that, to the extent that it is valid, it can be measured meaningfully only by the use of appropriate indices based upon a knowledge of the distinctive properties of different physiological response systems. It is necessary to conduct experiments to establish the relationship of activity in different physiological systems to the parameters of stress and the presumed total level of stimulus input with which the organism must cope. It will be shown in this paper that there is no one *true* relationship between two physiological measures, such as heart rate and skin conductance, but that, depending upon variations in the parameters of stress between and within the experiments in which correlations between measures were obtained, intraindividual correlations can be positive, negative, or of zero magnitude. The data can be understood in terms of adaptive functioning of the nervous system, and not in terms of error of measurement. Lacey *et al.*[9a] have made the same point, emphasizing the contrary impact on the cardiovascular system of task demands for cognitive elaboration as opposed to demands for attention to environmental events.

We will cite two experimental situations from work in our laboratory in which information was obtained on the covariation of heart rate and skin conductance under different conditions of stress. Their combined results will make it clear that the direction and magnitude of correlation between heart rate and skin conductance vary with such factors as the spacing of stressful episodes, the range of stress to which individuals are exposed, the points at which data are obtained following the onset of a stressful episode, and the rate at which stress mounts. It will be demonstrated that under conditions in which skin conductance provided a highly reliable and unambiguous index of stress, heart rate produced anomalous results. Selection of heart rate alone would have led to erroneous conclusions about the effect of stress upon arousal, while combining both measures would have resulted in a canceling-out process.

Intrasubject Correlations among Parachutists

The study reported here is one in a series on sport parachuting that we have been conducting in our laboratory over the past several years in order to investigate the experience and mastery of stress and conflict. In the present study, which was described in detail in an earlier issue of the JOURNAL,[4] we were interested in the physiological reactions of two groups of parachutists along a time dimension from before to after a parachute jump. One group consisted of 10 highly experienced parachutists for whom the stress produced by a jump could be assumed to be minimal, while the other group consisted of novice parachutists for whom the experience was manifestly highly threatening. The experienced parachutists had all made over 100 jumps, while no novice parachutists had made more than 5 jumps. Data on heart rate, skin conductance, and respiration rate were obtained for 14 points in time. Physiological activity was monitored on a control day on which the parachutist did not intend to jump; on the day of a jump at a few points before the parachutist entered the aircraft; continuously during ascent in the aircraft up to the point at which the electrodes had to be disconnected immediately before the parachutist exited the aircraft; and shortly after landing. With 14 readings for each of the three measures, simultaneously recorded, it was possible to obtain intrasubject correlations for each S on the three combinations of the measures. Table 1 presents a summary of the intrasubject correlations grouped according to the level of experience of the parachutist. The median intrasubject correlation for heart rate and skin conductance was $+.20$ for novices as compared to $+.68$ for experienced parachutists.

Only 2 out of 10 of the novices produced a correlation significantly greater than zero, and some produced negative correlations. The situation was consider-

TABLE 1. INTRASUBJECT CORRELATIONS AMONG BASAL CONDUCTANCE, HEART RATE, AND RESPIRATION RATE FOR 10 NOVICE AND 10 EXPERIENCED JUMPERS OVER THE ENTIRE JUMP SEQUENCE (POINTS 1–14)

	Novice parachutists			Experienced parachutists		
Variables correlated	Mdn. correl.	*N at .05	Range	Mdn. correl.	*N at .05	Range
Basal cond.–heart rate	$+.20$	2	$-.46-+.64$	$+.68$	8	$+.19-+.91$
Basal cond.–resp. rate	$+.21$	1	$-.51-+.60$	$+.65$	7	$+.30-+.83$
Heart rate–resp. rate	$+.56$	6	$-.05-+.66$	$+.83$	8	$+.34-+.93$

* Number of individual correlations significantly different from zero at the .05 level of confidence.

55

TAYLOR & EPSTEIN

ably different for experienced parachutists, all of whom produced positive correlations, eight of which were reliably
greater than zero. On the basis of such
data, what is one to conclude about the
true intrasubject correlation between
heart rate and skin conductance? While
the median correlation for the experienced parachutists is higher than the
+.54 reported by Lazarus *et al.*,[11] which
led them to express faith in the linear
covariation of physiological measures,
the correlations for the novices suggest
a complete lack of relationship. Obviously, the question as to which set of
correlations represents the true relationship between the variables is meaningless, as both sets of correlations describe
relationships within the different groups

equally well. The difference in correlations cannot be attributed to initial differences in basal rates, since initial as
well as final basal rates on both measures
were almost identical for the two groups.
Thus, it is unlikely that any form of
transformation could remove the difference.

In searching for an explanation, it is
useful to consider the relationship of
each measure taken individually to the
time dimension. Figure 1 presents basal
skin conductance data for novice and
experienced jumpers as a function of the
variations in stress associated with the
14 points in time. Figure 2 does the same
for heart rate. It is immediately evident
that both measures produce similar results. The novice and experienced parachutists show increasing physiological
activity up to a point, after which the
novices demonstrate a continuing increase and the experienced parachutists
a leveling-off followed by a decrease in
physiological activity. When each group
is examined separately to compare skin
conductance for novices (Fig. 1) with
heart rate in novices (Fig. 2), and to
make the same comparison for experienced jumpers, it is evident that within
both groups, the curves for heart rate
and skin conductance show a reasonably
high degree of correspondence. When
one measure is high, the other tends to
be high; when one is low, the other tends
to be low. This correspondence makes it
yet more puzzling as to why it was only
the experienced parachutists who produced reliable intrasubject correlations.
A clue is provided in the observation that
the range and upper limit of physiological activity on both measures is higher
for the novices than for the experienced
jumpers. The difference in range is of
particular interest, since, on the basis of
statistical considerations alone, range
should affect the magnitude of the correlations. Yet, on this basis, it would be
the novices and not the experienced
parachutists who would have the higher

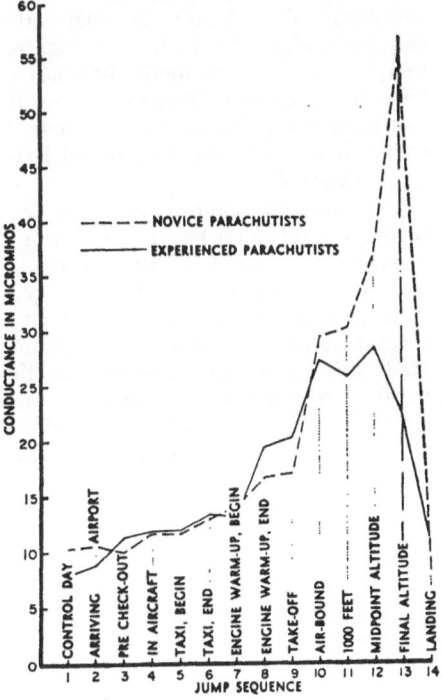

FIG. 1. Basal conductance of experienced
and novice parachutists as function of
sequence of events leading up to and following jump. (From Fenz and Epstein[4]).

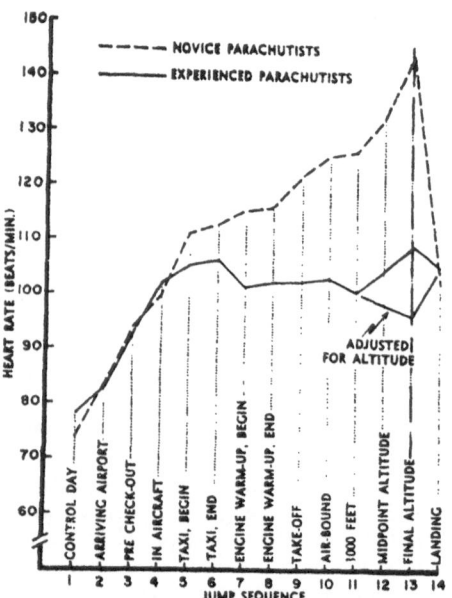

FIG. 2. Heart rate of experienced and novice parachutists as function of sequence of events connected with jump. "Adjusted for altitude" refers to correction for altitude based on values reported for mean heart rates at different simulated altitudes. (Novices jump at lower altitudes; no corrections are necessary.) All correlations were based on uncorrected values. That correlations were not markedly altered by altitude was confirmed by having experienced parachutists jump at same altitude as novices. (From Fenz and Epstein,[4] q.v.)

correlations. It must be assumed that some other factor is operating which more than compensates for the statistical bias produced by the effect of range. The possibility must be considered that the difference in correlations may be a result of the different levels of arousal reached by the two groups. This hypothesis can be tested by computing correlations using only the first 10 points, which eliminates the period of maximum stress for the novice parachutists, and makes their upper point of physiological activity more comparable with that of the experienced parachutists. When this

is done, the intrasubject correlations contributed by the two groups are highly similar (Table 2).

What has been noted about the correlation between heart rate and skin conductance holds equally true for the correlations between skin conductance and respiration rate, and between heart rate and respiration rate. It must be concluded that, even within a single stressful situation such as parachuting, there is no one true relationship between two physiological variables, such as heart rate and skin conductance; rather, the magnitude of the relationship is affected by the absolute level of the variables. As stress-produced arousal mounts, direct correlation between heart rate, skin conductance, and respiration rate within individuals gives way to asynchronous variation. The change in relationship can be understood if it is recognized that, in order to maintain homeostatic balance within and between systems, the relationship of physiological systems to each other and to general arousal is apt to be complex.

The situation might well have been further complicated had higher levels of stress been reached by the novices, or had the rate of increase been so great as to produce heart rate deceleration as a compensatory reaction to acceleration. Had this happened, considering that basal skin conductance shows no such reversal effects, it would follow that reliable negative correlations between heart rate and skin conductance would have been found. Given a mixed group of Ss who are threatened to different degrees by what an experimenter imagines to be a uniformly stressful experience, and also considering physiological differences in basic reactivity and homeostatic control mechanisms, it is possible for some individuals in the same situation to demonstrate reliable positive correlations, others reliable negative correlations, and others no relationship at all between certain physiological measures.

TABLE 2. Intrasubject Correlations Among Basal Conductance, Heart Rate, and Respiration Rate for 10 Novice and 10 Experienced Jumpers Only Until Airbound (Points 1-10)

Variables correlated	Novice parachutists			Experienced parachutists		
	Mdn. correl.	*N at .05	Range	Mdn. correl.	*N at .05	Range
Basal cond.-heart rate	+.36	4	+.13-+.72	+.60	5	+.05-+.96
Basal cond.-resp. rate	+.58	6	-.62-+.76	+.54	5	-.01-+.91
Heart rate-resp. rate	+.66	6	-.09-+.70	+.87	9	+.11-+.96

* Number of individual correlations significantly different from zero at the .05 level of confidence.

Covariation Between Measurements During Aggressive Competition

The two experiments to be reported here illustrate the manner in which the time relationships among a series of stressful events and the points in time at which physiological measurements are taken can radically affect the direction, as well as the degree, of relationship between two physiological measures.

First Study

The initial experimental situation (described in detail elsewhere[3]) consisted of an aggressive confrontation between S and a presumed opponent. Each S was informed that he would compete in a test of reaction time with a person in an adjoining room. He was told that at the beginning of a trial he was to set into an apparatus any of five levels of shock that he wished his opponent to receive if he defeated him, and that his opponent had the same privilege. If S lost, he was informed that he would receive information on the shock level his opponent had selected for him, and, at the same time, the corresponding shock. If he won, he would receive only the information. In reality, there was no opponent. Provocation, in the form of the opponent's shock settings, was varied according to the requirements of an experimental design. There were 37 trials in all. Recordings of heart rate and skin conductance were obtained at the following points: (1) at the very beginning of a session, during a

relaxation period; (2) immediately after establishing the threshold for shock experienced as unpleasant, by exposing S to a graded series of increasing shocks; (3) immediately following instructions for the experimental task; and (4) immediately after performance of the experimental task. Within each recording period, two readings were made, one at the beginning and one at the end of a 1.5-min. interval. The purpose of the two readings was to increase reliability and to provide a short-term measure of direction and rate of recovery.

Skin resistance from the dorsal and palmar sides of the left palm was recorded by silver-silver chloride electrodes[14] on a Grass Model 5 polygraph. For measuring heart rate, standard EKG plate electrodes were attached to the S's forearm and left calf. Electrical stimulation was delivered through a concentric disk electrode[16] on the left wrist, with a 60-cps constant current source. Sanborn Redux Jelly was used in applying all electrodes.

Data on S's behavioral aggression scores, or shock settings, will be published separately. Figure 3 presents the findings for heart rate and skin conductance plotted as a function of the four major events in the experiment. Skin conductance followed expected patterns. It was low during the relaxation period and rose very slightly during the recovery interval that followed, very likely as a result of mounting concern over the

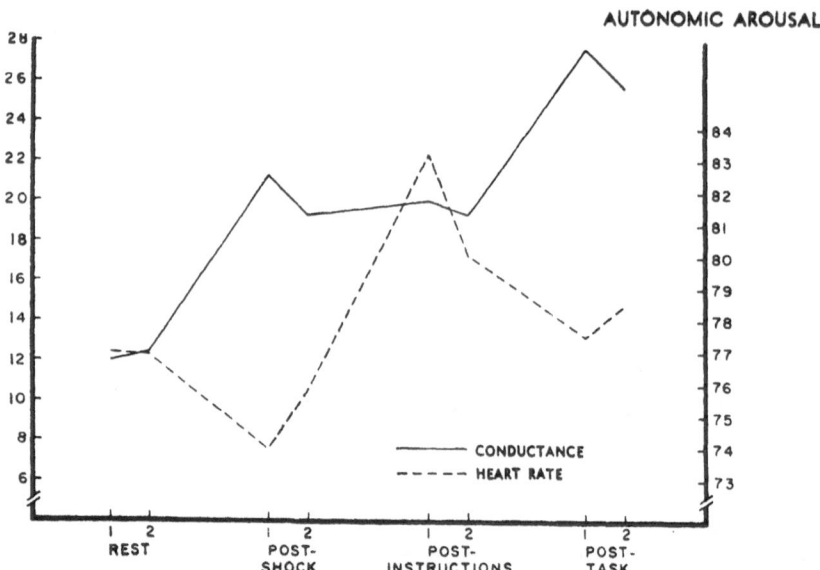

FIG. 3. Skin conductance *(scale at left)* and heart rate *(scale at right)* recorded at discrete points in experimental session.

task to come. There was a sharp rise associated with the period in which unpleasantness thresholds for shock were established, followed by a slight recovery during the recovery interval that followed. Following the instruction period, which was not manifestly stressful, skin conductance rose slightly, and the increase was all but eliminated in the recovery interval that followed. At the end of the experimental task, which *was* manifestly stressful, there was a sharp rise in conductance, followed by some recovery during the recovery interval. The situation is very different for heart rate, which, in most instances, reacted in a manner opposite from that expected. Following the two stressful periods during which shock was received, heart rate was relatively low. In the instruction period, at the end of which skin conductance had exhibited only a slight increase, heart rate exhibited its greatest increase. In the adaptation interval following each event, heart rate moved in the opposite direction from its preceding direction of movement—suggesting the operation of a compensatory control mechanism. In

short, heart rate and skin conductance varied in an opposite manner from each other as a function of stress, and heart rate produced anomalous results in relation to manifest stress. Considering the long time intervals between events, any rescoring by the "method of mean cyclic maxima" recommended by Malmstrom et al.[12] could make no essential difference. How is one to explain the strange findings on heart rate, which could lead to the interpretation that the instruction period was highly stressful, and that receiving noxious stimulation and competing in a threatening situation were relaxing? The direction of recovery following each event provides a clue. There is a strong tendency in this period for heart rate to reverse its previous direction of movement, suggesting the possibility that the anomalous findings at the end of each of the major events in the experiment were produced by reversals in the direction of reaction at stimulus onset. In the absence of continuous recording, this hypothesis could not be tested, and it was necessary to carry out a follow-up study.

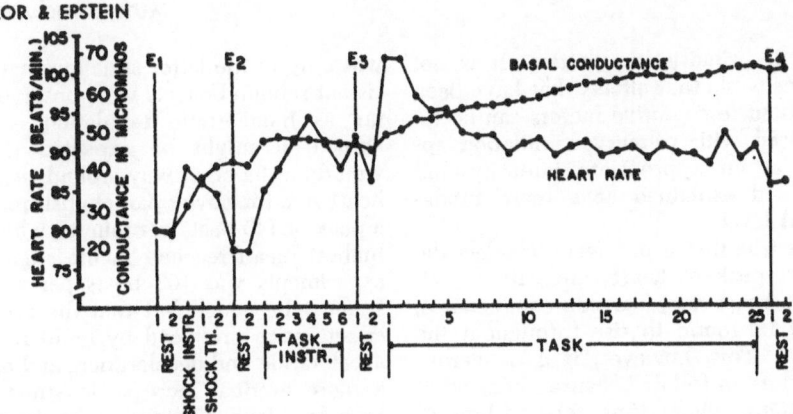

FIG. 4. Skin conductance and heart rate recorded continuously throughout experimental session.

Second Study

Thirteen male undergraduates enrolled in an introductory psychology course at the University of Massachusetts were tested in the same experimental situation as the one already described, except that physiological reactions were monitored continuously. Findings are summarized in Fig. 4, which includes the same points as in Fig. 3 plus a number of additional ones. The curves for skin conductance are no different from the curves in the previous experiment, and hence require no comment. The findings on heart rate support the hypothesis that the anomalous results in the previous study are partly a result of rebound effects produced by earlier, opposite reactions. The surprisingly low heart rate at the beginning of the "rest period" immediately *following* the determination of shock thresholds (where readings were taken in the first experiment to represent the reaction to the shocks) is seen to be preceded by high heart rate earlier in the period of shock-threshold determination. The low heart rate at the *end* of the aggressive-competitive task is seen to be preceded by a rapid rise in heart rate at the initiation of the task. It is of considerable interest that during both

periods of primary stress in which shocks were received, which included the aggressive-competitive task and the determination of shock thresholds, skin conductance rose and heart rate fell. While the fall in heart rate can be explained as a reaction to a high rate at the beginning of the period, it may be that heart rate is particularly sensitive to cognitive and anticipatory aspects of threat.[5, 6, 9a, 18] In this respect, it is noteworthy that heart rate during the period of instructions for establishing unpleasantness thresholds (as well as during the period of instructions for the aggressive-competitive task) was relatively high compared to skin conductance. Unfortunately, it is difficult to disentangle homeostatic compensatory effects from cognitive reactions associated with expectations, since the rate and final magnitude of stress build-up due to expectation in a particular situation is apt to be different from the rate and magnitude of stress build-up due to primary stimulation. Before one may assert with any confidence that heart rate is particularly sensitive to cognitive aspects of threat, it will be necessary to conduct experiments in which rate and intensity of stress input are systematically varied, once on the basis of expectancies and again on the basis of primary stimulation. It is not inconceivable that effects that have been attributed to cognitive factors can be reproduced with primary stimulation applied at an appropriate intensity and rate, and explained at a more fundamental level.

It is true that if one were to select the highest peak of heart rate within each period, heart rate, like skin conductance, would be found to rise throughout the session. This, however, is a dangerous procedure to follow because under other conditions, where time relationships or other features of the experiment were different, the effects of one event could easily cancel-out or otherwise distort the effects of another to a greater extent than in the present experiment. It is evident that heart rate is a far more complex measure than skin conductance, and its use as a measure of general arousal can be questioned in all but the simplest situations.

Comments and Conclusions

The studies described above make it clear that under certain circumstances heart rate and skin conductance vary directly, under others they are independent, and under yet others they are inversely related. These differences in correlation cannot be attributed to artifacts of measurement, but can be understood in terms of the physiological properties of the different systems. Heart rate is a highly labile system, which is subject to complex homeostatic controls and may also be particularly sensitive to cognitive aspects of threat and attention.[8] It was observed that some anomalous findings with heart rate could be explained by assuming they represented rebounds to earlier reactions. Thus, rapid acceleration was followed by marked deceleration and vice versa. It is interesting in this respect to contrast the findings from the study of parachutists with the findings from the studies of aggression, as it

was only in the latter situation that consistent rebound effects were observed. So far as homeostatic regulation is concerned, it might be expected that it would be the other way around, as mean heart rate for novice parachutists reached a peak of 145 beats per minute, while the highest mean reached in the aggression experiments was 103 beats per minute. It must be concluded that the rebound effects were produced by rapid rates of acceleration and deceleration, and not by a more gradual increase in stress to a high final level. This is not to deny that individual records of novice parachutists were more variable than the group data and that some novice parachutists did exhibit cyclic reactions; but it does indicate that rate of stimulus input—independent of intensity—is an important parameter of stress, which triggers homeostatic defenses in a consistent manner, across individuals.

What are the implications of the lack of correspondence among physiological measures for a concept of general arousal? According to Malmstrom et al.,[12] "the psychophysiological concept of arousal or activation depends on agreement between the autonomic variables." As was noted earlier, Lazarus et al.[11] stated that the absence of high correspondence among physiological measures ". . . is especially embarrassing to those who propose a general activation or arousal syndrome." It is our view that the widely held assumption that the concept of general arousal requires high levels of correspondence among different physiological measures rests upon a misconception. It follows the model of intelligence testing which requires high correlation among different abilities to support a concept of general intelligence. A model of arousal which is more in accord with physiological facts recognizes that as stress mounts, it triggers reactions at different points in time in different systems. Up to a point, one system may rise in activity and then be partially or fully inhibited[17] while another continues to rise.[4] It should be borne in mind that not only must the organism adjust to and control the over-all level of arousal produced by the total impact from all internal and external sources of stimulation to which the organism is sensitive, but it must also maintain homeostatic regulation within each of the subsystems.

It follows from the above that a practical solution to the measurement of general arousal, given the lack of correspondence among physiological measures, will not be found in transformations, in innovations in procedures of data reduction, or in combining measures. Pending the discovery of a practical measure that will tell us something about what is going on in the reticular activating system, or other integrating centers for arousal, the most practical solution appears to lie in learning more about the unique properties of the different physiological systems and thereby being able to select a measure that is well suited to the particular conditions that are being investigated. In this respect, it is important to acknowledge the existence of subsystems of arousal and their control, and to remain cautious about generalizing from one system to another until the principles relating each to the other and to the parameters of stress are carefully worked out. We need to know how variables such as rate of stimulus input, magnitude of input, and prestimulus basal level (singly and in interaction) are responded to throughout their range by different physiological systems. Cortical activation, autonomic arousal, striated muscle tension, and various indices of behavioral arousal—including measures of cognitive efficiency—all have unique features, and it will only add to confusion if they are used interchangeably.* Within each

broader functional system, each of the organs has its own unique features. Heart functioning understandably will react differently to the parameters of stress than skin conductance, which serves no vital function.

As a result of phasic and tonic homeostatic controls that can reverse the direction from acceleration to deceleration and vice versa, and evidence that it may be particularly sensitive to anticipation and attention, heart rate is apt to be a particularly poor measure of general arousal under many circumstances. This is not to deny that under other circumstances it may be an unusually sensitive and useful measure. Under most conditions where subjects can serve as their own controls, skin conductance is clearly to be preferred, as it increases monotonically with increasing stress. There is one exception of which we have recently become aware, and that occurs when stress is associated with induced muscle tension. Kaplan[7] reports that basal conductance usually falls while subjects maintain constant pressure on a dynamometer, and that the momentary response represented by GSR does not increase directly as a function of the momentary force that is exerted in discrete responses. Thus, skin conductance appears to be a good measure of arousal associated with stimulus input, but not response output. It is obvious that much work needs to be done on which measures of arousal best reflect increases in stimulus input and motor output, and under which circumstances. To accomplish this, it will be necessary to map out the parameters of stress, and to investigate them—singly and in combination—over a broad range for a number of presumed measures of general arousal.

Summary

One of the problems facing the researcher in the area of psychophysiology, given low correlations between physio-

---

*In a recent paper, published while the present report was still in press, Lacey[9] arrived at the same conclusion.

logical measures, is the selection of a physiological index of general arousal. Some researchers have attempted to solve this problem by using multiple measures. Others have attempted to improve correlations by innovations in data collection and data reduction, so that different single measures could be used interchangeably.

Results obtained on the covariation of heart rate and skin conductance under two markedly different conditions of stress are presented to demonstrate that the direction and magnitude of correlation between these measures vary with such factors as the spacing of stressful episodes, the range of stress to which Ss are exposed, the rate at which stress mounts, and the points at which the data are obtained following the onset of stimulation.

In a study of stress associated with parachute jumping, heart rate and skin conductance were monitored at various points up to the time of a jump for 10 novice and 10 experienced parachutists. The mean intra-S correlation was +.65 for experienced parachutists, but was not significantly different from zero for novice parachutists. The difference in correlations was found to be a result of different levels of maximum arousal reached by the two groups. When correlations were computed within a period of limited arousal only, both groups produced similar positive correlations.

In an investigation of aggression and physiological arousal, heart rate and skin conductance were monitored at discrete points in time while S participated in an aggressive, competitive task. Skin conductance was found to behave very much as expected. It was low during the relaxation period, rose sharply during the period in which unpleasantness thresholds for shock were established, rose only slightly in the instruction period that followed, and increased markedly during the aggressive confrontation. Heart-rate measurements followed an anomalous pattern. A follow-up study in which recording was continuous revealed that the anomalous findings for heart rate were associated with unique variations in time.

It was concluded that the solution to the measurement of general arousal and the selection of physiological measures will not be found in transformations, in innovations in data collection and reduction, or in combining measures, but in determining the unique properties of physiological systems as they relate to the parameters of stimulus input.

Department of Psychology
Kent State University
Kent, Ohio 44240

References

1. Ax, A. F. The physiological differentiation between fear and anger in humans. *Psychosom Med* 15:433, 1953.
2. Duffy, E. *Activation and Behavior.* Wiley, New York, 1962.
3. Epstein, S., and Taylor, S. P. Behavioral aggression and physiological arousal as a function of provocation and defeat. *J Personality* 35:265, 1967.
4. Fenz, W., and Epstein, S. Gradients of physiological arousal of experienced and novice parachutists as a function of an approaching jump. *Psychosom Med* 29:33, 1967.
5. Graham, F. K., and Clifton, R. K. Heart-rate change as a component of the orienting response. *Psychol Bull* 65:305, 1966.
6. Jenks, R. S., and Deane, G. E. Human heart rate responses during experimentally induced anxiety: A follow up. *J Exp Psychol* 65:109, 1963.
7. Kaplan, S. Skin resistance and memory. Progress Report, NIMH Research Grant MH 10310, 1966.
8. Lacey, J. I. "Psychophysiological Approaches to the Evaluation of Psychotherapeutic Process and Outcome." In *Research in Psychotherapy.* Rubinstein, E. A., and Parloff, M. B., Eds. American Psychological Association, Washington, D. C., 1959.

9. LACEY, J. I. "Somatic Response Patterning and Stress: Some Revisions of Activation Theory." In *Psychological Stress*, Appley, M. H., and Trumball, R., Ed. Appleton, New York, 1967.

9a. LACEY, J. I., KAGAN, J., LACEY, B. C., and MOSS, H. A. "Situational Determinants and Behavioral Correlates of Autonomic Response Patterns." In *Expression of Emotions in Man*. Knapp, P. H., Ed. International Universities Press, New York, 1963.

10. LACEY, J. I., and LACEY, B. C. Verification of the principle of autonomic response-stereotypy. *Amer J Psychol* 71:50, 1958.

11. LAZARUS, R. S., SPEISMAN, J. C., and MORDKOFF, A. The relationship between autonomic indicators of psychological stress: heart rate and skin conductance. *Psychosom Med* 25:19, 1964.

12. MALMSTROM, E., OPTON, E., and LA-ZARUS, R. Heart rate measurement and the correlation of indices of arousal. *Psychosom Med* 27:546, 1965.

13. OBRIST, P. A. Cardiovascular differentiation of sensory stimuli. *Psychosom Med* 25:450, 1963.

14. O'CONNELL, D. N., and TURSKY, B. Silver-silver chloride sponge electrodes for skin potential recording. *Amer J Psychol* 73:302, 1960.

15. SCHNORE, M. Individual patterns of physiological activity as a function of task differences and degree of arousal. *J Exp Psychol* 58:117, 1959.

16. TURSKY, B., WATSON, P. H., and O'CONNELL, D. N. A concentric shock electrode for pain stimulation. *Psychophysiology* 1:296, 1965.

17. WILDER, J. The law of initial value in neurology and psychiatry: facts and problems. *J Nerv Ment Dis* 125:73, 1957.

From A. Routtenberg (1968). Psychological Review, 75, 51-80, *by kind permission of the American Psychological Association.*

THE TWO-AROUSAL HYPOTHESIS:

RETICULAR FORMATION AND LIMBIC SYSTEM [1]

ARYEH ROUTTENBERG

Northwestern University

It is postulated that there are 2 major systems in the brain that maintain the ongoing behavior of the vertebrate organism. Arousal System I is related to the reticular activating system. It maintains the arousal of the organism, and provides the organization for responses. Arousal System II is related to the limbic system, and provides control of responses through incentive-related stimuli. The organization of these 2 mechanisms is postulated to be mutually inhibitory. It is shown how such an organization is of value in understanding reinforcement as part of a reciprocal relation between drive (Arousal System I) and incentive (Arousal System II). Memory is viewed as a consequence of this reciprocity.

The present paper grew out of an attempt to understand the relation between two recent major findings in neurobiology. The first was described by Moruzzi and Magoun (1949) and concerned itself with a medial core primarily in midbrain and hindbrain which was capable of activating or arousing the cerebral cortex. This system has often been referred to as the Ascending Reticular Activating System (ARAS). The second finding concerned the discovery (Olds & Milner, 1954) of a series of points primarily within the forebrain which when stimulated produced effects similar to "normal" reward.

The proposal offered here is that these two discoveries represent the description of two major brain mechanisms that are critical to the organism for the execution of appropriate behavior sequences. Because the two systems operate in such an intimate

fashion, much confusion has occurred in the analysis of certain data related to these systems. It is the purpose of the paper to show that an analysis of brain function assuming two arousal systems may be of value in the future to help correct this confusion. A second purpose is to organize a sufficient amount of information to point out where empirical facts appear necessary, and to stress certain special issues which have arisen in considering the information relevant to the two-arousal hypothesis.

THE NEED FOR TWO AROUSAL SYSTEMS

There has been much discussion concerning these two systems. The first, Arousal System I, was originally described by Moruzzi and Magoun (1949) with electrographic techniques. This system, which extends through the medial core of the brainstem, has been variously called the ascending reticular activating system, the reticular formation, or the arousal system. In theoretical or review articles concerning arousal and consciousness (Duffy, 1962; French, 1960; Hebb, 1955; Lindsley, 1960; Malmo, 1959; O'Leary

[1] The author wishes to thank Stanley A. Lorens and Benton J. Underwood for reading a preliminary draft of the manuscript, and to acknowledge his debt to P. Milner, S. Glickman, and J. Olds. During the preparation of the manuscript the author was supported by United States Public Health Service contract MH11991.

& Cohen, 1958; Rossi & Zanchetti, 1957; Samuels, 1959) it is to this structure that attention has been directed. The second, Arousal System II, has been suggested largely through studies of the limbic system by Nauta (1946), Anand and Brobeck (1951), Hess (1957), Nauta (1958), Olds (1962), and others. Although several workers have sought to describe the two systems as having common or identical properties (Glickman, 1960; Glickman & Schiff, 1967; Olds & Peretz, 1960; Sharpless, 1958), the purpose of the present paper is to show that distinctions between the two systems can be made, and that such distinctions assist in understanding certain aspects of the subcortical organization of reinforcement and learning. A similar distinction was drawn in a recent review of sleep literature (Routtenberg, 1966).

Since the pioneering work of Rheinberger and Jasper (1937) the activity of the electroencephalogram (EEG) was thought to correlate with level of consciousness. High frequency low voltage fast activity (LVF) represented arousal or alertness; low frequency high voltage slow waves (SW) represented decreased arousal or sleep. Within this context the data of Wikler (1952), Bradley and Key (1958), and Meyers, Roberts, Riciputi, and Domino (1964), that animals under atropine show slow wave activity, but yet are behaviorally awake, did not comport with the general view that EEG activity directly corresponded to various levels of consciousness. If reticular formation were important in the maintenance of waking behavior, and if waking behavior were indicated by reticular-produced LVF, how was it possible for an organism to be awake and yet demonstrate slow wave activity?

The work on reticular lesions and consciousness has also been difficult to understand. Lindsley, Schreiner,

Nolles, and Magoun (1950) showed that large lesions of the midbrain rendered cats comatose. The reported lesions extended from the dorsal aspect of the superior colliculus to the ventral areas of the midbrain including interpeduncular nucleus and surrounding regions. Subsequent work by Chow and Randall (1964), Chow, Randall, and Morrell (1966), Sprague, Levitt, Robson, Liu, Stellar, and Chambers (1963), and Adametz (1959) has shown that lesions restricted to the reticular formation itself do not necessarily render animals comatose, and that postoperative care of the animals and multiple-stage operations can assist in recovery from the brain lesion. It has been shown too that animals with reticular lesions were able to perform complex behavioral conditioning tasks (Doty, Beck, & Kooi, 1959). Again it would seem that a system of behavior that bases its critical mechanism in reticular formation would be hard-pressed to explain this result.

Data on reticular lesions are further complicated by the work of Feldman and Waller (1962) who reported that lesions in the midbrain reticular formation of cats which cause EEG synchronization do not cause somnolence. In fact, the animals were often alert and walking around. This is reminiscent of the atropine effect (e.g., Wikler, 1952). On the other hand, Feldman and Waller (1962) demonstrated that lesions restricted to the posterior hypothalamic-medial forebrain bundle region produced a sleeping or comatose animal capable of demonstrating low voltage fast EEG activity. These "dissociations" again make it difficult to understand consciousness in terms of a single arousal system.

Jouvet (1961), in studying the sleep mechanisms of the midbrain, pontine, and medullary systems, found that low voltage fast activity seen during sleep (S-LVF) with rapid eye movements (REM) still appeared following lesions of the reticular formation. This result has been confirmed by Carli, Armengol, and Zanchetti (1965) and Hobson (1965). It would appear that other structures may be involved in LVF.

In an effort to determine what structure or structures may be involved in producing S-LVF, Jouvet reported that certain limbic lesions eliminated S-LVF. This result comported well with the reports from Hernández-Peón (1965) that cholinergic stimulation of these same limbic regions reliably produced sleep behavior in cats implanted with chemical stimulation cannulae. Jouvet's finding concerning limbic lesions, however, was not replicated by Carli et al. (1965) nor by Hobson (1965). If the latter findings are supported by future research then the conclusion may be drawn that neither the reticular formation alone nor the limbic system alone is critical for LVF, but that either one may be capable of bringing about LVF.[2]

[2] It is premature, however, to draw any firm conclusions since methodological problems are numerous and hence interfere with accurate interpretation. In a study employing brain lesions it is difficult to characterize the extent of the lesion. Thus, two authors often describe the same lesion, but the extent and configuration of the fulguration in the two studies may be quite different. Second, many sample biases exist, both with respect to subject population and with respect to EEG analysis. The latter problem is well known among experimental electroencephalographers as Domino's question of Zanchetti (1967) well illustrates. The sample bias concerning subjects is particularly important when lesions are made in hypothalamic and reticular systems wherein wakefulness and autonomic activities are controlled. Thus, many subjects either become sick or die and subject populations consist of only those that survive. It then becomes an issue whether the animals that did not survive were, in

A recent study by Villablanca (1965) raises similar questions for a single-arousal-system view. This author has made precollicular *cerveau isolé* sections (transection between diencephalon and midbrain) and found low voltage fast activity to be present in cortex 7–11 days after the transection. How is LVF possible in the absence of RF? It is possible that the result is somehow related to denervation supersensitivity (Routtenberg, 1966; Sharpless, 1964; Sharpless & Halpern, 1962; Stavraky, 1961). Other possibilities exist. It would be tempting, at first blush, to ascribe the LVF to that generated by the thalamic reticular formation (Jasper, 1961). However, the work of Schlag and Chaillet (1963) precludes such a suggestion since they have shown that the arousing effect of high frequency midline thalamic stimulation is mediated downstream via the posterior commissure to reticular formation and then back up to cortex. Another possibility is that the subthalamic projection of the ARAS (Nauta & Kuypers, 1958) has taken over the function of LVF. Such a possibility does not readily explain why Villablanca found desynchronization with olfactory stimuli but not with visual stimuli. A third possibility is that medial forebrain bundle (MFB) system running through hypothalamus

fact, the only subjects with accurately placed lesions. Third, the number of stages in which the operation is performed may be critical. Thus, Jouvet reported that septal lesions reduce S-LVF markedly while Hobson was unable to confirm this finding. Jouvet performed his lesion in one stage, Hobson in two. Such a difference might account for the disparity in results. Thus, while tentative statements concerning the function of a structure may be made on the basis of lesion studies, the extent of lesion, sampling of subjects, and EEG data, stage of operation and recovery time usually vary from one study to the next, often rendering difficult accurate comparisons.

and telencephalon mediates the low voltage fast activity. This latter possibility would readily explain the obtained desynchronization following olfactory stimulation since this system is intimately related to the olfactory system (Scott & Pfaffman, 1967).

That this olfactory-related medial forebrain bundle system may be involved with arousal functions is suggested by the work of Kawamura, Nakamura, and Tokizane (1961), and by a confirming report of Torii and Wikler (1966). The former authors showed that stimulation of MFB at the level of posterior hypothalamus produced neocortical desynchronization and hippocampal theta. It should be recalled that theta activity has often been referred to as a "hippocampal arousal response." If a *cerveau isolé* transection was performed neocortical desynchronization disappeared but theta remained. Thus, the transection reduced neocortical "arousal" by virtue of cutting off midbrain RF; the same section, however, left hippocampal "arousal" intact. Such data suggest that the MFB system may be important in mediating one aspect of arousal. If a sufficient time for recovery of function is allowed (Villablanca, 1965), then this system might be able to produce neocortical desynchronization, perhaps via a septal-cingulate pathway suggested by Krnjvc and Silver (1965). It is clear, therefore, that in Villablanca's (1965) study, midbrain RF involvement in LVF seems unlikely. Posterior hypothalamic involvement in LVF represents one possible alternative.

These studies point out certain difficulties with a theory of consciousness based on a single arousal system. It would seem that the results of these studies, while difficult to explain in terms of a single arousal theory, may be less difficult to understand in terms

of the theory proposed here. According to this theory, Arousal System I is the primary system in producing neocortical desynchronization, although Arousal System II can produce neocortical desynchronization when Arousal System I is damaged. Elimination of Arousal System I would eliminate or reduce neocortical desynchronization; however, Arousal System II is sufficient to maintain the wakefulness of the organism. Elimination of Arousal System II may produce somnolence or severe disruption of primary vegetative activities but LVF may still persist. Arousal System I has a more sustaining—that is, tonic (Sharpless & Jasper, 1956), influence with respect to neocortical desynchronization. Arousal System II, on the other hand, appears to be more critical than Arousal System I for the maintenance of basic "vegetative" activities. Arousal System I occurs where stimulation-produced neocortical desynchronization is obtained; Arousal System II where stimulation-produced reward effects are obtained. Each may contribute, in the other's absence, to the function of the other.

While anatomical specification of the two systems is not yet possible (see concluding remarks) it should be stated that, at present, the current formulation identifies Arousal System I with the reticular formation (Nauta & Kuypers, 1958), and Arousal System II with the limbic-midbrain system (Nauta, 1958). The major ascending component of Arousal System I is Forel's tractus fasciculorum tegmenti. Descending pathways are complex; certain of these have been discussed by Glickman and Schiff (1967). The major component of Arousal System II is the MFB, which contains both ascending and descending components. Figure 1 shows the anterior midbrain location of Arousal Systems I and II.

Arousal System I at this level contains the axons of reticular cells of posterior midbrain, pons, and medulla origin. Arousal System II at this level contains axons of dorsal tegmental cells of posterior midbrain and pons which have coursed to this rostroventral position. These axons then ascend into, and form part of, the diencephalic component of the MFB.

How might the characterization of the two arousal systems assist in understanding the results that were apparently difficult to understand in terms of a single arousal hypothesis? The Lindsley et al. (1950) data may be contrasted with subsequent reports that did not find such profound impairments. According to the present view, the profound impairments resulting from their extensive lesions may have been caused by destruction of major components of *both* the Arousal I and Arousal II systems. Other studies which have employed less extensive lesions may have been restricted to the Arousal System I. The present view that lesions in Arousal System I *or* Arousal System II are not sufficient to cause permanent damage to the animal, but that lesions in both areas will have a profound effect, is open to empirical test.

The EEG dissociations have been discussed (Routtenberg, 1966), but bear repeating. It is assumed that a procedure such as atropine administration which may suppress Arousal System I activity directly (or indirectly via cortical suppression) will cause a reduction in low voltage activity, but will have less of an effect on observable behavior, although impairments in particular tasks exist (Carlton, 1963;

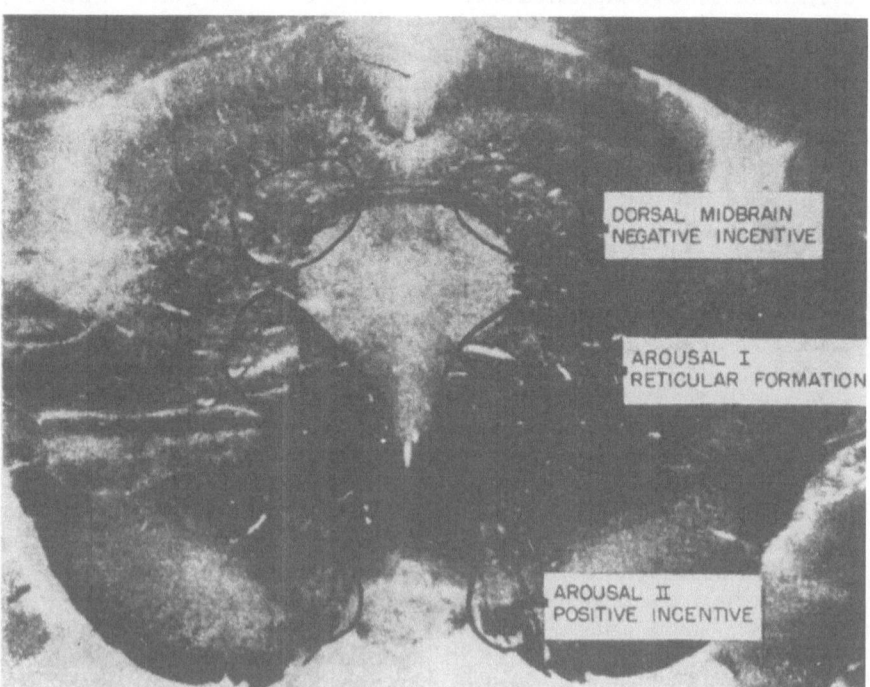

FIG. 1. Section of rat brain showing approximate location of dorsal midbrain, Arousal System I, and Arousal System II in anterior regions.

Whitehouse, Lloyd, & Fifer, 1964). What may be happening with respect to the effects of atropine and the reticular lesions of Feldman and Waller (1962), is that Arousal System I influence is reduced, but Arousal System II is still intact. The latter system is able to maintain the wakefulness of the animal. In situations where LVF appears in the absence of Arousal System I (Carli et al., 1965; Hobson, 1965; Jouvet, 1960; Villablanca, 1965) it is assumed that Arousal System II has some ability to bring about LVF. The critical structures involved may be near those areas ("wakefulness center") which when destroyed caused somnolence in the rat (Nauta, 1946).

In summary of this section, then, selected data have been reviewed, and an attempt has been made to show why the postulation of a second arousal mechanism may be necessary to understand brainstem functional organization adequately.

CERTAIN BEHAVIORAL COMPARISONS BETWEEN AROUSAL SYSTEM I AND AROUSAL SYSTEM II

In the present section an attempt will be made to show that Arousal System I is predominantly concerned with drive or organization for response, and Arousal System II primarily concerned with incentive or reward. Since Arousal System I's relation to drive has been discussed (e.g., Hebb, 1955; Malmo, 1959) and experimentally supported (e.g., Wilson & Radloff, 1967), it will not be detailed here.

The response organization function of Arousal System I may be understood in terms of a recent formulation by Glickman and Schiff (1967). The reticular formation of the midbrain (Arousal System I) is thought of as important in the integration of response mechanisms necessary for reinforcement. According to their view

the emitting of approach responses is positively reinforcing, withdrawal responses, negatively reinforcing. The present paper adopts a somewhat similar point of view as one important function of Arousal System I, that is, in the activation and organization of response sequences. In a more general sense, Arousal System I must be active for the production and the selection of the appropriate responses; thus, one might formulate the view that *response occurrence,* whether approach or withdrawal, *is more probable when Arousal System I is active and less probable when Arousal System I is inactive.* The specific ways in which this seems to occur are discussed, in detail, in Glickman and Schiff (1967).

The data concerning the view that Arousal System II is a reward system are primarily derived from literature on the self-stimulation phenomenon (Olds & Milner, 1954). Several authors (e.g., Lilly, 1958; Olds & Peretz, 1960; Olds, Travis, & Schwing, 1960; Ward, 1961) have implanted electrodes in the ventral midbrain areas and obtained self-stimulation behavior. Until recently, the majority of workers have attributed the reinforcement effect to stimulation of the interpeduncular nucleus. It appears quite clear from recent work (Routtenberg & Kane, 1966) that the interpeduncular nucleus is not important in the mediation of reward, but that an area immediately lateral to the interpeduncular nucleus is important. We have speculated that this area is the MFB component of the mammillary peduncle but more placements in this area are required before we can be sure of this statement.

Little data exist on the direct comparison between stimulation of Arousal System II and Arousal System I. In the Routtenberg and Kane study, high rates of self-stimulation were found in the ventral tegmental area of Tsai and moderate or low rates of self-stimulation in the dorsal tegmental region (some of these latter placements were in midbrain reticular formation). Highest rates of self-stimulation in the dorsal region were in the area of 300 presses in an 8-minute period. This figure agrees well with the report of Glickman (1960) concerning self-stimulation in the reticular formation of the midbrain. It is interesting that this rate of self-stimulation is not too disparate from that rate which Harrington and Linder (1962) demonstrated in rats for electrical stimulation of the feet. It is possible, therefore, that the rewarding effects of stimulation in reticular formation (Arousal System I) may be the result of the rewarding effect of moderate excitation or activation, and that such stimulation activates Arousal System II, permitting it to dominate Arousal System I activity. This problem will be discussed later in more detail (pp. 62 and 72).

Self-stimulation in the ventral area often reached the highest rates that we have ever obtained anywhere in the rat brain. We have several times seen over 1000 responses in an 8-minute period. It is felt that the disparity in self-stimulation rate reflects a more fundamental difference in these two areas in terms of their rewarding properties. While it is possible that the effects of stimulation may be as rewarding in one area as in the other, and rate of responding may not always be a good measure of the rewarding value of the area stimulated by the electrode (Hodos & Valenstein, 1962), other evidence still supports the view of a fundamental functional difference. Thus, lesions at the point of self-stimulation in the ventral tegmentum caused marked weight loss while lesions in the dorsal tegmentum caused a negligible weight loss. In addition, subjects with ventral lesions were continually active in an open field situation. This type of behavior was never seen in any of the animals with dorsally located lesions. One subject with ventral lesions kept its snout to the ground and would walk about the open field apparatus without pausing throughout the 5-minute test session. What was also clear was that this animal did not habituate in this activity. This can be contrasted with the work of Glickman, Sroges, and Hunt (1964) who found that lesions in the reticular formation of the midbrain (Arousal System I) did not impair habituation, although it did increase the activity level of their animals.

A recent report by Wyrwicka and Doty (1966) is of relevance to the present discussion. They found that feeding responses could be elicited by stimulation of the ventral tegmental area of Tsai, but rarely could such responses be elicited from reticular formation and more dorsal areas. Such a finding comports well with the weight-loss data reported by Routtenberg and Kane (1966).

Therefore, on the basis of differences in (a) rate of self-stimulation, (b) weight loss following lesions at the point of self-stimulation, (c) overt behavior following lesions in the two areas, (d) habituation of activity, and (e) stimulus-bound eating, it seems reasonable to presume that these two areas mediate different aspects of behavioral organization. In summary, the results that have been concerned with comparisons of the behavioral effects of lesions and stimulation in reticular formation (Arousal System I) and ventral tegmentum (Arousal System II) suggest that the two structures are important in mediating different aspects of behavior. As a working hypothesis it may be stated that Arousal System I is important in the organization of response aspect of behavior, and that Arousal System II is important in reinforcement, or increasing the probability that a particular response will occur again. While it is felt that the specific characterization of the distinction between the two systems is wanting in several respects, the data considered previously, as well as those to be considered in the remainder of this paper, make it clear that the distinction itself is a useful one.

SELF-STIMULATION DATA: SEPTAL-HYPOTHALAMIC COMPARISONS

In this section an attempt will be made to show how the two-arousal schema is of value in explaining certain data within the self-stimulation literature as well as showing how certain subcortical structures function within this schema.

Olds (1960) showed that rats would press a lever for hypothalamic stimulation but would not press a lever when dorsal midbrain (DM) stimulation was the available brain stimulus. In an escape situation where the animal was able to turn off intermittent brain stimulation, it was shown that subjects would turn off DM stimulation but would permit hypothalamic stimulation to remain on. These results showed quite conclusively that there were separate regions within the brain that could mediate positive and negative reinforcement.

In an effort to understand the relation between these two areas, Olds and Olds (1962) determined the effects of continuous background stimulation in one area on the self-stimulation or escape behavior of the other region. Two major results are of importance here. First, the animals self-stimulating for hypothalamic reward showed a diminution of this behavior only when continuous DM stimulation was present. When DM stimulation was not pres-

ent, self-stimulation occurred. Second, escape from DM stimulation was somewhat augmented by hypothalamic self-stimulation. The authors, impressed with the suppressing influence of DM stimulation on hypothalamic self-stimulation, viewed their results as suggesting a one-way inhibition of DM on posterior hypothalamus. The explanation of the slight augmentation of escape behavior was left open to several interpretations.

It seemed on a purely intuitive basis that rewarding stimulation should, if anything, diminish responding to aversive stimulation. That such was not the case in the Olds and Olds (1962) study was puzzling in the light of earlier brain reward experiments that would have predicted such a finding. For example, Brady (1958) found that animals pressing for rewarding brain stimulation would ignore the emotional or aversive properties of a signal previously paired with aversive foot shock; they would not ignore the signal when pressing for a "conventional" reinforcement. Brady's finding suggested that rewarding brain stimulation could attenuate certain aspects of a fear-producing or aversive situation. Such a view was additionally supported by the work of Heath and Mickle (1960) who showed that rewarding brain stimulation alleviated the symptoms of a severely depressed mental patient. These two studies suggested that rewarding stimulation of the brain can reduce, attenuate, or perhaps even eliminate, the "emotional" aspects of an aversive stimulus. How then can the Olds and Olds (1962) work be understood in terms of these data?

One rather obvious difference between the Olds and Olds (1962) work and that of both Brady (1958) and Heath and Mickle (1960) was that the Olds' used rewarding hypothalamic stimulation and the latter two studies used rewarding septal stimulation. The possibility that two rewarding sites (septal area and posterior hypothalamus) could produce essentially opposite effects with respect to aversive stimulation was investigated by Routtenberg and Olds (1963). It was shown that rewarding septal stimulation could reduce the escape responding to aversive dorsal midbrain stimulation. It was also shown, in the same animal, that one could increase escape responding with continuous, rewarding hypothalamic stimulation, and decrease escape responding with continuous, rewarding septal stimulation. These results suggested that rewarding brain stimulation was not a single entity varying only in intensity, since two rewarding loci in brain yielded opposite effects when related to aversive brain stimulation.

The view that important functional differences exist between posterolateral hypothalamus and septal area is supported by several studies which have shown different effects from septal and from hypothalamic stimulation. Olds (1958) showed that septal self-stimulation decreased after about 4 hours of responding on a schedule of continuous reinforcement, while hypothalamic self-stimulation continued for over 12 hours until the rat dropped from exhaustion. Perez-Cruet, Black, and Brady (1963) showed that self-stimulation in septal area reduced heart rate, while self-stimulation in hypothalamus increased heart rate. Meyers, Valenstein, and Lacey (1963) confirmed the finding that rewarding hypothalamic self-stimulation can increase heart rate, but these authors found both increases and decreases in heart rate as a result of septal self-stimulation.

Malmo (1964) has attributed the difference between the Perez-Cruet et al. (1963) and the Meyers et al. (1963) heart-rate data to the locus of stimulation within the septal area. Thus, according to Malmo, heart-rate decreases were obtained from the lateral septal nucleus, while mixed effects consequent to septal stimulation occurred following stimulation of the medial septal nucleus. It is interesting that different effects within the septal area have been reported by Brady (1961) in the conditioned emotion response (CER) situation, and in Routtenberg (1965; Experiment I), suggesting that there are functional differences within the septal region that may be more clearly understood, in the future, in relation to the cytoarchitectonic work of Andy and Stephan (1964).

Some recent experiments support the view that stimulation of septal area and stimulation of posterior hypothalamus yield markedly different and at times opposite effects. Brady (1961) showed that self-stimulation in septal area was not suppressed during the presentation of a conditioned stimulus known to elicit fear responses. Kasper (1964) found that stimulation of lateral septal area reduced avoidance of a water spout that delivered short shocks to the rat's mouth. Grossman (1964) reported that carbachol stimulation in septal area impaired performance in an active avoidance situation. In contrast, rewarding stimulation of hypothalamus facilitated a discriminated avoidance situation (Stein, 1965). Using a Sidman avoidance procedure, Sepinwall (1966) found that carbachol stimulation of septal area diminished performance, while carbachol stimulation of hypothalamus augmented performance. In a recent series of experiments, septal self-stimulation was reduced significantly less than hypothalamic self-stimulation by dorsal midbrain electrical and chemical (carbachol) stimulation (Routtenberg & Olds, 1966). These results show that, in general, septal stimulation tends to reduce the effects of aversive stimulation, while hypothalamic stimulation, in contrast, tends to augment these effects.

Studies on the autonomic system have tended to support the view that the septal region acts to quiet while hypothalamic stimulation activates the organism. With respect to the septal region, Kaada (1951) showed that stimulation of the subcallosal area and septal region lowered heart rate, reduced respiratory movements, lowered blood pressure, and reduced cortically induced movements. Stimulation also caused pupils to be constricted. Covian, Antunes-Rodrigues, and O'Flaherty (1964) showed that blood pressure was lowered by septal stimulation. It is of interest that this reduction lasted 3–5 minutes after the stimulus was terminated. Although not related to the blood pressure decline, bradycardia and inhibition of either inspiration or expiration were also noted. There were a few cases of increased blood pressure, one of which was definitely derived from stimulation of the medial septal area. Manning, Charben, and Cotten (1963) showed that stimulation of septal area produced bradycardia, decreased right ventricular force of contraction, and decreased systemic blood pressure. Both Covian et al. (1964) and Manning et al. (1963) have shown that the septal effect is the result of a depression of sympathetic tone rather than an increase in parasympathetic activity. With respect to posterior hypothalamus, Perez-Cruet, McIntire, and Pliskoff (1966) found that stimulation in hypothalamic areas yielding self-stimulation behavior led to hypertension.

Lesion data also support the notion that septal and hypothalamic areas are functionally quite distinct. For example, lesions in hypothalamus cause adipsia (Teitelbaum & Epstein, 1962), while lesions in the septal region cause hyperdipsia (Harvey & Hunt, 1965). Lesions in the septal area increase ACTH output as compared to lesions in hypothalamus or cingulate region (Usher, Kasper, & Birmingham, 1965). It appears well documented, therefore, that stimulation and lesion of septal area and hypothalamus yield clear differences and, at times, opposite effects.

In an effort to understand the functional differences between septal and hypothalamic areas, in view of the fact that both areas yield similar reward by stimulation, the schema presented in Figure 2 was constructed as an extension of the previous schema on the organization of brainstem mechanisms of sleep (Routtenberg, 1966). It will first be necessary to understand how the present schema can account for the differences between the effects of septal and hypothalamic self-stimulation. In subsequent sections the ability of the schema to deal with problems not specifically related to the theory's derivation will be discussed.

The schema presented in Figure 2 is an attempt to organize anatomical and physiological findings with respect to behavior in a summary form. Thus, particular arrows should not be taken as anatomical projections, although in the majority of cases such projections do exist. Nor should the direction of an arrow preclude the possibility of projections in the other direction. The schema is not strictly an anatomical diagram, therefore, but rather is a suggested model to help summarize the data considered here. It should be clear, too, that even if we were to draw all known anatomical connections of the system we would not understand the operation of the system since there would be no way (as yet) to determine from the anatomy whether the influence of the projection was inhibitory or excitatory. Finally, because this schema represents a summary of

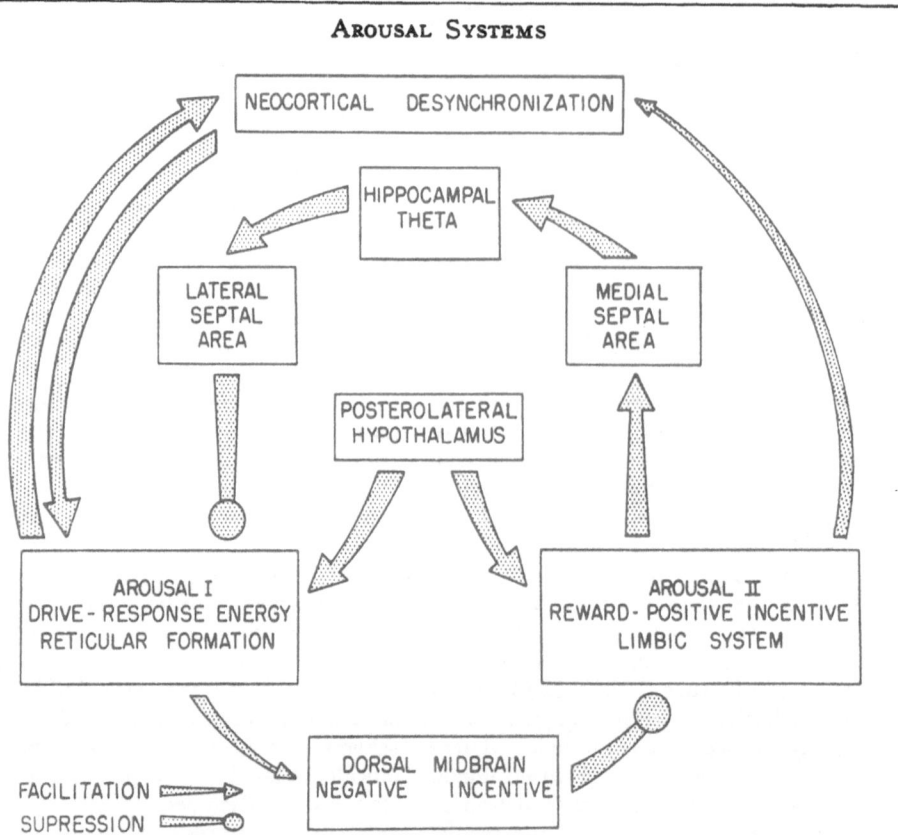

FIG. 2. Schema of major relations underlying the two-arousal hypothesis.

data, an attempt has been made to simplify the system as much as possible, with the view that the fundamental plan, overall operation of the system, and some of its complexity might still be retained.

According to the schema presented in Figure 2, septal area and hypothalamus are different with respect to their influence on Arousal System I. Posterolateral hypothalamus activates, septal area dampens Arousal System I activity. Thus, hypothalamic stimulation is rewarding because of both Arousal System I and Arousal System II activation.[3] Septal stimulation is reward-

ing because of Arousal System II activation and Arousal System I suppression. The former occurs indirectly as a consequence of the direct effect of the latter. One might therefore think of hypothalamic reward as exciting, septal reward as quieting. That Arousal System I suppression and Arousal System I excitation can both lead to rewarding effects may not be as difficult to understand as might first appear. Thus, such a view is not dissimilar from an optimal level of arousal theory (Hebb, 1966) which posits that reticular activity changes from high to medium and low to medium represent reward conditions. The present schema

[3] A somewhat similar view has been proposed by Deutsch (1960). It is important to note that this author does not distinguish between rewarding effects in septal area and rewarding effects in hypothalamus.

would posit that Arousal System II activation could accompany either increases or decreases in Arousal System I activity, depending on the nature (frequency, intensity, locus) of the input.

The present schema is helpful in understanding the experiments that show facilitation of escape and avoidance of both central and peripheral aversive stimulation with concurrent rewarding hypothalamic stimulation (Olds & Olds, 1962; Routtenberg & Olds, 1963; Sepinwall, 1965; Stein, 1965). Thus, hypothalamic stimulation would augment the activity in dorsal midbrain, and would make whatever aversive stimulus already present in the system still more aversive. It should be pointed out that aversiveness is, in part, the autonomic effects (e.g., blood pressure) which usually accompany a negative incentive situation and that the peripheral autonomic events that compose the configuration of an aversive response may overlap with those brought on by "rewarding" hypothalamic stimulation.

Why does continuous dorsal midbrain stimulation virtually shut off hypothalamic self-stimulation (Olds & Olds, 1962; Routtenberg & Olds, 1966)? According to the schema, dorsal midbrain stimulation is aversive, in part, because of its suppressing influence on Arousal System II. While hypothalamic self-stimulation would increase the activity of Arousal System II, it would also increase activity in Arousal System I, which would in turn maintain the already high level of activity in dorsal midbrain caused by continuous stimulation. This would more than compensate for the increase in Arousal System II brought about by hypothalamic self-stimulation. Thus, self-stimulation in hypothalamus would be, in this case, aversive. It will be recalled (p. 57) that Glickman (1960) found that self-stimulation in reticular

formation (Arousal System I) was obtainable from particular anatomical loci in anterior midbrain regions. Such a finding would appear to contradict the view that Arousal System I activity excites the region yielding aversive effects in dorsal midbrain. Although there is at present no definite resolution to this problem, it may be worthwhile to consider the possibility that moderate levels of arousal or activation activate Arousal System II to a greater extent than the DM system. Such a view is supported by the work of Stumpf (1965) and Ito (1966), who showed that moderate levels of reticular stimulation produced hippocampal theta (Arousal System II function), but higher voltage levels produced hippocampal desynchronization (Arousal System I function). This issue may also be related to the position of the stimulation electrode relative to nuclear groups in the two systems. Thus, one would expect that stimulation of "reticular formation" would not always produce theta activity (e.g., Petsche, Gogolak, & van Zwieten, 1965).

The present schema is also helpful in understanding the suppression of escape behavior elicited by aversive dorsal midbrain and peripheral stimulation with stimulation of the septal region (Brady, 1958; Heath & Mickle, 1960; Kasper, 1965; Routtenberg & Olds, 1963; Sepinwall, 1966). According to the present view, stimulation of the septal area reduces Arousal System I activity; this in turn would reduce the facilitation of dorsal midbrain activity. The activity of dorsal midbrain in the absence of Arousal System I activity may be analogous to the response of individuals with morphine who are able to describe the presence of pain but are in no way affected by it, that is, a painful stimulus which is not aversive.

Septal self-stimulation is reduced less than hypothalamic self-stimulation by dorsal midbrain stimulation (Routtenberg & Olds, 1966) because stimulation of the septal area tends to reduce activity of Arousal System I which would, in turn, reduce the activity of the dorsal midbrain region. According to the present model it should, in fact, be possible by arrangement of the current levels in septal area and dorsal midbrain to show that septal self-stimulation increases with the application of continuous dorsal midbrain stimulation.

CERTAIN FEATURES OF THE TWO-AROUSAL HYPOTHESIS

Positive Feedback by Disinhibition

Arousal System I and Arousal System II are arranged in a fashion so that each suppresses the activity of the other. Perhaps a more accurate view is that the two systems are in a constant state of activity, and that reciprocal suppression allows for Arousal System I and Arousal System II to be in a dynamic equilibrium; first one is active, then the other. One might assume, therefore, that *the organism regulates its behavior such that there exists a dynamic balance of activity between these two systems.*

But what happens when an imbalance occurs? According to the schema, activity in dorsal midbrain (for example) would lead to an increase in dorsal midbrain activity, that is, activity at any one point in the system would tend to augment the activity at that point, *unless* the system was provided with inputs that would alter that activity, perhaps by removal of the source (internal or external) of influence.

Although little data exist on the problem of time course of events, it seems necessary to discuss the issue. It can be seen in Figure 2 that stimulation in hypothalamus eventually results in the inhibition of Arousal System II through the dorsal midbrain system. Since dorsal midbrain activity is aversive, why should the animal press a bar for such stimulation? This is where a consideration of the time course of events appears important. Rewarding stimulation in hypothalamus causes an immediate augmentation of activity in both Arousal Systems I and II. As long as the stimulus is on, the two systems are both in balance (providing the electrode locus is stimulating the two systems equally), albeit in a high state of activity. The instant the stimulus is off, the aftereffect of Arousal System I stimulation is seen, that is, the cessation of hippocampal theta (Grastyan, Karmos, Vereczkey, & Kellenyi, 1966; Grastyan, Karmos, Vereczkey, Martin, & Kellenyi, 1965) and the occurrence of hippocampal desynchronization. The effects of Arousal System II compensation are then seen as the cessation of hippocampal desynchronization; the system is back at equilibrium (see concluding comments).

Septal Area

Up to this point little has been said concerning the differentiation between the medial and lateral septal area, shown in Figure 2, and the significance of the hippocampal theta generator. It is certainly not uncommon to view the septal area as an entity which when lesioned as an entity has certain behavioral effects (see, however, data on septal lesions, Kenyon & Krieckhaus, 1965). Unfortunately, this view does not approximate what, in fact, appears to be the case. The present formulation attempts to show a meaningful separation of the medial and lateral septal nuclei, although it is clear from the work of Andy and Stephan (1964) that further subdivisions exist, and likely have functional significance.

While acknowledging this fact, it should be sufficient for the present to differentiate between the medial and lateral septal nuclei if only as an illustration of the necessity for such divisions.

The anatomical connections between septal area and hippocampus have been described by many authors but the present schema leans heavily upon the work of Crosby (1917) and Votaw and Lauer (1963). These workers have shown in reptile and mammal, respectively, that medial septal region projects to the hippocampal formation, and that there are projections from Ammon's horn back to the lateral septal region. That medial septal region appears important in production of theta was demonstrated by Green and Arduini (1954), who showed that lesions of the septal region eliminate hippocampal theta, and by Petsche, Stumpf, and Gogolak (1962), who showed that cells of the medial septal region discharge with the positive going wave of the theta rhythm. Cells in lateral septal area did not show this behavior. To determine the causative relation between hippocampal theta and medial septal cellular activity, Stumpf, Petsche, and Gogolak (1962) applied various drugs and showed that whenever medial septal discharge was eliminated, theta was stopped. The reverse was not always true, however. LSD-25, for example, eliminated hippocampal theta, but did not alter the rhythmical beating of the septal cells. The conclusion was therefore drawn that the pathway for the generation of hippocampal theta is through the medial septal region.

The assumption of the output of hippocampal theta activity to the lateral septal region and the latter's suppression of Arousal System I rests on less firm physiological grounds, although presumptive evidence exists for the lat-

ter view. Of particular relevance here is the distinction drawn by Malmo (1964) between the effects of medial and lateral septal area and heart rate. He has noted that a decrease in heart rate alone is only found with lateral septal stimulation. Medial septal stimulation produces both increases and decreases in heart rate. Stimulation of lateral septal area, which causes a decrease in heart rate, also attenuates the effects of aversive stimulation (Kasper, 1964). This is consistent with the present formulation.

There is a paucity of data concerning the descending influence of lateral septal area on Arousal System I. Direct anatomical projections to Arousal System I, while existing (Powell, 1966), are not present in abundance; the major influence would likely be multisynaptic. There do exist, however, several studies which strongly support the view that a powerful subcortical suppressing influence on reticular formation is present (Adey, Segundo, & Livingston, 1957; Morrell, 1960; Sterman & Clemente, 1962; Sterman & Fairchild, 1966). For the present, and because of the absence of data, the lateral septal area—Arousal System I relation drawn in Figure 2 should be taken to represent a summary of this influence. Thus, while substantial evidence for a subcortical suppressing influence on Arousal System I exists, the anatomical and physiological evidence does not as yet permit precise specification of the way in which this suppression is brought about. This influence has been summarized by the lateral septal-Arousal System I relation depicted in Figure 2.

A recent report by Zucker (1965) is of interest with respect to discussion of the septal area function and its proposed role of Arousal System I suppression. Zucker notes that "one function of the septal limbic area is to dampen the increment in response strength which normally is induced by reinforcement [p. 351]." It is indeed interesting that we have assumed (a) that the septal area dampens the activity of Arousal System I, (b) that Arousal System I is primarily important for production of responses, and (c) that the septal area is activated by the positive incentive system.[4] The congruence of the two views derived from two disparate areas of investigation appears to strengthen the assumption that septal area is important in the inhibition of responses following reward. The discussion of Gerbrandt (1965) is also important in this regard.

The increased attack behavior and rage resulting from septal lesions (Brady & Nauta, 1953) may be due to the facilitation of responses as the result of the release of Arousal System I. It is interesting, too, that lesions of the septal area increase drinking behavior (Harvey & Hunt, 1965). It is possible, therefore, that lesions in the septal area increase drinking behavior in part because they increase the probability of responses mediated by the hypothalamic system. According to this view, lesions in the septal area should also increase eating behavior. This has been shown by Reynolds (1962), and by Pizzi and Lorens (1967).

A note of caution should be made concerning the effects of septal lesions on feeding and drinking. A recent report of Wolfman, Coon, and Schwartz (1966) has shown that septal lesions in monkeys have a profound effect on electrolyte balance such that urine becomes highly concentrated. Perhaps the animal with septal lesions is drink-

ing more to restore proper electrolyte balance. It is clear that caution is necessary in describing a feeding or drinking alteration produced by lesions solely in terms of "motivational" or "incentive" losses when metabolic or endocrine factors may be worth consideration.

Hippocampus

The relation of hippocampus to the present schema is primarily dependent upon the work of Grastyan and co-workers. He has shown (Grastyan et al., 1965, 1966) that stimulation in areas that yield reward causes hippocampal theta during stimulation, hippocampal desynchronization after stimulation. Stimulation of aversive areas yields desynchronization and "rebound" theta. The present schema makes use of these data and has been constructed so as to incorporate those results. Thus, theta indicates predominance of Arousal System II activity, desynchronization, Arousal System I. In both situations, however, neocortex most usually shows low voltage fast activity.

Grastyan (1959) maintains that the function of hippocampus is in the inhibition of the orienting reflex (a reflection of "reticular" activity). He has claimed that it is hippocampal desynchronization which inhibits arousal. Part of the problem with this formulation appears to be that there is no specification of what is meant by arousal. What can be gathered is that arousal is inferred from the presence of the orienting response, that is, the orienting response is seen when the animal is aroused. It is hard to understand what this means in terms of the present schema, although it is certainly true that stimulation in the part of Arousal Systems I or II, shown in Figure 1, can yield what Grastyan calls the orienting response.

The position supported here is that

[4] That reinforcement can dampen response strength is, in a sense, a contradictory statement. When memory is discussed in a later section, an attempt will be made to clarify this point.

ARYEH ROUTTENBERG

hippocampal theta appears during moderate levels of activation, and indicates that Arousal System II is dominant. Hippocampal desynchronization appears during high levels, indicating that Arousal System I is dominant. The suppression of Arousal System I by theta does not mean that System I is inactive but that Arousal System I is under hippocampal control. Thus, stimulation of Arousal System I can, in fact, bring about theta (Green & Arduini, 1954), perhaps because Arousal System II would likely be influenced by this stimulation (Kawamura et al., 1961) and would dominate until higher levels of stimulation were applied (Stumpf, 1965).

Grastyan (1959) has made the point that hippocampal theta appears when the environmental stimulus is of uncertain importance to the animal. It may be at a point when stimuli that are relevant are beginning to take on importance, but the animal is still not certain whether they are critical. It would seem appropriate to assume that when an uncertain stimulus is presented, organized response systems stop, and the animal attends to the properties of that stimulus as well as to its consequences. This is accomplished in the present formulation by assuming that hippocampal theta activity through the lateral septal region decreases the activity of Arousal System I, thus decreasing organized motor activity. This line of reasoning is supported both by the work of John and Killam (1960) and by that of Morrell (1960). They have shown that the hippocampus shows a particular type of activity during the initial stages of learning, but that once learning is established this type of activity disappears. The work of Grastyan seems important in implicating one function of hippocampus as critical for initial learning, but not important for the maintenance of learning.

We will return to this point when talking about learning and memory.

The inability of animals with hippocampal lesions to (a) suppress responses in a DRL situation (Clark & Isaacson, 1965), (b) habituate in an activity situation (Roberts, Dember, & Brodwick, 1962), and (c) suppress general motor responding (Teitelbaum & Milner, 1963) suggest that the hippocampus has an inhibitory function. In a recent summary of his work on hippocampus, Isaacson (1966) has suggested that this structure suppresses two components of an organism's natural response tendencies in an uncertain environment. One is the somatic action pattern, the other autonomic responses. It is assumed here that theta activity dampens the effects of these two responses which are energized by Arousal System I. These considerations support the view of the present schema that the hippocampus, when in theta activity, has an inhibitory function on Arousal System I, which is a response driving system. It is also possible that when hippocampus is in a desynchronized state, it inhibits Arousal System II activity. Thus, the function of the hippocampus may ultimately involve the modulation and control of the activity of the two arousal systems.

Medial Forebrain Bundle (MFB)

For those working in the field of self-stimulation it may be curious that little mention has been made of this fiber system in previous paragraphs nor has any mention been made of this system in the schema itself. Perhaps the major reason for this is that the precise role of this system in the operation of the schema is not clear. It is clear, however, that it does play a very important role, and that the projections between the posterolateral hypothalamus and Arousal System II, hypothalamus and medial septal area and lateral septal area, and parts of the afferents to Arousal System I, involve MFB. All of these projections are certainly involved in this system and it is necessary to mention them in consideration of the organization of this system. However, at the present the author feels that there are certain unresolved issues.

One of the complexities raised by Morgane (1961c) concerns the differentiation of MFB as it passes through the lateral hypothalamic region. Morgane (1961c) has found that lesions in the midlateral hypothalamus and lesions in the far lateral hypothalamus do not yield equivalent results. For example, lesions in the midlateral hypothalamus in the medial aspect of the lateral hypothalamus do not yield as severe an aphagia as do lesions in the far lateral hypothalamus. In addition, the effects of MFB lesions on these two systems are different (Morgane, 1961b). Lesions in MFB eliminate the stimulus-bound feeding caused by stimulation of the midlateral hypothalamus but such lesions do not eliminate the stimulus-bound feeding elicited by stimulation of the far lateral hypothalamus. The speculation which most adequately explains the Morgane data is that the far lateral system is more importantly involved with response mechanisms (Arousal System I) and the midlateral system is more importantly involved with positive incentive mechanisms (Arousal System II). The midlateral system appears to be more dependent upon the MFB.

The MFB appears to be a very important area for positive reinforcement effects by stimulation. Thus, lesions in the MFB reduce the effects of midlateral stimulation (Morgane, 1961b). One could also see how lesions in the midlateral system might be less effective in producing aphagia than far lateral lesions. The major component eliminated by midlateral lesions would be the incentive component whereas motor mechanisms would still be functioning. With far lateral lesions, the motor component would be destroyed and thus have a more severe effect. It has already been mentioned that Arousal System I is important in the production of responses necessary for reinforcement. That the far lateral system is associated with motor responses is further strengthened by the connection between the extrapyramidal structure, globus pallidus, and the far lateral hypothalamus (Morgane, 1961a). Baillie and Morrison (1963) have, in fact, suggested that the far lateral system is important in motor activity concerned with feeding. It should be mentioned, however, that Rodgers, Epstein, and Teitelbaum (1965) have pointed out certain deficiencies with this position. Rodgers et al. (1965) appear to support the notion that the effect of hypothalamic lesions is to reduce certain aspects of food-incentive motivation. Perhaps the Morgane work suggests that there is both a motor component and an incentive component. In summary, two aspects of the MFB as it passes through the lateral hypothalamic system have been speculated upon, and one possible relation to the two-arousal system suggested.

Drug-Brain Relations

The present schema has direct relevance to the understanding of drugs which act selectively at different sites. The example which will be considered here is the relation between chlorpromazine (CPZ) and pentobarbital (PBT). Pentobarbital is classified as a sedative hypnotic and CPZ is classified as a tranquilizer. Both of them depress the animal, but they have independent classification, which suggests that CPZ may have a different action than PBT. In this section an attempt will be made to show that CPZ acts on the Arousal System II and PBT has its primary action on the Arousal System I.

The depression of reticular activity by PBT is well known (Bradley, 1958). The activity of CPZ on the lateral hypothalamus is less certain, although recent microelectrode work (Zukauskas & Machne, 1964) has shown that CPZ does depress activity in hypothalamus. In addition, radioactively labeled CPZ selectively enters into the hypothalamic region (Wase, Christensen, & Polley, 1956).

Whatever the site of action, it is clear that these two drugs have different effects. Olds and Travis (1960) have shown that CPZ has a very marked depressant effect on hypothalamic self-stimulation, while Mogenson (1964) has shown that pentobarbital enhances self-stimulation. There is evidence from Kornetsky and Bain (1965) that CPZ and PBT have different actions on a task where the animal is required to make responses to one stimulus, and withhold responses when a second stimulus is presented. They found that PBT increased errors of commission whereas CPZ increased errors of omission. These differential behavioral effects suggest that CPZ and PBT have different modes of action. It is speculated here that the primary action of PBT is on Arousal System I, depressing reticular formation activity, and that the primary action of CPZ is to depress the activity of Arousal System II.

Killam and Killam (1958) have obtained results which appear difficult to understand in terms of traditional reticular theory, but which may be understandable in terms of the two-arousal hypothesis. In one experiment they found that evoked potentials in reticu-

lar formation (Arousal System I of the present schema) obtained as a result of sciatic stimulation were depressed by PBT and enhanced by CPZ. In another experiment they found that depression of click-evoked potentials in cochlear nucleus by reticular stimulation was reversed by PBT and enhanced by CPZ. That is, the potentials in the cochlear nucleus were restored following PBT administration, and even more reduced following CPZ administration. The authors conclude that "two different mechanisms may explain behavioral depression by the two compounds [p. 120]."

The present schema suggests the two mechanisms. Additionally, the hypothesized relation between the two is of value in interpreting the Killams' data. If PBT depresses Arousal System I, and CPZ Arousal System II, it may be seen from Figure 2 how PBT depresses RF function and how CPZ enhances it. The depression of RF by PBT is fairly straightforward, although the precise way in which this occurs is not clear. The enhancement of RF function by CPZ (enhanced sciatic-evoked potentials, increased depression of auditory evoked potentials in cochlear nucleus) may be brought about by the depression of Arousal System II. This would decrease hippocampal theta, and reduce the inhibitory activity of Arousal System II on Arousal System I. This would then lead to increased activity in Arousal System I. It would be of interest in this regard to determine whether CPZ depresses hippocampal theta.

THE RELATION OF THE TWO-AROUSAL SCHEMA TO MEMORY

Perhaps one of the difficulties with behavioral theories within psychology is that they have tended to stress one aspect of behavior to the exclusion of other aspects. There are theories of memory which do not deal with motivation (e.g., Underwood, 1957, 1964) and there are similarly theories of motivation which do not deal with memory (e.g., Skinner, 1938). The present account is put forward to show one way in which memory and motivation may be related. The details of the present approach must await empirical test. The point to be stressed is that the speculation is advanced primarily to bring memory and motivational mechanisms under the same roof (for further complaints on this issue, see Gleitman & Steinman, 1963).

According to the present view, one can assume that in the first stage of memory an internal or external event occurs which causes neural activity, and this neural activity persists for some time after the occurrence of the event. This is the first stage, the perseveration of neural activity. In the second stage, it is hypothesized that activity leads to some change on the postsynaptic membrane (PSM). Finally, in the third stage, if the changes that occur on the membrane persist for a long enough period of time, a biochemical change will take place on the PSM that will make permanent the sensitivity of the cell to a particular array of impulses. In terms of mechanism one could think of the neural activity and perseveration as an electrophysiological phenomenon subserving short-term memory, the synaptic membrane change as a neuropharmacological event subserving intermediate-term memory, and the changes within the PSM of a permanent nature as a biochemical effect subserving long-term memory.

While it would be worthwhile to go into more detail concerning the mechanisms underlying the three stages of memory at the neurophysiological, neuropharmacological, and neurobiochemi-cal levels, respectively, this discussion would be beyond the scope of the present paper. The data on perseveration have been reviewed (Glickman, 1961). Concerning neuropharmacological changes, the present author has considered the data of Axelsson and Thesleff (1959), and the speculations of Thesleff (1962) relevant to the second stage. Briefly, one could assume that continued perseveration would restrict the sensitivity of the postsynaptic membrane to those soma-dendritic areas where the perseveration was taking place. The greater the extent of the perseveration, the more likely the restriction of the membrane sensitivity to the point where perseveration was taking place. If perseveration stops, if the particular pattern of activity is reduced and other influences are present, then the effects of the perseveration will diminish, that is, the sensitivity of the PSM will become less restricted. What is important here is perseveration and repeated trials exciting a majority of the same sequence of nervous elements at particular loci on the PSM of each of these elements. It is the restriction of the sensitivity of the nerve cell membrane to particular areas that would be, in a sense, the function of the perseveration process.

The third stage of memory, long-term storage, is conceived of as a biochemical, perhaps irreversible, reaction occurring at the postsynaptic membrane. It is this biochemical change that is important in long-term storage. Although there has been much speculation and discussion on the biochemical nature of memory (Gaito, 1966), it is clearly beyond the scope of this paper to delve into those issues. The important point is that it seems necessary to account for long-term storage in terms of some chemical change, perhaps involving mucopolysaccharides on membrane (Bondareff, 1967; Brunngraber, 1966; Pease, 1966). It has been speculated here that there is some change occurring at the membrane as a result of the restriction of sensitivity at that particular point. The electron micrographs of Charlton and Gray (1966) showing thickenings of the PSM in a variety of vertebrates represents a possible structural substrate of the proposed mechanism.

How might the two-arousal schema be important in the development of memory? It is speculated that the schema plays a role in enhancing the probability of transition from short-term memory to intermediate-term memory. Thus, activation of Arousal System II (incentive) would reduce the activity in Arousal System I (response energy; drive) which would be disruptive of the consolidation process (Mahut, 1962; Walker, 1958). The neural activity occurring before the reward would be allowed to persist beyond the time of reward, because the disrupting influences of Arousal System I activity would be reduced by the activation of Arousal System II as a consequence of the rewarding stimulus. Activation of Arousal System II would reduce Arousal System I activity through the medial septal-hippocampus-lateral septal system (see Figure 2). In a typical animal learning situation, then, a rewarded response is reinforced because the drive that produced that response would be suppressed by the effects of the reward. Thus, incentive (Arousal System II) is viewed as suppressing drive (Arousal System I) and this suppression permits the maintenance of central activity that was previously made in a situation where reward occurred. The perseveration of impulses could then lead to a restriction of the sensitivity of the postsynaptic membrane (intermediate-term memory) and then biochemical change (long-term memory). That all

three stages of memory would occur should depend upon the extent of the perseveration and the number of trials in which some form of the reinforcement was presented.

The speculation concerning the role of Arousal Systems I and II in memory is indirectly supported by a report by Clemente et al. (1963) that following reward, synchronization (SW) appeared in cortical EEG tracings. According to the present schema, this "postreinforcement synchronization" represents the suppression of Arousal System I by reward activation of Arousal System II. That suppression of Arousal System I can lead to synchronization has been shown by Bremer (1935) and by Lindsley, Bowden, and Magoun (1949). Direct support comes from the Grastyan et al. (1966) study in which hippocampal theta appeared immediately following the ingestion of food reward.

In summary, memory is thought of as composed of three stages: short-term, intermediate-term, and long-term. The duration of the first stage is probably measured in seconds (Chorover & Schiller, 1966; Sprott & Waller, 1966), the second stage in minutes and hours (Chamberlin, Halick, & Gerard, 1963) and the final stage in days or weeks (Morrell, 1964). It should be emphasized that while these three stages may overlap temporally, they would be separable mechanistically.

The preceding schema of memory seems valuable for several reasons. First, it enables one to see how a nerve impulse can be translated to a permanent biochemical change and in addition how the biochemical change can be used subsequently in memory. Second, it is believed that the present formulation allows for a more clear understanding of the terms incentive (K) and drive (D). The confusion is apparent in Hilgard's (1956) discussion of the relation between the two where it is pointed out that "The incentive, in its role of enhancing drives, takes on qualities not suggested in its role as a drive reducer [p. 429]." In addition to the confusion of the relation between incentive and drive, there is also the problem of the definition of reinforcement. Thus, while the transitational nature of reinforcement and other measures not related to the experimenter's training may be used to indicate that a particular item or event is a reinforcer (Kimble, 1961), it still remains unclear precisely what a reinforcer is and what, in fact, it is doing.

The present schema offers a possible solution to this problem, by specifying the way in which a reward might act, and the way in which it is related to drive components of behavior. Thus, incentive or reward (Arousal System II-related) suppresses drive (Arousal System I-related) and this allows for the consolidation of those neural sequences that preceded the reward. In the other direction, drive suppresses incentive so that the energy for response may be made. It may be seen then that the two systems are in balance so as to permit the efficient execution of responses (Arousal System I), and then the retention of those responses (Arousal System II).

It should be stressed that the present schema does not view reinforcement and reward as equivalent. Thus, reward or incentive refers to the stimulus population which activates Arousal System II (Scott & Pfaffman, 1967) while reinforcement refers to the consequence of Arousal System II activity. According to the present view the consequence of Arousal System II activity would be the suppression of Arousal System I, and hence the reduction of Arousal System I interference with perseveration.

Concluding Remarks

Like the person who kept seeing a magic number (Miller, 1956), the author has found himself subjected to two arousal systems at every turn. Such consistent revelation suggests that a critical look at some of the issues raised but left unresolved might prove of value to author and reader alike.

Anatomical Description of the Two Functional Systems

It is clear that a precise spatial definition of the systems has not been made in the present paper. Such a situation was necessitated by the fact that information on function of individual tegmental nuclear groups in midbrain and hindbrain remains insufficient to warrant much more speculation than has been offered here. It has been the purpose of the paper to call attention to this lack and to suggest that precise anatomical brainstem localization of various physiological and behavioral correlates of the two systems would materially assist in the understanding of the more frequently explored subcortical forebrain structures. Some of the correlates that have been mentioned that clearly require anatomical precision may be mentioned:

Self-stimulation. While much evidence has accumulated concerning the localization of brain self-stimulation effects in certain subcortical forebrain structures, little evidence exists on the anatomical location of the phenomenon in posterior midbrain, pons, and medulla. In brief, it is not at all clear from the self-stimulation literature what are the "origins and insertions" of the reward phenomenon.

Hippocampal electrical activity. It has been argued that neocortical low voltage activity does not indicate whether an aroused individual is in moderate or high activation, but that hippocampal activity can differentiate between these two states. In the present paper, Arousal System I activity (high activation) has been associated with hippocampal desynchronization, while Arousal System II activity (moderate activation) has been associated with hippocampal theta. Because of lack of information concerning precise anatomical areas which mediate these two types of electrical activity seen in hippocampus, the author has found himself in the somewhat contradictory position of arguing that mild stimulation of Arousal System I can produce hippocampal theta. At this point data are needed to clarify this position. The present view would be that "reticular formation" as usually defined by neurophysiologists represents a wide variety of points in midbrain and pons that would represent components of both Arousal Systems I and II. Clarification must wait, therefore, until such data are forthcoming.

Neocortical desynchronization. Perhaps most surprising of all is the lack of anatomical specification of the brainstem structures involved in cortical low voltage fast (LVF) activity. Such work would necessarily involve the comparison of thresholds since it is clear that LVF may be obtained by any stimulus which is sufficiently intense. Such a study would be complicated by the habituation effects that occur following reticular stimulation (Glickman & Feldman, 1961). Nevertheless, it would be worthwhile to know what portions of the brainstem give the most intense EEG LVF response at the lowest level of stimulation.[5] In addition, it would be important to perform such studies in combination with lesions as, for example, in the work of Schlag and Chaillet (1963), Kawamura et al. (1961), and Torii and Wikler (1966). In this way, critical structures may be discerned.

Reticular lesions. One finding that has suggested the two-arousal hypothesis has been the appearance of LVF following lesions in midbrain reticular formation. The issue that has been dealt with but not answered definitely concerns the structure or system that has assumed the take-over of function (p. 53). Certainly an important research direction is to determine the structures and mechanism underlying the recovery of neocortical desynchronization function. A somewhat similar issue has arisen with respect to recovery of feeding (Teitelbaum & Cytawa, 1965).

Qualitative Nature of Schema

The schema depicted in Figure 2 suggests certain enhancing and suppressing relations between various anatomical and physiological mechanisms. As these relations are often speculative, their quantitative influence cannot be specified. An important direction for research would consist in attempting to model the type of system proposed here and determine whether there is any relation between the model and the biological system. Such an approach would permit possible quantification of influence. In this regard, the neuromine model proposed by Harmon (1964) is of interest in that he discusses the nature of the response of

[5] Recent reports by Kaada, Alnaes, and Wester (1967) and Bonvallet and Newman-Taylor (1967) represent recent attempts at discerning the functional organization within the reticular formation. The Kaada et al. (1967) report is particularly puzzling, since these investigators found that high frequency stimulation of reticular formation often caused synchronization. Such a result emphasizes our incomplete understanding of the classical phenomenon reported by Moruzzi and Magoun (1949).

two reciprocally inhibitory systems to the same input. Such a model may help specify the conditions under which the two arousal systems might oscillate in their ability to dominate or strongly influence patterns of brain activity.

Drug-Brain Relations

An attempt was made to understand the difference between the depressant action of chlorpromazine and pentobarbital in terms of the two-arousal hypothesis. Such a discussion points to several experiments that could test the adequacy of the suggestion. Subsequent to the initial formulation, other studies using pharmacological agents which desynchronized the EEG have appeared. Of particular relevance was a study by Barnes (1966) that showed that either eserine or amphetamine could cause a shift in EEG activity from slow waves to fast waves. Surprisingly, administration of both reinstated slow wave EEG activity. The author concluded that the reticular formation may contain "separate neuronal pools" and that those two systems might inhibit one another directly or indirectly.

The present view would be that eserine has a primary effect on Arousal System II, while amphetamine has a predominant effect on the Arousal System I. It is of interest in this regard that eserine potentiates S-LVF while amphetamine retards or reduces its appearance. Such a view is consistent with the views of the present paper as well as those offered previously (Routtenberg, 1966).

It should be stressed that the preceding comments represent suggested directions in understanding the neuropharmacology of the brainstem systems discussed here. Many questions, however, are difficult to answer at present. Why does amphetamine applied pe-

ripherally augment self-stimulation behavior (Stein, 1964), while related adrenergic compounds applied centrally reduce such behavior (Olds, Yuwiler, Olds, & Yun, 1964)? Eserine, in comparison with amphetamine, tends to achieve precisely the opposite effects both peripherally (Jung & Boyd, 1966) and centrally (Olds et al., 1964). Additionally, why does amphetamine augment self-stimulation behavior and reduce eating behavior elicited from the same electrode in lateral hypothalamus (Coons, 1964)? Such questions, while perhaps comprehensible in a most rudimentary fashion in terms of the present hypothesis, cannot be answered adequately at present.

Lesion and Stimulation Effects

While a good deal of the present schema is based on lesion and stimulation data, the author feels cautious towards data that lack support from other methodologies. Thus, it is typically thought that stimulation at a point X influences those areas to which X sends its outputs, and a lesion at X removes that influence. Unfortunately, it appears that the situation may, at times, be quite the reverse. Thus, stimulation may disrupt brain functions and act more like a lesion (Goddard, 1964; Schlag & Villablanca, 1967), and lesions may act more like stimulation by augmenting the excitability or lowering the threshold of denervated structures (Stavraky, 1961). It would seem advisable, therefore, to be cautious in the interpretation of data that lacks confirmation from other levels of analysis (e.g., electrophysiological).

Reinforcement

One derivation of the present paper is the definition of reinforcement in terms of certain neurological events. This concept is often used synonymously with reward, which is sometimes described as a reinforcer, sometimes as a reinforcement. In the present view, reward or positive incentive stimuli predominantly excites Arousal System II which normally leads to certain consequences, here called reinforcement. Thus, reinforcement is not viewed as rewarding, but rather as the consequence of the positive incentive leading to the enhanced probability of response reoccurrence. Therefore, reward does not necessarily lead to reinforcement, and reinforcement does not necessarily arise from reward. The latter case may arise when Arousal System II is activated, or Arousal System I suppressed in the absence of reward; the former when, upon presentation of reward, Arousal System I activity is in some way not reduced.

REFERENCES

ADAMETZ, J. H. Rate of recovery of functioning in cats with rostral reticular lesions. *Journal of Neurosurgery*, 1959, 16, 85–98.

ADEY, W. R., SEGUNDO, J. P., & LIVINGSTON R. B. Cortical influences on intrinsic brainstem conduction in cat and monkey. *Journal of Neuerophysiology*, 1957, 20, 1–16.

ANAND, B. K., & BROBECK, J. R. Hypothalamic control of food intake in rats and cats. *Yale Journal of Biology and Medicine*, 1951, 41, 123–140.

ANDY, O. J., & STEPHAN, H. *The septum of the cat.* Springfield, Illinois: Charles C Thomas, 1964.

AXELSSON, J., & THESLEFF, S. A study of supersensitivity in denervated mammalian skeletal muscle. *Journal of Physiology, London*, 1959, 147, 178–193.

BAILLIE, P., & MORRISON, S. D. The nature of the suppression of food intake by lateral hypothalamic lesions in rats. *Journal of Physiology, London*, 1963, 165, 227–245.

BARNES, C. D. The interaction of amphetamine and eserine on the EEG. *Life Sciences*, 1966, 5, 1897–1902.

BONDAREFF, W. An intercellular substance in rat cerebral cortex: Submicroscopic distribution of ruthenium red. *The Anatomical Record*, 1967, 157, 527–536.

BONVALLET, M., & NEWMAN-TAYLOR, A. Neurophysiological evidence for a differential organization of the mesencephalic reticular formation. *Electroencephalography and Clinical Neurophysiology*, 1967, 22, 54–73.

BRADLEY, P. B. The central action of certain drugs in relation to reticular formation of the brain. In H. H. Jasper (Ed.), *Reticular formation of the brain.* Boston: Little, Brown, 1958. Pp. 123–150.

BRADLEY, P. B., & KEY, B. J. The effect of drugs on arousal responses produced by electrical stimulation of the reticular formation of the brain. *Electroencephalography and Clinical Neurophysiology*, 1958, 10, 97–110.

BRADY, J. V. The paleocortex and behavior motivation. In H. F. Harlow & C. N. Woolsey (Eds.), *Biological and biochemical bases of behavior.* Madison: University of Wisconsin Press, 1958. Pp. 193–236.

BRADY, J. V. Motivational-emotional factors and intracranial self-stimulation. In D. E. Sheer (Ed.), *Electrical stimulation of the brain.* Austin: University of Texas Press, 1961. Pp. 413–430.

BRADY, J. V., & NAUTA, W. J. H. Subcortical mechanisms in emotional behavior: Affective changes following septal forebrain lesions in the albino rat. *Journal of Comparative and Physiological Psychology*, 1953, 46, 339–346.

BREMER, F. Cerveau isolé et physiologie du sommeil. *Comptes Rendus Societe de Biologie* (Paris), 1935, 118, 1235–1241.

BRUNNGRABER, E. Alternatives to the RNA memory hypothesis. Informal discussion presented at Illinois State Psychiatric Institute, 1966.

CARLI, G., ARMENGOL, V., & ZANCHETTI, A. Brainstem-limbic connections and the electrographic aspects of deep sleep in the cat. *Archives Italiennes de Biologie*, 1965, 103, 725–750.

CARLTON, P. L. Cholinergic mechanisms in the control of behavior by the brain. *Psychological Review*, 1963, 70, 19–39.

CHAMBERLIN, T. J., HALICK, P., & GERARD, R. W. Fixation of experience in the rat spinal cord. *Journal of Neurophysiology*, 1963, 26, 662–691.

CHARLTON, B. T., & GRAY, E. G. Comparative electron microscopy of synapses in the vertebrate spinal cord. *Journal of Cell Science*, 1966, 1, 67–80.

AROUSAL SYSTEMS

CHOROVER, S. L., & SCHILLER, P. H. Re-examination of prolonged retrograde amnesia in one-trial learning. *Journal of Comparative and Physiological Psychology*, 1966, **61**, 34–41.

CHOW, K. L., & RANDALL, W. Learning and retention in cats with lesions in reticular formation. *Psychonomic Science*, 1964, **1**, 259–260.

CHOW, K. L., RANDALL, W., & MORRELL, F. Effect of brain lesions on conditional cortical electropotentials. *Electroencephalography and Clinical Neurophysiology*, 1966, **20**, 357–369.

CLARK, C. V. H., & ISAACSON, R. L. Effect of bilateral hippocampal ablation on DRL performance. *Journal of Comparative and Physiological Psychology*, 1965, **59**, 135–140.

CLEMENTE, C. D., STERMAN, M. B., & WYRWICKA, W. Post-reinforcement EEG synchronization during alimentary behavior. *Electroencephalography and Clinical Neurophysiology*, 1964, **16**, 355–365.

COONS, E. E., JR. Motivational correlates of eating elicited by electrical stimulation in the hypothalamic feeding area. Unpublished doctoral dissertation, Yale University, 1964.

COVIAN, M. R., ANTUNES-RODRIGUES, J., & O'FLAHERTY, J. J. Effects of stimulation of the septal area upon blood pressure and respiration in the cat. *Journal of Neurophysiology*, 1964, **27**, 394–407.

CROSBY, E. C. The forebrain of Alligator mississippiensis. *Journal of Comparative Neurology*, 1917, **27**, 325–402.

DEUTSCH, J. A. *The structural basis of behavior.* Chicago: University of Chicago Press, 1960.

DOTY, R. W., BECK, E. C., & KOOI, K. A. Effect of brainstem lesions on conditioned responses of cats. *Experimental Neurology*, 1959, **1**, 360–385.

DUFFY, E. *Activation and behavior.* New York: Wiley, 1962.

FELDMAN, S., & WALLER, H. Dissociation of electrocortical activation and behavioral arousal. *Nature*, 1962, **196**, 1320–1322.

FRENCH, J. D. The reticular formation. In J. Field (Ed.), *Handbook of physiology*, Vol. II. Washington, D. C.: American Physiological Society, 1960. Pp. 1281–1305.

GAITO, J. *Macromolecules and behavior.* New York: Appleton-Century-Crofts, 1966.

GERBRANDT, L. K. Neural systems of response release and control. *Psychological Bulletin*, 1965, **64**, 113–123.

GLEITMAN, H., & STEINMAN, F. Retention of runway performance as a function of proactive interference. *Journal of Comparative and Physiological Psychology*, 1963, **56**, 834–838.

GLICKMAN, S. E. Reinforcing properties of arousal. *Journal of Comparative and Physiological Psychology*, 1960, **53**, 68–71.

GLICKMAN, S. E. Perseverative neural processes and consolidation of the memory trace. *Psychological Bulletin*, 1961, **58**, 218–233.

GLICKMAN, S. E., & FELDMAN, S. M. Habituation and arousal response to direct stimulation of the brainstem. *Electroencephalography and Clinical Neurophysiology*, 1961, **13**, 703–709.

GLICKMAN, S. E., & SCHIFF, B. B. A biological theory of reinforcement. *Psychological Review*, 1967, **74**, 81–109.

GLICKMAN, S. E., SROGES, R. W., & HUNT, J. Brain lesions and locomotor exploration in the albino rat. *Journal of Comparative and Physiological Psychology*, 1964, **58**, 93–100.

GODDARD, G. V. Amygdaloid stimulation and learning in the rat. *Journal of Comparative and Physiological Psychology*, 1964, **58**, 23–30.

GRASTYAN, E. The hippocampus and higher nervous activity. In M. A. B. Brazier (Ed.), *The central nervous system and behavior.* New York: Josiah Macy Jr. Foundation, 1959. Pp. 119–193.

GRASTYAN, E., KARMOS, G., VERECZKEY, L., MARTIN, J., & KELLENYI, L. Hypothalamic motivational processes as reflected by their hippocampal electrical correlates. *Science*, 1965, **149**, 91–93.

GRASTYAN, E., KARMOS, G., VERECZKEY, L., & KELLENYI, L. The hippocampal electrical correlates of the homeostatic regulation of motivation. *Electroencephalography and Clinical Neurophysiology*, 1966, **21**, 34–53.

GREEN, J. D., & ARDUINI, A. A. Hippocampal electrical activity in arousal. *Journal of Neurophysiology*, 1954, **17**, 533–557.

GROSSMAN, S. P. Effect of chemical stimulation of the septal area on motivation. *Journal of Comparative and Physiological Psychology*, 1964, **58**, 194–200.

HARMON, L. D. Neuromimes: Actions of a reciprocally inhibitory pair. *Science*, 1964, **146**, 1323–1325.

HARRINGTON, G. M., & LINDER, W. K. A positive reinforcing effect of electrical stimulation. *Journal of Comparative and Physiological Psychology*, 1962, **55**, 1014–1015.

HARVEY, J. A., & HUNT, H. F. Effect of septal lesions on thirst in the rat as indicated by water consumption and operant responding for water reward. *Journal of Comparative and Physiological Psychology,* 1965, **59,** 49–56.

HEATH, R. G., & MICKLE, W. A. Evaluation of seven years' experience with depth electrode studies in human patients. In E. R. Ramey & D. S. O'Doherty (Eds.), *Electrical studies on the unanesthetized brain.* New York: Hoeber, 1960. Pp. 214–241.

HEBB, D. O. Drives and the CNS. *Psychological Review,* 1955, **62,** 243–254.

HEBB, D. O. *A textbook of psychology.* Philadelphia: Saunders, 1966.

HERNÁNDEZ-PEÓN, R. Central neuro-humoral transmission in sleep and wakefulness. In K. Akert, C. Bally, & J. P. Schade (Eds.), *Sleep mechanisms.* Amsterdam: Elsevier, 1966. Pp. 96–117.

HESS, W. R. *Functional organization of the diencephalon.* New York: Grune and Stratton, 1957.

HILGARD, E. R. *Theories of learning.* New York: Appleton-Century-Crofts, 1956.

HOBSON, J. A. The effects of chronic brainstem lesions on cortical and muscular activity during sleep and waking in cat. *Electroencephalography and Clinical Neurophysiology,* 1965, **19,** 41–62.

HODOS, W., & VALENSTEIN, E. S. An evaluation of response rate as a measure of rewarding intracranial stimulation. *Journal of Comparative and Physiological Psychology,* 1962, **55,** 80–84.

ISAACSON, R. L. The limbic-midbrain system and behavior: Hippocampus. *American Psychologist,* 1966, **21,** 656.

ITO, M. Hippocampal electrical correlates of self-stimulation in the rat. *Electroencephalography and Clinical Neurophysiology* 1966, **21,** 261–268.

JASPER, H. H. Thalamic reticular system. In D. E. Sheer (Ed.), *Electrical stimulation of the brain.* Austin, Texas: University of Texas Press, 1961. Pp. 277–287.

JOHN, E. R., & KILLAM, K. F. Electrophysiological correlates of differential approach-avoidance conditioning of cats. *Journal of Nervous and Mental Disease,* 1960, **131,** 183–201.

JOUVET, M. Telencephalic and rhombencephalic sleep in the cat. In G. E. W. Wolstenholme & M. O'Connor (Eds.), *The nature of sleep.* (A Ciba Foundation symposium.) London: Churchill, 1961. Pp. 188–208.

JUNG, O. H., & BOYD, E. S. Effects of the cholinergic drugs on self-stimulation response rates in rats. *American Journal of Physiology,* 1966, **210,** 431–434.

KAADA, B. R. Somato-motor, autonomic, and electrocorticographic responses to electrical stimulation of rhinencephalic and other structures in primates, cat and dog. *Acta physiologica scandinavica,* 1951, **24** (Suppl. 83), 1—285.

KAADA, B. R., ALNAES, T. F. E., & WESTER, K. EEG synchronization induced by high frequency midbrain reticular stimulation in anesthetized cats. *Electroencephalography and Clinical Neurophysiology,* 1967, **22,** 220–230.

KASPER, P. Attenuation of passive avoidance by continuous septal stimulation. Paper presented at the meeting of the Eastern Psychological Association, Philadelphia, April 1964.

KAWAMURA, H., NAKAMURA, Y., & TOKIZANE, T. Effect of acute brain stem lesions on the electrical activities of the limbic system and neocortex. *Japanese Journal of Physiology,* 1961, **11,** 564–575.

KENYON, J., & KRIECKHAUS, E. E. Enhanced avoidance behavior following septal lesions in the rat as a function of lesion size and spontaneous activity. *Journal of Comparative and Physiological Psychology,* 1965, **59,** 466–468.

KILLAM, K. F., & KILLAM, E. K. Drug action of pathways involving the reticular formation. In H. H. Jasper (Ed.), *Reticular formation of the brain.* Boston: Little, Brown, 1958. Pp. 111–122.

KIMBLE, G. A. *Conditioning and learning.* New York: Appleton-Century-Crofts, 1961.

KORNETSKY, C., & BAIN, G. The effects of chlorpromazine and pentobarbital on sustained attention in the rat. *Psychopharmacologia,* 1965, **8,** 277–284.

KRNJVC, K., & SILVER, A. A histochemical study of cholinergic fibers in the cerebral cortex. *Journal of Anatomy,* 1965, **99,** 711–759.

LILLY, J. C. Learning motivated by subcortical stimulation: The "start" and "stop" patterns of behavior. In H. H. Jasper (Ed.), *Reticular formation of the brain.* Boston: Little, Brown, 1958. Pp. 705–721.

LINDSLEY, D. B. Attention, consciousness, sleep, and wakefulness. In J. Field (Ed.), *Handbook of physiology,* Vol. III. Washington, D. C.: American Physiological Society, 1960. Pp. 1553–1593.

LINDSLEY, D. B., BOWDEN, J. W., & MAGOUN, H. W. Effect upon the EEG of acute injury to the brain stem activating system. *Electroencephalography and Clinical Neurophysiology*, 1949, 1, 475–486.

Lindsley, D. B., Schreiner, L. H., Knowles, W. B., & Magoun, H. W. Behavioral and EEG changes following chronic brain stem lesions in the cat. *Electroencephalography and Clinical Neurophysiology*, 1950, 2, 483–498.

Mahut, H. The effects of subcortical electrical stimulation on learning in the rat. *Journal of Comparative and Physiological Psychology*, 1962, 55, 472–477.

Malmo, R. B. Activation: A neuropsychological dimension. *Psychological Review*, 1959, 66, 367–386.

Malmo, R. B. Heart rate reactions and locus stimulation within the septal area of the rat. *Science*, 1964, 155, 1029–1030.

Manning, J. W., Charben, G. A., & Cotten, M. deV. Inhibition of tonic cardiac sympathetic activity by stimulation of brain septal region. *American Journal of Physiology*, 1963, 205, 1221–1226.

Meyers, B., Roberts, K. H., Riciputi, R. H., & Domino, E. F. Some effects of muscarinic cholinergic blocking drugs on behavior and the electrocorticogram. *Psychopharmacologia*, 1964, 5, 289–300.

Meyers, W. J., Valenstein, E. S., & Lacey, J. I. Heart rate changes after reinforcing brain stimulation in rats. *Science*, 1963, 140, 1233–1235.

Miller, G. A. The magical number seven, plus or minus two: Some limits on our capacity for processing information. *Psychological Review*, 1956, 63, 81–97.

Mogenson, G. J. Effects of sodium pentobarbital on brain self-stimulation. *Journal of Comparative and Physiological Psychology*, 1964, 58, 461–462.

Morgane, P. J. Alterations in feeding and drinking behavior of rats with lesions in globi pallidi. *American Journal of Physiology*, 1961, 201, 420–428. (a)

Morgane, P. J. Distinct "feeding" and "hunger motivating" systems in lateral hypothalamus of rat. *Science*, 1961, 133, 887–888. (b)

Morgane, P. J. Medial forebrain bundle and "feeding centers" of hypothalamus. *Journal of Comparative Neurology*, 1961, 117, 1–25. (c)

Morrell, F. Microelectrode and steady potential studies suggesting a dendrite locus of closure. In H. H. Jasper & G. D. Smirnov (Eds.), The Moscow colloquium on electroencephalography of higher nervous activity. *Electroencephalography and Clinical Neurophysiology*, 1960 (Suppl. No. 13), 65–80.

Morrell, F. Modification of RNA as a result of neural activity. In M. A. B. Brazier (Ed.), *Brain function*. Vol. II. *RNA and brain function memory and learning*. Los Angeles: University of California Press, 1964. Pp. 183—202.

Moruzzi, G., & Magoun, H. W. Brain stem reticular formation and activation of the EEG. *Electroencephalography and Clinical Neurophysiology*, 1949, 1, 455–473.

Nauta, W. J. H. Hypothalamic regulation of sleep in rats: An experimental study. *Journal of Neurophysiology*, 1946, 9, 285–316.

Nauta, W. J. H. Hippocampal projections and related neural pathways to the midbrain in cat. *Brain*, 1958, 81, 319–340.

Nauta, W. J. H., & Kuypers, H. G. J. M. Some ascending pathways in the brain stem reticular formation. In H. Jasper (Ed.), *Reticular formation of the brain*. Boston: Little, Brown, 1958. Pp. 3–30.

Olds, J. Satiation effects in self-stimulation of the brain. *Journal of Comparative and Physiological Psychology*, 1958, 51, 675–678.

Olds, J. Approach-avoidance dissociations in rat brain. *American Journal of Physiology*, 1960, 199, 965–968.

Olds, J. Hypothalamic substrates of reward. *Physiological Reviews*, 1962, 42, 554–604.

Olds, J., & Milner, P. Positive reinforcement produced by electrical stimulation of septal area and other regions of rat brain. *Journal of Comparative and Physiological Psychology*, 1954, 47, 419–427.

Olds, J., & Peretz, B. A motivational analysis of the reticular activating system. *Electroencephalography and Clinical Neuropathy*, 1960, 12, 445–454.

Olds, J., & Travis, R. P. Effects of chlorpromazine, meprobamate, pentobarbital, and morphine on self-stimulation. In L. Uhr & J. G. Miller (Eds.), *Drugs and behavior*. New York: Wiley, 1960. Pp. 255–267.

Olds, J., Travis, R. P., & Schwing, R. C. Topographic organization of hypothalamic self-stimulation functions. *Journal of Comparative and Physiological Psychology*, 1960, 53, 23–32.

Olds, J., Yuwiler, A., Olds, M. E., & Yun, C. Neurohumors in hypothalamic substrates of reward. *American Journal of Physiology*, 1964, 207, 242–254.

ARYEH ROUTTENBERG

Olds, M. E., & Olds, J. Approach-escape interactions in rat brain. *American Journal of Physiology*, 1962, 203, 803–810.

O'Leary, J. L., & Cohen, L. A. The reticular core—1957. *Physiological Reviews*, 1958, 38, 243–276.

Pease, D. C. Polysaccharides associated with the exterior surface of epithelial cells: Kidney, intestine, and brain. *Journal of Ultrastructural Research*, 1966, 15, 555–588.

Perez-Cruet, J., Black, W. C., & Brady, J. V. Heart rate: Differential effects of hypothalamic and septal self-stimulation. *Science*, 1963, 140, 1235–1236.

Perez-Cruet, J., McIntire, R. W., & Pliskoff, S. S. Blood pressure and heart rate changes during hypothalamic self-stimulation. *Journal of Comparative and Physiological Psychology*, 1966, 60, 373–381.

Petsche, H., Stumpf, C. H., & Gogolak, G. The significance of the rabbit's septum as a relay station between the midbrain and hippocampus. I. The control of hippocampal arousal activity by the septum cells. *Electroencephalography and Clinical Neurophysiology*, 1962, 14, 202–211.

Petsche, H., Gogolak, G., & van Zwieten, P. A. Rhythmicity of septal cell discharges at various levels of reticular excitation. *Electroencephalography and Clinical Neurophysiology*, 1965, 19, 25–33.

Pizzi, W. J., & Lorens, S. A. Effect of lesions in the amygdala-hippocampo-septal system on food and water intake in the rat. *Psychonomic Science*, 1967, 7, 187–188.

Powell, E. W. Septal efferents in the cat. *Experimental Neurology*, 1966, 14, 328–337.

Reynolds, D. V. A preliminary study of changes in food consumption following lesions in the septum and tegmentum in the albino rat. Unpublished doctoral dissertation, Stanford University, 1962.

Rheinberger, M. B., & Jasper, H. H. Electrical activity of the cerebral cortex of the unanaesthetized cat. *American Journal of Physiology*, 1937, 119, 186–196.

Roberts, W. W., Dember, W. N., & Brodwick, M. Alternation and exploration in rats with hippocampal lesions. *Journal of Comparative and Physiological Psychology*, 1962, 55, 695–700.

Rodgers, W. L., Epstein, A. N., & Teitelbaum, P. Lateral hypothalamic aphagia: Motor failure or motivational deficit? *American Journal of Physiology*, 1965, 208, 334–342.

Rossi, G. F., & Zanchetti, A. The brainstem reticular formation. Anatomy and physiology. *Archives Italiennes de Biologie*, 1957, 95, 199–435.

Routtenberg, A. Certain effects of stimulation in septal area and hypothalamus. Unpublished doctoral dissertation, University of Michigan, 1965.

Routtenberg, A. Neural mechanisms of sleep: Changing view of reticular formation function. *Psychological Review*, 1966, 73, 481–499.

Routtenberg, A., & Kane, R. S. Weight loss following lesions at the self-stimulation point: Ventral midbrain tegmentum. *Canadian Journal of Psychology*, 1966, 20, 343–351.

Routtenberg, A., & Olds, J. Attenuation of response to an aversive brain stimulus by concurrent rewarding septal stimulation. *Federation Proceedings*, 1963, 22, 515. (abstract)

Routtenberg, A., & Olds, J. The effect of dorsal midbrain stimulation on septal and hypothalamic self-stimulation. *Journal of Comparative and Physiological Psychology*, 1966, 62, 250–255.

Samuels, I. Reticular mechanisms and behavior. *Psychological Bulletin*, 1959, 56, 1–25.

Schlag, J. D., & Chaillet, F. Thalamic mechanisms involved in cortical desynchronization and recruiting responses. *Electroencephalography and Clinical Neurophysiology*, 1963, 15, 39–62.

Schlag, J., & Villablanca, J. Thalamic inhibition by thalamic stimulation. *Psychonomic Science*, 1967, 8, 373–374.

Scott, J. W., & Pfaffman, C. Unit activity in medial forebrain bundle following olfactory stimulation. Eastern Psychological Association, Boston, April 1967.

Sepinwall, J. Cholinergic stimulation of the brain and avoidance behavior. *Psychonomic Science*, 1966, 5, 93–94.

Sharpless, S. K. Designated discussion. In H. H. Jasper (Ed.), *Reticular formation of the brain*. Boston: Little, Brown, 1958. Pp. 722–723.

Sharpless, S. K. Reorganization of function in the nervous system—use and disuse. *Annual Review of Physiology*, 1964, 26, 357–388.

Sharpless, S. K., & Halpern, L. M. The electrical excitability of chronically isolated cortex studied by means of permanently implanted electrodes. *Electroencephalography and Clinical Neurophysiology*, 1962, 14, 244–255.

SHARPLESS, S. K., & JASPER, H. Habituation of the arousal reaction. *Brain*, 1956, 79, 665–680.

SKINNER, B. F. *The behavior of organisms*. New York: Appleton-Century-Crofts, 1938.

SPRAGUE, J. M., LEVITT, M., ROBSON, K., LIU, C. N., STELLER, E., & CHAMBERS, W. W. A neuroanatomical and behavioral analysis of the syndrome resulting from midbrain lemniscal and reticular lesions in the cat. *Archives Italiennes de Biologie*, 1963, 101, 225–295.

SPROTT, R. L., & WALLER, M. B. An experimental analysis of retrograde amnesia. *Journal of the Experimental Analysis of Behavior*, 1966, 9, 663–669.

STAVRAKY, G. W. *Supersensitivity following lesions of the nervous system*. Toronto: University of Toronto Press, 1961.

STEIN, L. Self-stimulation of the brain and the central stimulant action of amphetamine. *Federation Proceedings*, 1964, 23, 836–850.

STEIN, L. Facilitation of avoidance behavior by positive brain stimulation. *Journal of Comparative and Physiological Psychology*, 1965, 60, 9–19.

STERMAN, M. B., & CLEMENTE, C. D. Forebrain inhibitory mechanisms: Cortical synchronization induced by basal forebrain stimulation. *Experimental Neurology*, 1962, 6, 91–102.

STERMAN, M. B., & FAIRCHILD, M. D. Modification of locomotor performance by reticular formation and basal forebrain stimulation in the cat: Evidence for reciprocal systems. *Brain Research*, 1966, 2, 205–218.

STUMPF, C. The fast component in the electrical activity of the rabbit's hippocampus. *Electroencephalography and Clinical Neurophysiology*, 1965, 18, 477–486.

STUMPF, C., PETSCHE, H., & GOGOLAK, G. The significance of the rabbit's septum as a relay station between the midbrain and hippocampus. II. The differential influence of drugs upon both the septal cell firing and the hippocampus theta activity. *Electroencephalography and Clinical Neurophysiology*, 1962, 14, 212–219.

TEITELBAUM, H., & MILNER, P. M. Activity changes following partial hippocampal lesions in rats. *Journal of Comparative and Physiological Psychology*, 1963, 56, 284–289.

TEITELBAUM, P., & CYTAWA, J. Spreading depression and recovery from lateral hypothalamic damage. *Science*, 1965, 147, 61–63.

TEITELBAUM, P., & EPSTEIN, A. N. The lateral hypothalamic syndrome: Recovery of feeding and drinking after lateral hypothalamic lesions. *Psychological Review*, 1962, 69, 74–90.

THESLEFF, S. A neurophysiological speculation concerning learning. *Perspectives in Biology and Medicine*, 1962, 5, 293–295.

TORII, S., & WIKLER, A. Effects of atropine on electrical activity of hippocampus and cerebral cortex in cat. *Psychopharmacologia*, 1966, 9, 189–204.

UNDERWOOD, B. J. Interference and forgetting. *Psychological Review*, 1957, 64, 49–60.

UNDERWOOD, B. J. Forgetting. *Scientific American*, 1964, 210, 91–99.

USHER, D. R., KASPER, P., & BIRMINGHAM, M. K. Influence of the limbic-system on pituitary-adrenal function. Paper presented at the Meeting of the Canadian Federal Biological Science, Ottawa, June 1965.

VILLABLANCA, J. The electrocorticogram in the chronic *cerveau isolé* cat. *Electroencephalography and Clinical Neurophysiology*, 1965, 19, 576–586.

VOTAW, C. L., & LAUER, E. W. An afferent hippocampal fiber system in the fornix of the monkey. *Journal of Comparative Neurology*, 1963, 121, 195–206.

WALKER, E. L. Action decrement and its relation to learning. *Psychological Review*, 1958, 65, 129–142.

WARD, H. P. Tegmental self-stimulation after amygdaloid ablation. *Archives of Neurology and Psychiatry*, 1961, 4, 657–659.

WASE, A. W., CHRISTENSEN, J., & POLLEY, E. The accumulation of S⁸⁵—chlorpromazine in brain. *Archives of Neurology and Psychiatry*, 1956, 75, 54–56.

WHITEHOUSE, J. M., LLOYD, A. J., & FIFER, S. A. Comparative effects of atropine and methylatropine on maze acquisition and eating. *Journal of Comparative and Physiological Psychology*, 1964, 58, 475–476.

WIKLER, A. Pharmacologic dissociation of behavior and EEG "sleep patterns" in dogs: Morphine, n-allylmorphine, and atropine. *Proceedings of the Society of Experimental Biology* (New York), 1952, 79, 261–265.

WILSON, G. T., & RADLOFF, W. P. Degree of arousal and performance: Effects of reticular stimulation on an operant task. *Psychonomic Science*, 1967, 7, 13–14.

WOLFMAN, E. F., COON, W. W., & SCHWARTZ, S. Sodium retention following experimental lesions ot the precommissural septum in the monkey. *Journal of Surgical Research,* 1966, **6**, 2–18.

Wyrwicka, W., & Doty, R. W. Feeding induced in cats by electrical stimulation of the brain stem. *Experimental Brain Research,* 1966, **1**, 152–160.

Zanchetti, A. Brain stem mechanisms of sleep. *Anesthesiology,* 1967, **28**, 81–99.

Zucker, I. Effect of lesions of the septal-limbic area on the behavior of cats. *Journal of Comparative and Physiological Psychology,* 1965, **60**, 344–352.

Zukauskas, E., & Machne, X. Effect of chlorpromazine on the response patterns of hypothalamic units. *International Journal of Neuropharmacology,* 1964, **3**, 341–352.

(Received February 17, 1967)

Section Two

Pavlov and Strength of the Nervous System

Editorial Commentary

on

Pavlov and Strength of the Nervous System

One of the earliest Eastern pioneers in the area of nervous system activity level, and the one who first proposed the concept of endurable ranges for stimulation, was Ivan Pavlov. Pavlov's reasoning derived from the conditioning literature, where it had been demonstrated that the magnitude of a conditioned reflex increases with the intensity of the conditioned stimulus *up to a ceiling value* for that intensity. Beyond this ceiling value, increases in intensity produce decreases in response magnitude. The maximum possible stimulus strength relative to the response strength is the 'law of strength'. The rationale for such a protective mechanism, at the microscopic level, is that cellular tissue would be damaged if forced to respond to ever-increasing stimulus intensities*. Thus,

there is an inhibitory process which is both protective as well as 'transmarginal' (beyond the limit). The higher an organism's threshold (of response prior to decrement), the greater the strength of cerebral cellular tissue and the greater the strength of the nervous system. The two ways in which the threshold may be reached are through intensity and through frequency or duration of stimulus. The more intense the stimulus before response decrement, the stronger the nervous system. The greater the frequency or longer the duration of the stimulus before response decrement, the stronger the nervous system. Both cases may be plotted as the classic inverted-U function:

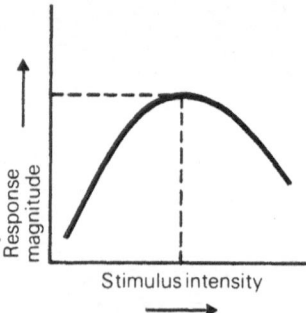

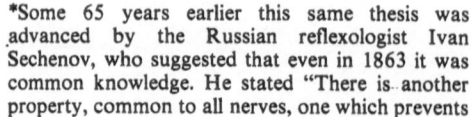

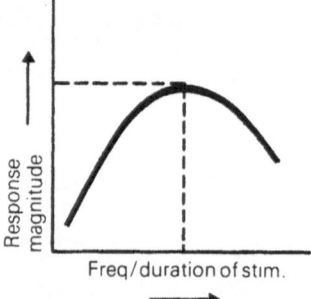

*Some 65 years earlier this same thesis was advanced by the Russian reflexologist Ivan Sechenov, who suggested that even in 1863 it was common knowledge. He stated "There is another property, common to all nerves, one which prevents the child from concentrating too long on a single impression; this is fatigableness of the nerve, i.e. its property to become dulled as a result of protracted activity in one direction. These are, of course, well-known facts."

Pavlov posited a functional relationship between strength of nervous system and the tendency to focalize or distribute stimulus input. Since it would appear to be evolutionarily adaptive to distribute the load of stimulation over the cortex, Jeffrey Gray (1964) proposed that there were two additional thresholds passed *before* reaching 'Pavlov's threshold', (Pavlov's threshold being the one just mentioned as protective and transmarginal). With stimulus intensity plotted on the abscissa, increasing from the origin, and excitation or arousal plotted on the ordinate, increasing from the origin, the first threshold is that of simple adaptation level (the absolute sensory threshold). This is the 'reiz limen' or twilight zone, with stimulus intensity just great enough to be perceived or not perceived (not all senses have 'terminal limens' or upper limits). The greater the strength of nervous system, the higher the absolute sensory threshold. Gray argued that a higher threshold is encountered when stimulation remains focalized on a part of the cortex. This is the Threshold of Concentration of Excitation. Gray's second Threshold of Irradiation of Excitation derives from Pavlov's notion that the cortical excitatory process may irradiate over the entirety of the cortex. This 'distri-

bution of stimulation' would, of course, be adaptive in the event of intense or prolonged input. Gray has argued that the greater the stength of the nervous sytem the *higher* the threshold of irradiation and the *lower* the threshold of concentration. The reasoning here has precisely to do with Pavlov's theory relating nervous system strength to focalization of stimulation. Since it is adaptive to distribute the load, stronger nervous systems will begin to irradiate at lower stimulus intensities. Again, according to Pavlov, a concentrated cortical focus of either excitation or inhibition 'induces' the opposite process in the surrounding cortical zone. In other words, concentrated inhibition induces excitation (positive induction), while concentrated excitation induces inhibition (negative induction). Beyond the threshold of irradiation, the ceiling value is reached. This is the protective threshold or Pavlov's Threshold of Transmarginal Inhibition. Strictly speaking, it is an inhibitory process that shuts down the processing of input when that input has become too intense or too prolonged. Thus, the higher the threshold of transmarginal inhibition the greater the strength of nervous system.

The readings in this section are intended to

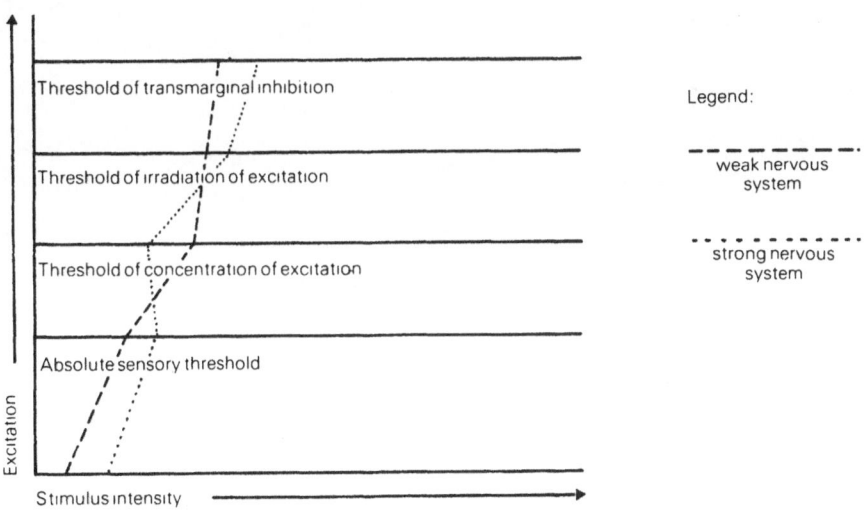

supply some advanced theoretical understanding of the Pavlovian notion of strength of nervous system, as well as provide examples of recent laboratory research in this area. In

addition, a sample of the research of Sales and his colleagues on augmenting and reducing has been included. Individuals with strong nervous systems resist incoming stimuli. This tendency has been called 'dampening' and such individuals are called reducers. Those with weak nervous systems who are overly sensitive to stimuli tend to 'blow-up' or magnify input and are called augmenters. The reader is advised that the Pavlov–Gray thresholds discussed herein are entirely of a 'theoretico-empirical' nature. There has been no formal empirical integration between nervous sytem strength and cortical thresholds. If, at this point, there is any question in the reader's mind as to what strength of nervous system has to do with personality, hold the reins momentarily. The following companion section on introversion/extraversion will hopefully make clear many of the implications.

References

Gray, J. (1964). *Pavlov's Typology.* (Oxford: Pergamon Press)

Pavlov, I. (1927). *Conditioned Reflexes.* (Oxford: Oxford University Press)

Sechenov, I. M. (1965). *Reflexes of the Brain.* (trans. S. Belsky) p. 54. (Cambridge, Mass.: The M.I.T. Press)

From P. S. Kupalov (1961). Annals of the New York Academy of Sciences, *92,* 1046-1053, *by kind permission of the New York Academy of Sciences.*

SOME NORMAL AND PATHOLOGICAL PROPERTIES OF NERVOUS PROCESSES IN THE BRAIN

P. S. Kupalov

Institute of Experimental Medicine, Leningrad, U.S.S.R.

Suppose it were possible to insert microelectrodes into all the nerve cells of the brain without injuring them or altering their normal condition, and to record their resting potentials and action potentials. Could we then, on the basis of our recordings, obtain a picture of the activity of the brain as a whole and relate it to the outward behavior of the animal? Could we say what sorts of conditioned reflexes have been formed in this animal, what stimuli from the internal organs and the external world are acting upon it at a given moment, what its response reactions to these influences will be (and accurately describe these reactions), and when they will occur? It is clear that all these questions must be answered in the negative. That is why the methods of investigation that were introduced by Pavlov, and to which we adhere, not only retain their importance today but will continue to be important in the future.

The physiology of higher nervous activity that Pavlov created has as its purposes the study of the mechanisms of nervous processes and the functional organization of the brain, the study of those brain functions that ensure the animal's (appropriate) interrelations with the surrounding world (the animal's behavior), and the utilization of physiological knowledge for the understanding of subjective phenomena: all these under both normal and pathological conditions.

The irradiation of nervous processes plays an important role in the activity of the brain. Excitation initiated by an external stimulus spreads extensively through the brain, selectively involving different regions of the brain to different degrees, and thereby promoting coordinated and unified functioning. As it pertains to the hemispheres, this property was studied by Pavlov under the name of "the law of irradiation and concentration of the processes of excitation and inhibition." We need not dwell on facts that are known to everyone, although they have been the object of sharp criticism from certain authors who have misinterpreted them.

Let me begin by setting forth some recent data of ours pertaining to the irradiation of excitation under the influence of unconditioned stimuli. General patterns established for lower nervous centers always are reflected in the function of the brain as a whole.

It was of interest to choose two secretory centers and show the effect they have on each other as a result of the irradiation of excitation. For this purpose we selected the salivary and lacrimal nervous centers. Dogs with externalized salivary and lacrimal ducts were used in the experiments; the operation on the lacrimal glands was developed by K. S. Abuladze.

If we feed a dog or irrigate its mouth with an acid solution, we observe that tears are secreted as well as saliva. The reverse is also true; stimulation of the

Kupalov: Properties of Nervous Processes in the Brain

conjunctiva with a weak acid solution or mechanically with a wad of cotton results in secretion of saliva as well as of tears. This shows that the process of excitation evoked by the corresponding stimuli not only irradiates in the brain within the immediate centers of the given stimulus, but also involves other centers that do not bear a direct relation to these stimuli.

The fact that this is a matter of irradiation, that specific excitation from the primary nervous center reaches the second center, may be seen from the following.

When the conjunctiva is stimulated mechanically, lacrimation begins after two seconds, but salivation begins after 5 sec. If a meat-biscuit powder is eaten, salivary secretion is observed after 2 to 3 sec., but lacrimation is not seen until after 20 sec. When the oral cavity is irrigated with an acid solution, salivation begins after 2 to 4 sec., but lacrimation begins only after 40 sec. The conclusion is that when the oral cavity is stimulated a comparatively weak excitation reaches the lacrimation centers; more time is required before the weak impulses summate sufficiently to give a distinct secretory reaction.

Moreover, the chemical composition of the tears is different, depending on whether they are secreted in response to stimulation of the oral cavity with food or acid. The concentration of proteins in the tears secreted in response to eating food is several times greater than that in response to acid. That is, tears secreted in response to eating the meat-biscuit powder contain about 15 mg. of protein per milliliter, whereas tears secreted upon stimulation of the oral cavity with acid contain only 5.7 mg./ml. of protein (I. A. Lapina's experiments). We may conclude that a qualitatively different excitation process irradiates to the centers for the lacrimal glands in these two cases: a fact of considerable importance for our understanding of brain activity.

The irradiation of excitation is determined not only by the properties of the nervous process evoked in the primary center, but also by the functional state of the nervous centers to which the excitation spreads. If before the oral cavity is stimulated we first stimulate the conjunctiva, the secretion of tears increases approximately twofold. Therefore, after stimulation of the conjunctiva a state of elevated excitability or latent excitation remains for some time in the lacrimation center. Some of the nerve cells of this center, which were already subliminally excited, send forth a wave of propagated nerve impulses as a result of summation. This is one of the phenomena that Pavlov called the summation reflex.

There is reason to think, however, that this is not just a matter of simple summation, but that the excitation process irradiates preferentially to the focus whose excitability is increased, or to the center of stronger excitation. This rule is of great importance for the formation of conditioned reflex connections. The interrelationships that obtain may be schematically depicted as follows. Let us suppose that six single waves of excitation irradiate from center A to centers B and C. Of these units, four represent intense waves of excitation—two going to B and two to C—and two waves are weak, dying out along the way before reaching these centers. If we first create a state of elevated excitability in center B by stimulating it directly, the weak wave will now reach it, and B will receive three units of excitation, while C receives only two, as before. If the excitation in center *B* is made stronger still, it is possible that a diversion will result, and that some of the waves of excitation that had previously gone to center *C* will now be directed to *B*.

Here are some of our results. When a dog is fed, the resulting parotid secretion is approximately equal on the two sides. Before the dog had eaten, however, one of the externalized areas of the tongue (for example, on the right side) was painted with an acid solution and we waited until salivation in response to this stimulation stopped completely and the nervous center returned to the resting state; after this we again gave food to the animal, and salivation from the right parotid was significantly increased.

We have not performed experiments of this type on decorticate dogs, and we still do not know how much of this summation reflex can be attributed to lower centers and how much to the hemispheres (that is, how much can be ascribed to the so-called cortical representation of these unconditioned reflexes). But the same pattern can be seen in motor reactions of an animal in which there is no doubt that the cortex participates.

We can often observe such behavior in the formation of motor conditioned reflexes in which a dog is supposed to go to one table in response to the first of the conditioned stimuli and to another table in response to the second. If food is given at table *A* after the conditioned stimulus is applied, and this is repeated several times in succession, the dog will subsequently go to table *A* even in response to the application of a second conditioned stimulus followed by the presentation of food at table *B*. This happens in the initial period of formation of conditioned reflexes, while they are not yet stabilized.

Concentration of the excitation process is also closely related to irradiation of the process. If no other conditions interfere, then upon repeated application of the unconditioned stimulus the extent of irradiation diminishes and the excitation process becomes more concentrated. For example, following acid stimulation of an externalized area of the tongue on the left side, salivation occurs chiefly from the left parotid gland, but there is also a small amount of secretion contralaterally, from the right gland. In response to repeated stimulation, the secretion from the right parotid gradually diminishes and then completely disappears. The excitation process becomes more concentrated and affects only the centers of the left parotid. Once created, this state of concentrated excitation remains for many hours.

Unconditioned reflexes are based on the innate functional organization of the nervous system. This innate functional organization is also the basis of the property of irradiation and concentration of nervous processes and the phenomenon of the summation reflex. In turn, these properties promote the formation of the new functional organizations of the brain that arise during the development of conditioned reflexes. As for the summation reflex, it undoubtedly constitutes the first step in the formation of a conditioned, temporary nervous connection.

The intimate mechanism of formation of a temporary connection is still unknown, and it is my impression that the latest investigations in the area of brain physiology have not brought about any radical change in this respect. However, we do have some important information as to the functional organization of nervous processes in conditioned reflex activity.

Kupalov: Properties of Nervous Processes in the Brain

Some time ago we showed that the nervous processes in the brain may be divided into processes resulting in external reactions and processes that establish only the over-all tone of the brain, that is, processes of general activating significance, both positive and negative (leading to elevation or reduction of tone). We were unable to localize the processes of the second type, to ascribe their occurrence to any definite morphological structure in the brain, or to establish their fundamental mechanism. Now, however, since the brilliant work that has come primarily from the laboratory of Horace W. Magoun, disclosing the function of the reticular system, this whole problem has entered a new phase of development.

The essential fact we were able to establish at the very outset, which is our contribution to the physiology of the brain, consists in our discovery that these processes of a general activating character can be reproduced by conditioned reflex means: that they can be elicited by influences in the experimental situation that had no such effect prior to the formation of the temporary connection. It follows that we may speak of particular conditioned reflexes in which the reaction to the external stimulus culminates not in a definite external reaction but, on the whole, only in a change in the functional state of the brain, a change in the tone of certain divisions, or mechanisms, of the brain. We therefore called such conditioned reflexes "truncated" conditioned reflexes.

Reflexes of this type, both of a general and of a more local character, constantly take part in conditioned reflex activity. In the formation of a conditioned reflex, the excitation process evoked by a given conditioned stimulus first begins to irradiate preferentially to the centers of the unconditioned reflex and finally fuses with the process of unconditioned excitation in a single combined nervous process. This is primarily shown by the fact that the conditioned stimulus activates the centers of the unconditioned reflex and affects its execution, increasing its magnitude, speed, and accuracy. These data of ours have recently been substantiated in the work of J. P. Segundo of Montevideo, Uruguay (personal communication).

The particular conditioned stimulus that directly elicits the conditioned reaction is not the only stimulus connected with the unconditioned reflex; various extraneous stimuli and numerous components of the experimental situation are also connected with it. These factors increase the excitability of the unconditioned centers even before the conditioned stimuli are applied, preparing these centers for the subsequent action of the unconditioned stimulus and for the most effective unconditioned reaction. This also happens by the mechanism of truncated conditioned reflexes.

At present we still do not have accurate data concerning the question of the sequence of occurrence of the nervous processes in the various divisions of the brain in conditioned reflex activity, or how they are united in a single complex nervous process, or the final functional organization of this process. However, it is possible to isolate a few fundamental elements in this organization: the activity of the cortical portions of the analyzers (that is, cortical projection zones); the activity of the cortical representation of the unconditioned reflexes; the activity of the unconditioned centers; the activating mechanism of the reticular system, located in various subcortical divisions of the brain; and possibly also an analogous mechanism within the cortex itself. A special

Annals New York Academy of Sciences

position is occupied by the activity of the central nervous elements of the motor apparatus responsible for the execution of the so-called voluntary movements. In man, finally, all of this is crowned, according to Pavlov, by the function of the second signal system, which ensures the function of speech. All of this operates as a coordinated whole.

If conditioned reflex experiments are conducted day after day and the conditioned stimuli are applied in a definite constant sequence, there results that organized functional structure of temporally correlated nervous processes that Pavlov called the dynamic stereotype. I spoke of this in greater detail at the Moscow Colloquium on the Electroencephalography of Higher Nervous Activity in 1958.

When a coordinated system of conditioned reflexes is developed on this basis, the nervous processes that are generated during the application of the conditioned and unconditioned stimuli and those that occur in the intervals between the applications of the conditioned stimuli constitute a complex nervous process that is temporally integrated and proceeds in an orderly fashion. In this case, even before the recurrent application of the conditioned stimulus an elevation of the excitability of the centers of the conditioned stimulus occurs. This elevation of excitability may be so great that spontaneous reactions occur, motor as well as secretory. In the case of conditioned food reflexes the dog may persist in looking in the direction from which the conditioned stimulus ought to be heard. Obviously this is the phenomenon that psychologists call attention and expectancy. First there is a general alimentary excitation, a general preparation for future alimentary activity, the expectation of feeding in general that is supposed to follow. Then the reaction is concretized, and the animal awaits the definite conditioned stimulus that is followed by feeding, and focuses its attention on this stimulus.

Everything I have said so far is only a schematic representation, of course, but it can be regarded as correct since it has been confirmed by experiments of many sorts. For example, Jiurgea in our laboratory was able to form a conditioned reflex to stimulation of the visual cortex by implanted electrodes, combining this stimulation with stimulation of the motor cortex, also with implanted electrodes. He repeated these experiments in the United States, working with Doty. Here, the fundamental condition for the successful formation of a conditioned reflex is that a definite interval be allowed between successive combinations of conditioned and unconditioned stimuli: a definite, sufficiently long interval of time. If the time interval between two successive trials is too short, the first stimulation of the visual cortex (conditioned stimulation) will be connected with the second stimulation of the motor cortex (unconditioned stimulation) to the same extent as the second with the first, and the necessary directedness in the total nervous process will not develop. For this reason it is impossible to obtain a distinct conditioned reflex under such conditions. This fact itself, therefore, is an illustration of the formation of a complex, long-lasting nervous process during the development of a conditioned reflex.

By making use of the fact that during the formation of a conditioned reflex the excitability of the centers of the conditioned stimuli increases until a

Kupalov: Properties of Nervous Processes in the Brain

spontaneous reaction occurs, we have been able to obtain an active reproduction of involuntary reactions as conditioned "excitators" of the alimentary reflex: specifically, to obtain a conditioned shaking-off reflex. If the dog is given food every time it shakes itself during the experiment as a result of whatever skin stimulations may have arisen, it begins to shake itself more and more frequently in this experimental situation. The general alimentary excitation, irradiating to the centers of the shaking-off reflex, will elevate their excitability; and weak skin stimulations (irritations) that are always present and do not normally elicit the shaking-off reflex become supraliminal and adequate to elicit the reflex. Eventually the dog begins to shake itself actively, so effortlessly, so accurately, and so often that this essentially involuntary act cannot be distinguished from voluntary movements.

We believe that voluntary movements arise by the same mechanism when they become the first components of motor alimentary conditioned reflexes.

Currently, we are studying the completely normal behavior of animals when their freedom of movement in a large experimental room is not restricted, with the experimenter being isolated from the dog. This behavior can be satisfactorily explained, without artificiality, on the basis of our concepts of the properties and organization of the nervous processes of the brain.

In conclusion, I propose to discuss certain data on the irradiation of nervous processes in pathological conditions.

In various difficult nervous problems—particularly cften during overstrain of internal inhibition in cases of delayed conditioned reflexes—we have repeatedly obtained extreme, abnormal irradiation of inhibition. The first deviation from normal is a marked reduction in the magnitude of the secretory conditioned reflex; in the next stage the secretory response is absent throughout the entire application of the conditioned stimulus. Inhibition, normally present only in the first phase of a delayed reflex, remains throughout the entire second phase of the reflex. Later, secretion begins to disappear even in response to the unconditioned stimulus. The dog may eat for 20 seconds without secreting a drop of saliva. If this pathological state is intensified, the dog does not take the food presented to it immediately, but hesitates for a few seconds, that is, the inhibition now spreads to the motor centers as well. Finally, the inhibitory process irradiates to such an extent that the dog absolutely refuses to eat.

We have called this phenomenon pathological irradiation of the inhibitory process, since the inhibitory process spreads abnormally and very extensively. The whole phenomenon is undoubtedly initiated by the cerebral cortex, since delayed conditioned reflexes cannot be obtained in the decorticate animal. However we ought not to represent the inhibitory process, as such, as spreading from any individual cortical point, involving other divisions of the cortex and the subcortex. The inhibitory influences spread from the cortex, but such influences may have several starting points.

We ought to add that in the animal's subsequent behavior not everything will depend on pathological irradiation of inhibition. All pathology of higher nervous activity is permeated by the mechanism of formation of pathological conditioned connections. Various pathological functional states and reactions

Annals New York Academy of Sciences

are stabilized and reproduced under particular external influences. They may be very persistent and hard to remove. In some instances such pathological connections remain for years. We have a striking example of this in the case of attempts to form a defense motor conditioned reflex to acid stimulation of an exposed area of the tongue (I. A. Lapina).

Another example of pathological irradiation of nervous processes can be illustrated by the following experiments. A dog is taught to lie quietly in its stand with small electric lights fastened close to its eyes. At 5-min. intervals these lights are permitted to flash for periods of 20 sec. One eye is stimulated by light flashes at a frequency of three per second, and the other at a frequency of seven per second. From M. N. Livanov's data we know that it is difficult for an animal to tolerate stimulation of the eye with light flashes in a rhythm that differs from the normal discharge rhythm of cortical cells. W. Grey Walter has shown that, in man, stimulation by flickering lights is accompanied by unpleasant sensations and, in persons with a tendency to epilepsy, it may provoke epileptic seizures. According to I. V. Danilov's experiments, stimulation of the eyes by asynchronous light flashes is an even greater challenge to the animal's nervous system. Asymmetry of cortical potentials in the two hemispheres develops. Then wave-spike discharges appear, which are characteristic for epilepsy, as Jasper has shown. Furthermore, when such experiments are carried on day in and day out over a long period of time, the dogs develop clonic and tonic contractions of the hind-limb muscles. Such hyperkinesias become very stubborn; they arise not only upon stimulation with light, but spontaneously as well, and they should be considered pathological.

Thus a nervous process of abnormal organization, generated in the visual cortex, irradiates to the motor cortex and produces a picture of hyperkinesia with the presence of nerve cell discharges of an epileptiform character.

I have been describing to you certain properties of nervous processes, established through the use of the fundamental method developed by Pavlov. I have tried to show how a knowledge of these properties makes it possible to study the complex organization of nervous processes that occurs in conditioned reflex activity, and to explain various facts about animal behavior. In our work we have followed our own path, which differs from the direction of the investigations that are being carried on in the United States. It is my hope that the exchange of views will increase mutual understanding and will promote further productive development of our knowledge of the activity of the brain.

References

ABULADZE, K. S. 1958. Izucheniie reflektornoi deiatel'nosti sliunnykh i sleznykh zhelez (Study of Reflex Action of Salivary and Lachrymal Glands), Izdatel'stvo Akademii Meditsinskikh Nauk SSSR (Publ. by Academy of Medical Sciences of USSR), Moscow. : 3–104.

DANILOV, I. V. 1958. Narusheniia vysshey nervnoi deiatel'nosti sobak pri asinkhronnom svetovom razdrazhenii (Disturbance of Higher Nervous Activity of Dogs upon Asynchronous Light Stimulation) Zhurnal vysshei nervnoi deiatel'nosti imeni I. P. Pavlova (I. P. Pavlov, J. Higher Nervous Activity). 8: 537–545.

GIURGEA, C. 195.. Obrazovaniie uslovnogo refleksa pri priamom razdrazhenii kory bol'shikh polusharii (Function of Conditioned Reflex with Direct Stimulation of the Cerebral Cortex), Dissertatsiia (Dissertation). Leningrad, USSR.

Kupalov: Properties of Nervous Processes in the Brain

DOTY, R. W. & C. GIURGEA. Conditioned Reflexes Established by Coupling Electrical Excitation of Two Cortical Areas. Brain Mechanisms and Learning. E. Delafresnaye, Ed. In press.

KUPALOV, P. S. 1960. The organization of the nervous processes of the brain during the conditioned reflex activity. Suppl. No. 13 of Electroencephalog. Clin. Neurophysiol. : 3–11.

LAPINA, I. A. 1959. Obrazovaniie zastoinoi dvigatel'noi reaktsii sgibaniia lapy u sobak (Formation of Fixed Motor Flexion Reaction of the Dog's Paw), Ezhegodnik. Trudy Instituta Eksperimental'noi Meditsiny (Ann. Publ. Trans. Inst. Exptl. Med.), Leningrad, USSR. : 32–38.

LIVANOV, M. N. 1952. Nekotoryie itogi elektrofiziologicheskikh issledovanii uslovnoreflektornykh sviazei. (Some Results of Electrophysiologic Investigations of Conditioned-Reflex Connections), Trudy 15-go soveshchaniia po problemam vysshei nervnoi deiatel'nosti. (Trans. 15th Conference on Problems of Higher Nervous Activity), Izdatel'stvo Akademii Nauk SSSR (Publ. by Academy of Sciences of USSR). Moscow-Leningrad, USSR. : 248–261.

PENFIELD, W. & H. JASPER. 1954. Epilepsy and the Functional Anatomy of the Human Brain. Little, Brown. Boston, Mass.

WALTER, V. J. & W. GREY WALTER. 1949. The central effects of rhythmic sensory stimulation. EEG and Clin. Neurophysiol. 1: 57–86.

From B. M. Teplov (1967). Biological Bases of Individual Behavior, 1-10, *by kind permission of Academic Press*

The Problem of Types of Human Higher Nervous Activity and Methods of Determining Them*

B. M. TEPLOV

Institute of Psychology, Moscow, U.S.S.R.

The concept of types of higher nervous activity (or, synonymously, types of nervous system) was introduced into science by Pavlov. It was used by Pavlov in two different ways. On the one hand, type of higher nervous activity denoted a certain combination of the basic characteristics of excitatory and inhibitory processes, while on the other hand it denoted a particular "picture" or "pattern" of animal or human behaviour.

At first these two meanings of the concept "type" were assumed to coincide, i.e., certain properties of the nervous system must correspond to certain forms of behaviour. It was supposed that dogs (in Pavlov's laboratories, experimental work was always done on dogs) with weak nervous processes are always timid, and that dogs with great mobility of nervous processes are sociable and "mobile" in their behaviour. However, even in Pavlov's time evidence against this supposition was being accumulated. No precise distinction between the two meanings of the term "higher nervous activity type" was made by Pavlov, though in the basic studies of his later period he usually defined the types of nervous activity as certain "combinations of basic properties of the nervous system". For 15–20 years after Pavlov's death, the confusion between the two meanings of the term "type of higher nervous activity" caused great misunderstandings in studies of this problem, particularly as applied to Man.

In recent years a number of investigations have produced convincing enough proof that behaviour forms are to a great extent dependent on the conditions of life and early environment of the animal, whereas the

* A paper delivered at the VII International Congress of Anthropological and Ethnographical Sciences, Moscow, 1967.

108

properties of the nervous system are very little changed, except during early ontogeny.

It is clear from the above that there may not be any simple relationship between type as a combination of nervous system properties, and type as a specialized "picture" of behaviour, i.e. temperament. But this certainly does not mean that there is no interrelation between them at all. The properties of the nervous system do not predict any definite behaviour forms, but create conditions which are favourable for some forms and unfavourable for others.

At present in the physiology of higher nervous activity only the meaning of the term "type" as a combination of properties of the nervous system is of strictly scientific significance. Interpretation of the term "type" as a characteristic form of behaviour is, to my mind, psychological, and the principles of classification of these latter are to be studied by psychology. For the time being this task has no universally accepted solution. This report will deal only with types as combinations of properties of the nervous system.

The properties of the nervous system are understood as its natural innate characteristics. In this respect we support Pavlōv. We cannot yet consider it as proven that a combination of basic properties of the nervous system can be called the "genotype" as it was by Pavlov. The terms "innate" and "hereditary" are not synonymous. Innate properties are not only hereditarily dependent ones, but also those formed in embryonic development and even during early ontogeny (formation of a child's nervous system continues for several years after its birth). As for animals, significant evidence proving that certain properties of the nervous system are inherited has recently been presented (Krasuskii, 1953; Fedorov, 1953). In some cases basic properties of the nervous system seem to be determined genetically in humans. However, it does not follow from the above that properties of the human nervous system always have a genetic basis.

From Pavlov there come two ideas which have become very popular: the theory of three basic properties of the nervous system (strength of the nervous system, equilibrium of the excitation and inhibition processes, mobility of the nervous processes) and the theory that there are four basic types of nervous system.

The theory of four types by no means comes from Pavlov's theory of the three basic properties of the nervous system. Originally, Pavlov built his type classification on the principle of equilibrium between the excitation and inhibition processes; later, he based his classification on the strength of the nervous system, assigning the equilibrium principle to second place; in his final variant of the classification he intentionally

1. TYPES OF HIGHER NERVOUS ACTIVITY

used the last of the proposed properties of the nervous system, i.e., mobility of the nervous processes. However, although the major principle of classification was changed several times, the number *four* remained in the list of basic types of nervous system. We shall not go into details of what made Pavlov retain the number four in this list (the classical theory of four temperaments probably played an important role). But it is necessary to stress that this preference did not come from the theory of the basic properties of the nervous system. In the last and most detailed of Pavlov's papers on this problem, he himself said that there may be at least 24 possible combinations of the basic properties of the nervous system, but he never rejected the idea of four types.

After Pavlov's death the theory of four types began to be considered by many physiologists and psychologists as the essence of Pavlov's theory of types and this obscured Pavlov's real discovery, i.e., the discovery of the basic properties of the nervous system. This considerably delayed the development of knowledge of this aspect of the physiology of higher nervous activity.

There is neither theoretical nor experimental reason to believe that the number of basic types of nervous system is four. Recently, authors free from the prejudices of the "four types" theory who have attempted to build an orderly classification of types have obtained quite different numbers of types. For instance, Krasusky (1963), working on data obtained in Koltushy on the typological characteristics of 116 dogs, found 48 variants of nervous system types. It is hardly feasible to indicate the traditional four types as basic.

I consider that as yet it is impossible to formulate an orderly classification of the types of nervous system or to determine scientifically the number of basic types. In order to solve these problems it is necessary to have several questions answered. They are: which properties of the nervous system are to be taken as basic? What are the interrelations between these properties? What combinations of properties of the nervous system are possible and which of them are most natural, most typical? No data have yet been collected (at least for Man) to indicate any definite combinations of properties as typical or even predominant.

Pavlov not only introduced the concept of the basic properties of the nervous system into science, but also put forward a great number of far-reaching and well founded ideas as to the nature of these properties. But since Pavlov's death many new methods of experimental investigation have been introduced, and a number of new phenomena have been discovered. Besides that, one must not forget that Pavlov carried out experimental work only on dogs, and his assertions as to Man were mostly made by analogy. Thus, the task of the scientist studying the properties of the human nervous system is to continue the creative work begun by Pavlov, and not repeat as irrefutable truth everything formulated by Pavlov.

The leading method of studying the human nervous system is the experimental one, as only this makes it possible to distinguish manifestations of innate properties of the nervous system from the behaviour forms developed during life. Methods based on observation and interpretation of "life indices" are of great practical importance, but only on condition that, as an essential preliminary, by means of laboratory experiment the physiological significance of each of the basic properties is worked out, and the behaviour to which it gives rise investigated.

Various experimental methods are used to investigate the properties of the nervous system. The following list (not claiming to be exhaustive) may give an idea of the variety of these methods.

1. Methods of the conditioned-reflex alteration of visual sensitivity. This phenomenon was discovered by Dolin in Pavlov's laboratory in 1936 and named the "photochemical reflex". It has been widely used to study nervous system properties in our laboratory. Using this method we have succeeded in obtaining a great deal of replicable and orderly data. The chief shortcoming of this method lies in its extreme laboriousness and the long periods of time necessary for work with each subject.

2. Method of galvanic skin reactions (GSR). Lately, together with other methods, this has been frequently used in our laboratory.

3. Measurement of the absolute visual and auditory thresholds under both the usual and special conditions. "Special" conditions means: (a) measurement of absolute visual thresholds affected by auditory stimuli, and of absolute auditory thresholds affected by visual stimuli; (b) measurement of visual thresholds in the presence of another visual stimulus ("induction method"); and (c) measurement of visual and auditory thresholds after administration of caffeine.

4. Measurement of other sensory functions: adequate optic chronaxie (AOC), critical frequency of flicker-fusion (CFF), critical frequency of flashing phosphene (CFP) at different intensities of electric current, etc. (Schwarz, 1963; Turovskaya, 1963).

5. The EEG method, which has lately assumed greater and greater significance. It offers a number of significant indices of nervous system properties: some indices of "background" EEG (alpha-index, frequency and amplitude of alpha-rhythm); indices of dynamics of orienting and conditioned-orienting blockade of alpha-rhythm produced by acoustic and photic stimuli; and particularly the reaction of driving of EEG rhythms under conditions of rhythmic light stimulation (Golubeva, 1963).

1. TYPES OF HIGHER NERVOUS ACTIVITY

6. Motor reaction methods (Leites, Gurevich). Many scientists use only methods of this kind. They occupy an important though not the central place in our laboratory. Their chief shortcoming is the voluntary nature of the reactions which are studied. This causes extreme complications in the investigation of the nature of stable physiological characteristics of the nervous system, and makes it difficult to obtain precise and reliable results. We try to take into account those indices in the motor methods which are less dependent on the subject's will, i.e., mainly reaction time and its alterations under certain conditions. Recording the electrical activity of the muscles in these experiments is of great value—the person can voluntarily avoid movement, but he cannot voluntarily stop the muscles' electrical activity if there is the slightest tendency towards making a movement.

Each of the above methods may be more or less efficient in giving indices of the separate properties of the nervous system. We aim at the expression of these indices in as strict a quantitative form as possible. According to our experience in work performed during recent years, this is quite possible with most of the methods.

The chief method of proving that some index characterizes a definite property of the nervous system is correlation of different experimental indices. If we obtain two or more indices which, according to theoretical hypotheses, may express one and the same property of the nervous system, and their comparison after experiments on a sufficient number of subjects gives some significant correlation, in that case there is some evidence for the correctness of our hypotheses. The analysis of the physiological meaning of these indices in total can answer the question of the nature of the given property. For statistical treatment of the results of the comparisons we use correlational and factor-analytic methods.

The results of our investigations show that manifestations of each of the basic properties of the nervous system form a kind of "syndrome", i.e., a combination of correlated indices. One of the indices is the basic, or informative one—it most directly characterizes the property under investigation and presents the distinctive feature characterizing it.

The difficulty of research which aims to discover indices of the basic properties of the nervous system is increased by the fact that one and the same index may be dependent on two or more nervous system properties, that is, it can be included in two or more different syndromes. This circumstance makes the results of factor analysis especially useful in a mathematical treatment.

What are to be taken as the basic properties of the nervous system? The answer to this question may be given only in schematic form and must to a certain degree be dogmatic. Some of the statements making up this answer may be considered as proven, others are as yet hypothetical.

The first property and the one studied in most detail is the strength of the nervous system with regard to excitation. The basic distinctive feature of this property is the capacity of the nervous system to endure prolonged or frequently repeated excitation without displaying transmarginal inhibition. The main experimental method is to elicit repeatedly a conditioned reflex with reinforcement at short intervals. Hence, this property may be defined as the endurance of the nervous system in the face of continuous (or frequently repeated) excitation.

Our investigations have proved that this basic property of the nervous system with regard to excitation correlates with the following group of indices:

1. Resistance to the inhibitory effect of extraneous stimuli. The chief experimental test consists of comparison of the value of the absolute visual threshold in silence and with a metronome ticking, or comparison of the value of the absolute auditory thresholds in darkness and under the effect of flashing light (Yermolayeva-Tomina, 1959).

2. Certain characteristics of concentration (or, *vice versa*, irradiation) of the excitatory process. The experimental test is the "induction method", which compares the value of the absolute visual threshold for a point stimulus in an empty dark visual field and in the presence of additional point stimuli of various intensities. Use of special conditions (administration of caffeine, fatigue of visual analyser by means of repeated determination of the threshold, etc.) make it possible to obtain several intercorrelated indices (Rozhdestvenskaya, 1955).

3. The nature of manifestation of the law of strength. With low stimulus intensities, an increase of stimulus intensity brings about an increase of the intensity (or speed) of reaction, which is more marked if the nervous system is weak, and less marked if it is strong. With moderate and high intensities this is reversed: the strength law is more clearly expressed if the nervous system is strong. The simplest experimental test is measurement of reaction time to stimuli of different intensities (Nebylitsyn, 1960).

4. Value of absolute visual and auditory thresholds: the greater the strength of the nervous system, the higher the thresholds, or in other words, the lower the sensitivity of the nervous system. The weak nervous system is a nervous system of high sensitivity (Teplov, 1955; Nebylitsyn, 1959).

This point needs special attention. A lot of work has been done to test it. It may now be considered as proved, as it has been tested on a sufficient

1. TYPES OF HIGHER NERVOUS ACTIVITY

number of subjects. There are also a number of supporting observations obtained from experiments on animals.

We consider that this finding, which contradicts earlier opinions, refutes the idea that it is possible to evaluate some types of nervous system as "good" and others "bad". The weak nervous system, i.e., the nervous system which is of low endurance but high sensitivity, is not in all cases to be considered "worse" than the strong nervous system which is of high endurance but low sensitivity. For certain kinds of work a weak nervous system may be preferable, for other kinds the strong nervous system is preferable. It is necessary to reject the evaluative approach towards such properties as strength or weakness, mobility or inertness, excitation or inhibition of the nervous system.

The second property of the nervous system seems to be its strength with regard to inhibition. The main feature of this property is the capacity of the nervous system to endure continuous or frequently repeated inhibitory stimuli. The experimental material we have at our disposal, which is not yet extensive (Rozhdestvenskaya, 1963), shows that the experimental test of this property may be prolongation or numerous repeated presentations of the differential stimulus at short intervals. We do not yet know any other manifestations of this property and therefore are not able to describe completely the corresponding syndrome. The strength of the nervous system with regard to excitation has been studied in detail, but the investigation of the strength of the nervous system with regard to inhibition has only just begun. This is the reason for the absence of any data on the question of equilibrium or balance of the nervous processes with respect to strength.

Only recently has our laboratory made any attempt to compare the two basic tests used for this purpose—numerous repeated presentations at short intervals of conditioned stimuli with reinforcement and numerous repeated presentations of differential stimuli. When this lengthy work is finished we shall be able to provide the first data on the third property of the nervous system—the equilibrium of the nervous processes as regards their strength.

This does not mean, however, that we do not know anything about equilibrium or balance of the nervous processes. On the basis of a number of experimental investigations we can describe the syndrome of experimental indices which, no doubt, characterizes the balance of the nervous processes. This syndrome includes the following indices:

(1) the speed of formation of conditioned reflexes; (2) the speed of formation of differentiations; (3) the relative numbers of "positive" and "inhibitory" errors (i.e. cases of positive reactions to inhibitory stimuli and absence of reaction to positive stimuli); (4) the speed of extinction

without reinforcement of the conditioned reflex; (5) the speed of extinction of the orientation reflex; (6) the amplitude of the orientation reflex; (7) certain features of the formation of conditioned inhibition; and (8) some features of the alpha rhythm in the EEG in the absence of stimuli (mainly alpha-index, i.e., percentage of time engaged by the alpha rhythm).

No doubt, the above indices characterize the equilibrium of the nervous system, but not equilibrium as to the strength (endurance) of the nervous processes. Nebylitsyn has advanced a hypothesis that the above indices correspond to some property of the nervous system independent of strength. It can be called "dynamism" of the nervous processes. First of all it is characterized by the ease and speed with which the nervous system generates the processes of excitation or inhibition. The basic features of this property are the speed of formation of conditioned reflexes as well as of differentiations. The nervous system which is "dynamic" as to excitation rapidly forms positive conditioned associations, and one "dynamic" as to inhibition rapidly forms inhibitory associations. The comparative ease of formation of both associations characterizes balance or equilibrium as to dynamism. There are certain grounds for believing that what is usually called equilibrium of the nervous system is equilibrium as to dynamism rather than equilibrium as to strength.

The most obscure property is Pavlov's third one, namely, mobility of the nervous processes. The experimental evidence goes decidedly against recognition of mobility as a unitary property of the nervous system, including such different manifestations as the speed of transformation of the signs of stimuli and the speed of initiating or terminating the nervous processes. The indices of these manifestations do not correlate with one another (Borisova et al., 1963). The term "mobility" seems suitable for denoting the property characterized by the speed of transformation (it is used in this way by physiologists experimenting on animals). Data obtained in these experiments indicate that the mobility of excitation and that of inhibition may be different. But the indices of the speed of initiation and termination of the excitatory process show good correlation with each other, and no correlation with the speed of transformation. The property of the nervous system characterized by them may be named, we suggest, "lability" (Teplov, 1963). The indices of the speed of initiation and termination of the inhibitory process have not yet been studied, nor, in consequence, has equilibrium of the nervous processes as to their lability.

Thus, at present the following structure of the properties of the nervous system may be proposed: (1) strength (endurance), (2) dynamism (the

1. TYPES OF HIGHER NERVOUS ACTIVITY

ease of generation of the nervous process), (3) mobility (the speed of transformation), and (4) lability (the speed of initiation and termination of the nervous process). Each of these properties may be different as regards the excitatory process or the inhibitory process. Consequently, it is advisable to discuss the equilibrium of nervous processes by treating each of these properties separately.

As is clear from the above, a great deal of this scheme is as yet hypothetical, but it can at least serve as a programme for future investigations.

REFERENCES

Borisova, M. N., Gurevich, K. M., Yermolayeva-Tomina, L. B., Kolodnaya, A. Y ., Ravich-Shcherbo, I. V. and Schwarz, L. A..(1963). Material for the Comparative Investigation of Different Indices of Mobility of the Human Nervous System. *In* Teplov, B. M. (Ed.), "Typological Characteristics of Higher Nervous Activity in Man", Vol. III. RSFSR Academy of Pedagogical Sciences, Moscow.

Fedorov, V. K. (1953). Effects of Parents' Nervous System Training upon Lability of Nervous Processes in Descendants (Mice). Papers of Pavlov Institute of Physiology, Vol. II.

Golubeva, E. A. (1963). An Attempt to Investigate Reorganization of Brain Biocurrents as an Index of Individual Differences in Nervous Processes Equilibrium. *In* Teplov, B. M. (Ed.) "Typological Features of Higher Nervous Activity in Man", Vol. III. RSFSR Academy of Pedagogical Sciences, Moscow.

Gurevich, K. M. (1963). After-effect of Positive and Inhibitory Stimuli in the Motor-Reaction. *In* Teplov, B. M. (Ed.) "Typological Features of Higher Nervous Activity in Man", Vol. III. RSFSR Academy of Pedagogical Sciences, Moscow.

Krasusky, V. K. (1953). Methods of Studying Nervous System Types in Animals. Papers of Pavlov Institute of Physiology, Vol. II.

Krasusky, V. K. (1963). Methods of evaluation of nervous processes in dogs. *J. of Higher Nervous Activity*, **13**.

Leites, N. S. (1956). The Problem of Typological Differences in the After-effects of Excitatory and Inhibitory Processes. *In* Teplov, B. M. (Ed.), "Typological Features of Higher Nervous Activity in Man", Vol. I. RSFSR Academy of Pedagogical Sciences, Moscow.

Nebylitsyn, V. D. (1959). Investigation of the Connection between Sensitivity and Strength of the Nervous System. *In* Teplov, B. M. (Ed.), "Typological Features of Higher Nervous Activity in Man", Vol. II. RSFSR Academy of Pedagogical Sciences, Moscow. English translation in Gray, J. A. (Ed.) (1964). "Pavlov's Typology". Pergamon, Oxford.

Nebylitsyn, V. D. (1960). Reaction time and Nervous System Strength. Communications 1 and 2. Dokl. RSFSR Acad. Pedagog. Sci. Moscow. Nos. 4 and 5.

B. M. TEPLOV

Nebylitsyn, V. D. (1963). On the structure of the basic properties of the nervous system. *Vop. Psikhol.*, No. 4.

Rozhdestvenskaya, V. I. (1955). An attempt to determine the strength of the process of excitation through features of its irradiation and concentration in the visual analyzer. *Vop. Psikhol.* No. 3. English translation in Gray, J. A. (Ed.) (1964). "Pavlov's Typology", p. 379. Pergamon, Oxford.

Rozhdestvenskaya, V. I. (1963). Determination of Human Inhibitory Process Strength in Experiments with Increment of Duration of Differentiated Stimulus. *In* Teplov, B. M. (Ed.), "Typological Features of Higher Nervous Activity in Man", Vol. III. RSFSR Academy of Pedagogical Sciences, Moscow.

Schwarz, L. A. (1963). Speed of Recovery of Absolute Visual Sensitivity after Illumination as an Index of Nervous Processes Lability and Other Tests as to Mobility. *In* Teplov, B. M. (Ed.), "Typological Features of Higher Nervous Activity in Man", Vol. III. RSFSR Academy of Pedagogical Sciences, Moscow.

Teplov, B. M. (1955). On notions of weakness and inertness of the nervous system. *Vop. Psikhol.*, No. 6.

Teplov, B. M. (1963). New Data on Investigation of Human Nervous System Properties. *In* Teplov, B. M. (Ed.), "Typological Features of Higher Nervous Activity in Man", Vol. III. RSFSR Acad. Pedagog. Sci. Moscow.

Turovskaya, Z. G. (1963). Correlation Between Some Indices of Human Nervous System Strength and Mobility. *In* Teplov, B. M. (Ed.), "Typological Features of Higher Nervous Activity in Man", Vol. 3. RSFSR Academy of Pedagogical Sciences, Moscow.

Yermolaeva-Tomina, L. B. (1959). Concentration of Attention and Strength of the Nervous System. *In* Teplov, B. M. (Ed.), "Typological Features of Higher Nervous Activity in Man", Vol. II. RSFSR Academy of Pedagogical Sciences, Moscow. English translation in Gray, J. A. (Ed.) (1964). "Pavlov's Typology". Pergamon, Oxford.

From H. J. Eysenck and A. Levey (1967). Biological Bases of Individual Behavior, 206-220, *by kind permission of the authors and Academic Press*

Conditioning, Introversion–Extraversion and the Strength of the Nervous System*

H. J. EYSENCK and A. LEVEY

Institute of Psychiatry, University of London, England

Teplov's main contribution to psychology consisted of the systematic working out of the relations obtaining between personality, on the one hand, and the concepts of excitation and inhibition, on the other (Gray, 1964). The work carried out in our laboratories, too, has concerned itself very much with these relations (Eysenck, 1957), and in spite of obvious differences in approach there have also been certain interesting similarities. In particular, it would seem that the Pavlovian notion of "strong" and "weak" nervous systems, which has formed the basis for most of Teplov's experimental work, bears a striking similarity to the notions of extraverted and introverted personality types, as they emerge from our own. The "weak" personality type appears to resemble the introvert, the "strong" personality type the extravert. Even if it is admitted that similarity does not imply identity, it is certainly striking that two quite independent approaches should issue in such closely related concepts (Eysenck, 1967).

This similarity becomes even more apparent when we consider these personality types in terms of physiological and neurological concepts. Gray (1964) has translated the concepts used by Pavlov and Teplov into the language of modern neurophysiology, and has shown that different degrees of arousal of the reticular formation can mediate all or most of the experimentally ascertained differences between "weak" and "strong" nervous systems. In a similar manner, Eysenck (1967) has suggested a close relationship between reticular formation arousal thresholds and introversion–extraversion. According to these theories, low thresholds of the ascending reticular activating system would be characteristic of the "weak" nervous system and the introvert, high thresholds of the

* Thanks are due to the M.R.C. for the support of this investigation.

13. CONDITIONABILITY AND EXTRAVERSION

"strong" nervous system and the extravert. Again, the synchronizing part of the reticular formation exerts an inhibitory influence on cortical activity, and it may be supposed that low thresholds of this system characterize the extravert and the "strong" nervous system. Unfortunately, little direct evidence is available relating to these theories, but work on the EEG (Savage, 1964), on critical flicker fusion (Gray, 1964) and in particular on drugs known to affect the reticular formation (Killam, 1962) has on the whole borne out the general theory in a rather striking manner (Eysenck, 1963b).

Among the similarities resulting from experimental work perhaps the most impressive is that relating to sensory thresholds. The lower thresholds found in persons possessing a "weak" nervous system constitute one of the most important proofs of the Teplov school for the correctness of their theories. As a direct consequence of their work, and the hypothesis relating introversion to a "weak" nervous system, several studies have recently been carried out in England to study sensory thresholds in introverts and extraverts. Using the Maudsley Personality Inventory (Eysenck, 1959) as the measure of personality, Haslam (this volume) has several times found a significantly lower pain threshold in introverts as compared with extraverts, and Smith (1968) has similarly discovered lower auditory thresholds in introverts using the usual psychophysical methods as well as a forced-choice technique. These and other experiments, too numerous to mention, make it likely that the conceptions of our two schools are in fact closely related, and that empirical work directly devoted to a verification of this hypothesis would be of considerable value.

One interesting contrast between the Russian and the English work has been the comparative neglect of direct measures of conditioning by Teplov, as compared with the large body of work reported on this topic by the Maudsley group (Eysenck, 1965b). We have used in the main the eyeblink conditioning experiment, in which a puff of air to the eye is the unconditioned stimulus (UCS), and a tone delivered over ear-phones the conditioned stimulus (CS). A summary of the work on this test and on GSR conditioning, carried out by us and also by various other experimenters, has shown that different investigators have reported very divergent results, some producing the predicted positive correlation between introversion and conditionability, others failing to find such a correlation. The failure of so many experiments to duplicate the results of our early studies, which gave very positive results, would appear to be due to their failure to duplicate the exact conditions of the tests carried out; as will be shown below, the general theory linking introversion with greater cortical arousal ("excitation") predicts in some detail the exact choice of parameters which alone would be expected to generate positive correlations between introversion and conditioning. In particular, it is proposed that the following three parameters are crucial, and must be carefully selected and controlled in order to obtain positive results. (1) Partial reinforcement favours introverts; 100% reinforcement does not. (2) Weak unconditioned stimuli favour introverts; strong UCS do not. (3) Small CS–UCS intervals favour introverts; large US–UCS intervals do not.

Partial reinforcement. Pavlov has already pointed out that unreinforced trials produced inhibition, and if we link the growth of inhibition with extraversion in particular, then clearly partial reinforcement will impede conditioning more in extraverts than in introverts (Eysenck, 1957). Furthermore, there is direct evidence to link partial reinforcement with cortical inhibition along neurophysiological lines; as Magoun (1963) has pointed out, "in each of the several categories of conditioned reflex performance in which Pavlov found internal inhibition to occur . . . recent electrophysiological studies have revealed features of hyper-synchronization and/or spindle bursting in the EEG".

UCS strength. It is well known that conditioning is in part a function of the strength of the UCS (and possibly of the CS also—Kimble, 1961). Given that introverts have lower sensory thresholds (and probably smaller difference thresholds as well) than extraverts, then objectively identical UCS would be subjectively stronger for introverts, and should therefore produce stronger conditioned responses. UCS of too great strength, on the other hand, should produce "protective inhibition" much earlier in introverts than in extraverts. It may further be surmised that UCS of low strength adapt quickly, and thus produce inhibition; this growth of inhibition again should be stronger in extraverts than in introverts. There is direct experimental backing for the inhibitory action of weak UCS and of partial reinforcement in the work of Ross and Spence (1960) who conclude that "inhibition of performance is more readily accomplished under conditions of low puff strengths . . . The differences between the 100% and 50% reinforcement groups at high levels of puff strength require that considerable 'inhibition' still be present with such puffs".

CS–UCS interval. It is well known that optimal CS–UCS intervals in eye-blink conditioning centre around 500 msec, but no work appears to have been done on individual differences in this respect. The concept of reaction time is clearly relevant here; Gray has summarized the work of the Teplov school by saying that "at stimulus intensities below that at which asymptotic reaction time is reached, the weaker the nervous system, the faster the reaction time". By going below the 500 msec

13. CONDITIONABILITY AND EXTRAVERSION

mark, we can ensure that we go below the asymptotic value for conditioning, and under those conditions, particularly when allied with weak UCS, we would expect introverts to react better to short CS–UCS intervals than extraverts. Gray (1964) has reviewed the whole literature on these relations quite exhaustively, including the work of Fuster (1958) and of Isaac (1960) on the association with the reticular formation, and there seems little doubt that the experimental findings mediate a relationship such as that proposed.

It follows from what has been said that the very divergent findings with respect to the proposed relationship between introversion and eyeblink conditioning which form such a prominent feature of the literature, including the Russian, are only to be expected, considering that many different variations of type of reinforcement, CS–UCS interval and strength of UCS and CS have been employed. The experiment to be reported here, which was carried out by Levey in the Maudsley laboratory, was specially designed to throw light on the hypotheses outlined above, relating to the change in the relation between conditioning and introversion with change in the conditions of the experiment. Subjects were tested under all possible combinations of two conditions of reinforcement, two CS–UCS intervals, and two UCS strengths; for each pair of conditions a prediction was made (this has already been outlined) as to which condition would favour the introverts as compared with the extraverts. The detailed conditions of testing were as follows: *Reinforcement schedule*—100% reinforcement against 67% reinforcement. *CS–UCS interval*: 400 msec vs. 800 msec. *UCS strength*: 6 lb/in^2 vs. 3 lb/in^2.

Subjects were selected on the basis of the Maudsley Personality Inventory, and categorized as extraverted, introverted, or intermediate (ambivert); they were also categorized as high, low or average on neuroticism. Equal numbers were then chosen from each of these categories, until 18 subjects had been included in each of the eight experimental groups (combinations of reinforcement schedule, CS–UCS interval, and UCS strength), making a total of 144 subjects in all; all of these were male. Figure 1 shows the growth, over 48 acquisition trials, of conditioned habit strength for the extraverted, introverted and ambivert groups; there is a slight superiority of the introvert group over the extravert group in this overall comparison, amounting to some 20% on the last few trials; the ambivert group is situated in between the other two groups most of the time, although it overlaps with both other groups on occasion. The differences are not significant on an analysis of variance, largely because of the tremendous size of the variances; this of course is not unexpected because of the variations in testing conditions imposed by our general scheme. Figures 2a and 2b show the results for weak and strong UCS respectively; as expected the weak UCS shows introverts much more conditionable, while the strong UCS shows extraverts more conditionable. Ambiverts are intermediate between the two extreme groups. This reversal is quite dramatic and supports the prediction.

The results for the 400 and 800 msec CS–UCS interval show, as expected, that the short interval favours the introverts; for the long interval there is very little difference between the groups (Figs. 3a, b). The results for partial and continuous reinforcement show that there is a slight tendency for partial reinforcement to favour the introverts, but

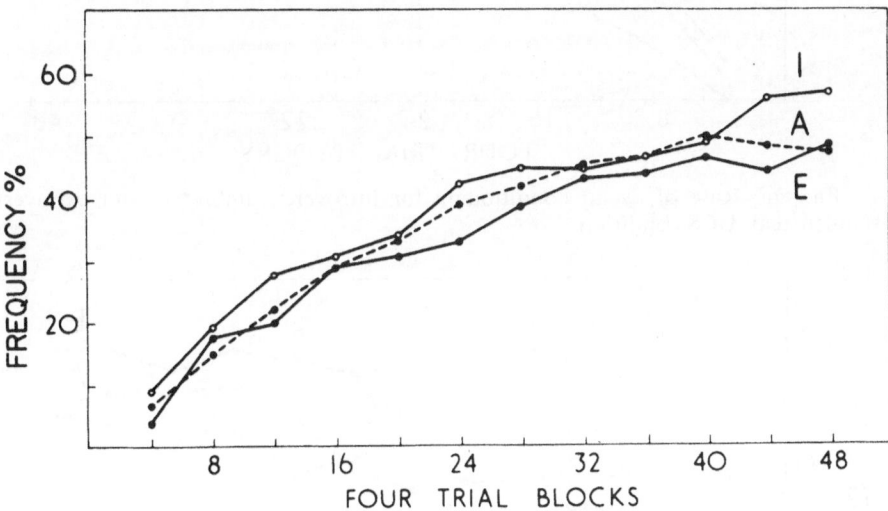

FIG. 1. Rate of eyelid conditioning in extraverts, introverts and ambiverts under combination of all parameters.

this tendency is not strong enough to give much support to our hypothesis (Figs. 4a, b). If the results of this experiment can be taken as representative, we might conclude that strength of UCS was the most important parameter, followed by CS–UCS interval, with reinforcement schedule last. However, any such generalization would of course be restricted to the values of UCS strength, interval duration, and reinforcement schedule adopted in this experiment; there is no reason to suppose that these are in any sense optimal. It seems very likely that much greater differences between introverts and extraverts could be demonstrated with better choice of parameter values. In particular, pressures of less than 3 lb/in² as UCS strength, and intervals even shorter than 400 msec. present good prospects of improving discrimination.

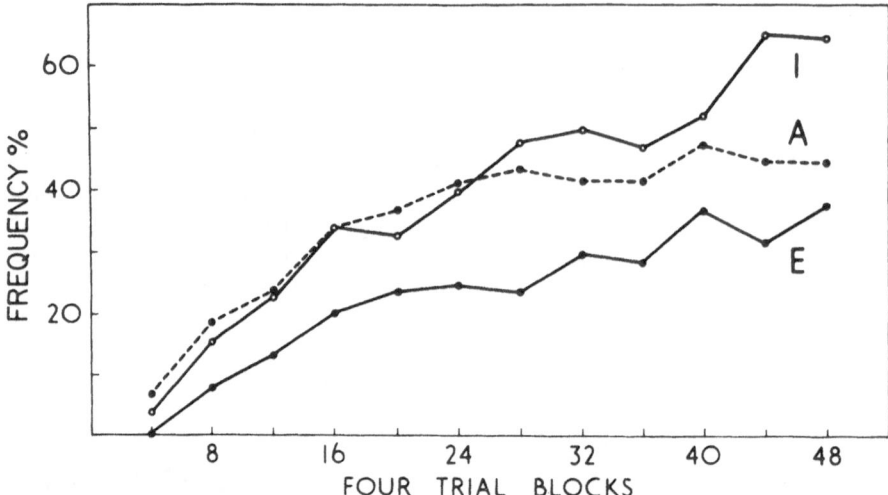

FIG. 2a. Rate of eyelid conditioning for introverts, ambiverts and extraverts under weak UCS conditions.

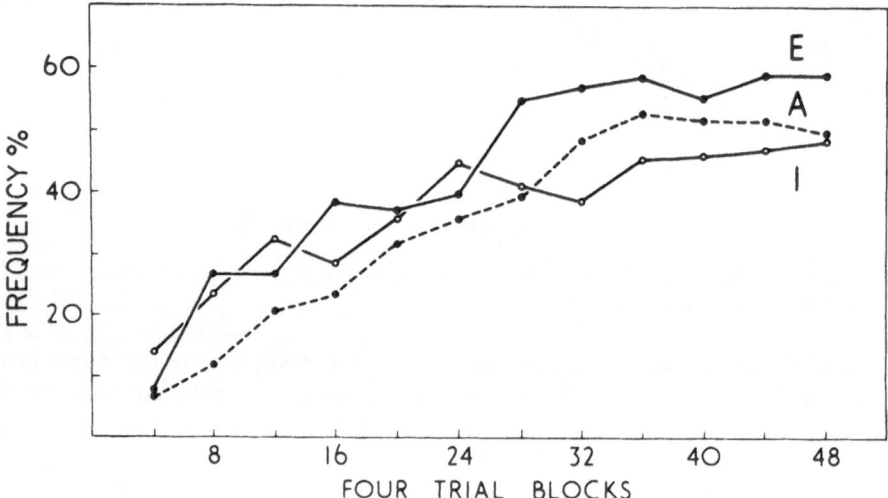

FIG. 2b. Rate of eyelid conditioning for extraverts, ambiverts and introverts under strong UCS conditions.

Figures 5a and 5b present results for optimal and worst combinations of conditions respectively, i.e., weak UCS, short CS–UCS interval, and partial reinforcement (Fig. 5a) as against strong UCS, long CS–UCS interval, and continuous reinforcement (Fig. 5b). The difference is

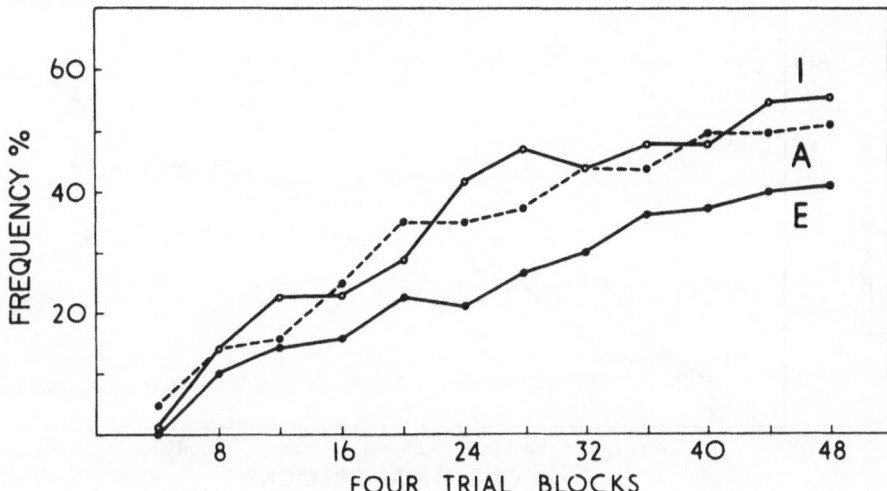

FIG. 3a. Rate of eyelid conditioning for introverts, ambiverts and extraverts under short CS–UCS interval conditions.

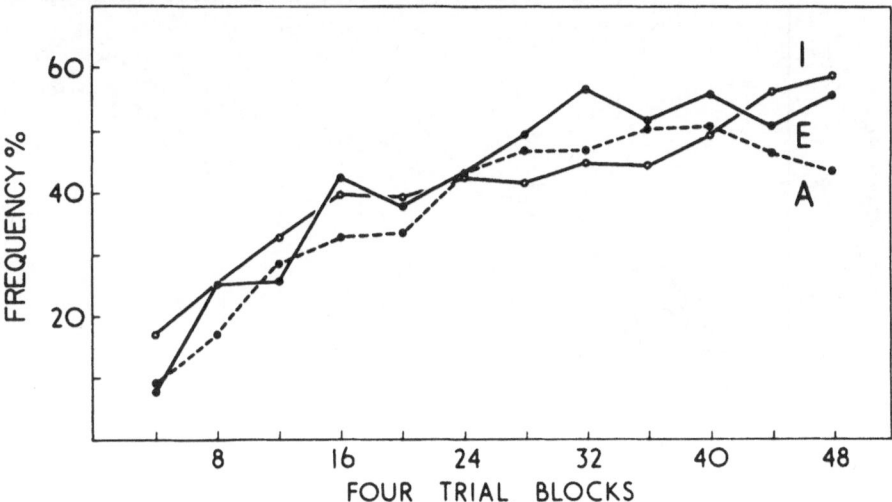

FIG. 3b. Rate of eyelid conditioning for extraverts, ambiverts and introverts under long CS–UCS interval conditions.

obvious, and may be summed up in the intra-group correlations. For the optimal conditions, the correlation between introversion and conditioning is $+0.40$, while for the worst conditions it is -0.31; this difference is significant at the 1% level on a one-tail test. In the combination of

13. CONDITIONABILITY AND EXTRAVERSION

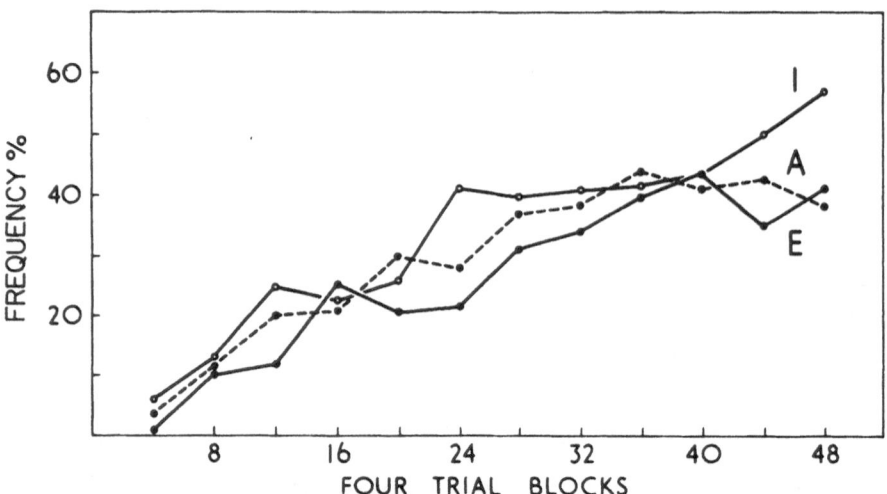

FIG. 4a. Rate of eyelid conditioning for introverts, ambiverts and extraverts under partial reinforcement conditions.

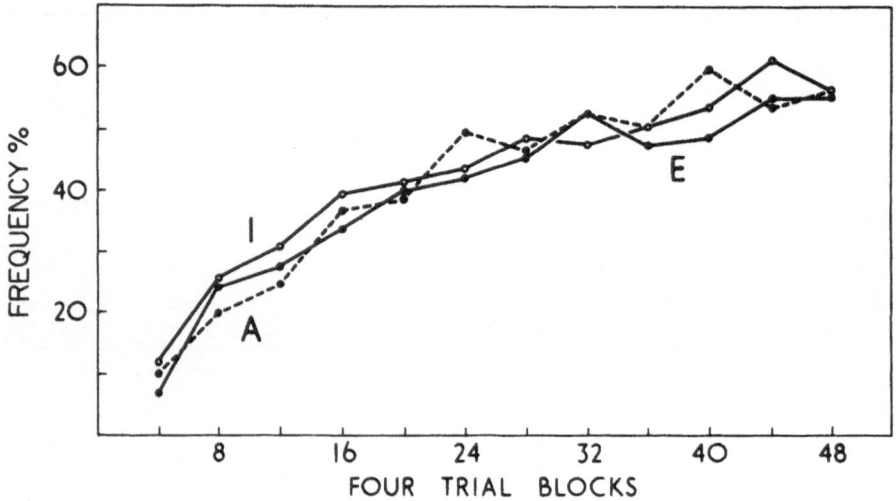

FIG. 4b. Rate of eyelid conditioning for extraverts, ambiverts and introverts under 100% reinforcement conditions.

conditions favourable, according to theory, to the introverts, we find that after 30 trials the extraverts show no evidence of any conditioning at all, while the introverts have reached a level of conditioning at which 46% of responses are in fact conditioned. Conversely, under conditions

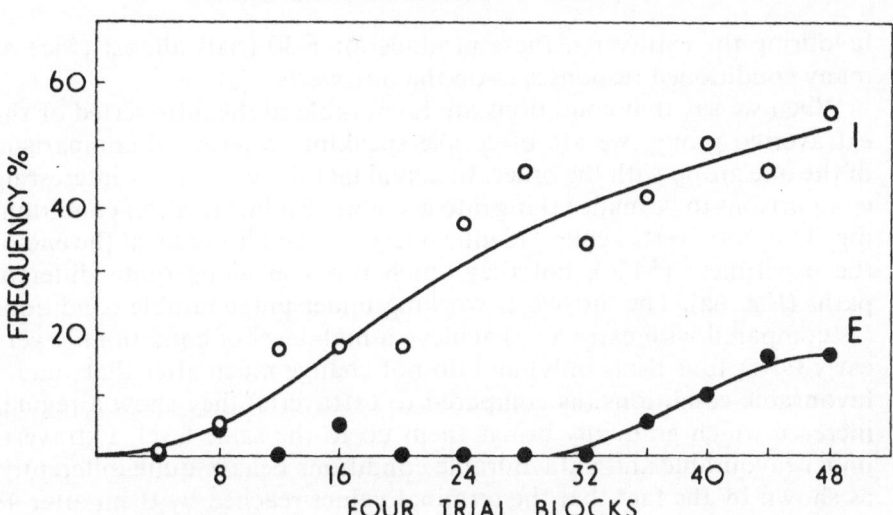

FIG. 5a. Rate of eyelid conditioning for introverts and extraverts under conditions of partial reinforcement, weak UCS, and short CS–UCS interval.

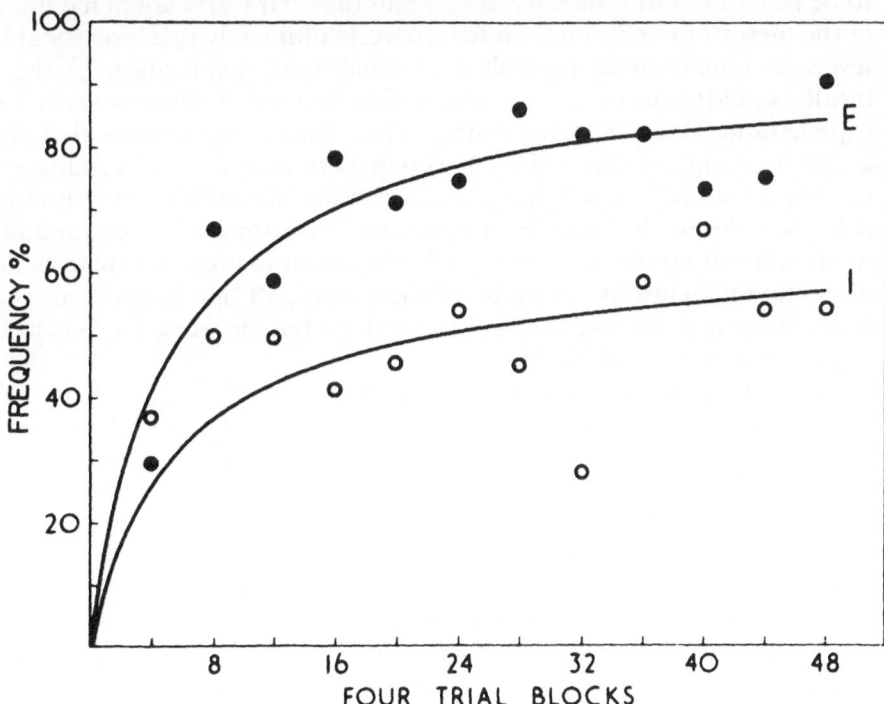

FIG. 5b. Rate of eyelid conditioning for extraverts and introverts under conditions of 100% reinforcement, strong UCS, and long CS–UCS interval.

13. CONDITIONABILITY AND EXTRAVERSION

favouring the extraverts, these produce after 30 trials almost twice as many conditioned responses as do the introverts.

When we say that conditions are favourable to the introverted or the extraverted group, we are of course speaking in terms of comparison of the one group with the other. In actual fact there are many interesting comparisons to be made taking into account absolute levels of conditioning. Thus introverts achieve identical levels of conditioning at the end of the experiment (54%), but they reach this end along quite different paths (Fig. 6a). The introverts working under unfavourable conditions (as compared with extraverts) achieve a high level of conditioning very early (after four trials only) and do not change much after that; under favourable conditions (as compared to extraverts) they show a regular increase which gradually brings them up to the same level. Extraverts under favourable and unfavourable conditions behave quite differently, as shown by the fact that the terminal values reached by them after 48 trials differ sharply; under unfavourable conditions, only 12% condition, under favourable conditions, 92% (Fig. 6b). If these data can be assumed to be generally valid, then it would seem that extraverts are much more at the mercy of conditions, while introverts ultimately reach reasonable levels of conditioning regardless of conditions. Replication of these results would seem to be desirable before too much effort is spent on explanations along theoretical lines. [It is interesting to note that the ambivert group shows very similar growth patterns under both conditions, namely the usual gradual increment in number of conditioned responses (Fig. 6c). As might have been expected the strong UCS–continuous reinforcement conditions result in better conditioning, but there is no dramatic difference in the shape of the curves; all that is apparent is a lower starting point and a less marked slope for the weak UCS–partial reinforcement conditions.]

In this case conditions may be said to be *overall* favourable or unfavourable according to the total amount of conditioning that takes place under these conditions for the total population tested. Thus strong UCS intensity produces quicker conditioning than does weak UCS intensity; 800 msec CS–UCS intervals are somewhat better than 400 msec intervals; continuous reinforcement is better than partial reinforcement. The results clearly show that the conditions which are favourable for the formation of conditioned responses *on the whole* are, in this experiment at least, also those which are favourable to extraverts and unfavourable to introverts, respectively. One might be tempted to argue from these facts towards some general law of the following kind: introverts form conditioned responses even under objectively unfavourable conditions, whereas extraverts only form conditioned responses

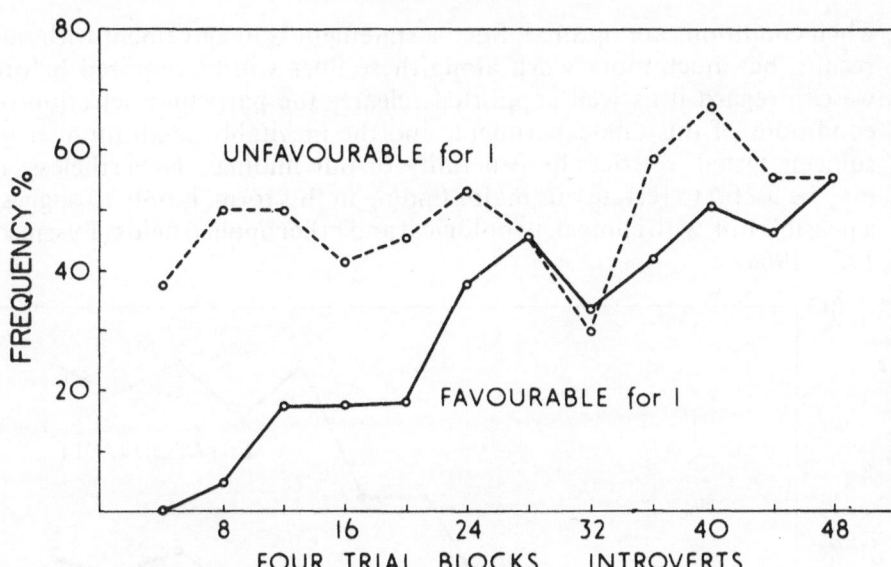

FIG. 6a. Rate of eyelid conditioning for introverts under conditions favourable and unfavourable for introverts.

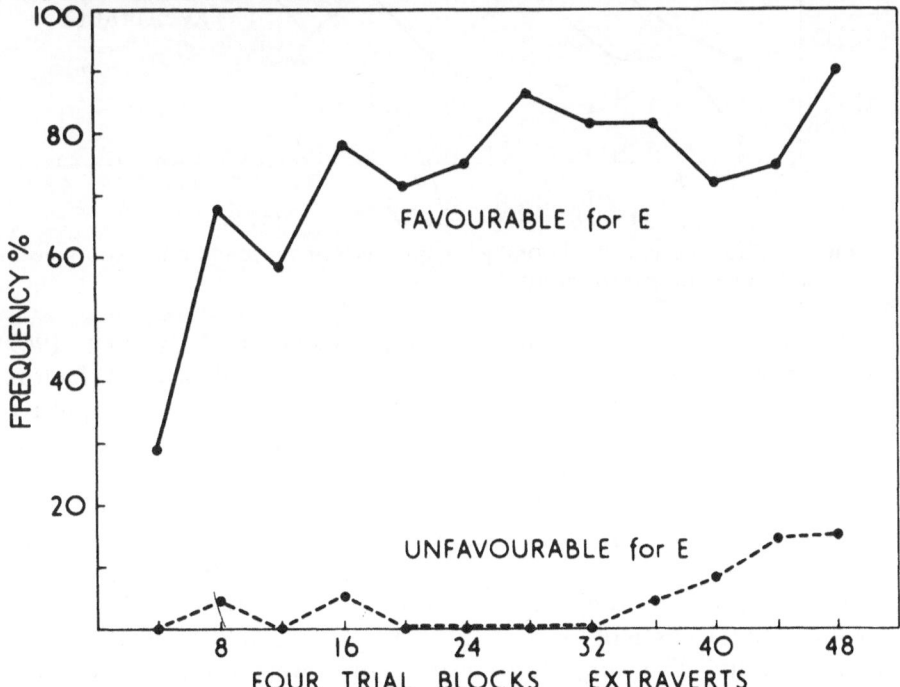

FIG. 6b. Rate of eyelid conditioning for extraverts under conditions favourable and unfavourable for extraverts.

13. CONDITIONABILITY AND EXTRAVERSION

when conditions are optimal. Such a statement is in agreement with our results, but much more work along these lines will be required before we can regard it as well supported; clearly the particular selection of conditions of this one experiment, and the inevitably small number of subjects tested, restrict the generality of our findings. Nevertheless, it may be useful to restate our major finding in this form, if only to suggest a possible link with clinical, penological and other applied fields (Eysenck, 1957, 1964).

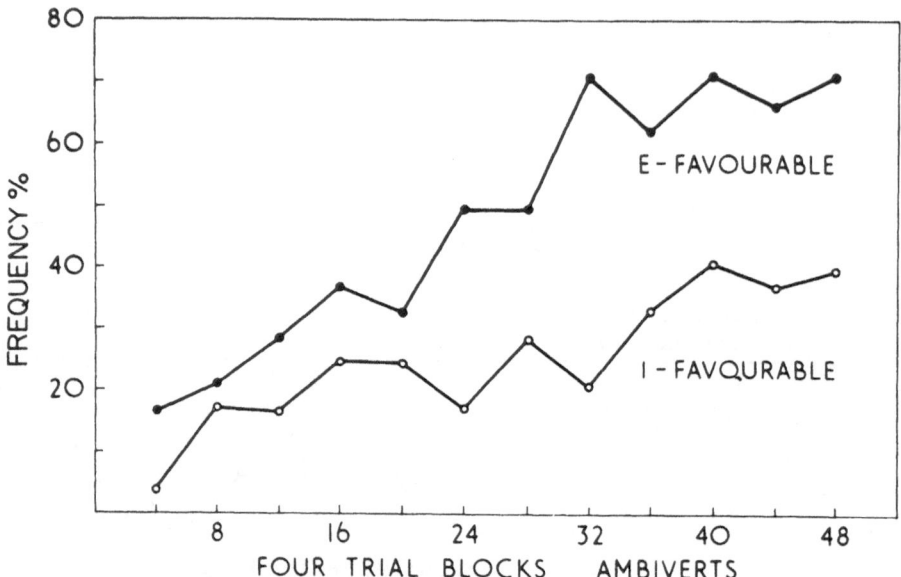

FIG. 6c. Rate of eyelid conditioning for ambiverts under conditions favourable for introverts and extraverts, respectively.

One last point requires investigation. Eysenck and Eysenck (1969) have shown that extraversion is made up of several primary factors, themselves of course intercorrelated, of which Sociability and Impulsiveness are the main ones. The possibility exists that the correlation between eyeblink conditioning and extraversion is mediated by only one of these factors, and it seemed likely to us that the Imp. factor would reflect more directly than the Soc. factor the intensity of ongoing cortical activation; we might expect, therefore, that subjects differing in Impulsivity would show more clearly the differences in conditioning performance owing to the strength of the nervous system than would subjects differing in Sociability. The subjects' questionnaires were therefore re-scored for Imp. and Soc., and divided into high and low respectively on these two sub-factors. Conditioning scores for the weak UCS, short CS–UCS interval and partial reinforcement condition were calculated for high- and low-scorers on these two factors, and are plotted in Figs 7 and 8; Fig. 7 shows the comparison between extraverts and introverts when scored only for Imp., and Fig. 8 shows the comparison between extraverts and introverts when scored only for Soc. It will be clear that any differentiation between extraverts and introverts on eyeblink conditioning is due entirely to Imp., and not at all to Soc. The data are only suggestive, and the original experiment was not planned with this analysis in mind, but the results clearly agree well with our finding that criminals are differentiated from normals only on Imp., not at all on Soc.; this would seem to follow from our hypothesis linking criminal behaviour causally with an inability to form conditioned responses readily.

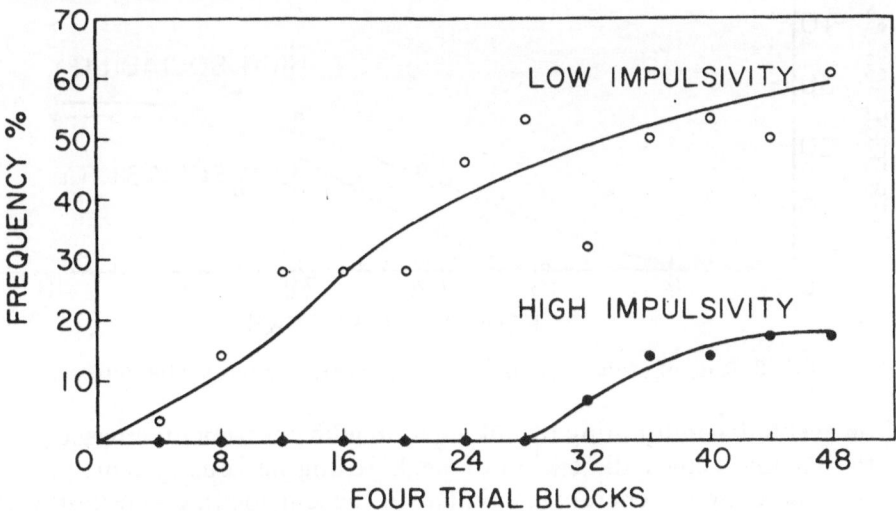

FIG. 7. Rate of eyelid conditioning for high impulsive and low impulsive subjects.

It is now time to summarize the results obtained. As has been stressed before (Eysenck, 1962), it is meaningless to compare groups of persons on a test of conditioning unless parameters are precisely specified, and if individual differences are the subject matter of the experiment, then such parameters must be chosen in accordance with a specific theory. The fact that the literature is full of contradictory results, achieved with apparently random selection of parameters, reinforces this point. Our data show that it is possible to choose conditions which give results favouring introverted subjects or extraverted subjects; what is interesting and important is that these conditions could be formulated and stated on theoretical grounds, so that the experimental results serve to support

13. CONDITIONABILITY AND EXTRAVERSION

and verify the theory. The overall failure of the experiment to show differences between introverts and extraverts at a reasonable level of significance is also in line with the hypothesis: when conditions are evenly balanced between favouring one group or the other, then averaging results over all conditions should not give results strikingly favouring one side. It should be noted that the conditions chosen were by no means extreme; it will be interesting to continue experimentation with more extreme conditions, and thus render the differentiation of introverts and extraverts even more clear-cut and obvious than has been possible in the present experiment. It should also be interesting to continue work

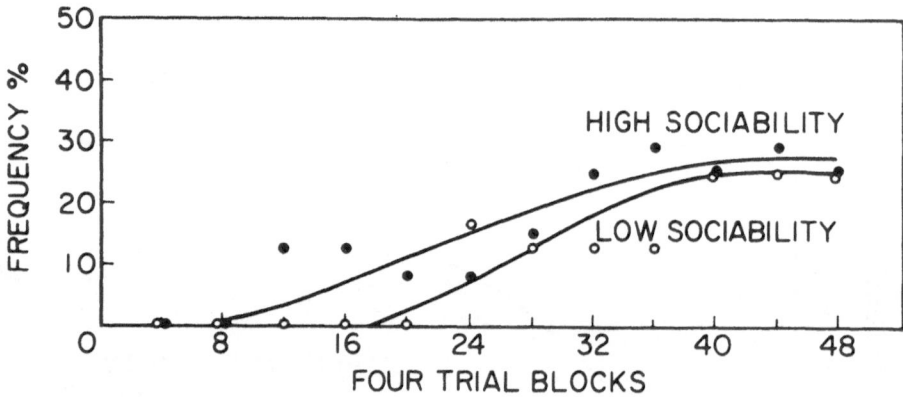

FIG. 8. Rate of eyelid conditioning for sociable and unsociable subjects.

on eyeblink conditioning by linking it up with experimental measures of the Pavlov–Teplov dimension of weak–strong nervous system; predictions here are in general very similar to those made in connection with introversion–extraversion. Altogether it is believed that Pavlov was right in pointing out the fact that individual differences in conditioning are extremely prominent in work in this field, and that these differences hold much promise in mediating predictions and explanations of human conduct, neurosis and crime. Efforts to do so (Eysenck, 1957, 1965b; Eysenck and Rachman, 1965) can only benefit from more intensive study of the relation between personality and different parameters of eyeblink conditioning.

REFERENCES

Eysenck, H. J. (1957). "The Dynamics of Anxiety and Hysteria." Routledge and Kegan Paul, London.
Eysenck, H. J. (1959). "The Maudsley Personality Inventory". University of London Press.

H. J. EYSENCK AND A. LEVEY

Eysenck, H. J. (1962). Conditioning and personality. *Br. J. Pyschol.*, **53**, 299.

Eysenck, H. J. (1963a). The biological basis of personality. *Nature*, **199**, 1031.

Eysenck, H. J. (Ed.) (1963b). "Experiments with Drugs". Pergamon, Oxford.

Eysenck, H. J. (1964). "Biological factors in neurosis and crime." *Scientia*, **1**.

Eysenck, H. J. (1965a). Extraversion and the acquisition of eyeblink and GSR conditioned responses. *Psychol. Bull.*, **63**, 258.

Eysenck, H. J. (1965b). "Crime and Personality". Routledge and Kegan Paul, London.

Eysenck, H. J. (1967). "The Biological Basis of Personality". C. C. Thomas, Springfield, Ill.

Eysenck, H. J., and Eysenck, S. B. J. (1969). "Personality Structure and Measurement". Routledge and Kegan Paul, London.

Eysenck, H. J. and Rachman, S. (1965). "The Causes and Cures of Neurosis". London.

Fuster, J. M. (1958). Effects of stimulation of brain stem on tachistoscopic perception. *Science, Lond.* **127**, 150.

Gray, J. A. (1964). "Pavlov's Typology". Pergamon, Oxford.

Isaac, W. (1960). Arousal and reaction times in cats. *J. comp. physiol. Psychol.*, **53**, 234.

Killam, E. K. (1962). Drug action on the brain stem reticular formation. *Pharmacol. Rev.*, **14**, 175.

Kimble, C. A. (1961). "Conditioning and Learning." Appleton, Century Croft, New York.

Magoun, D. W. (1963). Central Neural Inhibition. *In* Jones, M. R. (Ed.), "Nebraska Symposium on Motivation 1963." Lincoln, Nebraska.

Ross, L. E. and K. W. Spence, (1960). Eyelid conditioning performance under partial reinforcement as a function of UCS intensity. *J. exp. Psychol.*, **59**, 379.

Savage, R. D. (1964). Electro-cerebral activity, extraversion and neuroticism. *Br. J. Psychiat.* **110**, 98.

From J. A. Gray (1967). Behaviour Research and Therapy, *5*, 151-169, *by kind permission of the author and Pergamon Press*

STRENGTH OF THE NERVOUS SYSTEM, INTROVERSION–EXTRAVERSION, CONDITIONABILITY AND AROUSAL

JEFFREY A. GRAY

Institute of Experimental Psychology, Oxford, England

Summary—The Soviet work on the dimensions of personality known as 'Strength of the Nervous System' and 'Equilibrium in Dynamism' is compared with the Western work on introversion–extraversion, in the light of the suggestions that have been made that each of these three dimensions is related to level of arousal. Two particular hypotheses are discussed in relation to existing data: (1) that introversion–extraversion is identical to strength of the nervous system; (2) that introversion–extraversion is identical to equilibrium in dynamism. Some general theoretical implications of these two hypotheses are considered.

IN THE last decade a group of workers under the direction of the late Professor Teplov in Moscow have made considerable progress in the development of Pavlov's theory of the physiological basis of personality so that it may be applied to Man. The Pavlovian background is reviewed in exhaustive detail by Teplov (1964). In addition, I have reviewed elsewhere (Gray, 1964a) the work done by Teplov's group in applying to Man one particular aspect of Pavlov's theory, namely that dealing with a dimension of personality termed "strength of the excitatory process" or "strength of the nervous system". Table 1 lists some of the major differences which have been found to exist between individuals who are at the extreme "strong" or extreme "weak" ends of this continuum; though it should be emphasised that it is only by consulting the full review that the reader will be able to discover the experimental procedures (which are in some cases extremely complex) associated with these findings as well as their theoretical significance. In general, I have summarised the difference between the srong and weak nervous systems (taking these terms to refer to the two extremes of a continuum, not to two different types of nervous system) as follows

> The weak nervous system is more *sensitive* than the strong: it begins to respond at stimulus intensities which are ineffective for the strong nervous system; throughout the stimulus–intensity continuum its responses are closer to its maximum level of responding than the responses of the strong nervous system; and it displays its maximum response, or the response decrement which follows this maximum, at lower stimulus intensities than the strong nervous system.
> These same differences may be expressed by saying that the strong nervous system is more *stable* than the weak—it is better able to withstand extreme intensities of stimulation, better able to continue responding appropriately and without decrement at high stimulus intensities (Gray, 1964a, p. 281).

In an attempt to put these findings of the Moscow group in a theoretical context which would be less unfamiliar than the strictly Pavlovian framework used in Teplov's laboratory, I have suggested (Gray, 1964b) that it is possible to re-interpret the data on strength of the nervous system as showing that this dimension of personality is a dimension of levels of arousal or 'arousability'. In other words, it is suggested that the individual with a weak nervous system is more highly aroused than a strong individual when both are exposed to objectively identical physical stimulation. This re-interpretation may be taken on a purely behavioural level, using the kind of theoretical framework developed by such workers as Duffy (1962) and Freeman (1948). Alternatively, we may give the notion of arousal level a physiological substrate by supposing that it is dependent on the degree to which the cerebral cortex is bombarded by impulses from the non-specific reticular activating system (RAS) discovered by Moruzzi and Magoun (1949) and linked with notions of arousal in the psychological sense by a number of writers (Lindsley, 1957; Hebb, 1955; Malmo, 1959;

TABLE 1. DIFFERENCES BETWEEN STRONG AND WEAK NERVOUS SYSTEMS (GRAY, 1964a)

	Strong nervous system	Weak nervous system
Response decrement due to 'extinction with reinforcement' ('transmarginal inhibition')	Low	High
Absolute sensory thresholds	High	Low
Reaction time at low stimulus intensities	Slow	Fast
Threshold of 'concentration of excitation' as tested by the 'induction method' (Gray, 1964a, p. 183 et seq.)	Low	High
Threshold of 'irradiation of excitation' in the 'induction method' (Gray, loc. cit.)	High	Low
Critical frequency of flashing phosphene (see footnote on p. 196)	Low	High
Change in absolute sensory threshold due to heteromodal stimulation	Lowered	Raised
Susceptibility to effects of stimulant drugs (caffeine)	Low	High
Dependence of EEG photodriving effect on stimulus intensity (Nebylitsyn, 1966)	Low	High

Berlyne, 1960; Samuels, 1959). In either case, the hypothesis that weak and strong individuals differ from one another in arousability remains to a large degree a re-interpretation of the Pavlovian theory, rather than a rival theory. For, as pointed out elsewhere (Gray, 1964b, pp. 296–300), the key concept in the Pavlovian theory used by Teplov's group—'the intensity of the excitatory process' (which, under most conditions, is said to be higher, the weaker the nervous system)—bears very considerable similarities to the Western concept of arousal.

If there is any merit in the hypothesis that strength of the nervous system is a dimension of arousability, one obvious and important line of experimental advance would be to compare measures of strength of the nervous system with measures of the various Western dimensions of personality which are believed to have some connection with level of arousal. When I wrote my review of the work of Teplov's group, it seemed that the most obvious candidates for this role were the dimensions of neuroticism (Eysenck, 1957) or manifest anxiety (Taylor, 1953, 1956). However, in the last few years there have been a number of suggestions (Corcoran 1961; Claridge 1960, 1967; Eysenck, 1963) that the dimension of introversion–extraversion (Eysenck, 1957) may be, in part or in its entirety, dependent on differences in arousability. This view is dealt with most thoroughly by Eysenck (1967), who makes out a strong case for it, while not abandoning the belief that other physiological differences also underlie this dimension of personality. Since there are sufficient data to hand to make it worth taking this view seriously, the present paper will be devoted to a consideration of the hypothesis (*Hypothesis* 1) that *the dimensions of strength of the nervous system and introversion–extraversion are identical, with the weak nervous system corresponding to the introvert.* We shall not consider here the possibility of identifying neuroticism with strength of the nervous system, largely because there are few data relevant to this hypothesis, but also because such data as do exist run counter to it at one key point: it is *not* the case that neurotics have lower sensory thresholds (see below) than normals (Granger, 1957). We shall, however, consider a second alternative hypothesis, namely, that introversion–extraversion corresponds to the dimension described by the Moscow group as 'equilibrium in dynamism' (Nebylitsyn, 1966).

Since there is no account in English of the work of the Moscow group on 'dynamism', it will be necessary to indicate the salient features of this work. The account that follows is largely based on the writings of V. D. Nebylitsyn (1963a, 1964, 1966; Teplov and Nebylitsyn, 1963a, 1963b), an outstanding young Soviet psychologist who succeeded to Teplov's chair after the latter's untimely death in 1965.

The concept of 'dynamism' ('dinamichnost' in the Russian) is very close to the notion of 'conditionability', as this term is used in Western writings, with the exception that in the work of the Moscow school it is thought that there are two independent forms of dynamism: dynamism of the excitatory process (roughly, the ability to form positive conditioned reflexes rapidly) and dynamism of the inhibitory process (the ability to form inhibitory conditioned reflexes rapidly). The term 'dynamism' was introduced by Nebylitsyn (1963a), after he had shown in a historical and theoretical review that the Soviet literature contained a serious ambiguity[*] in its use of the notion of 'equilibrium of the nervous processes'. This ambiguity took the following form.

It has been customary to measure 'equilibrium' in Soviet work on typology by comparing the speed of formation of positive and negative conditioned reflexes. At the same time, it has been usual to describe 'equilibrium' as 'equilibrium in the *strength* of the nervous processes'. Yet, as the reader will see from Table 1, the more basic dimension of strength of the *excitatory* process is not measured by the speed of formation of positive conditioned reflexes, nor is the dimension of strength of the *inhibitory* process measured by the speed of formation of inhibitory conditioned reflexes. [Indeed, work from Teplov's laboratory suggests that, contrary to the views expressed by earlier Soviet workers, there are no differences in speed of conditioning between individuals of different degrees of strength of the excitatory process (see Gray, 1964b, p. 299). This is a point to which we return below.] In that case, Nebylitsyn rather naturally asks, what is the equilibrium that is measured by the relative speed of formation of positive and negative conditioned reflexes equilibrium *between*? As he shows, there is no reason to suppose that speed of formation of conditioned

[*] This ambiguity probably has its origin in the gradual change in Pavlov's theory of types from a system based on the notion of equilibrium to one in which the concept of strength of the nervous system played the leading role (see Teplov, 1964, pp. 5–27) for a detailed account of this change.

JEFFREY A. GRAY

reflexes depends on either of the two basic Pavlovian dimensions—strength and mobility of the nervous processes (Pavlov, 1955, p. 313; Teplov, 1964)—and from this he concludes that there must be some other basic property of nervous functioning of which the dimension of 'equilibrium', as this has traditionally been understood in the Soviet literature, is a derivative. It is this basic property which he proposes to call 'dynamism'.

Another important conclusion which flows from Nebylitsyn's (1963a) analysis is that, since the equilibrium usually measured in Soviet laboratories is not equilibrium in *strength* of the opposing processes of excitation and inhibition, there should also be a dimension of equilibrium in strength which it *is* possible to measure. In fact, he proposes that, in general, a complete description of an individual's type, in the sense of his position along a number of independently varying dimensions of personality, should involve the determination of a value on any given dimension *separately* for the processes of excitation and inhibiton, followed by the calculation of a derived value for equilibrium between the two processes with respect to that dimension (see Table 2).

TABLE 2. GENERAL METHOD FOR CLASSIFICATION OF PROPERTIES OF THE
NERVOUS SYSTEM AND FOR EVALUATING EQUILIBRIUM (FROM NEBYLITSYN, 1963a)

	Strength	Dynamism	Mobility
Excitation	2	4	3
Inhibition	2	1	5
Equilibrium	0	+3	−2

In this connection, it should be pointed out that the dimension of strength of the nervous system discussed in this paper and reviewed elsewhere (Gray, 1964a) is, strictly speaking, a dimension of strength of the *excitatory* process only. As discussed by Teplov (1964, pp. 95–97), it is also possible to measure, in principle, a dimension of strength of the inhibitory process and, consequently, equilibrium with respect to strength of the nervous processes. Efforts are being made by the Moscow group to develop methods of measuring the strength of the inhibitory process (Rozhdestvenskaya, 1963; Nebylitsyn, 1966, pp. 201–205), notably by increasing the duration or frequency of presentation of an inhibitory conditioned stimulus and observing any consequent disruption of the inhibitory conditioned reflex. However, it is too early to say whether these efforts are likely to bear fruit. Concerning the remaining Pavlovian dimension, 'mobility' of the nervous processes (see Teplov, 1964, pp. 73–94), Pavlov himself pointed out at a 'Wednesday' meeting in 1935 (Nebylitsyn, 1966, p. 24) that it is necessary to test the degree of mobility of both the excitatory process and the inhibitory process separately in each experimental subject.

'Dynamism of the excitatory process', then, refers to that property of the nervous system which underlies the ability to form positive conditioned reflexes with more or less rapidity; while 'dynamism of the inhibitory process' refers to that property of the nervous system which underlies the ability to form inhibitory conditioned reflexes with more or less rapidity. Furthermore, there is, in the Russian view, a third, derived, dimension of nervous functioning, namely, 'equilibrium in dynamism'. This is the property of the nervous system which underlies the relative superiority in speed of conditioning which is shown, in a given individual, by either positive or negative conditioned reflexes: where positive conditioned reflexes are formed relatively more rapidly, we speak of a 'predominance of excitation with respect to dynamism'; where inhibitory conditioned reflexes are formed with relatively greater rapidity, we speak of a 'predominance of the inhibitory process with respect to dynamism'.

Now there are rather obvious similarities between the concept of equilibrium in dynamism and Eysenck's (1957) view of the excitation–inhibition balance which he believes to underlie the personality dimension of introversion–extraversion. Indeed, Eysenck has explicitly connected this dimension with conditionabiilty, introverts being supposed to develop positive conditioned reflexes more rapidly than extraverts. There is, however, one important difference between Eysenck's approach and that of the Moscow group which should be brought out. As Nebylitsyn (1966, pp. 308–309) points out, once it is admitted that for any given property of nervous functioning, it is necessary to investigate the excitatory process and the inhibitory process separately, it follows that there are, in principle, three possible forms of relation between variation in the resulting two dimensions. These may be totally unrelated to one another; they may be related positively, in the sense that high values along the dimension relating to the excitatory process are accompanied by high values along the corresponding dimension relating to the inhibitory process; or they may be negatively related, in the sense that high values on the one dimension correspond to low values on the other*. The latter relationship is assumed in Eysenck's hypothesis as to the physiological substrate of introversion–extraversion: introverts are said to generate excitatory potentials more easily *and* inhibitory potentials less easily than extraverts (Eysenck, 1957). Yet it is clearly an empirical question whether this is indeed the correct relationship to assume. Nebylitsyn (1966, pp. 314–323) discusses the data obtained in his laboratory relevant to the relationship between dynamism in excitation and inhibition and concludes that no final decision is yet possible. He appears, however, to incline to the view that there is a great deal of independence between the two dimensions. My own view of the data he adduces is that they leave open a strong possibility that the relation between the two forms of dynamism, or speed of conditioning, is in fact of the kind postulated by Eysenck. If we assume that this *is* the case, it makes it easier to compare the Soviet work on dynamism with Eysenck's work on introversion–extraversion, and we shall therefore do so. However, the empirical and theoretical issues involved in this question of the general relationship between measures of positive conditioning and of inhibitory conditioning are clearly of very great importance, and it is to be hoped that they will receive more explicit experimental attention in the future than has been the case to date†.

The general similarity between the Russian concept of equilibrium in dynamism and Eysenck's view of the excitation–inhibition balance is reinforced by the fact that, just as Eysenck (1967) has proposed that this balance is critically dependent on the activity of the reticular activating system, so Nebylitsyn (1964) has proposed that dynamism in excitation is dependent on activity in this same system. On the assumption that dynamism in excitation and dynamism in inhibition‡ are negatively related to one another, it follows that Nebylitsyn's

* Similar arguments are advanced by Claridge (1967).

† See Appendix, where some of Nebylitsyn's data are briefly presented and this genarel problem is considered further.

‡ Nebylitsyn (1964) also suggests that dynamism in inhibition depends on 'regulating cortical influences'. There is not space here to consider the implications of this part of his theory.

JEFFREY A. GRAY

proposal amounts to the suggestion that a high level of activity in the reticular activating system is conducive to a predominance of excitation in dynamism. There are therefore grounds for proposing, as an alternative way of linking the work of the Moscow group with the dimension of introversion–extraversion, a second hypothesis—*Hypothesis* 2: *the dimensions of introversion–extraversion and equilibrium in dynamism are identical, the introvert corresponding to the individual with a predominance of excitation in dynamism*. For the reader to be able to evaluate this hypothesis it is necessary for him to have some idea of the way in which individuals at the extreme poles of the 'equilibrium in dynamism' dimension have been shown to differ from one another. The most important findings made by the Moscow group are set out in Table 3.

TABLE 3. DIFFERENCES BETWEEN INDIVIDUALS WITH A PREDOMINANCE OF EXCITATION
AND THOSE WITH A PREDOMINANCE OF INHIBITION IN DYNAMISM*

	Predominance of excitation	Predominance of inhibition
Speed of conditioning (EEG)	High	Low
Duration of a-depression to novel stimulus, whether auditory or visual	Long	Short
Duration of conditioned a-depression	Long	Short
Speed of habituation of a-depression to novel stimulus	Slow	Fast
Speed of extinction of conditioned a-depression	Slow	Fast
Speed of formation of differentiation in EEG conditioning	Slow	Fast
Amount of a-depression during presentation of CS for delayed CR (EEG)	High	Low
Speed of formation of delayed CR (EEG)	Slow	Fast
a-index	Low	High
a-amplitude	Low	High
a-frequency	High	Low
β-index	Low	High
β-amplitude	Low	High
β-frequency	Low	High
θ-frequency	Low	High
EEG photo-driving effect	Small	Large

* Based on data—all obtained from EEG experiments—from Nebylitsyn (1963b, c, 1966).

Before we turn to a consideration of the data relevant to our two hypotheses, one general point must be made. We have *two* hypotheses (introversion=weakness of the nervous system, and introversion=predominance of excitation in dynamism) only because of the data from Teplov's laboratory suggesting that the dimension of equilibrium in dynamism is orthogonal to the dimension of strength of the nervous system. These data were obtained from carefully conducted factor-analytic studies, one of which is reviewed by Gray (1964a, pp. 267–274); see also Nebylitsyn (1963b) and Nebylitsyn et al. (1965). However, only the last of these studies has simultaneously used a fairly large number of tests of strength and of dynamism, as well as further tests unrelated to either of these dimensions. It remains possible that a really large-scale study of this kind might show that strength of the nervous system and equilibrium in dynamism are not so completely unrelated as it is at present believed. It might turn out, for example, that, although to some degree distinct from one another, they constitute two subfactors both related to a single major factor, perhaps the factor uncovered in Western studies as that of introversion–extraversion, or the factor described by Claridge (1967) as 'dysthymia–hysteria'. This is a possibility which should be borne in mind in what follows.

Now the obvious way to settle the issues raised by our two hypotheses is by experiment. What is needed, of course, is a large-scale study in which a group of subjects is tested on the Western measures of introversion–extraversion and on the Russian tests of strength and dynamism. Not only has no such experiment yet been conducted, but the fact that the situations used by the Russians are very different from most of the procedures used in the work on introversion–extraversion makes it difficult to bring data to bear on our two hypotheses in any but the most general way. This situation, however, has one big advantage: the difference in procedures means that, if future research does show that one of the Russian dimensions can be identified with one of the Western ones, we would be justified in putting much more confidence in its reality. The purpose of this article is to suggest the lines of research in this field which, in the light of existing data, are likely to prove most fruitful.

To these data we now turn. We shall consider first those points which are in favour of the introversion = weakness of the nervous system hypothesis; and then those points which are in favour of the alternative hypothesis and therefore offer some difficulty for the identification of introversion with weakness.

1. *Sensory thresholds*

One of the most important findings of Teplov's group is that individuals with a weak nervous system have low absolute sensory thresholds in both the visual and auditory modalities (Gray, 1964a, pp. 207–230). It is therefore of considerable significance that it has also been shown in recent experiments that introverts have lower auditory (Smith, 1967) and pain (Haslam, 1966) thresholds than extraverts. The possible connection between lowered sensory thresholds and heightened arousal has been discussed by Gray (1964b, pp. 308–314).

2. *The effects of distraction*

Yermolayeva-Tomina (1959; see Gray, 1964a, pp. 248–260) has shown that sensory thresholds are lowered in the strong nervous system but raised in the weak by the simultaneous presentation of a distracting heteromodal stimulus. Elsewhere (Gray, 1964b, pp. 330–332) it has been suggested that this result is due to the effect of the additional stimulation on level of arousal, this being taken closer to the optimum for this particular task in the less highly aroused (strong) individual but beyond the optimum in the more highly aroused (weak) individual. A number of similar findings have been reported for the effects of distraction on introverts and extraverts. Bakan, Belton and Toth (1963) and Colquhoun and Corcoran (1964), using vigilance-like tasks, found that introverts perform more efficiently in isolation, extraverts in a group. Claridge (1960), also using a vigilance task, found the same result when he introduced the simultaneous performance of a second task as the additional source of stimulation. Furthermore, Corcoran (1965) has presented data to support the view that these effects of additional stimulation are due to the fact that introverts start off with a chronically higher level of arousal than extraverts.

JEFFREY A. GRAY

3. *Stimulus intensity and transmarginal inhibition*

Both weak individuals (Gray, 1964a) and introverts (Eysenck, 1967) have been conceived as, relative to their opposite numbers, *amplifying* stimulation. (The connection between this view and notions of arousability will be obvious.) Thus it is expected that any change in performance which can be produced by increasing stimulus intensity will be reached at a lower stimulus intensity in the more highly aroused (weak, introvert) than in the less highly aroused (strong, extravert) individual. I have reviewed the data on strength of the nervous system from this point of view elsewhere (Gray, 1964a). In the case of introversion-extraversion, the evidence for this hypothesis is not yet so firm, but there are nevertheless some interesting pointers. Thus Corcoran (1964) found that unconditioned salivation to an acid stimulus was higher in introverts than in extraverts, as it is, of course, if the acidity is increased. Furthermore, Eysenck and Eysenck (1967 a, b) have reported that, if the stimulus (lemon juice) is made extremely strong by getting the subjects to *swallow* it, this relation may be reversed, introverts now salivating significantly less than extraverts, though both show an increase relative to the situation in which the lemon juice is *not* swallowed. This may be an example of transmarginal inhibition, that is, a performance decrement which occurs when stimulus intensity is raised to a very high level. If further studies support this view, we would have an extremely important piece of evidence in favour of the introversion = weakness hypothesis; for the greater susceptibility of the weak nervous system to transmarginal inhibition is the cornerstone of the theory of strength of the nervous system (Gray, 1964a).

From the hypothesis that introverts amplify stimulation it may also be deduced that introverts will prefer lower levels of stimulation than extraverts (Eysenck, 1967). In accordance with this deduction Weisen (1965) found that extraverts (psychopaths) would work to turn stimulation of high intensity *on*, introverts (anxiety neurotics) to turn it *off*. Other studies have shown greater tolerance for pain in the extravert (Lynn and Eysenck, 1961; Petrie *et al.* 1960). Finally, Eysenck (1967) discusses a number of experiments which suggest that introverts have greater tolerance for sensory deprivation than extraverts.

4. *Flicker phenomena*

There is a very confused situation at present in the Russian work on flicker phenomena as a function of personality. A curious discrepancy exists between the arguments that are applied to the critical frequency of flashing phosphene* (CFP) and the critical frequency of flicker-fusion (CFF). The former is taken as a measure of strength of the nervous system (Nebylitsyn, 1960; see Gray, 1964a, pp. 242–248), the weak individual having a higher CFP than the strong. This is because CFP varies positively with stimulus intensity, and the dependence of this measure on strength of the nervous system fits the familiar pattern of weak individuals reacting as though to a higher intensity stimulus than strong individuals. Furthermore, it has been shown that, over a critical range of voltages, CFP does indeed correlate with other measures of strength (Nebylitsyn, 1960; Gray, 1964a, p. 244). CFF, on the other hand, which varies in the same way with stimulus intensity (Granger, 1960) has never been used in experiments on strength of the nervous system. Instead, it is taken to be a measure of "lability of the nervous processes" (Nebylitsyn, 1966; Teplov, 1964, pp.

---

* When the frequency of an electric current, which is passed through the eye so as to produce the visual sensation known as a 'phosphene', is increased, a threshold is reached beyond which no further visual sensation is produced: this is the 'critical frequency of flashing phosphene'.

73–94)*. However, the logical parallels between CFP and CFF are reinforced by a number of experimental findings proceeding from Teplov's group (Borisova *et al.*, 1963; Turovskaya, 1963; Golubeva, 1966) which suggest that high lability and high weakness are intimately connected with one another. It seems possible, therefore, that the weak individual, relative to the strong, is characterised by high thresholds both of CFP and CFF. Elsewhere (Gray, 1964b, pp. 314–318) I have discussed the possibility that, in general, the ability to resolve a train of high-frequency stimuli into its discrete components will be facilitated by a high level of arousal.

The importance of these findings in our present context is that there is evidence from a number of studies (Simonson and Brožek, 1952) that CFF is higher in introverts than in extraverts. Thus, *if* CFF is higher in the weak nervous system, as is CFP, we have another piece of evidence favouring the identification, introversion = weakness.

5. *Drug effects*

There is a striking similarity between the role played by caffeine in the theory of strength (Gray, 1964a) and the role played by stimulant drugs in the theory of introversion propounded by Eysenk (1963, 1967): caffeine moves people towards the weak end nf the dimension of strength, and stimulant drugs are said to have an introverting effect. (There is no reason to suppose that the effects attributed to caffeine in the Russian work would not equally be expected of other representatives of the class of stimulant drugs.) Another important similarity is that in both cases stimulant drugs appear to have a relatively greater effect in the more aroused (introverted, weak) individual (Gray, 1964a, p. 279 and *passim*; Eysenck, 1967). The data supporting these statements are reviewed in the articles by Gray and Eysenck cited above. It is clear that the parallel treatments accorded to stimulant drugs in the two bodies of work is a powerful argument in favour of the identification, introversion = weakness, as well as being in good agreement with the view that both these dimensions are functions of arousal level.

In the Western work on introversion–extraversion an important role is also played by depressant drugs, which are supposed to have an extraverting effect (Eysenck, 1963, 1967). This view has been supported empirically, notably by the work on the sedation threshold pioneered by Shagass and his colleagues (e.g. Shagass and Jones, 1958; see Eysenck, 1967, for review). It would be of great value to obtain similar data for the effects of depressant drugs on individuals varying in strength of the nervous system.

6. *Susceptibility to fatigue*

One of the interesting things about the work on fatigue as a function of personality is that, in this instance (in the absence of any linkage with notions of arousal), the theory of strength and the theory of introversion, which usually make their predictions in somewhat similar ways, come up with different predictions. On the basis of the notion that the weak nervous system is one with a low "working capacity" (a term which is defined by Teplov, 1959, as "the capacity to endure stimulation which is extreme in its duration or intensity") it is predicted that weak individuals will show a decline over time in their efficiency of performance which is greater than the comparable decline shown by strong individuals. On the basis of the notion that extraverts are more susceptible to reactive inhibition than

* Recent work from the Moscow laboratory (Nebylitsyn, 1966) shows clearly the complex nature of the functions described by Teplov (1964) under the heading 'mobility of the nervous processes'. One group of these functions is now regarded as separate from the others and is collectively described as 'lability'. Among the tests being tried out as measures of 'lability' are—apart from CFF—the adequate optic chronaxie, and the relation between the ascending and descending psychophysical thresholds. However, it is too soon to say whether a genuinely unitary function is being measured by these tests.

introverts, it can be predicted from Eysenck's theory that it is the former who will show a greater decline in efficiency as a result of fatigue. In other words, contrary to the general form of the identification we are examining, this time *extraverts* are expected to behave in the same way as the weak nervous system. In some ways, then, the relation between these two personality dimensions, on the one hand, and susceptibility to fatigue, on the other, makes a particularly good test both of the identification of weakness with introversion and of the hypothesis that each of these dimensions of personality is a function of arousal level.

Before turning to the relevant data, let us consider what changes we would make in our predictions if we based ourselves on an arousal view of the two personality dimensions. Clearly, our prediction will depend on whether continuation at the particular task leads to a gradually *decreasing* or a gradually *increasing* level of arousal*. In the former case, we would predict that the individual high on arousal (weak, introvert) would show less of a decline in efficiency than the individual low on arousal (strong, extravert). In the latter case, however, we would predict that the individual *low* on arousal (strong, extravert) would be more resistant to fatigue. In other words, both the Teplovian and the Eysenckian prediction would be made, but under different conditions. Furthermore, since continuation at the same task must involve some degree of monotonous stimulation, it is likely that a gradual *decrease* in arousal level over the duration of the experiment will more often be encountered in work on fatigue than the converse; thus we would expect it to be more difficult to arrange conditions so as to make the Teplovian observation than to make the Eysenckian observation†.

What, then, are the facts? Data supporting Eysenck's prediction that the extravert is more susceptible to fatigue have been presented by Broadbent (1958), by Bakan, Belton and Toth (1963), and by Halcomb and Kirk (1965), all using vigilance tasks, in which overall stimulus intensity is relatively low and monotony great—conditions which should lead to a decreasing level of arousal. Early data from Teplov's laboratory (Yermolayeva-Tomina, 1960; see Gray, 1964a, pp. 260–262) also seemed to support the Teplovian prediction, that the weak nervous system would be more highly susceptible to fatigue. Here the task used was a mental arithmetic task, in which it is extremely difficult to estimate what is likely to be happening to arousal level; but there is certainly no obvious reason to suppose it should be increasing to any great extent. However, recent work conducted by Rozhdestvenskaya and Yermolayeva-Tomina (1966) failed to confirm these results and, indeed, found that individuals with a *strong* nervous system showed greater physiological signs of fatigue in a vigilance-like situation. Thus, in the only case where both Russian and Western work has used the same type of situation (a vigilance task) the results support the identification of introversion with weakness—results which are particularly convincing inasmuch as the expectation of the experimenters was exactly the opposite of what was obtained.

It should not be thought, however, that it is always the highly aroused subject (weak, introvert) who is more susceptible to fatigue; and of course our analysis in terms of arousal does not lead us to expect that this will be the case. As well as the Yermolayeva-Tomina (1960) finding referred to above, there are also indications in the literature on introversion-extraversion that there are conditions in which the greater susceptibility to fatigue of the

* This is probably the same distinction as that made by Rozhdestvenskaya (1964, p. 371) between conditions leading to 'exhaustion of the nerve cells' (transmarginal inhibition or high arousal) and those leading to 'the onset of a hypnotic state' (low arousal). The introduction to Rozhdestvenskaya's paper contains interesting data obtained in classical conditioning experiments relevant to this distinction.

† It has been suggested to me by S. Rachman that it might be possible to use a gradually increasing administration of a stimulant drug for this experiment.

introvert can be abolished or even reversed (e.g. Claridge, 1960; Corcoran, 1965; Colquhoun and Corcoran, 1964). It is clear that much more detailed findings are needed, especially from experiments in which overall level of stimulus intensity is deliberately varied. Nevertheless, it seems possible that our analysis in terms of level of arousal is not too far from the truth, and, if this could be established, it would be a strong argument in favour of the view that both introversion and weakness are consequences of high arousability.

7. *Reactive inhibition*

Hull's (1943) concept of 'reactive inhibition' has played a considerable role in Eysenck's treatment of introversion–extraversion (Eysenck, 1957). However, in the last decade or so the difficulties involved in this concept have become increasingly clear (e.g. Gleitman, Nachmias and Neisser, 1954). At the same time, more and more of the data once explained in terms of reactive inhibition have been dealt with in other ways. We have just seen an example of this, in the alternative account proposed for susceptibility to fatigue in terms of changing levels of arousal. Other examples are the treatment of extinction of instrumental behaviour in terms of a theory based on 'frustration' (Amsel, 1962; Gray and Smith, 1967), or the revised account of certain aspects of the 'reminiscence' phenomenon in terms of consolidation proposed by Eysenck (1965). Again, it would seem relatively easy to deal with the disruptive effects of massed practice on learning in terms of a lowered level of arousal due to the greater monotony of stimulation produced by this procedure; though obviously this hypothesis stands in need of experimental test.

The question therefore arises whether there is still any need, either in general learning theory or in the theory of introversion–extraversion, for the concept of reactive inhibition. This question is of particular relevance in the present context because there is considerable similarity between 'reactive inhibition' and 'transmarginal inhibition' as the latter is used in the Russian theory of strength of the nervous system. For example, the phenomenon of extinction with reinforcement is attributed to reactive inhibition in the Western literature (Kendrick, 1958) and to transmarginal inhibition in the Russian literature (Gray, 1964a). Again, both massing of trials and increased stimulus intensity (which leads to increased response magnitude) are thought to lead to a growth in both forms of inhibition. Yet in Eysenck's (1957) theory it is the extravert who is most susceptible to reactive inhibition, while in the theory of strength of the nervous system (Gray 1964a) it is the weak individual who is more susceptible to transmarginal inhibition. This would lead to an identification of the weak individual with the extravert, the reverse of the identification which we have considered throughout this paper.

This dilemma is, of course, the general form of which the problem of susceptibility to fatigue in the two theories of personality, considered in the preceding section, is a special case. A tentative resolution of the dilemma was reached there by re-analysing the problem in terms of level of arousal. Is it possible to extend this solution to all the situations in which Eysenckian theory predicts greater susceptibility to reactive inhibition in the extravert?

An analysis of the general Hullian treatment of reactive inhibition suggests that there are two separate ideas mixed up in this concept. One is a tendency to cease making a specific response which has just been made; this is the way in which the term is formally defined by Hull (1943), and we can call it 'reactive inhibition proper'. The other is a general fall (i.e. *not* specific to any particular response) in the organism's level of functioning; it is this that corresponds to 'de-arousal', and, although never so defined, it is often this that is

JEFFREY A. GRAY

meant by 'reactive inhibition'*. Now, if there were no evidence for a process corresponding to reactive inhibition proper, we could abandon the concept of reactive inhibition entirely and substitute for it that of de-arousal. At the time that Hull introduced the concept, there was indeed very little evidence for the existence of such a process. It was introduced, rather, as a theoretical postulate which, it was hoped, would account for the phenomena which Pavlov had subsumed under the heading 'internal inhibition'. [In fact, as Gleitman, Nachmias and Neisser (1954) have shown, it does not do this job at all well.] Recently, however, good evidence has been obtained in Eysenck's laboratory (Spielman, 1963; Eysenck, 1964) that there is indeed an empirical phenomenon which corresponds very closely to reactive inhibition proper. This evidence was obtained from a simple tapping task in which it was possible to measure the number and duration of involuntary rest pauses, the assumption being that such pauses are produced by the accumulation of reactive inhibition proper. Furthermore—and this is the important point for our present purposes—extraverted subjects were considerably more susceptible to reactive inhibition measured in this way, in accordance with the prediction from Eysenck's (1957) theory.

It appears, then, that it is not possible entirely to abandon the concept of reactive inhibition in favour of a concept of de-arousal. It remains unclear how significant reactive inhibition proper is, and how the extravert's greater susceptibility to it relates to his lower arousal level. It is also difficult to see what structure or process in the central nervous system is likely to be responsible for the phenomenon. Furthermore the relations between 'reactive inhibition proper' and 'transmarginal inhibition', assuming that both these terms correspond to real processes, remain to be worked out. It is clear that, if the general identification of weakness of the nervous system with introversion is correct, these two forms of inhibition cannot be the same. In that case, it is going to require considerable experimental ingenuity to distinguish clearly between them. With regard to our general theme—the relation between strength of the nervous system and introversion–extraversion—it is obviously very important to find out whether individuals classified by the Russian tests as 'strong' show a greater susceptibility to reactive inhibition proper, as measured by the Spielmann tapping test for involuntary rest pauses. There are at present no data available on this point.

8. *EEG measures*

We come now to the most serious difficulty for the identification of weakness with introversion, and at the same time evidence for the identification of introversion with predominance of excitation in dynamism. Both Savage (1964) and Marton and Urban (1966) have reported lower indices of α-activity in introverts as compared to extraverts. Claridge (1967) reports similar findings in a population mainly composed of diagnosed neurotics. On the other hand, Nebylitsyn (1963b, 1966) found that predominance of excitation in dynamism was correlated with low α-index, low α-amplitude and high α-frequency, and that none of these measure related to strength of the nervous system. Moreover, Marton and Urban reported that introverts showed slower EEG habituation than extraverts, as was the case for Nebylitsyn's subjects with predominance of excitation in dynamism. If it can be confirmed both that introverts have lower α-indices than extraverts and that there is no relation between α-activity and strength of the nervous system, it would be impossible to maintain that the dimensions of introversion–extraversion and strength of the nervous system are identical.

* See Appendix.

9. Speed of conditioning

One of the most important elements in Eysenck's (1957) theory of introversion–extraversion has been the supposition that introverts condition better than extraverts. It is clear that this places the dimension of introversion–extraversion very close to the dimension of equilibrium in dynamism, since this dimension is actually defined in terms of speed of conditioning. Furthermore, there is no evidence to date of any systematic differences in speed of conditioning between weak and strong individuals (see Gray, 1964b, p. 299). On the face of it, then, this offers another serious difficulty for the identification of introversion with weakness of the nervous system. However, Eysenck's (1966) more recent statements on the relation between introversion–extraversion and speed of conditioning show that his general theoretical system predicts that introverts will condition better than extraverts only under certain conditions. Furthermore, empirical data obtained by Eysenck and Levey (Eysenck, 1966) from studies of the conditioned eyelid response in introverts and extraverts suggest that the most important of these conditions would probably also favour individuals with a weak nervous system as compared to those with a strong nervous system: namely, a weak UCS (given the established difference in sensory thresholds between weak and strong individuals) and a short CS–UCS interval (given the established difference in reaction time between weak and strong individuals). Thus, although much more work clearly remains to be done in this important field, the evidence from speed of conditioning for the hypothesis is not as negative as it at first appears. Nevertheless, it remains true, that, if introversion is indeed equivalent to weakness, and if the Moscow group is correct in supposing that it is possible to define a dimension of conditionability which is orthogonal to that of strength of the nervous system, then the effect of degree of extraversion on speed of conditioning must be a comparatively minor one, occurring only under special conditions.

It will be clear that no final conclusion as to the merits of the various hypotheses discussed in this paper is possible. Indeed, we have raised far more questions than we have offered answers. Nevertheless, there appears to be sufficient evidence for it to be worth devoting serious attention to the hypothesis that the dimensions of strength of the nervous system and introversion–extraversion are identical, both being based upon level of arousal.

Acknowledgements—My thanks are due to H. J. EYSENCK, with whom I had the benefit of discussing many of the issues mentioned in this paper, and to S..RACHMAN for his comments on the manuscript.

REFERENCES

*References marked * are in Russian*

AMSEL A. (1962) Frustrative nonreward in partial reinforcement and discrimination learning: some recent history and a theoretical extension. *Psychol. Rev.* **69,** 306–328.

BAKAN P., BELTON J. A. and TOTH J. C. (1963) Extraversion–introversion and decrement in an auditory vigilance task. In *Vigilance: a symposium.* (Eds. BUCKNER D. N. and MCGRATH J. J.), McGraw-Hill, New York.

BERLYNE D. E. (1960) *Conflict, Arousal and Curiosity.* McGraw-Hill, New York.

*BORISOVA M. N., GUREVICH K. M., YERMOLAYEVA-TOMINA L. B., KOLODNAYA A. YA., RAVICH-SHCHERBO I. V. and SHVARTS L. A. (1963) A comparative study of different indices of mobility of the nervous system in man. In *Typological Features of Higher Nervous Activity in Man.* (Ed. TEPLOV B. M.), pp. 180–201. Akad. pedagog. Nauk RSFSR, Moscow.

BROADBENT D. E. (1958) *Perception and Communication.* Pergamon Press, Oxford.

BROADHURST P. L. (1960) Applications of biometrical genetics to the inheritance of behaviour. In *Experiments in Personality.* Vol. I *Psychogenetics and Psychopharmacology.* (Ed. EYSENCK H. J.), pp. 3–102. Routledge & Kegan Paul, London.

JEFFREY A. GRAY

CLARIDGE G. S. (1960) The excitation–inhibition balance in neurotics. In *Experiments in Personality.* Vol. 2. (Ed. EYSENCK H. J.), Praeger, New York.
CLARIDGE G. S. (1967) *Personality and Arousal.* Pergamon Press, Oxford.
COLQUHOUN W. P. and CORCORAN D. W. J. (1964) The effects of time of day and social isolation on the relationship between temperament and performance. *Br. J. soc. clin. Psychol.* 3, 226–231.
CORCORAN D. W. J. (1961) Individual differences in performance after loss of sleep. Unpublished Doctoral dissertation, University of Cambridge.
CORCORAN D. W. J. (1964) The relation between introversion and salivation. *Am. J. Psychol.* 77, 298–300.
CORCORAN D. W. J. (1965) Personality and the inverted-U relation. *Br. J. Psychol.* 56, 267–274.
DUFFY E. (1962) *Activation and Behaviour.* John Wiley, New York.
EYSENCK H. J. (1957) *The Dynamics of Anxiety and Hysteria.* Praeger, New York.
EYSENCK H. J. (1963) *Experiments with Drugs.* Pergamon Press, Oxford.
EYSENCK H. J. (1964) Involuntary rest pauses in tapping as a function of drive and personality. *Percept. mot. Skills* 18, 173–174.
EYSENCK H. J. (1965) A three-factor theory of reminiscence. *Br. J. Psychol.* 56, 163–181.
EYSENCK H. J. (1966) Conditioning, introversion–extraversion, and the strength of the nervous system. *Proc. Eighteenth Int. Congr. exp. Psychol.* Moscow. Ninth Symposium, pp. 33–44.
EYSENCK H. J. (1967) *The Biological Basis of Personality.* Harper & Row, Springfield, Illinois (in press).
EYSENCK S. B. G. and EYSENCK H. J. (1967a) Salivary response to lemon juice as a measure of introversion. *Percept. mot. Skills* (in press).
EYSENCK S. B. G. and EYSENCK H. J. (1967b) Physiological reactivity to sensory stimulation as a measure of personality. *Percept. mot. Skills* (in press).
FREEMAN A. L. (1948) *The Energetics of Human Behavior.* Cornell University Press, Ithaca.
GLEITMAN H., NACHMIAS J. and NEISSER U. (1954) The S–R reinforcement theory of extinction. *Psychol. Rev.* 61, 23–33.
GOLUBEVA E. A. (1966) Photo-driving brain potentials and typological characteristics of the nervous system. *Proc. Eighteenth int. Congr. exp. Psychol.* Moscow. Ninth Symposium, pp. 127–132.
GRANGER G. W. (1957) Night vision and psychiatric disorders. *J. ment. Sci.* 103, 48–79.
GRANGER G. W. (1960) Abnormalities of sensory perception. In *Handbook of Abnormal Psychology.* (Ed. EYSENCK H. J.), pp. 108–166. Pitman, London.
GRAY J. A. (1964a) Strength of the nervous system as a dimension of personality in man: a review of work from the laboratory of B. M. Teplov. In *Pavlov's Typology.* (Ed. GRAY J. A.), pp. 157–287. Pergamon Press, Oxford.
GRAY J. A. (1964b) Strength of the nervous system and levels of arousal: a reinterpretation. In *Pavlov's Typology.* (Ed. GRAY J. A.), pp. 289–364. Pergamon Press, Oxford.
GRAY J. A. (1967) Disappointment and drugs in the rat. *The Advancement of Science* 23, (595–605).
GRAY J. A. and SMITH P. (1967) An arousal–decision model for partial reinforcement and discrimination learning. Paper delivered to the *Symposium on Discrimination | Learning*, Experimental Analysis of Behaviour Group, Brighton, April 5–6, 1967.
HALCOMB C. G. and KIRK R. E. (1965) Organismic variables as predictors of vigilance behavior. *Percept. mot. Skills* 21, 547–552.
HASLAM D. R. (1966) Individual differences in pain threshold and the concept of arousal. Unpublished Ph.D. thesis, Bristol University.
HEBB D. O. (1955) Drives and the c.n.s. (conceptual nervous system). *Psychol. Rev.* 62, 243–254.
HULL C. L. (1943) *Principles of Behaviour.* Appleton–Century, New York.
KENDRICK D. C. (1958) Inhibition with reinforcement (conditioned inhibition). *J. exp. Psychol.* 56, 313–318.
LINDSLEY D. B. (1957) The reticular system and perceptual discrimination. In *Reticular Formation of the Brain.* (Eds. JASPER H. H. et al.), *Henry Ford Hospital International Symposium.* pp. 513–534. Churchill, London.
LYNN R. and EYSENCK H. J. (1961) Tolerance for pain, extraversion and neuroticism. *Percept. mot. Skills* 12, 161–162.
MALMO R. B. (1959) Activation: a neuropsychological dimension. *Psychol. Rev.* 66, 367–386.
MARTON M. and URBAN YA (1966) An electroencephalographic investigation of individual differences in the processes of conditioning. *Proc. Eighteenth int. Cong. exp. Psychol.* Moscow. Ninth symposium, pp. 106–109.
MORUZZI G. and MAGOUN H. W. (1949) Brain stem reticular formation and activation of the EEG. *Electroenceph. clin. Neurophysiol* 1, 455–473.
*NEBYLITSYN V. D. (1960) The correlation between certain indices of the electrical excotability of the eye and strength of the nervous system. *Dokl. Akad. pedagog. Nauk RSFSR* No. 2, 99–102.
*NEBYLITSYN V. D. (1963a) The structure of the fundamental properties of the nervous system. *Vopr. Psikhol.* No. 4, pp. 21–34.

STRENGTH OF THE NERVOUS SYSTEM

*Nebylitsyn V. D. (1963b) An electroencephalographic investigation of the properties of strength of the nervous system and equilibrium of the nervous processes in man using factor analysis. In *Typological Features of Higher Nervous Activity in Man.* (Ed. Teplov B. M.), Vol. 3, pp. 47–80. Akad. pedagog. Nauk RSFSR, Moscow.

*Nebylitsyn V. D. (1964) Cortico-reticular relations and their place in the structure of the properties of the nervous system. *Vopr. Psikhol.* No. 1, 3–24.

*Nebylitsyn V. D. (1966) *Fundamental Properties of the Human Nervous System.* Akad. pedagog. Nauk RSFSR, Moscow.

*Nebylitsyn V. D., Golubeva E. A., Ravich-Shcherbo I. V. and Yermolayeva-Tomina L. B. (1965) A comparative study of rapid methods for determining the basic properties of the nervous system in man. In *Typological Features of Higher Nervous Activity in Man.* (Ed. Teplov B. M.), Vol. 4, pp. 60–83. Akad. pedagog. Nauk RSFSR, Moscow.

Osgood C. E. (1953) *Method and Theory in Experimental Psychology.* Oxford University Press, New York.

Pavlov I. P. (1928) *Lectures on Conditioned Reflexes: Twenty-five Years of Objective Study of the Higher Nervous Activity (Behaviour) of Animals.* Vol. 1. (Trans. and Ed. Gantt W. H.), International Publishers, New York.

Pavlov I. P. (1955) *Selected Works.* (Trans. Belsky S.), Foreign Languages Publishing House, Moscow.

Petrie A., Collins W. and Solomon P. (1960) The tolerance for pain and for sensory deprivation. *Am. J. Psychol.* 123, 80–90.

*Rozhdestvenskaya V. I. (1963) The determination of strength of the inhibitory process in man by extending the duration of action of a differential stimulus. In *Typological Features of Higher Nervous Activity in Man.* (Ed. Teplov B. M.), Vol. 3, pp. 108–116. Akad. pedagog. Nauk RSFSR, Moscow.

Rozhdestvenskaya V. I. (1964) The strength of the nervous system as shown in the ability of nerve-cells to endure protracted concentrated excitation. In *Pavlov's Typology.* (Ed. Gray J. A.), pp. 367–378. Pergamon Press, Oxford.

Rozhdestvenskaya V. I. and Yermolayeva-Tomina L. B. (1966) A study of mental capacity for work in relation to typological characteristics of the nervous system. *Proc. Eighteenth int. Congr. exp. Psychol.,* Moscow, Ninth symposium, pp. 51–59.

Samuels Ina (1959) Reticular mechanisms and behaviour. *Psychol. Bull.* 56, 1–25.

Savage R. D. (1964) Electro-cerebral activity, extraversion and neuroticism. *Br. J. Psychiat.* 110, 98–100.

Shagass C. and Jones A. L. (1958) A neurophysiological test for psychiatric diagnosis: results in 750 patients. *Am. J. Psychiat.* 114, 1002–1009.

Simonson E. and Broezk J. (1952) Flicker fusion frequency: background and application. *Physiol. Rev.* 32, 349–378.

Smith S. L. (1967) The effect of personality and drugs on auditory threshold when risk-taking factors are controlled. Submitted to *Psychom. Med.*

Spielman J. (1963) The relation between personality and the frequency and duration of involuntary rest pauses during massed practice. Unpublished Ph.D. thesis, University of London.

Stein L. (1964) Reciprocal action of reward and punishment mechanisms. In *The Role of Pleasure in Behaviour.* (Ed. Heath R. G.), pp., 113–139. Harper & Row, New York.

Taylor Janet A. (1953) A personality scale of manifest anxiety. *J. abnorm. Soc. Psychol.* 48, 285–290.

Taylor Janet A. (1956) Drive theory and manifest anxiety. *Psychol. Bull.* 53, 303–320.

*Teplov B. M. (1959) Some results of the study of strength of the nervous system in man. In *Typological Features of Higher Nervous Activity in Man.* Vol. 2. Akad. pedagog. Nauk RSFSR, Moscow.

Teplov B. M. (1964) Problems in the study of general types of higher nervous activity in man and animals. In *Pavlov's Typology.* (Ed. Gray J. A.), pp.3–153. Pergamon Press, Oxford.

*Teplov B. M. and Nebylitsyn V. D. (1963a) The study of the basic properties of the nervous system and their significance for the psychology of individual differences. *Vopr. Psikhol.* No. 5, 38–47.

*Teplov B. M. and Nebylitsyn V. D. (1963b) The experimental study of the properties of the nervous system in man. *Zh. vyssh. nervn. Deyat.* 13, 789–797.

*Turovskaya Z. G. (1963) The relation between some indices of strength and of mobility of the nervous system in man. In *Typological Features of Higher Nervous Activity in Man.* (Ed. Teplov B. M.), Vol. 3, pp. 248–261. Akad. pedagog. Nauk RSFSR, Moscow.

Wagner A. R. (1966) Frustration and punishment. In *Currnet Research on Motivation.* (Ed. Haber R. N.). Holt, Rinehart & Winston, New York.

Weisen A. (1965) Differential reinforcing effects of onset and offset of stimulation on the operant behavior of normals, neurotics and psychopaths. Unpublished Ph.D. thesis, University of Florida.

Yermolayeva-Tomina L. B. (1959) Concentration of attention and strength of the nervous system. Translated in *Pavlov's Typology.* (Ed. Gray J. A.), pp. 446–464. Pergamon Press, Oxford (1964).

*Yermolayeva-Tomina L. B. (1960) Individual differences in the ability to concentrate attention and strength of the nervous system. *Vopr. Psikhol.* No. 2, 184–195.

JEFFREY A. GRAY

APPENDIX

Inhibition and Excitation

It seems worth commenting at a little more length on certain general issues which were touched upon in the body of this paper. These issues arise out of the problem posed by the relationship between measures of positive and of inhibitory conditioning—that is, the problem described by Nebylitsyn (1966) as the relationship between dynamism in excitation and dynamism in inhibition. Before considering these issues themselves, we must be clear about the sense in which 'inhibition' is meant in the phrase 'dynamism in inhibiton'. A general examination of the most important ways in which the term 'inhibition' has been used in Pavlov's and Hull's theories of learning may also clarify some of the problems which, as we have seen, are involved in the Hullian construct of 'reactive inhibition'. We begin, then, with a general examination of this kind.

In general it is possible to distinguish three main kinds of phenomenon which have been subsumed under various inhibitory constructs. First, there is a specific response decrement which occurs when the contingencies of reinforcement are changed in such a way that a particular response is no longer followed by the consequences which used to follow it; this is the kind of response decrement which Pavlov regarded as being due to 'internal' inhibition. Second, there is a specific response decrement which is due to causes other than changes in the contingencies of reinforcement; examples of this are various phenomena which Pavlov attributed to 'transmarginal' inhibition or Hull to 'reactive' inhibition. Third, there is a non-specific response decrement, i.e. a response decrement which affects all forms of the organism's functioning simultaneously; in modern theories this might well be called 'de-arousal'*.

Now, in both Pavlov and Hull, concepts of inhibition which are of one of the first two kinds (i.e. specific to a particular response) are apt to change, often unnoticed, into concepts of the third kind. This occurs most explicitly in Pavlov's paper *Inhibition and Sleep— One and the Same Process* (1928, p. 305). Pavlov justifies the change on the grounds that the repeated presentation of an inhibitory CS leads often to sleep. However, he does not consider the possibility that the causes of internal inhibition and of sleep, even though these are both observed in the same experiment, might be different—namely, the omission of reinforcement in the first case and the monotonous conditions of stimulation which result from the omission of reinforcement in the second case.

In Hull, the transition from inhibition as specific response decrement to inhibition as non-specific fall in level of functioning is more insidious. Perhaps the most revealing case is his application of the concept of inhibition to serial learning phenomena (see Osgood, 1953, p. 502 *et seq.*). Hull attempts to use this concept to account both for the typical bow-shaped curve of errors obtained in serial learning experiments and for the fact that the number of errors is increased under conditions of massed practice. To cope with the shape of the error curve, it is pointed out that each item in the series can be considered at once as stimulus for every item that follows it and response for every item that precedes it. It is then proposed that each of the resulting S–R bonds (except the one which, at any particular point in the series, is correct) will be under inhibition of delay and that the greatest number of responses inhibited in this way will be in the middle of the list. So far, the analysis is logical enough, and it will be observed that it depends on a form of inhibition which is specific to a particular

---

* Claridge (1967) uses the term inhibition in yet another way—as the process which underlies suppression of response to certain stimuli during selective attention to others.

response and to a particular stimulus. However, in order to link the shape of the error curve with the effects of distribution of practice, it is said that the inhibition generated during a trial *dissipates with time* during the inter-trial interval, thus producing the superiority of spaced practice. It is here that the transition to a non-specific kind of inhibition takes place. It is clear that 'inhibition of delay' cannot dissipate in time, for the whole function of such an inhibitory process is to adjust the time of response so that it coincides with the arrival of the reinforcing stimulus. Thus, at the end of a trial in a serial learning experiment, there can be *no* inhibition of delay remaining to be dissipated. Evidently, Hull is now thinking rather of some general fall in the organism's level of functioning which can be reversed by a rest pause or by a change of stimulation.

It is hoped that these general comments on the uses—*and* abuses—of 'inhibition' by Pavlov and Hull will help unravel some of the tangles we discovered in our attempt to survey the possible relations between strength of the nervous system and introversion–extraversion. In the case of reactive inhibition—which plays such an important role in Eysenck's treatment of extraversion—it would seem that the process of "de-arousal" could equally well account for many of the phenomena which have often been attributed to reactive inhibition. As we have seen, vigilance decrement is one case in point. 'Reactive inhibition proper', however— that is, a response decrement contingent upon making a response and specific to the response made—is clearly beyond the scope of the concept of de-arousal. Finally, the inhibition involved in 'dynamism in inhibition', or 'inhibitory conditionability', is obviously inhibition in the first sense distinguished above—that process which underlies response decrement due to the omission of reinforcement.

With this preamble, we turn to the problem of how 'dynamism in excitation' and 'dynamism in inhibition' relate to each other. There are in fact a number of different but interlocked issues in this problem.

First, there is the question whether the same relationship will be found to hold in both classical and instrumental conditioning. In other words, suppose it is the case that individual differences in speed of formation of *classical* positive conditioned reflexes relate in one of the three ways distinguished by Nebylitsyn (positively, inversely, or not at all) to individual differences in speed of formation of classical inhibitory conditioned reflexes; will individual differences in speed of acquisition of rewarded *instrumental* behaviour relate in the same way to individual differences in speed of extinction of unrewarded instrumental behaviour?

Secondly, at the instrumental level, it is possible that the problem of the relationship between individual differences in the speed of acquisition and the speed of extinction of rewarded behaviour is the same as the problem of the relationship between sensitivity to reward and sensitivity to punishment; for there is evidence that the same physiological mechanism is involved in the *extinction* of *positively* reinforced behaviour and the *acquisition* of *negatively* reinforced behaviour (Wagner, 1966; Gray, 1967). The extent of our ignorance in this field may be shown by the following example. The Maudsley Reactive and Nonreactive strains of rats (Broadhurst, 1960) have been selectively bred to be, respectively, highly sensitive and highly insensitive to the effects of punishment. Much is known about the behaviour patterns of these two strains; yet there are no grounds to predict whether there will be any differences in their sensitivity to reward and, assuming such differences do exist, whether they will take the form of the Reactive strain being *more* or *less* sensitive to reward than the Nonreactive strain.

Thirdly, if it is generally true that the response decrement which occurs when reinforcement is discontinued is due to the operation of a punishment system, then the similarity

JEFFREY A. GRAY

which sometimes appears to exist between concepts of "inhibition" and of "de-arousal" (see e.g. Pavlov, 1928, p. 305 *et seq.*; or remarks by Claridge, 1960, pp. 136–137) can be misleading; for the operation of the punishment system will often lead to an *increase* in arousal (Gray and Smith, 1967).

Finally, there is the extremely important question of the role played by drug effects in Eysenck's treatment of introversion–extraversion (Eysenck, 1963). He regards stimulant drugs, such as amphetamine, as having an introverting effect, and depressant drugs, such as sodium amylobarbitone, as having an extraverting effect. If introversion–extraversion is linked with level of arousal, these drugs are seen as having, respectively, an arousing and de-arousing effect. But there is an alternative possibility. There is evidence (Gray, 1967) that, in instrumental conditioning situations amylobarbitone reduces the effects of both punishment and frustrative nonreward, and also evidence (Stein, 1964) that amphetamine increases sensitivity to reward. It is possible, therefore, that introverts are relatively more sensitive to the effects of both reward and punishment: amphetamine would then mimic introversion by increasing sensitivity to reward; amylobarbitone would mimic extraversion by decreasing sensitivity to punishment; and the arousing and de-arousing effects of these drugs would be a secondary phenomenon, due to increased input from the reward system or decreased input from the punishment system, respectively, to the arousal system (Gray and Smith, 1967). In that case, it should be noted, we would be treating introversion–extraversion, to put the matter in the Russian terminology, as a dimension of dynamism in which high values of both excitation and inhibition coincide at the introverted pole.

All these possibilities remain open, awaiting experimental attack.

So that the reader may judge for himself the correctness of Nebylitsyn's (1966) conclusion that dynamism in excitation and in inhibition are relatively independent of each other (contrary to the Eysenckian assumption that they are inversely related to each other), Tables 4 and 5 show some of the data upon which he bases this conclusion. In Table 5 are

TABLE 4. CORRELATION MATRIX OF EEG MEASURES OF DYNAMISM

Measures	1	2	3	4	5	6	7
1. Duration of a-depression to first presentation of auditory stimulus		493*	334	447*	437	709‡	440
2. No. of stimulations to extinction of a-depression to auditory stimulus			665†	700‡	363	358	600†
3. Duration of a-depression to first presentation of visual stimulus				855‡	531*	334	622†
4. Mean duration of a-depression to ten presentations of visual stimulus					561†	449*	697‡
5. Mean duration of a-depression to 25 joint presentations of auditory CS and visual UCS						509*	513*
6. Mean conditioned a-depression to isolated presentation of auditory stimulus							411
7. No. of stimulations to extinction of a-depression							

Zeroes and decimal points omitted. $*P < 0.05$; $†P < 0.01$; $‡P < 0.001$; Data from twenty Ss reported by Nebylitsyn (1966, p. 318).

STRENGTH OF THE NERVOUS SYSTEM

shown two alternative factor-analytic solutions to the matrix of correlations between various EEG measures (presumed to be related to dynamism) shown in Table 4. On the left of Table 5 is shown the centroid solution; Nebylitsyn interprets Factor A as 'dynamism of the excitatory process' and Factor B as 'dynamism of the inhibitory process'. (Factor C, interpreted as 'α-reactivity', is of no importance in the present context.) On the right is shown a solution involving a general factor (g)—perhaps a general factor of equilibrium in dynamism—and two group factors (c_1 and c_2) which correspond, respectively, to Factors B and A in the centroid analysis.

TABLE 5. FACTOR ANALYSIS OF EEG MEASURES OF DYNAMISM

Measures	Centroid analysis							Bifactorial analysis			
	Factors							g	c_1	c_2	h^2
	Centroid			After rotation			h^2				
	I	II	III	A	B	C					
1. Duration of a-depression to first presentation of auditory stimulus	685	−430	−240	**823**	190	075	72	583		608	71
2. No. of stimulations to extinction of a-depression to auditory stimulus	745	261	−285	397	**731**	094	70	485	682		70
3. Duration of a-depression to first presentation of visual stimulus	806	394	218	193	**693**	**573**	85	709	593		85
4. Mean duration of a-depression to ten presentations of visual stimulus	875	309	149.	318	**700**	**536**	88	749	542		85
5. Mean duration of a-depression to 25 joint presentations of auditory CS and visual UCS	667	−151	248	469	206	**515**	53	749			56
6. Mean conditioned a-depression to isolated presentation of auditory stimulus	668	−516	026	**789**	026	278	71	680		497	71
7. No. of stimulations to extinction of conditioned a-depression	761	151	−076	398	**574**	345	61	684	479		70

Zeros and decimal points omitted. Factor-loadings higher than 0·50 are in bold type. Data from twenty Ss reported by Nebylitsyn (1966, p. 319).

From S. M. Sales, R. M. Guydosh and W. Iacono (1974). Journal of Personality and Social Psychology, *29*, 16-22, *by kind permission of the American Psychological Association*

RELATIONSHIP BETWEEN "STRENGTH OF THE NERVOUS SYSTEM" AND THE NEED FOR STIMULATION [1]

STEPHEN M. SALES, RAYMOND M. GUYDOSH, AND WILLIAM IACONO [2]

Carnegie-Mellon University

Research has suggested a relationship between the need for stimulation, as measured by the kinesthetic aftereffects task, and tendencies to "reduce" or "augment" incoming stimuli. Unfortunately, previous results are unclear. In Study I, college students with high auditory thresholds (who presumably reduce incoming stimulation) were particularly unresponsive to simple stimuli. In *both* simple and moderately complex stimulus situations, high-threshold subjects were more bored and expressed less enjoyment and interest than did low-threshold subjects, presumably because neither situation involved truly complex stimuli. These "insensitive" subjects also were particularly likely to drink coffee (a stimulant) and to have been born and raised in urban settings. In Study II, high-threshold college students appeared earlier for the experiment during the quiet summer session than did low-threshold subjects. They also placed especially many figures in a highly interactive model social setting compared to the number of figures they placed in a less interactive setting, relative to the numbers placed by more sensitive subjects, before judging the setting overcrowded. These results suggest that high-threshold subjects have a greater desire for social stimulation.

Recently, Sales (1971) has proposed a theory to explain differences among persons in the need for stimulation that involves three assumptions:

1. Exposure to a stimulus does not affect all individuals in the same way. Some subjects' nervous systems "damp down" (reduce) objective stimulus inputs, while other subjects' nervous systems "augment" these inputs.

2. Individuals have an "optimum" level of internal, received stimulation. If current stimulation evokes an internal response which is either "too small" or "too large," subjects attempt to change their input and react negatively to the current input. If current stimulation evokes an internal response which is "just right," subjects attempt to maintain this input and react positively to it.

3. The optimum level of internal, evoked stimulation tends to be similar for all individuals.

While not an intuitively obvious theory, it has led to a variety of testable propositions, and these have generally been confirmed. For instance, employing the kinesthetic aftereffects task as his measure of augmentation/reduction, Sales (1971) has observed that reducers (*a*) talk a great deal during group discussions, (*b*) exhibit high levels of activity in a deprived stimulus situation, (*c*) attend closely to complex verbal communications, and (*d*) react favorably to complex visual patterns. Eysenck (1955) and Petrie (1967) have independently shown that reducers on the kinesthetic aftereffects procedure are likely to be extraverts. Petrie (1967) has reported that kinesthetic aftereffects reducers tend to smoke, drink alcohol, and have large numbers of friends; she has also shown that double-blind ratings of campers' "activity level" are related to kinesthetic aftereffects performance, with reducers being rated as

[1] Stephen M. Sales died on October 8, 1972. Joel W. Goldstein assisted in the preparation of the final manuscript. The authors are indebted to Kenneth E. Friend for his assistance in programming the computer-controlled aspects of this experiment and to Esther G. Sales for her helpful comments on an earlier draft of this article. The laboratories in which this research was conducted were supported by Research Grant MH 07722 from the National Institute of Mental Health and Grant GU 1118 from the National Science Foundation. Raymond M. Guydosh was supported by a National Institute of Mental Health traineeship.

Requests for reprints should be addressed to Joel W. Goldstein, Department of Psychology, Carnegie-Mellon University, Pittsburgh, Pennsylvania 15213.

[2] Now at the University of Minnesota.

more active. Petrie, McCulloch, and Kazdin (1962) have reported that juvenile delinquents, who perhaps were led to their delinquency by a desire for "thrills," were more likely than control subjects to reduce on the kinesthetic aftereffects task, while Ryan and Foster (1967) have demonstrated that contact athletes (who presumably enjoy the intense stimulation of contact sports) also tend to reduce on this procedure. Finally, Sales (1972) has reported that kinesthetic aftereffects reducers respond particularly favorably to novel auditory and visual inputs and that they are particularly likely to seek out complex and interesting social situations.

However, certain problems attend the use of the kinesthetic aftereffects procedure. In particular, the assumption underlying use of this task (i.e., that it measures individuals' tendencies to reduce or augment incoming stimulation) rests on a very shaky data base. On the one hand, Petrie (1967), Ryan and Foster (1967), and Spilker and Callaway (1969) have reported findings which support this interpretation of the kinesthetic aftereffects measure. However, other investigators (Buchsbaum & Silverman, 1968; Morgan, Lezard, Prytulak, & Hilgard, 1970) have provided generally negative results.

If the kinesthetic aftereffects procedure does not measure tendencies to augment or reduce stimulation, of course, then the proper interpretation of findings involving this task becomes ambiguous. For this reason, it seems appropriate to search for other measures of augmentation and reduction, for only alternate measures can provide unambiguous support for the contention that variations in the need for stimulation are based on individuals' tendencies to reduce or to augment incoming stimuli.

Research directed toward the Pavlovian typology of nervous systems has suggested a number of potential alternate measures. Pavlov believed that dogs (and by extension, people) differed in the "strength of excitation" of their nervous systems. "Strong" individuals, Pavlov felt, were relatively insensitive to faint stimuli but were effective in dealing with intense stimulation; "weak" individuals, he believed, were relatively sensitive to faint stimuli but could not cope with

intense or massed stimulation. Gray (1964), in describing this aspect of Pavlov's typological system, argued that weak subjects augment incoming stimuli, while strong subjects reduce such inputs. Thus, any measure of strength should be appropriate for the present purposes. Fortunately, Russian research (e.g., Nebylitsyn, 1964) has suggested a number of fairly simple measures of this construct. And recently, Sales and Throop (1972) have reported significant (and reasonably large) correlations between three such indices of strength and the kinesthetic aftereffects measure.

If it is true that variations in the need for stimulation are based on individual's tendencies to reduce or augment incoming stimuli, then subjects with strong nervous systems should be high in this need, while weak subjects should be low. And while hardly conclusive, some data which support this prediction do exist. Specifically, Pavlov observed that strong dogs were extremely active when at liberty, as if they were attempting to expose themselves to a constantly varying (and therefore complex) environment. However, he noted that these same dogs exhibited a pronounced somnolence when placed on the experimental stand, as if the uniform stimuli present in this situation so bored these animals that they quickly fell asleep. (In addition, Siddle, Morrish, White, and Mangan, 1969, reported that extraverted humans tend to be strong, but they suggested that this relationship can be disrupted by high levels of neuroticism.) The present investigations were attempts to provide more conclusive evidence regarding the question: Is there a relationship between the need for stimulation and "strength of the nervous system"?

Study I

Method

Subjects

Thirty-nine male and 12 female undergraduates at Carnegie-Mellon University were subjects, and all received required experimental credit for their participation. (The usual equipment failures and misunderstood instructions resulted in slightly smaller Ns for many of the analyses reported below.)

Procedure

On entering the laboratory, the subject was taken to a dimly lighted, 76×72 inch soundproof cham-

S. SALES, R. GUYDOSH, AND W. IACONO

ber. The room was completely paneled in off-white acoustical tile and contained only a small table, a chair, a pair of headphones, and a stimulus board hidden by a beige cloth. All further instructions were delivered to the subject through an inter-communication system.

The subject's absolute loudness threshold was then determined using the method of limits procedure (Corso, 1967). Four series of tones were presented in an ascending, descending, descending, ascending order in 2-decibel steps. All tones were 1 kilohertz and lasted for three seconds; all were generated by a Hewlett-Packard signal generator (Model 200AB), fed through a Hewlett-Packard sound attenuator (Model 350B), and delivered to the subject binaurally through Lafayette stereophonic headphones (Model 99 0204).[3] Following Nebylitsyn (1964), we have employed this measure of threshold as the index of strength.[4] Subjects with high thresholds (e.g., insensitive subjects) are considered strong (and thus presumably high in the need for stimulation); subjects with low thresholds are considered weak (and thus presumably low in the need for stimulation). There was no particular difference between males and females in the threshold measure, nor did sex appear to affect any of the relationships to be reported below.

The subject's attention was then directed to a small response button. He was informed that, for each button press during the next 20 minutes, he would receive two seconds of auditory and visual stimulation; he was encouraged to press the response key as many or as few times as he wished. The subject's questions, if any, were answered. He then was asked to press the response key once "for practice" and then to respond as he wished. The practice trial ensured that all subjects were exposed to the experimental stimuli; it also initiated the 20-minute free-response period. The subject's responses during the entire 20-minute period, and during each of the 10-minute halves, were automatically recorded.

Two experimental conditions were employed. In the first, both the auditory and the visual stimuli were kept as simple as possible. The visual stimulus was a two-second presentation of a single 7½-watt, white light bulb placed in the center of a 17 × 17 inch board, while the auditory stimulus was a two-second presentation of a 60-decibel, 1-kilohertz tone. Twenty-four subjects were used in this condition.

[3] Presentation of these stimuli, and all other stimuli employed in Study I, was controlled by a DDP-116 computer.

[4] Prior to the administration of the threshold procedure, Nebylitsyn's $\Sigma(t)/t_{min}$ measure was obtained from all subjects following the procedure outlined by Sales and Throop (1972). It was originally hoped that this measure would be related to threshold and that these two independent indices of strength could be combined into a single measure. However, the $\Sigma(t)/t_{min}$ index related neither to threshold nor to any of the present dependent variables. Because of this apparent lack of validity, discussion of this measure has been omitted.

In the second condition, the two displays were somewhat more complex. The visual stimulus was presented via a 36 × 27 inch board containing 24 randomly placed, 7½-watt light bulbs; a combination of red, white, green, blue, and orange bulbs was employed. The apparatus provided a two-second presentation of either (a) 8 lights or (b) 16 lights after each response; the display which followed each response was randomly determined and varied over responses. The auditory stimulus was a two-second series of 1-kilohertz, 60-decibel tones. To create this display, two variables were separately randomized: a dichotomous signal variable (off–on) and a three-value temporal variable (¼ second, ½ second, and one second). These two variables were then paired to create a long series of tones which sounded somewhat like a transmission of Morse code. This series was broken into two-second segments, and one of these was transmitted to the subject after each response. Twenty-seven subjects were used in this condition.

Following the free-response period, the subject was asked to complete a short postexperimental questionnaire including a three-item scale of interest in and enjoyment of the free-response period (coefficient alpha was .925 for this scale in the present sample) and a one-item measure of boredom during the free-response period. Appropriately anchored 7-point scales followed each question in these parts of the questionnaire. The questionnaire also asked the subject to indicate whether or not he drank coffee and to describe the setting in which he had been born and raised (six response categories, from farm to city/suburb, were included). After the experiment, all subjects were thoroughly debriefed.

Results and Discussion

Effectiveness of the Manipulation

The data indicated that the experimental conditions generally achieved the desired impact. The stimuli presented in the simple condition evoked an average rating of 2.13 on a 7-point manipulation check (a rating of 7 indicated that the stimuli were perceived as "very complex"); those presented in the more complex condition evoked an average rating of 3.96 ($t = 4.64$, $df = 46$, $p < .001$).[5] However, neither the simple nor the complex situation was viewed as particularly complex (i.e., both mean values were below the midpoint on the 7-point response scale). Thus, the two experimental conditions used here seem to involve "simple" and "moderate" stimuli (rather than "simple" and "complex"

[5] Two-tailed significance tests have been employed for all statistics except the Spearman rank correlations, all of which tested directional hypotheses.

displays), and they shall be so labeled here-after.

Operant Responses

The two experimental conditions clearly evoked different response rates when compared for all subjects. Subjects in the simple condition gave an average of 140.4 responses during the entire experimental period, while subjects in the moderate condition gave an average of 297.3 responses ($F = 17.60$, $df = 1/43$, $p < .001$). This result replicated previous research and requires no particular discussion here. More interesting for the present concerns was the relation between strength of nervous system and response rate. In the simple condition, a Spearman correlation between strength and response rate yielded an r value of $-.41$ ($p = .03$) indicating significantly less responses for strong subjects than for weak subjects.[6] In the moderate condition, the Spearman correlation indicated a similar trend although at a less satisfactory level of significance ($r = -.26$, $p = .11$). Examination of Table 1 suggests that these results were due primarily to differences in the responsiveness to the two conditions of strong subjects who were presumably high in the need for stimulation ($t = 7.87$, $p < .001$), rather than to differences in the responsiveness of weak subjects ($t = 1.59$, ns). Further, the associated interaction between strength (categorized as above or below median threshold) and condition is significant ($F = 9.85$, $df = 1/43$, $p < .001$), supporting the present expectation that strong subjects are more affected by varying stimulation levels. Presumably, had it been possible to create a truly "complex" condition, strong subjects would have given more responses than weak subjects and a Spearman correlation would have been significant in the positive direction. Evidence for the latter supposition is discussed below.

Over both conditions of the experiment, there was a highly significant tendency for subjects' responses to decrease over time ($F = 19.78$, $df = 1/44$, $p < .001$), and this tendency was somewhat stronger in the sim-

[6] An apparent nonlinear but monotone relation between strength and response measures suggested the use of the Spearman correlation.

TABLE 1

NUMBER OF RESPONSES AS A FUNCTION OF STRENGTH AND EXPERIMENTAL CONDITION

Strength	Experimental condition	
	Simple	Moderate
Strong	22.7 (10)	292.8 (14)
Weak	238.4 (12)	303.0 (11)

Note. Cell *n*s are given in parentheses.

ple condition than in the moderate condition ($F = 3.58$, $df = 1/44$, $p < .10$). However, while there appeared to be some tendency for strong subjects to satiate more quickly than weak subjects, the Strength $\times$ Blocks interaction failed to approach accepted levels of significance.

Questionnaire Data

There was slightly greater interest and slightly less boredom in the moderate condition than in the simple condition; however, the differences in the two conditions did not approach customary significance levels for either measure. The more important consideration for the present issue is the relation between these two measures and strength of nervous system. In each condition, strength correlated negatively with interest and enjoyment (simple condition: Spearman $r = -.26$, $p = .11$; moderate condition: Spearman $r = -.38$, $p = .03$). Similarly, as expected, in each condition, strength correlated positively with boredom (simple condition: Spearman $r = .49$, $p = .01$; moderate condition: Spearman $r = .36$, $p = .04$). Thus, in both conditions, strong subjects perceived the situations as less interesting and more boring than their weak counterparts. These results were in accord with the prediction that strong subjects, being presumably high in the need for stimulation, require greater external stimulation to reach an optimum internal level.

Some question might be raised as to whether strong subjects should be more favorable to the somewhat more interesting condition. As previously mentioned, neither condition was perceived as very complex. Since strong subjects are presumably high in the

S. Sales, R. Guydosh, and W. Iacono

need for stimulation, one might expect them to be relatively negative toward both of the fairly simple conditions used in this experiment. In any event there is no evidence that strong subjects are negative toward experimental settings in the abstract. In an earlier study (Sales, 1972), kinesthetic aftereffect reducers, who are presumed to be strong (Sales & Throop, 1972), responded more favorably than kinesthetic aftereffects augmenters to a highly complex experimental manipulation which involved "an experimental movie, a strobe light, a celestial light, a black light (with appropriate posters), and . . . a taped program of song fragments, motorcycle noises, and other miscellany [Sales, 1972, pp. 57–58]." Apparently, then, strong subjects (who are presumably high in the need for stimulation) are relatively negative toward both simple and moderate stimuli (such as those employed in the two conditions of the present investigation) but are quite positive toward extremely complex stimuli.

In addition to the above results, subjects' responses to the questionnaire indicated a significant relationship between strength and tendencies to drink coffee (a stimulant). A majority (62%) of the strong (i.e., high need for stimulation) subjects reported that they did drink coffee, while a majority (68%) of the weak subjects reported that they did not ($\chi^2 = 4.46$, $p < .05$). This finding replicates earlier results (e.g., Petrie, 1967), although previous research employed the kinesthetic aftereffects task. Finally, the data indicated a mild tendency for strong subjects to have been born and raised in urban settings (city or suburb) and for weak subjects to have been born and raised in environments which can perhaps be conceptualized as less intense ($\chi^2 = 2.93$, $p < .10$). This result was a replication of an earlier (but unpublished) finding of the first author. It was particularly important since it suggests an experiential basis for strength and thus for the need for stimulation. However, the relationship between childhood environment and strength is neither highly significant (in a statistical sense) nor clearly understood, and therefore this finding remains a suggestion for further research rather than a definitive observation in itself.

Study II

Further evidence for a relation between strength of nervous system and the need for stimulation may be investigated using situations involving social types of stimulation. Social situations might create greater complexity, and stimulation from social sources probably forms the largest proportion of stimulus input a person receives in a natural environment. Thus, it would be important to consider such sources in theorizing about possible experiential bases of strength. Finally, observations discussed previously which relate to such phenomena as extraversion, activity level, or delinquency seem based on social sources of stimulation.

One possible source of social stimulation consists of input received from those people in one's immediate vicinity. Desor (1972) has proposed that such stimulation constitutes a basis for one's perception of overcrowding and has suggested that such perceptions may depend on individual differences. Personal differences in the need for stimulation as based on strength of nervous system would seem to offer an obvious explanation for differing perceptions of "too much" stimulation.

Method

Subjects

Seventeen males and 13 females were recruited by campus newspaper advertisements and notices posted on the Carnegie-Mellon University campus during a summer session. All subjects were college-age students who had never taken advanced psychology courses. Each subject was paid $1.50 for about 30 minutes of participation.

Procedure

Immediately on the subject's arrival at the lab, the experimenter made note of the exact time on a watch set from time given by a commercial radio station. These data were for use in a time of arrival measure. The subject was then greeted, asked some preliminary questions including occupation and background in psychology, and then directed to a seat in one corner of the lab and given instructions for the determination of absolute loudness threshold. The experimenter then left the room, and threshold was determined using the method described in Study I. After the threshold determination, the subject's attention was directed to two model rooms in an opposite corner of the lab. These models and the accompanying instructions and equipment were constructed according to the methodology of Desor (1972). The subject was asked to imagine that the models represented rooms and that an accompanying set of figures constructed of clothes pins and pipe cleaners represented people. He was then told to read the accompanying instructions, follow them, and to signal the experimenter (who again left the room) when he had completed the task. The instructions required the subject to imagine that one of the model rooms represented an airport waiting room and the other, a lounge area in which a cocktail party was being held. He was instructed to place in the rooms "as many people as you can without making it too crowded." After the task, the subject was debriefed and paid.

Results and Discussion

Arrival Time

Arrival time (except for four subjects who arrived unnoticed) was compared with the scheduled time on the subject's appointment. Because the experiment took place during a comparatively quiet summer session with few activities and diversions on campus, it was hypothesized that participation in the experiment itself would serve as a source of social stimulation. Strong subjects, who are presumably high in the need for stimulation, should have felt particularly deprived of social stimulation during the summer session and consequently should demonstrate a greater desire for a possible source of stimulation by arriving early for their experimental appointment. Weak subjects should have felt somewhat less deprived and thus not arrive as early. In accordance with the hypothesis, the Spearman correlation between strength and number of minutes early indicated a significant positive relation between the two measures (Spearman $r = .34$, $p = .04$), demonstrating that strong subjects were more attracted to a potential source of social stimulation.

Environmental Settings

Since strong subjects are presumably more desirous of social stimulation, it was expected that they would place more figures in each of the two social settings before admitting to overcrowding than would weak subjects. As expected, there was a positive relation between strength and number of

TABLE 2
NUMBER OF "PEOPLE" PLACED IN EACH SOCIAL SETTING AS A FUNCTION OF STRENGTH

Strength	Setting	
	Airport	Cocktail party
Strong	26.5	37.9
Weak	20.7	23.5

Note. $n = 15$ subjects in each cell.

people placed in both the airport waiting room and the cocktail party setting (airport: Spearman $r = .24$, $p = .10$; cocktail party: Spearman $r = .51$, $p = .002$). Thus, it appears that strong subjects welcome the greater social stimulation accompanying a greater number of people present in social settings.

In addition, there was a significant main effect in the analysis of variance due to social setting ($F = 13.16$, $df = 1/28$, $p < .001$) which duplicates previous findings and needs no further discussion here. Of further interest is the significant Strength (again categorized by dividing the subjects at the median threshold) × Setting interaction ($F = 4.83$, $df = 1/28$, $p < .05$). As indicated in Table 2, strong subjects appeared to be differentially affected by changing social settings ($t = 3.18$, $p < .01$), while weak subjects were not ($t = 1.59$, ns). This result agreed with those of Study I and with the supposition that strong subjects, being high in the need for stimulation, are particularly sensitive to changes in stimulation levels.

CONCLUSION

The results of these two studies offered reasonable support for the hypothesized relation between strength of nervous system and the need for stimulation. Strong subjects (i.e., those with high auditory thresholds) were much more responsive to relatively more complex stimuli than they were to simple stimuli; weak subjects exhibited no particular difference in this respect. Strong subjects were somewhat more bored by both a simple and moderately complex situation and enjoyed each of the situations (neither of which was viewed as complex) less than

S. Sales, R. Guydosh, and W. Iacono

weak subjects. Strong subjects were more likely than weak ones to use a stimulant (coffee) voluntarily; strong subjects were somewhat more likely than weak subjects to have been born and raised in (presumably stimulating) urban environments. Strong subjects tended to demonstrate a greater desire to experience a possible source of social stimulation by arriving earlier for experimental appointments than did weak subjects. Finally, strong subjects placed greater numbers of figures in social settings before judging them too crowded, suggesting that they prefer greater social stimulation than do weak subjects. These results were all congruent with the contention that strength of nervous system is related to the need for stimulation, and they supported the hypothesis (Sales, 1971) that nervous systems which reduce incoming stimuli provide the basis for this need.

REFERENCES

Buchsbaum, M., & Silverman, J. Stimulus intensity control and the cortical evoked response. *Psychosomatic Medicine*, 1968, 30, 12–22.

Corso, J. F. *The experimental psychology of sensory behavior.* New York: Holt, Rinehart & Winston, 1967.

Desor, J. A. Toward a psychological theory of crowding. *Journal of Personality and Social Psychology*, 1972, 21, 79–83.

Eysenck, H. J. Cortical inhibition, figural aftereffect, and theory of personality. *Journal of Abnormal and Social Psychology*, 1955, 51, 94–106.

Gray, J. A. (Ed.) *Pavlov's typology.* New York: Macmillan, 1964.

Morgan, A. H., Lezard, F., Prytulak, S., & Hilgard, E. R. Augmenters, reducers, and their reaction to cold pressor pain in waking and suggested hypnotic analgesia. *Journal of Personality and Social Psychology*, 1970, 16, 5–11.

Nebylitsyn, V. D. An investigation of the connection between sensitivity and strength of the nervous system. In J. A. Gray (Ed.), *Pavlov's typology.* New York: Macmillan, 1964.

Petrie, A. *Individuality in pain and suffering.* Chicago: University of Chicago Press, 1967.

Petrie, A., McCulloch, R., & Kazdin, P. The perceptual characteristics of juvenile delinquents. *Journal of Nervous and Mental Disorders*, 1962, 134, 415–421.

Ryan, E. D., & Foster, R. Athletic participation and perceptual augmentation and reduction. *Journal of Personality and Social Psychology*, 1967, 6, 472–476.

Sales, S. M. Need for stimulation as a factor in social behavior. *Journal of Personality and Social Psychology*, 1971, 19, 124–134.

Sales, S. M. Need for stimulation as a factor in preferences for different stimuli. *Journal of Personality Assessment*, 1972, 36, 55–61.

Sales, S. M., & Throop, W. F. Relationship between kinesthetic aftereffects and "strength of the nervous system." *Psychophysiology*, 1972, 9, 492–497.

Siddle, D. A. T., Morrish, R. B., White, K. D., & Morgan, G. L. Relation of visual sensitivity to extraversion. *Journal of Experimental Research in Personality*, 1969, 3, 264–267.

Spilker, B., & Callaway, E. 'Augmenting' and 'reducing' in averaged visual evoked responses to sine wave light. *Psychophysiology*, 1969, 6, 49–57.

(Received May 24, 1972)

From J. -Y. Frigon (1976). British Journal of Psychology, *67*, 467-474, *by kind permission of the author and the British Psychological Society*

EXTRAVERSION, NEUROTICISM AND STRENGTH OF THE NERVOUS SYSTEM

By JEAN-YVES FRIGON

Department of Psychology, University of Montreal, Canada

The hypothesized identity of the dimensions of extraversion–introversion and strength of the nervous system was tested on four groups of nine subjects (neurotic extraverts, stable extraverts, neurotic introverts, stable introverts). Strength of the subjects' nervous system was estimated using the electroencephalographic (EEG) variant of extinction with reinforcement. Introverted subjects were found to have weak nervous systems, according to the EEG index, while extraverted subjects had strong nervous systems, thus confirming the hypothesis. It was also found that the dimension of strength of the nervous system was unrelated to differences in neuroticism. The results are interpreted as adding support to Eysenck's theory relating differences in extraversion–introversion to differences in cortical arousal.

Since the publication of Gray's book (1964) on the dimension known in Russia as 'strength of the nervous system (NS)' and his reinterpretation of it as a dimension of arousability, few studies have tried to relate that dimension of individual differences to measures of personality. According to Gray (1967) and Eysenck (1966, 1967), the dimension of personality that would best correspond to the dimension of strength of the NS is that of extraversion–introversion since they both seem to be dependent on differences in arousability. Gray (1967), in an excellent analysis, has argued that the most plausible hypothesis is that 'the dimensions of strength of the nervous system and introversion–extraversion are identical, with the weak nervous system corresponding to the introvert' (p. 153), an hypothesis which is also adopted by Eysenck (1967).

Despite the fact that the hypothesis relating introversion–extraversion to strength of the NS is theoretically well founded, studies which have tried to validate it experimentally have produced discouragingly deceptive and contradictory results (Mangan, 1967; Mangan & Farmer, 1967; Zhorov & Yermolayeva-Tomina, 1972). Considering that these results all failed to confirm the correspondence between introversion–extraversion and strength of the NS, Zhorov & Yermolayeva-Tomina (1972) conclude 'that either (1) the hypothesis of the relation between introversion and weakness is, despite its plausibility, wrong, or (2) the method of determining strength employed in these experiments was not adequate for the task of measuring the strength of the nerve cells of the brain structures...' (p. 267) and they add that 'the latter assumption is probably closer to the truth'.

It is also our opinion that this latter assumption reflects the truth. The relationship between extraversion–introversion and strength of the NS has been studied with an estimation of nervous system strength obtained by the reaction time (RT) method (Mangan & Farmer, 1967; Zhorov & Yermolayeva-Tomina, 1972). This method, however, does not seem appropriate to such a study for two main reasons.

First, the RT method provides only an indirect index of nervous system strength. According to Nebylitsyn (1972, p. 165), there are now two well-validated methods which yield a direct index of the strength of the NS. These are the 'induction' and

JEAN-YVES FRIGON

the 'extinction with reinforcement' methods, and the most feasible of the two is the electroencephalographic (EEG) variant of extinction with reinforcement (Teplov & Nebylitsyn, 1969; Nebylitsyn, 1972, pp. 157–168). It should be noted that Soviet researchers, when exploring the relationship between nervous systems differing in strength and their characteristic reactions to varying conditions, such as absolute sensitivity or sensory stimulation, have always used one or more direct referent indices of nervous system strength. However, those studies relating strength of the NS to introversion–extraversion (Mangan & Farmer, 1967; Zhorov & Yermolayeva-Tomina, 1972) have not employed a direct referent index of nervous system strength. This is unfortunate since the indirect index provided by the RT method may not be sensitive enough to differences in strength.

Second, although the index of nervous system strength obtained with the RT method is said to correlate positively with other indices of strength, this correlation has not been very well validated. Nebylitsyn (1972, pp. 191–208) has argued that the RT method can be used to estimate the strength of the NS, provided that one uses the ratios of latency for a given intensity to latency to the highest stimulus intensity, rather than the absolute magnitudes of response latency. This conclusion is based on two studies in which the RTs of two groups of subjects (strong and weak NSs) are measured under six levels of stimulus intensity and two conditions – non-caffeine and caffeine – (Nebylitsyn, 1960: see Nebylitsyn, 1972, p. 192). Using experimental design terminology, these situations define a $P \times Q \times R$ split-plot factorial design with repeated measures on the last two factors (Kirk, 1968, p. 298). However, it is evident, from the analysis of variance table presented by Nebylitsyn (1972, p. 200), that a $P \times Q \times R$ factorial design for independent measures on all three factors was used (Kirk, 1968, p. 217), and this analysis is inappropriate for these data.

The sums of squares of the main and interaction effects would be identical under both techniques of analysis. But, with the analysis of variance appropriate to this type of repeated measures design, the error term would be divided into four parts, the partitioning of the degrees of freedom would be different, and the F ratios would accordingly be computed differently. Without the raw data it is difficult to evaluate exactly how the use of the appropriate analysis design would have modified Nebylitsyn's results. Nevertheless, it is very likely that the between-subjects F ratio has been inflated due to the improper analysis. Consequently, the significant strength effect reported by Nebylitsyn may not really be significant. This inappropriate analysis may not invalidate completely the RT method. But it surely reveals an inadequate validation procedure and puts some doubts on its appropriateness as a measure of nervous system strength. Therefore, the use of this method may account for the contradictory results which have been obtained in studies on the relationship between extraversion–introversion and strength of the NS.

The term 'extinction with reinforcement' refers to a temporary decrement of a conditioned response (CR) which occurs through multiple presentations of the conditioned stimulus–unconditioned stimulus (CS–UCS) in rapid succession, a procedure which theoretically has an exhausting effect on the nerve cells. Briefly, the method consists in presenting subjects with a number of CS–UCS combinations in which the intertrial interval is shorter than under normal conditions. A decrease

Extraversion, neuroticism and strength of nervous system

in the magnitude of the CR at the end of this series of rapid presentations of CS–UCS is taken as an indication of weakness of the NS; the absence of such a decrease or an increase in the magnitude of the CR is an indication of strength of the NS (cf. Gray, 1964; Nebylitsyn, 1972; and Teplov & Nebylitsyn, 1969, for a thorough discussion of the theoretical basis and a more detailed account of the method of extinction with reinforcement). Two types of CRs have usually been used with this method: the first is what the Soviet psychologists call the photochemical reflex (photochemical variant of extinction with reinforcement); the second is based on the conditioned EEG desynchronization of alpha waves (EEG variant of extinction with reinforcement). The latter variant is less time consuming and is preferred by Teplov & Nebylitsyn (1969) and Nebylitsyn (1972).

The purpose of the present study was to test the hypothesis of the correspondence between introversion–extraversion and strength of the NS. The referent index of nervous strength was the EEG variant of extinction with reinforcement. It was hypothesized that introverts would show a decrease in the magnitude of the CR during extinction with reinforcement, and as such have a weak nervous system, while extraverts would show a stability or an increase in the magnitude of the CR, and thus have a strong nervous system. In statistical terms, we predicted an interaction between extraversion–introversion and measures of the magnitude of the CR during extinction with reinforcement.

METHOD

Subjects

The subjects were 36 male volunteers who were divided into four equal groups. They were all undergraduate students and were paid $3.00 for their participation. They were selected from a pool of 145 possible subjects on the basis of their scores on the Eysenck Personality Inventory (EPI), form A. The EPI was administered to all of the 145 students. Total mean scores and standard deviations were 11·75 and 3·10 respectively on the Extraversion (E) scale, and 9·68 and 3·85 respectively on the Neuroticism (N) scale. Experimental subjects were selected so that their scores on the test differed by more than one standard deviation from the mean on each of the four possible configurations of personality: high and low Extraversion (scores of 15 or more or 9 or less on the E scale) and high and low Neuroticism (scores of 14 or more or 6 or less on the N scale). There was no significant difference in N score between the two groups who differed significantly on E score ($t = 0·348$; d.f. $= 34$, n.s.); similarly, there was no significant difference in E score for the subjects high and low on N score ($t = 0·579$; d.f. $= 34$, n.s.).

Apparatus

Electroencephalographic activity was recorded on a Beckman–Offner Type R dynograph with AC/DC couplers. Two derivations were taken from the occipital region with Beckman–Offner silver/silver chloride skin electrodes (8 mm in diameter) filled with Beckman–Offner electrode paste.

During the experiment, subjects were seated in a dark soundproof room. Tones were presented through a speaker by a Heathkit sound generator. The intensity of the tones was measured by a Bruël and Kjaer sound level meter (meter model 2203; octave filter type 1613; microphone 4131).

Visual stimuli were presented from the exterior on a white screen superimposed on a one-way mirror that was fitted in one wall of the soundproof room. Grason–Stadler electronic timers and programming apparatus were used to control the duration of the CS, UCS, and interstimulus interval (ISI). Intertrial intervals (ITIs) were programmed on a film strip which activated the timers controlling the presentation of the stimuli.

The experimenter could communicate with subjects at all times through a two-way intercom.

Jean-Yves Frigon

The experimenter also monitored the subject and the stimuli from the outside, throughout the experiment, with a videoscope camera that was located inside the soundproof room.

Design and procedure

Upon entering the laboratory, the subject was seated in a comfortable armchair inside the soundproof room. General information about the apparatus and instructions about the nature of the experiment were given during the application of the electrodes. No information was given about the relationship between the CS and UCS. The subjects were tested in random order. The experimenter did not know, during testing, to which personality group they belonged.

Eleven of the subjects (six extraverts and five introverts) were tested in the morning and the remaining 25 subjects (12 extraverts and 13 introverts) in the afternoon. The effects of time of day on performance differences between introverts and extraverts are well known (Colquhoun & Corcoran, 1964). Since, however, an approximately equal number of extraverts and introverts were respectively tested in the morning and in the afternoon, any systematic effect of time of day on the conditioning data should have been prevented. Moreover, although time of day effects have been established with regard to subjects' performance, it is dubious whether alpha conditioning and indices of nervous system strength would be affected by this variable.

As usual in alpha conditioning studies, some subjects (four introverts and two extraverts) had to be rejected for various reasons, such as for not showing sufficient alpha waves or for being under heavy medication. These subjects were replaced with subjects from the original pool. They all met the criteria for subjects' selection set forth above.

The conditioning parameters were the following: the CS was a tone, 1000 Hz, 70 dB, of 5 sec duration. In most alpha-blocking conditioning studies, the UCS is usually a flash of light. The CR thus obtained, however, is very labile and the disappearance of the CR may be due to a decrease in novelty of the UCS, instead of being the result of extinction with reinforcement. To solve this problem, Teplov & Nebylitsyn (1969) and Nebylitsyn (1972) presented subjects with reinforcing stimuli which they called 'activating' stimuli. These stimuli were not merely lights, but slides of pictures with instructions to remember the details shown and to be prepared to answer questions in a post-experimental inquiry. Nebylitsyn reported that, with this type of reinforcement, alpha-blocking CRs were found to be very stable for most subjects. One can either use the same or different slides throughout the trials with comparable results (Nebylitsyn, 1972, p. 165). In the present study, such an 'activating' UCS was used and the same slide was presented in all trials. This slide was a representation of a pyramid in the Teotihuacan Valley (Mexico). The interval between CS onset and slide onset (ISI) was 1·5 sec. The slide was presented for 3·5 sec and both the CS and UCS ended simultaneously.

The conditioning and extinction with reinforcement paradigm called for the following conditions.

Habituation. First, the orienting reaction to the CS was extinguished with the tone presented alone until there was no alpha-blocking on three consecutive trials. The ITIs varied from 15–20 sec. A random number table was used to generate the sequence of ITIs. Sequences of ITIs also ranging from 15–20 sec were used during conditioning, differential conditioning, and CR baseline conditions, as well.

Conditioning. The conditioning paradigm consisted of 50 trials. On 45 occasions, CS–UCS were paired with an ISI of 1·5 sec. To observe the development of the CR, five CS-alone test trials were given on trials 10, 14, 22, 28 and 45. All 50 trials were given, even though the criterion of conditioning was an anticipatory response to the CS on three consecutive trials.

Differential conditioning. After the 50 conditioning trials, which in all cases were more than necessary to produce a stable CR, differential conditioning was begun, with a 500 Hz, 50 dB tone. Reinforced (CS–UCS) and unreinforced (differential stimulus) trials were presented according to the Gellerman table (Stevens, 1951, p. 533) and were continued until the differential stimulus did not produce alpha-blocking on three consecutive trials.

CR baseline. Before proceeding with the extinction with reinforcement series, 15 trials were given, 12 of these being reinforced trials (CS–UCS), and the other three being CS-alone test trials (trials 3, 11, 15). The mean duration of alpha-blocking in seconds on those three test trials was taken as the CR baseline prior to extinction with reinforcement. This measure of CR baseline is the only departure from Nebylitsyn's procedure, which measured it on the first three test trials of the extinction with reinforcement series. Since the ITI during that series of trials

Extraversion, neuroticism and strength of nervous system

Table 1. *Mean number of trials to reach the criterion of habituation,
of conditioning and of differential conditioning*

Group	Habituation		Conditioning		Differential conditioning	
	$\overline{X}$	s	$\overline{X}$	s	$\overline{X}$	s
E N	11·67	3·81	8·44	2·01	9·11	2·98
E S	15·22	6·94	8·22	2·22	10·00	5·36
I N	15·89	2·47	8·00	3·08	8·67	3·08
I S	13·56	4·61	8·56	2·01	8·44	2·88

is different from the ITI used during conditioning, it seemed preferable to have a measure of CR baseline with conditions identical to those prevailing during conditioning.

Extinction with reinforcement. In the extinction with reinforcement trials, subjects were presented with 48 CS–UCS pairings at ITIs of 4–5 sec, compared with 15–20 sec ITIs during conditioning. To observe the evolution of the CR, 12 test trials (CS-alone) were given. These occurred after trials 3, 10, 12, 19, 21, 24, 31, 34, 36, 39, 41 and 48. It should be noted that the ratio of reinforced/unreinforced trials by blocks of three successive test trials was the same here as it was during the measure of CR baseline. The ordering of the test trials also prevented the development of a temporal anticipation of CS-alone.

CR magnitude was the mean duration of alpha-blocking in seconds during the action of CS on blocks of three successive test trials (means of test trials 1–3, 4–6, 7–9, 10–12). Following Nebylitsyn's procedure, the mean of three successive test trials was taken to assure a more stable measure of CR magnitude, since there is always considerable trial-to-trial variability in EEG conditioning.

RESULTS

As reported by Teplov & Nebylitsyn (1969) and Nebylitsyn (1972), habituation, conditioning and differential conditioning, were fairly easy to obtain in all subjects. Means and standard deviations of the number of trials necessary to reach the criterion in each of these conditions are shown in Table 1. A 2×2 (high and low E and N) analysis of variance was performed on this variable, on each of the conditions of habituation, conditioning and differential conditioning. Neither of the F ratios computed in these three analyses revealed a significant effect of E or N. This indicates that the rates of habituation, of conditioning and of differential conditioning were approximately equivalent for all groups.

The main hypothesis of the present study predicted a significant E × blocks of trials interaction. This was tested with a $2 \times 2 \times 5$ analysis of variance with repeated measures on the last factor. This analysis compared CRs magnitudes of the four personality groups (two levels of E and two levels of N) on the five successive blocks of three test trials (baseline was labelled as block 1). On the basis of the *a priori* hypothesis about the E × blocks interaction, a direct linear trend analysis of that interaction was performed (Kirk, 1968, p. 190). This analysis is presented in Table 2.

It can be seen that the linear trend of the E × blocks of trials interaction is significant. The CRs magnitudes over blocks of three test trials for E and I subjects are shown in Fig. 1. It appears that introverts are more cortically aroused than extraverts at the beginning of the blocks of test trials.

An analysis of the simple effects of blocks of test trials at each level of E reveals that introverts show a gradual decrease of the magnitude of the CR from blocks

Jean-Yves Frigon

Table 2. *Analysis of variance of CR magnitude (sec)*

Source	d.f.	m.s.	F
Between subjects	35		
E	1	26·07	7·22*
N	1	1·20	< 1
E × N	1	7·57	2·10
Subj w. groups	32	3·61	—
Within subjects	144		
Blocks	4	10·36	8·93**
E × blocks	4		
linear	1	6·32	4·42*
residual	3	0·43	< 1
Blocks × subj			
w. groups (linear)	32	1·43	—
N × blocks	4	2·54	2·19
E × N × blocks	4	0·55	< 1
Blocks × subj w. groups	128	1·16	—

$* P < 0.05; \quad ** P < 0.01.$

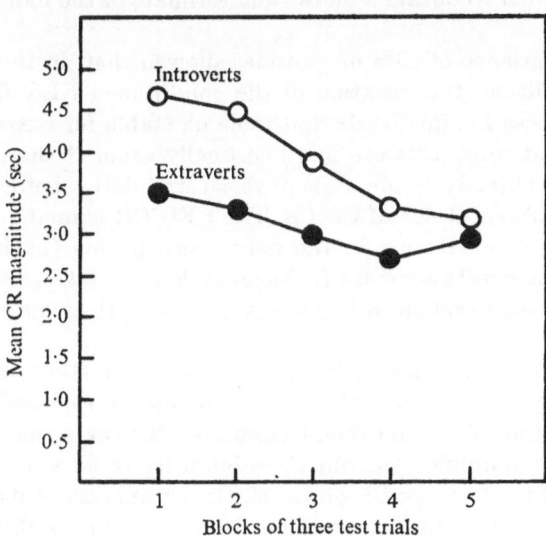

Fig. 1. Mean CR magnitudes over blocks of three test trials for extraverts and introverts.

1 to 5 ($F = 8.47$, d.f. $= 4, 128$, $P < 0.001$). However, the small decrease of the magnitude of the CR for extraverts is not significant ($F = 2.10$, d.f. $= 4, 128$, $P > 0.05$), thus explaining the significant linear trend of the E × blocks of trials interaction.

Table 2 also shows that Neuroticism did not affect CRs magnitudes either alone or in interaction with other factors.

DISCUSSION

The fact that extraverts and introverts did not differ in their rate of conditioning should not be taken as an argument against Eysenck's well-known view on the positive correlation between introversion and conditionability (Eysenck, 1965,

Extraversion, neuroticism and strength of nervous system

1967; Eysenck & Levey, 1972). Indeed, Eysenck (1967) and Eysenck & Levey (1972) have shown that, in conditioning studies, the parameters of stimulation must be carefully chosen, since it is possible to have conditions favouring introverted or extraverted subjects. The purpose of the present study was not to test the conditionability of the subjects, and it may be that the particular conditions of the experiment did not favour the better conditioning of one group or the other.

On the other hand, rates of habituation, of conditioning and of differential conditioning are related to another dimension of the neo-Pavlovian typology of individual differences, namely 'dynamism of the nervous system' (Gray, 1967; Teplov & Nebylitsyn, 1969; Nebylitsyn, 1972). Gray (1967) has already suggested that the dimensions of extraversion–introversion and dynamism of the NS are independent and the present results also lead us to this conclusion. It should be noted, however, that rates of habituation, of conditioning and of differential conditioning are only some of the many EEG indices of the dynamism of the NS (cf. Nebylitsyn, 1972, pp. 86–112). Therefore, it would be important to measure more of these indices in order to obtain a more valid estimate of the independence of these two dimensions.

The analysis of variance of CRs magnitudes showed that, in the 'extinction with reinforcement' condition, the duration of the conditioned EEG desynchronization progressively decreases for introverts and remains stable for extraverts. It is clear from the results that introverts are more cortically aroused than extraverts when both are exposed to objectively identical physical stimulation before proceeding with the series of rapid presentations of the CS. The EEG CR is unaffected in extraverts by the building up of excitation in the nerve cells during 'extinction with reinforcement', while introverts show a CR decrease. This is taken as an indication of weakness of the nervous system in introverts and strength of the nervous system in extraverts.

This finding suggests that Gray's (1967) and Eysenck's (1967) hypothesis on the identity between the dimensions of extraversion–introversion and strength of the NS is empirically sound. It should then be expected that extraverted subjects react, in general, as if they amplified the objective intensity of all stimulation and introverted subjects as if they damped it down (cf. Gray's analysis, 1964). Moreover, this indicates that most of the differences found between subjects differing in nervous system strength (cf. Gray, 1964; Nebylitsyn, 1972; Nebylitsyn & Gray, 1972) also apply to the extraversion–introversion dimension of personality. It has already been shown that introverts have lower auditory thresholds than extraverts (Smith, 1968). Shigehisa & Symons (1973) have also established that auditory sensitivity decreases in introverts, in reaction to an increase of the intensity of visual stimulation, and increases in extraverts. These results are consistent with data on the differences between individuals with strong and weak nervous systems. Gray (1964) suggests that the reactions of the weak vs. strong nervous systems individuals in relation to drugs, susceptibility to fatigue, etc., should also apply to the introversion–extraversion dimension of personality. These predictions are theoretically plausible, but they have yet to be empirically validated.

The results of this experiment may be interpreted as giving some support to Eysenck's theory linking differences in extraversion–introversion to differences in

JEAN-YVES FRIGON

cortical arousal. Furthermore, these results also confirm Gray's (1967) view that the dimension identified in Russia as 'strength of the nervous system' is not related to Eysenck's measure of neuroticism.

As indicated earlier, the discrepancy between the present results and those obtained in previous studies could be attributed to the indirect nature of the index of nervous system strength, which probably does not allow a good discrimination among subjects on the dimension of strength of the NS. Thus, it can be seen that it is important to use a direct referent index of this dimension when exploring its relationship to other individual differences characteristics.

REFERENCES

COLQUHOUN, W. P. & CORCORAN, D. W. J. (1964). The effects of time of day and social isolation on the relationship between temperament and performance. *Br. J. soc. clin. Psychol.* **3**, 226–231.

EYSENCK, H. J. (1965). Extraversion and the acquisition of eyeblink and GSR conditioned responses. *Psychol. Bull.* **63**, 258–270.

EYSENCK, H. J. (1966). Conditioning, introversion–extraversion and the strength of the nervous system. In V. D. Nebylitsyn (ed.), Symposium 9, *18th Int. Congr. Psychol., Moscow,* 33–44.

EYSENCK, H. J. (1967). *The Biological Basis of Personality.* Springfield, Ill.: Thomas.

EYSENCK, H. J. & LEVEY, A. (1972). Conditioning, introversion–extraversion and the strength of the nervous system. In V. D. Nebylitsyn & J. A. Gray (eds), *Biological Bases of Individual Behavior.* New York: Academic Press.

GRAY, J. A. (ed.) (1964). *Pavlov's Typology.* Oxford: Pergamon Press.

GRAY, J. A. (1967). Strength of the nervous system, introversion–extraversion, conditionability and arousal. *Behav. Res. Ther.* **5**, 151–169.

KIRK, R. E. (1968). *Experimental Design: Procedures for the Behavioral Sciences.* Belmont, Cal.: Brooks/Cole.

MANGAN, G. L. (1967). Studies of the relationship between Neo-Pavlovian properties of higher nervous activity and Western personality dimensions: IV. A factor analytic study of extraversion and flexibility, and the sensitivity and mobility of the nervous system. *J. exp. Res. Person.* **2**, 124–127.

MANGAN, G. L. & FARMER, R. G. (1967). Studies of the relationship between Neo-Pavlovian properties of higher nervous activity and Western personality dimensions: I. The relationship of nervous strength and sensitivity to extraversion. *J. exp. Res. Person.* **2**, 101–106.

NEBYLITSYN, V. D. (1972). *Fundamental Properties of the Human Nervous System.* New York: Plenum Press.

NEBYLITSYN, V. D. & GRAY, J. A. (eds) (1972). *Biological Bases of Individual Behavior.* New York: Academic Press.

SHIGEHISA, T. & SYMONS, J. R. (1973). Reliability of auditory responses under increasing intensity of visual stimulation in relation to personality. *Br. J. Psychol.* **64**, 375–381.

SMITH, S. L. (1968). Extraversion and sensory threshold. *Psychophysiology* **5**, 293–299.

STEVENS, S. S. (ed.) (1951). *Handbook of Experimental Psychology.* New York: Wiley.

TEPLOV, B. M. & NEBYLITSYN, V. D. (1969). Investigation of the properties of the nervous system as an approach to the study of individual psychological differences. In M. Cole & I. Maltzman (eds), *A Handbook of Contemporary Soviet Psychology.* New York: Basic Books.

ZHOROV, P. A. & YERMOLAYEVA-TOMINA, L. B. (1972). Concerning the relation between extraversion and strength of the nervous system. In V. D. Nebylitsyn & J. A. Gray (eds), *Biological Bases of Individual Behavior.* New York: Academic Press.

(Manuscript received 17 June 1975; revised manuscript received 12 September 1975)

Section Three

Introversion/Extraversion

Editorial Commentary

on

Introversion/Extraversion

In 1955 Hans Eysenck first published what was to become one of the most controversial theories of individual differences in psychology. The two original tenets of the theory integrated aspects of the earlier writings of Pavlov, Hull and Jung. The first tenet pertained to differences in the rate at which individuals develop reactive inhibition in response to stimulation. The second tenet reinterpreted Pavlov's theory of nervous types in terms of Western typologies of personality, particularly that of Jung (1923). The classic statement of inhibition theory remains that of Hull (1943), wherein he defined reactive inhibition (I_R) or inhibitory potential as:

Whenever any reaction is evoked in an organism there is left a condition or state which acts as a primary negative motivation in that it has an innate capacity to produce a cessation of the activity which produced the state (p.278)

The theoretical ancestry of Hull's reactive inhibition hypothesis (as well as Kohler's 'satiation' or perceptual inhibition hypothesis) is Spearman's General Law of Fatigue (1927), which states that 'the occurrence of any cognitive event produces a tendency opposed to its occurrence afterwards'. The interplay between inhibition and personality was first proposed by Eysenck, who conceived of inhibition as a central cortical process rather than a peripheral one as Hull had (Eysenck, 1967, p. 82). In *The Dynamics of Anxiety and Hysteria* Eysenck (1957) set forth the two fundamental postulates relating cortical inhibition to personality:

(1) Postulate of Individual Differences
    Human beings differ with respect to the speed with which excitation and inhibition are produced, the strength of the excitation and inhibition produced and the speed with which inhibition is dissipated. These differences are properties of the physical structures involved in making stimulus-response connections.

(2) Typological Postulate
    Individuals in whom reactive inhibition is developed quickly, in whom strong reactive inhibitions are generated, and in whom reactive inhibition is dissipated slowly, are thereby predisposed to develop extraverted patterns of behaviour and to develop hysterical-psychopathic disorders in case of neurotic breakdown; conversely, individuals in whom reactive inhibition is developed slowly, in whom weak reactive inhibitions are generated, and in whom reactive inhibition is dissipated quickly, are thereby predisposed to develop introverted patterns of behaviour and to develop dysthymic disorders in case of neurotic breakdown.

In brief, cortical inhibition develops more rapidly in hysterics than in dysthymics (anxiety, reactive depression, obsessionality). Hysterics and dysthymics were thus regarded as the prototype groups for examining personality correlates of cortical inhibition. Since cortical inhibition extends beyond the realm of pathology, Eysenck adopted Jung's typology of introversion/extraversion to describe normal behaviour. Simply stated, extraverts are more prone to develop cortical inhibition than introverts. The pathological counterpart of extraversion is hysteria, while the pathological counterpart of introversion is dysthymia. The following two tables provide characteristic psychophysiological and behavioural differences between extraverts and introverts. The tables present theoretical predictions that should *not* be construed as empirically reliable. Additionally, the predictions pertain to extremes on a continuum, usually designated by cut-off scores on the Eysenck Personality Inventory. Most individuals are neither extraverted nor introverted but ambiverted.

Eysenck has placed the physiological substrate for introversion/extraversion in the ascending reticular activating system (ARAS). Degree of introversion or extraversion is determined by level of ARAS activity. Introverts possess high ARAS activity and therefore high arousal. With a high internal level of arousal, the individual avoids external (environmental) stimulation, thus appearing behaviorally 'introverted'. The opposite is true of the extravert: low ARAS activity and low internal arousal. Two important sets of experimental data bear upon this hypothesis and, indirectly, relate ARAS activity to Eysenck's postulates regarding cortical inhibition.

Pharmacological studies indicate that depressant drugs (especially sodium amobarbital) and alcohol have an extraverting effect on behaviour (Eysenck, 1967). The barbiturates, with the minor exception of those methylated derivatives having convulsant properties, are central nervous system depressants; however, the drugs have their *extraverting* effect in doses *short* of that required to achieve sedation. Gray (1970) argues that barbiturates effect the medial septal area and hippocampus *before* producing even mild incoordination or disorientation. The relevance of Gray's proposition will be addressed momentarily.

Table 1

Behavioural	Introverts	Extraverts
Conditionability	good: hypersensitive to stimulus cues	poor: response hierarchies fail to develop because discrimination between stimulus cues is lacking
Group behaviour	as group size increases talkativeness tends to decrease	as group size increases talkativeness tends to increase
Risk taking behaviour	poor	good
Driving behaviour	tend to have good driving records	tend to have poor driving records
Sexual behaviour	lower sex drive	higher sex drive: report engaging in sex more often & with more people
Drug effects	sensitive to stimulants: coffee tends to make anxious while alcohol has little effect	sensitive to depressants: coffee has little effect while alcohol intoxicates relatively quickly
Reaction to pain	low threshold: report discomfort at lower levels of intensity	high threshold: report discomfort at higher levels of intensity
Sleep habits	tend to wake up earlier in the morning and retire earlier in the evening	tend to wake up later in the morning but are alert later into the evening

Table 2

Physiological indices*	Introverts	Extraverts
Strength of nervous system	weak	strong
Cortical inhibition	develops slowly	develops rapidly
Satiability (perceptual inhibition)	builds up slowly and to a lower level	builds up quickly and to a higher level
EEG	low alpha	high amplitude alpha, slow wave activity
EMG	high muscle tension	low muscle tension
Blood pressure (systolic)	higher	lower
Heart rate	higher	lower
Skin temperature (digital)	higher	lower
Skin potential	high negative potential	low negative potential
Skin conductance	high conductance	low conductance
Spontaneous fluctuations (mean number of fluctuations in skin conductance during habituation)	higher	lower
Absolute sensory thresholds (visual & auditory)	lower	higher
Optic rheobase (threshold of electrical sensitivity of the eye)	lower	higher
Sedation threshold (amount of sodium amobarbital necessary to induce slurred speech)	higher	lower
Mecholyl test (Funkenstein Test) (blood pressure response to acetyl-beta-methylcholine chloride, a parasympathomimetic)	brisk interplay: quick correction mixed with slight rises and falls in blood pressure	profound and prolonged drop in blood pressure
Two-flash threshold (threshold for fusion of brief paired flashes of light)	lower threshold	higher threshold
Critical frequency of flicker-fusion (measure of nervous system lability)	higher threshold	lower threshold
Critical frequency of flashing phosphene (measure of nervous system strength) (measured only at *low* intensities of stimulation)	higher threshold	lower threshold

Visual (spiral) after-effect	long: persistence of excitation after the removal of evoking stimulus	short: rapid decay of excitation after removal of evoking stimulus
Necker cube	higher frequency of reversals	lower frequency of reversals
Vigilance & signal detection †	good: decline is slow	poor: may do well initially but decay is rapid
Stroop (colour word) Test (test of distractability)	fewer errors	more errors

---

* A number of indices are included which are not physiological measures *per se* but are assumed to reflect underlying physiological processes, such as temporal inhibition in the case of the spiral after-effect and the Necker cube.

† Diurnal variation tends to alter this prediction, that is, introverts excel in the morning, extraverts in the afternoon.

It should be kept in mind that many of these physiological indices bear little correlational relationship with one another (such as sedation threshold and spiral after-effect) and may well be reflecting different characteristics of the nervous system. Additionally, time-of-day effects, sex differences, pre-test fatigue or stress and other sources of variation all contribute to anomalies in prediction.

The second bit of experimental evidence concerns the behavioural effects of frontal lobe lesions. Animals so lesioned appear to behave more extraverted. Over 40 years ago Wilder Penfield (1935) noted that significant lesioning or ablation of the frontal lobe impaired 'capacity for planned initative'. More recently, Penfield (1975) labelled the 'interpretive cortex' those areas which, from an evolutionary standpoint, are recent additions: prefrontal and temporal enlargements. According to Penfield, some of these added convolutions *'will be devoted to interpretation of present experience in the light of past experience.'* He goes on to say that *'These new areas of cerebral cortex, both frontal and temporal, are employed in the mechanisms of mind-action after the early period of what may be called conditioning or programming,"* p.19.

To return to what may seem like a long-lost point, the initial goal was to provide a theoretical bridge between cortical inhibition/excitation and the presumed substrate of introversion/extraversion in the ARAS. In brief, drugs that depress the central nervous system also produce extraverted behaviour. Gray argues that the locus for barbiturate-induced extraversion lies in the hippocampus and medial septal area. It also appears that frontal lobe lesioning produces extraverted behaviour. Penfield attributes to recent con-

volutions in the frontal lobe early developmental conditioning. The notion of conditionability is fundamental to introversion/extraversion theory. Extraverts are said to possess poor conditionability.

Gray (1970, 1972) modified Eysenck's ARAS theory by incorporating several of the just mentioned findings. He adopted the frontal cortex–medial septal area–hippocampal system (FCHS) as the governing physiological mechanisms for introversion/extraversion. The FCHS may be viewed as three-tiered: (1) ARAS, (2) septo-hippocampal system, (3) orbital-frontal cortex. Stimulation of the hippocampus inhibits upward conduction from the midbrain to the thalamic part of the ARAS. The result is a negative feedback loop: (1) increased hippocampal activity, (2) producing inhibition of ARAS activity. Thus, there is an equilibrium between reticular activation (Tier 1) and hippocampal inhibition (Tier 2). Tier 3, the orbital-frontal cortex, is the higher cortical centre responsible for controlling the septo-hippocampal system (Tier 2). The effect of a drug like sodium amobarbital can thus be explained in the following manner: it depresses medial septal cells (duplicating the effect of an orbital-frontal lesion), which blocks (or disrupts) hippocampal theta rhythm. It is interesting to note at this point that hippocampal inhibition of conduction from the midbrain to the thalamus can be reduced by doses of barbiturate too small to directly affect the ARAS. Thus, one might consider adding to Mark's (1969) spectrum of barbiturate effects "extraversion": *extraversion* ↔ sedation ↔ hypnosis ↔ anaesthesia ↔ poisoning → death.

The readings in this section are specific to introversion/extraversion research. However, a deliberate attempt was made to provide a broad survey that would reflect several theoretical viewpoints. Whereas Section 2 focused on the predominantly Russian-researched area of strength of nervous system, this section looks at the more Western dimension of introversion/extraversion. While there appears to be a compatible marriage between the two areas (introverts possessing weak nervous systems and extraverts strong nervous systems), there is as yet no one-to-one correspondence. Gray (1964) has pioneered efforts to achieve such a union at the conceptual and empirical levels.

At the outset of this introduction it was mentioned that Eysenck's theory was uniquely controversial. To provide balance and permit the reader some insight into drawbacks of this research two particularly noteworthy criticisms are included. The first concerns focal attention to one parameter – introversion/extraversion. At the *causal* level many important sources of variation in human behaviour may be omitted. While at the descriptive level the theory has generated a prodigious amount of research, it may be quite academic whether hysterics and dysthymics are extraverted and introverted if the latter (descriptive) dimension accounts for little of the variance of the former (causal) dimension. In that case the descriptive part of the theory (introversion/extraversion) has little utility, other than to generate research on personality correlates of introverted and extraverted behaviour, with no legitimate extrapolation to aetiology. The second, related, and most critical drawback concerns the proliferation of terms which ostensibly mean the same thing and very few of which are clearly operationally defined. Eysenck himself uses the terms excitation–inhibition, introversion/extraversion and dysthymia–hysteria interchangeably. Introversion/extraversion stands on its own merit as a clearly delineated dimension of personality. It is only a *behavioural* dimension however and

may be quite different from the *physiological* dimension of excitation–inhibition or the *psychopathological* dimension of dysthymia–hysteria. Additionally, Eysenck's use of cortical excitation appears to be synonymous with other terms such as activation, energy mobilization, and stimulation, all four of which refer to arousal. Arousal is, of course, no more cogent a concept than any of the others. In most general terms, arousal usually refers to variation in *intensity* of behaviour. However, at the very least, arousal carries two distinct meanings, one tonic and the other phasic, a distinction made by Sharpless and Jasper (1956) over 20 years ago. From the physiological standpoint, it would make research in this area more credible and less ambiguous if one term was employed and that term firmly attached to one physiological mechanism. Presently, *high* arousal is an umbrella that includes elevations on half a dozen different psychophysiological measures, good vigilance and signal detection, long spiral aftereffects, a high sedation threshold, a low pain threshold, a high threshold for the critical frequency of flashing phosphene, high sensitivity scores (slope of the psychophysiological ogive), lower absolute sensory thresholds for audition and perception and extreme scores on several paper and pencil tests (Eysenck's Personality Inventory, Zuckerman's Sensation Seeking Scale, Guilford's S (social introversion) and R (rhathymia) scales, etc.). Surely, all of these indices do not assess the same physiological mechanism. One problem is that arousal is typically conceptualized or defined centrally (ARAS) and measured peripherally (electrodermal activity, heart rate, blood pressure, muscle tension, etc.). In human research techniques of measurement are non-intrusive but could be standardized. It is not within the scope of this introductory statement to delve into these issues, however, they are crucial enough that even the casual reader should be superficially acquainted with them.

References

Eysenck, H. (1955). A dynamic theory of anxiety and hysteria. *J. Ment. Sci.,* **101,** 28–51

Eysenck, H. (1957). *The Dynamics of Anxiety and Hysteria.* (New York: Praeger)

Eysenck, H. (1967). *The Biological Basis of Personality.* (Springfield: Charles C. Thomas)

Gray, J. (1964). *Pavlov's Typology.* (New York: Pergamon Press)

Gray, J. (1970). The psychophysiological basis of introversion-extraversion. *Behavioural Research and Therapy*, **8**, 249–266

Gray, J. (1972). The psychophysiological nature of introversion-extraversion: A modification of Eysenck's theory. In Nebylitsyn, V. D. and Gray, J. (eds.), *Biological Basis of Individual Behavior*. (New York: Academic Press)

Hull, C. L. (1943). *Principles of Behaviour*. (New York: Appleton-Century-Crofts)

Jung, C. G. (1923). *Psychological Types*. Trans. H. Godwin Baynes. (New York: Harcourt, Brace & Company)

Mark, L. C. (1969). Archaic classification of barbiturates. *Clin. Pharmacol. Ther.*, **10**, 287–291

Penfield, W. and Evans, J. (1935). The frontal lobe in man: A clinical study of maximum removals. *Brain*, **58**, 115–138

Penfield, W. (1975). *The Mystery of the Mind*. (Princeton: Princeton University Press)

Sharpless, S. and Jasper, H. (1956). Habituation of the arousal reaction. *Brain*, **79**, 655–680

Spearman, C. (1927). *Abilities of Man*. (London: Macmillan)

From W. McDougall (1929). Journal of Abnormal and Social Psychology, *24,*
293-309, *by kind permission of the American Psychological Association*

THE CHEMICAL THEORY OF TEMPERAMENT APPLIED TO INTROVERSION AND EXTROVERSION

By WILLIAM McDOUGALL
DUKE UNIVERSITY

W E CAN hardly hope to make progress in the understanding
of the differences between one personality and another
until we shall have achieved some agreement as to the
main classes of constituent factors of personality and some consistency in the terminology we employ in discussing them. We
have seen in recent years a number of interesting attempts to
distinguish types of personality from the psychiatric point of
view. These have, I think, thrown some light on the problems of
genesis, especially of psychogenesis, and on the problems of treatment. But all the efforts in this direction with which I am
acquainted seem to me to suffer from neglect to distinguish clearly
between the main classes of factors that enter into the make-up of
personality. They seem to assume that certain types of personality
of significance for psychiatry may be distinguished and defined
on a single basis, without any prior analysis of the chief classes of
constituent factors. In so far all the theories of types seem to me
to be at fault.

Personality is extremely complex; it comprizes factors of many
distinguishable classes. It seems very improbable that individual
differences in respect to any one class of factors should be of such
overwhelming influence as to swamp the influence of factors of
other classes and to render possible a useful scheme of types drawn
up on the basis of that one class alone.

I suggest[1] that, if we are to avoid confusion and many cross
divisions of types, at least five great classes of factors of personality must be distinguished. For these five classes seem to be, in
great measure, though not entirely, independent variables in the
make-up of personality; that is to say, the factors of any one of
these five classes may be combined in any one personality with
any combination of factors of the other four classes. These five
classes are:

---

[1] In accordance with the scheme which I have long used in teaching and which is
indicated in my *Outline of Psychology*.

(1) The factors of *intellect* (under which head I include intelligence and knowledge and such peculiarities as retentiveness of memory, types of imagery, etc.).

(2) The factors of *disposition* (which I conceive to be the array of innately given conative or affective tendencies varying widely in their relative strengths from one individual to another).

(3) The factors of *temper*. These are the least recognized and the most woefully confused and obscured of all by our present chaotic psychological terminology and theory. Yet they are of prime importance in the make-up of personality. I conceive them as general peculiarities of the mode of working of all the conative tendencies or "drives";[2] such peculiarities as persistency, urgency or intensity, high affectability by success and failure, and the opposites of these.

(4) Factors of *temperament*. These may be broadly defined as the influences, direct or indirect, of bodily metabolism (more especially of the endocrine secretions) upon the psycho-physical processes of the nervous system.

(5) Factors of *character*. These are matters of acquired organization of the affective tendencies in sentiments and complexes, which in turn are organized in great systems or (in well developed character) in one hierarchical system.

These five classes of factors of personality are, it seems to me, largely independent of one another; thus any type of intellect may go with any type of temper, temperament, disposition, or character; and so of each of the others; hence, in order to characterize a personality, we must state its type of intellect, of disposition, of temper, of temperament, and of character. When it is attempted to set up types of personality, as so many have done, without first distinguishing these five main classes of factors, the result inevitably is a mass of false generalizations, exceptions to which are at least as easy to find as conforming instances.

Such inevitable confusion is well illustrated, I suggest, by the efforts of Dr. C. G. Jung to define two types called by him the introvert and the extrovert types. That Jung is attempting by the use of these terms to point to some deep-lying and very important peculiarities of personality I have no doubt. I have found the distinction between introversion and extroversion extremely useful, both in theory and in the practical handling of cases of neurotic disorder, and also in understanding normal personalities.

---

[2] I am driven to use this unsatisfactory word because it is the only one which will serve to indicate to many possible readers what I am driving at.

And many other workers in the field of abnormal psychology seem to have accepted the distinction and made much use of the terms. Yet I feel sure that Jung has attempted to give too rich a content to the terms. He seems to regard the peculiarities which he seeks to define as temperamental; yet, in describing the two types, he assigns to them peculiarities which are peculiarities of intellect, of disposition, of temper, and of character, as well as of temperament proper.

Jung, accepting William James' famous classification of thinkers as tender minded and tough minded, identifies his introverts with the former and his extroverts with the latter. He thus commits himself to the view that introverts are rationalists and system-makers, who care little for facts and forcibly fit data into their ideal constructions in accordance with their *a priori* premises; that the extrovert, on the other hand, cannot construct a system, is interested not at all in the inner life of man, but only in objective facts, is positivist, determinist, fatalist, irreligious and a sceptic. Jung further identifies his introverts with the "classics" of Ostwald and his extroverts with Ostwald's romantics; and thus adds to the characteristics of the former as follows: "They produce with much difficulty, are little capable of teaching or of exercising direct personal influence, and, lacking enthusiasm, are paralyzed by their own severe criticism, living apart and absorbed in themselves, making scarcely any disciples, but producing works of finished perfection."

Jung then chooses as illustrative examples of his two types, Dr. Sigmund Freud and Dr. Alfred Adler, seeking to explain the peculiarities of their psychological teachings as expressions of extroversion and introversion respectively. Could anything be more unfortunate? Freud, with his lifelong intense interest in the inner life of man and his highly elaborated system, is classed with those who are not interested in the inner life and cannot make a system. Adler, who has a large popular following and whose voluminous writings are peculiarly lacking in system and order, with those who cannot exert personal influence and who are paralyzed by their severe self-criticism and who produce works of finished perfection.

While the extrovert is said by Jung to be interested only in the outer world, the introvert is said to shrink from it; "the objective world suffers a sort of depreciation, or want of consideration, for the sake of the exaltation of the individual himself, who then, monopolizing all the interest, grows to believe no one but himself worthy of consideration.'' And in many other passages Jung insists on the introvert's lack of interest in the world of sense-perception. It is further implied that the introvert is but little given to bodily exertion and little interested in physical activities. Let us see how this fits with the facts in the case of a great writer of whom we have very full accounts; I mean the late Count Tolstoy. Tolstoy's vivid interest in the inner life of men and especially his own, his seclusiveness, his difficulty in ''getting on'' with other men, his prolonged internal conflicts and perpetual self-examination, all these traits mark him unmistakably as strongly introverted; yet the author of a recent study [3] insists that ''his purely sensory life was unusually vivid and clearly defined. . . . Any description in Tolstoy's work is apt to be striking for the minuteness and accuracy of the detail; his powers of simple observation are probably unrivalled in literature.'' Again we are told: ''He was very fond of eating and drinking, of hunting, riding, walking and outdoor sports of all kinds, of dancing, carousing and gambling.'' We see here very clearly how the interests and intellectual traits refuse to conform to Jung's demands and to exhibit the alleged correlation with the temperamental trait of introversion. Many other such instances may easily be found.

In one passage Jung ascribes to the extrovert a high degree of docility or suggestibility, a peculiarity which seems to me to be one of disposition rather than of temperament, and one perfectly compatible with marked introversion; and one might ask whether his chosen example of extroversion, Dr. Freud, exhibits high suggestibility. In another passage he ascribes to the extrovert as a distinctive trait great sensitiveness to the regards of other men, a peculiarity which, I submit, belongs to character rather than to temperament.

If we inquire how Jung conceives his introvert and extrovert traits to be founded in the structure of personality, the answer is very unsatisfactory. Although he speaks of the distinction as one of temperament, he cannot regard it as founded in any general chemical influence affecting the nervous system; for he asserts that the conscious and the unconscious parts of the personality are always opposites in this respect, that where the conscious is introverted, the unconscious in extroverted, and *vice versa.* He falls back upon the common but extremely unsatisfactory expedient of postulating two mechanisms, an introverting and an

---

[3] ''Tolstoy and Nietzsche,'' by H. E. Davis, N. Y., 1929.

extroverting mechanism possessed by all subjects, the one pre-dominating in the conscious life of the introvert, the other in his unconscious (and *vice versa* for the extrovert).

There is in all Jung's discussions of this topic only one state-ment that seems to me at once illuminating and altogether accept-able, if we are to define introversion and extroversion as pure temperamental peculiarities. This is the passage [4] in which he writes that "hysteria is characterized by a centrifugal tendency of the libido, whilst in dementia praecox its tendency is cen-tripetal".

I suggest that, accepting the cue given in this passage, we can single out of the complexities of the traits to which Jung applies the terms extroversion and introversion, a simple personality factor which is purely one of temperament in the proper or strict sense, the possession of which in various degrees of intensity is an im-portant constitutional factor in every personality. I suggest that all personalities can be ranged in a single linear scale according to the degree to which this factor is present in their constitutions. Those who stand near one end of the scale are the marked extro-verts; those near the other are the well-marked introverts; and the greater part of mankind, possessing this factor in moderate degree, stand in the middle region of the scale. [5]

Such a distribution of a temperamental trait is most naturally explained by the influence of some one chemical factor generated in the body and exerting a specific influence upon all the nervous system in proportion to the quantity that is produced and liberated into the blood stream.

Let me illustrate by reference to the internal secretion of the thyroid gland. Each of us seems to have a natural or normal rate of thyroid secretion which plays an important rôle in determining his position in the scale of rapidity of general metabolism. In morbid conditions the rate may be gravely increased or diminished. At or near the one end of the scale stands the sufferer from Graves' disease; at or near the other the victim of myxoedema or thyroid insufficiency. In this case we know that the one end of the scale represents excess of an endocrine, the other end a defect of the same secretion. In the case of the extroversion-introversion scale we have no such clear indication as to which end of the scale represents excess, which defect, of the postulated chemical sub-

---

[4] "Analytical Psychology," p. 288, London, 1917.

[5] It seems probable that the distribution of degrees of this factor may follow a normal curve; but this is a matter for future research.

stance (presumably an endocrine secretion of some one gland, or possibly a more widely secreted product of the metabolism of various tissues). But I suggest that in all probability extroversion is the positive state, introversion the negative; that is to say, extreme introversion represents a defect, a minimal quantity or minimum rate of secretion of the postulated substance—(let us call it X); and extroversion in its various degrees is the consequence of correspondingly large quantities or rapid rates of secretion of X. My ground for preferring this view will be stated in a later paragraph.

Let me first try to define the difference between what I take to be simple extroversion and simple introversion, the pure temperamental traits as I conceive them. And since introversion is the simpler state, while extroversion (according to the view I am putting forward) is the consequence of the additional constitutional factor X, or if its presence in larger quantity, I begin with introversion.

The marked introvert is the man in whom the inhibition normally exerted by activity of the cerebral cortex on all lower nervous functions is manifested in high degree. We are most familiar with this inhibitory influence of cortical activity in the case of the spinal reflexes. We know that cortical activity depresses or inhibits the spinal reflexes, and that destruction or impairment or arrest of cortical function releases the cord from this inhibitory influence. We do not know how this inhibitory influence is exerted; though it is, I believe, capable of explanation in terms of the drainage hypothesis. Yet the fact is well established in the case of the spinal reflexes; and we have similar though less abundant evidence that the activity of the cortex depresses or partially inhibits in a similar way the functions of the thalamus or of the mid-brain structures in general. I refer here chiefly to the observations of Dr. Henry Head, which show that the protopathic functions of the thalamus are intensified as a consequence of certain lesions of the cortex or of the cortico-thalamic paths.

We may, I think, go further and point to evidence that the cortical regions of highest function (the so-called silent areas) exert similar inhibition upon the cortical areas of lower function, the sensori-motor areas. I refer to the fact, first pointed out by Francis Galton, that children and primitives seem to use imagery in their thinking more freely and copiously than do civilized adults; and that, with the development of powers of reflective and

William McDougall

abstract thinking, the use of imagery seems to decline, to become less free, less abundant, less vivid.

The introvert, then, is the man in whom the lower levels of the nervous system are constantly subject to a high degree of inhibition by the higher cortical activities; and of these lower inhibited functions the most important are the affective or emotional-conative functions of the thalamic region. I have long accepted and taught in my books [6] the view that the emotional functions have their principal seat in the thalamus, and Professor W. B. Cannon has recently adduced evidence which seems to put this view beyond doubt. We may confine our attention to them. Now if my view of inhibition is correct (namely, that it is effected by drainage of the energy liberated in one system of neurones into some other system more actively functioning), inhibition of the affective centers of the thalamus by the cortex does not mean that their excitation is prevented.[7] It means only that the energies liberated in the affective centers is diverted from its normal channels of expression, from all those efferent channels which directly lead to the bodily expressions of emotion; it is diverted or long-circuited to and through the cortex, where it coöperates in sustaining the activities of reflective thinking, a process which results in the simultaneous excitation of various affective tendencies which partially check or neutralize one another so far as external expression is concerned.

Thus the introvert, by reason of the free dominant activity of his cortex and in virtue of its restraining or inhibitory effect on the outflow of thalamic excitation in its normal or direct channels of emotional expression, is a man in whom thought seems to flourish at the expense of emotion. It is not that he is incapable of emotion or strong affects; but his affects do not readily find outward expression; they are absorbed in and disguised by the supervenient cortical activities and the consequent arousal of conflicting tendencies. He seems relatively cold and expressionless; he cannot easily let himself go; his emotional expressions, in word or gesture or other bodily forms, are very moderate and restrained even when he is strongly moved. He tends to be over self-conscious and introspective; and that adds to his general inhibitedness.

Introversion seems then to be the natural consequence of the

[6] *Eg.* in my *Social Psychology*, London, 1908.
[7] Cf. appended note on Inhibition by Drainage.

great development and free activity of the cortex. Hence children in general grow more introverted as they grow up, *i.e.*, as the cortex assumes its full rôle; and primitives on the whole are less introverted than the civilized. The grown dog is more introverted than the puppy; and if we deprive him of his cortex in part or whole by surgical interference, we remove in part this restraining influence on the thalamic levels; he becomes emotional and restless, perpetually on the move so long as he is awake; he regresses to puppyhood.

As the cortex developed its enormous proportions in the human species, there was danger of excessive introversion; danger that the life of phantasy, of reflection, of deliberation, should render men unfit for the life of action and unfit for social intercourse, for maintaining that sympathetic rapport with their fellows which is the basis of all social life and is rendered possible only by a certain freedom of emotional expression. Man's increasing capacity for thinking threatened to diminish unduly his capacity for action and for social life.

Hence nature has provided an antidote against such increasing and excessive introversion. It has generated in the tissues, or in some tissue unknown, an extroverting hormone or endocrine substance X, the function of which is to prevent, to diminish in some measure, this inhibiting paralyzing influence of the cortex upon the more primitive lower-level functions of the nervous system. And the man who is constitutionally provided with a large amount of this antidote to cortical inhibition is the extrovert.

The extrovert, then, is the man who, though he may possess, and commonly does possess, a cortex developed just as highly as that of the introvert, nevertheless does not suffer in the same degree the inhibition of all emotional expressions that characterizes the introvert. Every affect, every emotional-conative excitement, readily flows out from the subcortical levels into outward expression, instead of being largely drained off to and absorbed into the cortex. His emotional stirrings find immediate expression in action, save only on the occasions when some real difficulty or problem compels him to stop to think, or when he makes a voluntary effort to deliberate before action.

Individuals certainly differ widely in respect to this freedom of outflow of affective excitement into action and expression, and I suggest that we shall do well to restrict the terms introversion and extroversion to denote the various degrees of this one simple temperamental peculiarity. For these degrees seem to be the most essential feature of the highly complex traits to which Jung and others have applied these names.

How, then, may we conceive the postulated internal secretion X to work upon the brain to maintain various degrees of extroversion, to antagonize and moderate the inhibiting influence of the cortex? I suggest that we may find the clue to a simple, intelligible and adequate hypothesis in consideration of the influence of alcohol upon the brain functions (and of ether and chloroform), and that the phenomena of alcoholic intoxication go very far to justify the hypothesis.

I have observed in a number of cases that the markedly extroverted personality is very susceptible to the influence of alcohol. A very small dose deprives him of normal self-restraint and control and brings on the symptoms of intoxication, all of which are essentially expressions of diminished cortical control over the lower brain-levels. The introvert on the other hand is much more resistant to alcohol. He can take a considerable dose without other effect than that he becomes extroverted; that is to say, the predominance of his higher cortical processes over those of lower levels is diminished; he becomes less inhibited in action and expression; he enjoys for the time being the advantages of the extrovert; he talks freely and expresses his emotions in action, gesture, tears and laughter. Alcohol, in short, seems to be an extroverting drug pure and simple so far as its influence on the nervous system is concerned. What exactly, then, is the mode of action of alcohol on the nervous system? In articles published as long ago as 1898 [8] I suggested that alcohol acts directly upon the synapses of the brain to increase their resistances to the passage of the nervous current. In a later publication [9] I have elaborated this view, showing that we have only to conceive that alcohol acts upon the synapses of the various brain-levels, increasing their resistances in the order from above downwards (in the inverse order of their fixity of organization) in order to have a simple and perfectly adequate explanation of all the stages of intoxication. Since this scheme met with the approval of the several eminent physiologists and pharmacologists with whom I coöperated in writing that little book, it may be said to be pretty well founded.[10]

---

[8] "Contribution towards an Improvement of Psychological Method," *Mind*, 1928.

[9] "Alcohol and Its Effects on the Human Organisms." H. M. S. Stationery Office, London, 1924.

[10] I have further supported this view by showing (by the aid of a special and very delicate laboratory procedure) that alcohol and ether are precise antagonists of strychnine in its influence upon cerebral process; and the probability is great that strychnine works upon synapses to diminish their resistances.

In order to explain extroversion, I make, then, the simple assumption that in the extrovert some tissue (or tissues) normally and constantly secretes the extroverting substance X, a substance whose action upon the nervous system is very similar to that of alcohol (ether and chloroform); that is to say, I assume that the extroverting internal secretion X acts directly upon all synapses raising their resistance to the passage of the nervous current or discharge from neurone to neurone. I make also the highly probable assumption that the synapses of the various levels of the nervous system are in the main solidly and stably organized in proportion to the phylogenetic and ontogenetic age of the levels in which they occur. In other words, I assume that the synapses of the higher levels are the less solidly organized, have higher resting resistances and are less stable, more subject to variation of their resistances by a variety of influences, including the chemical influences of strychnine, alcohol, and the postulated substance X.

According to this view, then, the marked extrovert is he whose metabolism constantly or normally furnishes and throws into the blood-stream enough of the substance X to keep the subject in a state of mild or incipient intoxication. And the position of each individual in the introvert-extrovert scale is a direct and simple function of the amount of X normally secreted by his tissues; the extreme introvert being the man with a well developed cortex and a minimum of X.

I find support for this view in the relation of introversion and extroversion to the incidence of nervous and mental disorder. Jung has expressed the opinion that the introvert is the more liable to neurasthenia and schizophrenia, the extrovert to hysterical and manic-depressive disorder. My own small experience leads me to accept this view. And I would add insomnia to the list of characteristic introvert troubles. The introvert mind or brain does not easily come to rest. The introvert in many cases finds the need of a night-cap in the shape of a stiff peg of whiskey in order to pass quickly into sleep. Further, he cannot easily be hypnotized.

To the list of extrovert peculiarities I would add susceptibility to hypnosis, to crystal visions, trances and automatic actions of all kinds. All these differences seem to mean the greater liability of the extrovert to suffer dissociative effects in the nervous system whether local, as in local functional paralyses and anesthesia, or general, as in general amnesia, trance, hypnosis and sleep. And this is to be expected; for, just as alcohol is a dissociating drug which acts first and most intensely upon those most delicately

William McDougall

organized synapses that are involved in the latest acquired and highest-level processes of the cortex subserving self-conscious control and self-criticism, and involving the reciprocal play of one cortical system of highest level neurones upon another; so also the extroverting substance X may be supposed to affect most markedly these higher level synapses, maintaining during waking life an incipient state of dissociation and rendering easier the onset of all more pronounced states of cerebral dissociation, from normal sleep and alcoholic intoxication to hypnosis and functional paralyses and amnesias. In short, the introvert is the more liable to disorders of continuing conflict, because conflict cannot readily be oviated by dissociation; while the extrovert readily finds relief from internal conflict through the onset of some complete dissociation between conflicting systems and tendencies.

A last point in support of this view may be made by contrasting the British [11] and the American people in respect to introversion-extroversion. It seems beyond question that position in the scale is in the main determined by hereditary constitution, and varies from race to race; some races, like the Negro, being predominantly extrovert, others, like the red men of this country, predominantly introvert. If this is so, how explain the notorious fact that, by and large, Americans are decidedly more extroverted than the British? I do not suggest that all Americans are extrovert. The typical Yankee is perhaps hardly on the extrovert side of the scale. Yet the difference is on the whole considerable. The difference may be perhaps in part explained by the more expansive surroundings of the American. But it seems likely that in the main it is due to the influence of climate on our metabolism. On coming to America we all notice a marked difference of climate which renders it easy to keep running about maintaining social contacts of all sorts. And the Britisher hardly feels the need of the alcohol to which he is accustomed to resort for the relief of his introversion. I suggest that the essence of this climatic effect is the stimulation of the tissue that produces the extroverting substance X, and a more rapid secretion of it into the blood.[12]

---

[11] British introversion is well illustrated by a recent advertisement labelled "Chatter-boxes." Two Britishers foregather for a friendly chat, both smoking in their pipes tobacco of a famous brand. One says: "Good stuff this!" After a silence of five minutes the other replies: "Yes, not bad!"

[12] The observations reported by Dr. C. A. Neymann (at the Atlanta meeting of the American Psychiatric Association, May, 1929) to the effect that active tubercular disease seems to conduce to increase of extroversion, fits very well with this simplified view of the nature of introversion and extroversion and with the chemical theory here maintained.

According to the usage I propose, the words extroversion and introversion would imply solely the two opposite and extremer degrees of a purely temperamental peculiarity, one that is simple, fully intelligible in terms of our knowledge of the nervous functions, and profoundly important from the points of view of education, psychiatry and mental hygiene.

I conclude by drawing attention to the fact that Pavlov describes very clearly two types of temperament in the dogs that served in his experiments on the conditioned reflex.[13] His descriptions of the two types might well serve as definitions of the human introvert and extrovert. If, then, introversion and extroversion are well marked in dogs, the fact indicates that they are based on some relatively simple physiological factor such as is here postulated.

APPENDED NOTE ON THE THEORY OF INHIBITION ON WHICH THE FOREGOING ARTICLE IS FOUNDED

In an article in the *Journal of General Psychology* (April, 1929), I have argued that the work on conditioned reflexes of Professor Pavlov and his colleagues gives strong support to the hypothesis of inhibition by drainage as formulated in my article in *Brain*, 1903. It is the renewal of my confidence in that hypothesis that has led me to apply it in this article to the problem of the neural basis of introversion and extroversion and thus to give more definite form to the view propounded in my *Outline of Abnormal Psychology*.

It seems worth while in this connection to refer to the excellent review of the present state of knowledge of the nervous functions by Dr. J. F. Fulton (*Muscular Contraction and the Reflex Control of Movement*, N. Y., 1926). Fulton summarily rejects the hypothesis of inhibition by drainage on the ground that no positive evidence for it exists. Now the only direct positive evidence of it we can hope to discover is evidence that the inhibiting process gains in intensity at the expense of the inhibited process. Such evidence is afforded by my observations on graded visual contrast;[14] but this evidence is ignored by Fulton. He proceeds to state two theories of the inhibitory process, the interference theory of Wedensky and the chemical theory of Sherrington. He finds sufficient grounds for rejecting the interference theory, and thus leaves only the chemical theory in the field. Yet Fulton reports a number of facts which go far to justify the drainage hypothesis; and in the end he seems to come very near to it. In the first place, he shows that even though the all-or-none principle be accepted for peripheral nerve-processes, it does not follow that it

---

[13] Compare my condensed account of these observations in article in *Journ. of General Psychology*, April, 1929, ''The Bearing of Prof. Pavlov's Work on the Problem of Inhibition.''

[14] *Journ. of Physiology*, March and July, 1903.

holds for the central processes. Secondly, he seems to accept the view that energy liberated in one neurone may be discharged into another. Such discharge (which I postulated under the phrase, the vicarious usage of nervous energy) is, of course, an essential assumption of the drainage hypothesis. He writes: ''The extent of after-discharge, therefore, may be taken as a measure of the 'size' of the excitatory 'charge' existing in individual motoneurone; the size may also be measured by the ease with which it may be inhibited, that is to say, by stimulus intensity. In the early part of the stimulation plateau an inhibitory stimulus of given strength is less effective than in a later part, and in the 'after-discharge plateau' it is very much more effective than in any part of the 'stimulation-pleateau'. The charge, or the amount of excitatory substance—in any given motoneurone tends to diminish progressively during the stimulation plateau and diminishes very rapidly during the after-discharge plateau.'' (Pp. 326.) Here Fulton recognizes that the stimulated central neurone acquires a charge of *something* which it gradually discharges across synapses into efferent-lying neurones. Following Sherrington, he speaks of this *something* as a chemical substance. I can find no good reason for preferring to regard this excitatory charge as a chemical substance rather than as some form of energy (presumably electrical). But the main point is that the facts compel us to believe that stimulation of a neurone generates in it a ''charge'' which is more or less gradually discharged into other neurones.

There follow a number of statements which are perfectly compatible with the drainage theory but hardly compatible with the chemical theory of inhibition; *e.g.*, ''Prolonged stimulation of the cortex not infrequently gives rise to localized epileptiform convulsions of various parts of the musculature. And, as in typical Jacksonian epilepsy, the convulsion may occur simultaneously in antagonistic muscles.'' (P. 452.) Of similar significance are the phenomena of double reciprocal innervation. ''When two afferent nerves, one of which causes flexor contraction and extensor relaxation, the other causing the converse of this—flexor relaxation and extensor contraction—are stimulated simultaneously, the strength of the respective stimuli may be so adjusted that contraction occurs in both flexor and extensor muscles without movement. By slightly altering the relative strength of stimuli either the flexor contraction or the extensor contraction may be made to predominate.'' (P. 453.) Further: ''This result [balanced excitation of the antagonistic muscle-groups] is sometimes difficult to demonstrate experimentally because unless the balance is perfect (and the stimulation brief) the usual result of opposing inhibitory and excitatory stimuli is rhythmic contraction similar in every way to reflex walking. In other words, when the spinal centers of the hind limb are subjected synchronously to excitatory and inhibitory stimulation, the extensor ('half') centers on one side first become dominant and then the extensor 'half-centers' on the other side and so on. But the excitatory dominance of one or the other is always associated with simultaneous inhibition of the symmetrical 'half-center'. The usual effect of opposing stimuli, therefore, is rhythmicity. . . . The fact that the rhythmic stepping occurs in a pair of isolated knee extensors excludes the possibility that the antagonistic muscles and their nerves are necessary in so far as generation through them of secondary reflexes is concerned. Moreover, reflex walking is observed in response to concurrent stimulation of both peroneals after the two isolated extensors have been de-afferented.'' (P. 468.) That is to say, continued stimulation of the two afferent nerves, in the absence of all other afferent impulses, may cause in the antagonistic muscles either balanced equal contractions or rhythmic alternation of contraction and relaxation, the contraction of the one coinciding in time with the relaxation of the other. All this seems perfectly compatible with the view that we have to do here with a simple switching or deflection of afferent streams of energy from the one efferent path to the other. But it is very difficult to reconcile with the chemical theory, which postulates that central inhibition is due to the production at some point in the stimulated tract of an inhibitory substance. For it would seem that the longer the action of an inhibitory stimulation producing such a chemical effect, the greater must be the store of inhibitory substance produced. How then should continuation of a stimulation which produces such inhibitory substance do other than prolong the inhibition and render excitation more difficult. And in the phenomena of successive spinal induction we have evidence that such cumulative inhibitory effect of stimulation of an afferent nerve (such as the chemical theory would seem to demand) does not occur. Not only does it not occur, but rather the opposite effect occurs. ''In a reflex center during inhibition there occurs an intrinsic change, which within limits as it proceeds, renders the inhibitory influence less effective and favors the effect upon it of excitatory influence.'' (P. 470.) Here, it seems to me we have, in the words of the author of the chemical theory of inhibition (Sherrington), a direct refutation of it. The inhibiting stimulus is assumed to inhibit by way of causing the production of an inhibitory substance at some point in the nerve path; yet it is also assumed to cause in the same path ''an intrinsic change'' which progressively renders its own inhibitory influence less effective and favors excitation. Are not the two assumptions mutually incompatible? They can be reconciled only by making the complicated assumption that the stimulus has two local effects, the production of both inhibitory and excitatory substances, and that under constant stimulation the production of the former begins at a maximum rate which declines, while the production of the second begins at a slow rate which increases; so that the effect is at first an excess of the inhibitory substance, and, at a later stage, such accumulation of excitatory substance as will suffice to overcome the influence of the inhibitory substance. Such complicated assumptions seem very improbable. If, on the other hand, as I pointed out long ago (supporting the suggestion with an array of indirect evidence) we suppose the synaptic transmission-process to be subject to a rapidly oncoming fatigue, we have an adequate interpretation of the phenomena of rhythmic alternation and of successive spinal induction, in terms of a simple switching of the current from one path to the other as the balance of resistances in the two paths concerned tips from one to the other.

Finally, in discussing the inhibition exerted on the spinal reflexes by the cerebral functions, Fulton assumes that the cortex sends down inhibitory impulses to spinal internuncial neurones, and that the direct path across the cord from afferent to efferent neurone is thus blocked. "In view of the extensive bifurcation of the incoming posterior root fibers, the end-result of operation of such a mechanism would be that while the local reflex path across the cord would become obliterated, the ascending paths to the mid-brain would remain functional, and in this way incoming impulses would be *deflected* up the cord for higher integration. . . . It would appear, moreover, that so long as a given controlling higher center is present the majority of afferent impulses are *long-circuited* in this way. When, however, the higher centers are cut away, the majority of impulses pursue the phylogenetically older paths across the cord." [15] Fulton cites experiments made by Amsler which show that a similar relation obtains between the cortical and the thalamic functions; and this is of especial interest in connection with the present paper, because my argument is based on the assumption of just this relation. "Amsler concluded from these observations that so long as the cerebral cortex remained intact the pain impulses were long-circuited through this organ [the cortex]. . . . When these higher centers were removed, the nociceptive impulses then immediately traversed the phylogenetically older reflex paths of the thalamus." (P. 532.) This long-circuiting of impulses from thalamus to cortex, together with the inhibition of the efferent discharge from the thalamus, is the principle upon which I have chiefly relied in the body of this article. But it remains a question of great interest—Does the long-circuiting from lower to higher levels take place because, as Fulton believes, the higher level sends down inhibitory impulses that block the efferent discharge at the lower level, so that the afferent impulses of the lower level thus find a path of least resistance through the higher level? Or does the long-circuiting take place because the higher levels when active (*i.e.*, in the waking state) are intrinsically paths of lower resistance than the more direct lower-level paths of efferent discharge, the inhibition of the efferent discharge of those lower-level paths following upon the long-circuiting or diversion of the afferent impulses to the higher level? Here, as in all other cases, the conception of inhibition by drainage offers a simple and adequate interpretation of the facts in place of the highly complicated assumptions rendered necessary by the chemical theory.

That the activity of the cortex should modify the nature of the spinal reflexes by direct action through the pyramidal tract would remain consistent with the drainage theory; but according to that theory this would be affected through excitatory impulses descending the pyramidal tract

---

[15] Italics mine.

and modifying the relative resistances of the efferent spinal synapses by favoring some synapses as against others.

Fulton accepts the view that the immediate effect of light upon the retina is the liberation of an excitatory chemical substance in rods and cones; a substance which continues to excite the nerve-fibers after the light-ray ceases to act; and he takes this as a model of excitatory processes in general. Now (as described in my "Observations in Support of T. Young's Theory of Light- and Color-Vision", Mind, Vol. X, 1900) the after-image thus generated normally undergoes a steady decline of intensity which may be prolonged during many seconds or even minutes. During this period of decline the after-image may be inhibited many times (by intenser stimulation of any other part of the retina). At each inhibition it disappears suddenly and completely, and returns equally suddenly and completely; and the normal curve of decline of intensity is not appreciably affected by these periods of inhibition.* This seems to be good evidence that the inhibition is not dependent upon the production of an inhibitory substance that antagonizes the excitatory substance; for, if it were of that nature, one should expect all grades of neutralization of the excitatory effect. Instead, we find that the inhibitory effect occurs according to the all-or-none principle. Again, an inhibitory phenomenon perfectly consistent with the drainage theory, but very difficult to reconcile with the chemical theory of inhibition.

Fulton, then, shows good reason to believe that excitation of the neurone produces suddenly within it a charge of *something* which is discharged more gradually across the synapse into the efferent neurone, and that, where there is more than one synapse with efferent neurones, the discharge follows the path of least resistance. These are the essential postulates of the drainage theory. Only one other is necessary, namely, that the synaptic resistance is a variable function, which can be diminished by excitation of any neurone taking part in the structure of the synapse. If these postulates be granted, inhibition by drainage follows as the inevitable consequence. Fulton admits the variability of synaptic resistances, but assumes that they can be varied only in the direction of increase of resistance by means of excitatory impulses which, in virtue of their impingement upon some peculiarly constituted part of the neurone, produce an inhibitory substance. By implication he denies *facilitation;* I find no discussion of facilitation, and the word does not occur in the very full index. Yet is not facilitation a fact? Facilitation is the third postulate of the drainage theory. If facilitation be granted, I do not see how inhibition by drainage can be denied.

Why then so much resistance to this hypothesis? Fulton adduces no facts or reasonings that rule it out; he rejects it on the ground that there is no direct evidence supporting it. Well, my observations on graded

---

* My description of these phenomena, of fundamental importance to the understanding of the retino-cerebral processes, have been ignored for nearly thirty years. They have recently been described anew in detail by Prof. Abbecke of Bonn.

contrast were made through using it as a working hypothesis; and they provide direct evidence in its support. And it is not likely that other such evidence can be found, until observations are directed by the working hypothesis to the discovery of further evidence of this nature, evidence that the intensity of the inhibiting excitation gains at the expense of the inhibited excitation. It seems not unlikely that Pavlov and his colleagues, if they had used this working hypothesis, might, by means of their very delicate methods, have obtained abundant evidence of this nature.

From H. J. Eysenck (1955). Journal of Abnormal and Social Psychology, *51*, 94-106, *by kind permission of the author and the American Psychological Association.*

CORTICAL INHIBITION, FIGURAL AFTEREFFECT, AND THEORY OF PERSONALITY[1]

H. J. EYSENCK

Institute of Psychiatry, Maudsley Hospital, London

THE formulation of a complete theory of personality must be based on the discovery of invariances of two rather different types. In the first place, what is required is *static* or *descriptive* invariance, i.e., the taxonomic, nosological, or dimensional analysis of personality. Work of this kind would result in a descriptive system of personality in terms of a limited number of abilities, traits, and attitudes; in the exact sciences the most obvious analogue to this system would be the discovery of the Periodic Table of Elements. The statistical methods involved in studies of this kind would be those making use of analysis of interdependence (correlational analysis, component analysis, association and contingency analysis, factor analysis).

In the second place, what is required is *dynamic*, or *sequential* invariance, i.e., the analysis of lawful sequences of behavior and the discovery of their causes. Work of this kind would result in a causal system of laws in terms of concepts such as conditioning, inhibition, oscillation, etc.; in the exact sciences the most obvious analogue to this would be the discovery of the laws' of motion. The statistical methods involved in studies of this kind would be those making use of analysis of dependence (analysis of variance and covariance, regression analysis, and confluence analysis).

As has been pointed out elsewhere (5), a logical case can be made out for maintaining that the *static* type of analysis should precede the *dynamic*; before we can discover dynamic laws responsible for extraversion, say, or neuroticism, we must demonstrate that these

concepts do in fact refer to measurable and operationally definable entities. Work summarized in *The Structure of Human Personality* has shown that many different investigators holding divergent points of view and making use of a great variety of test procedures can be found to agree with respect to their main conclusions in the taxonomic field. The following six points present a brief summary of the main areas of agreement:

1. Human conduct is not specific, but presents a certain amount of *generality*; in other words, conduct in one situation is predictable from conduct in other situations.

2. Different degrees of generality can be discerned, giving rise to different levels of personality organization of structure. It follows that our view of personality structure must be *hierarchical*.

3. Degrees of generality can be operationally defined in terms of correlations. The lowest level of generality is defined by test-retest correlations; the next level (trait level) by intercorrelations of tests purporting to be measures of the same trait, or the same primary ability; the highest level by correlations between different traits defining second-order concepts like g in the cognitive field and "neuroticism" in the orectic field, or type concepts like extraversion-introversion.

4. Mental abnormality (mental deficiency, neurosis, psychosis) is not qualitatively different from normality, in the sense that a person with a broken arm, or a patient suffering from haemophilia, is different from someone not ill; different types of mental abnormality constitute the extreme ends of continuous variables which are probably orthogonal to each other.

5. It follows from the above that psychiatric diagnostic procedures are at fault in diagnosing categories, such as "hysteria" or "schizophrenia;" what is required is the determination of the main dimensions involved, and a quantitative estimate of the patient's position on each of these dimensions. (See example below.)

6. The main dimensions involved in the

[1] The writer is indebted to the Bethlem Royal Hospital and the Maudsley Hospital Research Committee for a grant which made this study possible. Dr. L. Minski, Superintendent of Belmont Hospital, and Dr. M. Desai, Chief Psychologist, gave permission for patients to be tested and very kindly helped in the selection of patients, as did various psychiatrists at Belmont Hospital, to all of whom thanks are due. Numerous discussions with Mr. M. B. Shapiro clarified many theoretical problems, and the writer is indebted to Mr. A. E. Maxwell for statistical help and advice.

analysis of personality for which sufficient experimental data are available to make possible a theoretical formulation are neuroticism and extraversion-introversion.

While the congruence of empirical findings in this field is welcome, it should not be allowed to disguise from us the fact that the task of personality theory cannot stop halfway. We would be well advised to regard traits, types, abilities, attitudes, and "factors" generally not as the end products of our investigation, but rather as the starting point for a more causal type of analysis. Thurstone (44) has pointed out that a coefficient of correlation is a confession of ignorance; it indicates the existence of a relation but leaves the causal problem quite indeterminate. Much the same is true of a statistical factor; based, as it is, on an analysis of a set of correlations, it still does not in itself reveal to us anything about the causal relations at work. In this paper, therefore, an attempt is made to go beyond the purely descriptive studies which have so far engaged the main attention of our laboratory and to attempt the construction of a causal hypothesis with respect to at least one of the main personality dimensions.

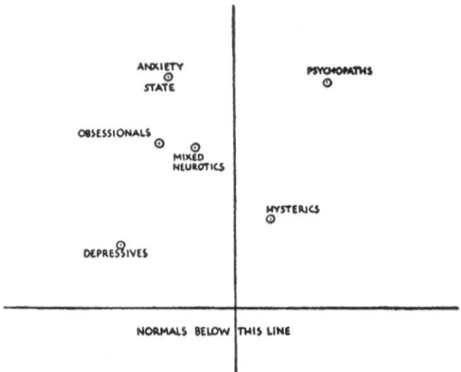

FIG. 1. EMPIRICALLY DETERMINED POSITIONS OF GROUP MEANS FOR NEUROTIC PATIENTS DIAGNOSED AS REACTIVE DEPRESSION, OBSESSIONAL, ANXIETY STATE, MIXED, HYSTERIC, AND PSYCHOPATH, RESPECTIVELY

EXTRAVERSION AND THE CORTICAL INHIBITION HYPOTHESIS

A brief summary of an experimental investigation will indicate the type of fact calling for an explanation. Proceeding on the hypothesis that the test differences between hospitalized neurotics and nonhospitalized "normals" (i.e., people without psychiatric involvement) would provide us with an outside criterion of "neuroticism," and that test differences between hysterics (Jung's prototype group for the concept of "extraversion") and dysthymics (patients suffering from anxiety, Jung's prototype group for the concept of "introversion") would provide us with an outside criterion of "extraversion-introversion," a battery of objective tests of persistence, suggestibility, and other traits was administered to groups of hysterics, psychopaths, reactive depressives, obsessionals, anxiety states, mixed neurotics, and normals (13). Retaining the hysterics, anxiety states, and normals as criterion groups, intercorrelations were calculated between tests for the subjects in the remaining groups, and a

Lawley-type factor analysis was performed. Three clear-cut simple structure factors emerged, corresponding to intelligence, neuroticism, and extraversion. Intelligence tests had high loadings on the intelligence factor; the tests differentiating between the normal and neurotic groups had high loadings on the neuroticism factor; the tests differentiating between the hysterics and anxiety states had high loadings on the extraversion-introversion factor.

Factor scores on the introversion-extraversion factor were then calculated for the persons in the various groups. Figure 1 gives a diagrammatic indication of the results obtained. The line separating the neurotic groups from the normal subjects was drawn so as to put 10 per cent of the normal group on the neurotic side, this being the percentage found by R. Fraser (8) to show debilitating neurotic tendencies in a normal working-class population. It will be seen that psychopaths are slightly more extraverted than hysterics, and that obsessionals and depressives are about as introverted as anxiety states. Differences between extraverted groups and introverted groups are fully significant. Mixed neurotics are intermediate between the other groups; normals are very significantly lower on "neuroticism" than any of the neurotic groups. These results allow us to use the hysteric-psychopath group on the one hand and the dysthymic group (anxiety state, reactive depression, obsessionals) on the other as criteria for any predictions made in terms of a theory of extraversion-introversion.

One further fact is relevant in connection with any hypothesis regarding extraversion-introversion. In a study of monozygotic and dyzygotic twins, McLeod (24) has shown that a factor of extraversion-introversion (in addition to other factors) could be obtained from the intercorrelation of a large number of objective tests; he also found that the intercorrelation of factor scores was very much higher for the monozygotic than for the dyzygotic twins. This indicates that extraversion is strongly based on an inherited disposition. If we are willing to use Holzinger's coefficient h^2 as a very rough index of the contribution of heredity to the variance of our extraversion measure in this sample, we would have to conclude that the contribution of heredity is very much stronger than that of environment.

This finding suggests that our search for a causal factor responsible for extraverted behavior should be concentrated on properties of the central nervous system, and more particularly the cortex, as it is unlikely that peripheral factors could be responsible for the far-reaching and complex differences observed between extraverts and introverts. Historically there have been several attempts in this direction; we need only mention the work of Gross (10, 11) on the primary and secondary function, and that of Spearman (41) on perseveration. Experimental evidence is not lacking to show that these early attempts were quite unsuccessful; the recent work of Rim (34), for instance, has shown not only that there is no one general factor of perseveration, but also that none of the twenty or so tests of perseveration used by him succeeded in differentiating at a reasonable level of significance between hysterics and dysthymics.

More acceptable, perhaps, is a theory proposed by Pavlov (26), who considered the phenomena of hysteria to be closely linked with his concept of *inhibition*. Postulating excessive concentration of excitation in a weak nervous system, Pavlov argues that in the hysteric the process of negative induction should give rise to intense inhibition effects. His theory is difficult to follow in detail, and testable deductions cannot easily be made with any confidence. Further, Pavlov did not extend his tentative hypothesis to the typological field, nor did he himself carry out any experimental work on human beings to support or refute it. Nevertheless, the theory here presented is essentially a development and simplification of his. It bases itself on the concept of *reactive inhibition* developed by Hull (17), rather than on that of *negative induction* developed by Pavlov (27), because the evidence in favor of the former appears more conclusive than the evidence in favor of the latter, and also because the former seems to lend itself more easily to the formulation of exact and testable predictions.

We may state this theory in three parts, dealing respectively with the general law, the postulation of individual differences, and the typological postulate. The general law reads as follows:

A. Whenever any stimulus-response connection is made in an organism (excitation), there also occurs simultaneously a reaction in the nervous structures mediating this connection which opposes its recurrence (inhibition). This hypothesis is a more general formulation of Hull's first submolar principle; it states in effect, as he puts it, that

all responses leave behind in the physical structures involved in the evocation, a state or substance which acts directly to inhibit the evocation of the activity in question. The hypothetical inhibitory condition or substance is observable only through its effect upon positive reaction potentials. This negative action is called *reactive inhibition*. An increment of reactive inhibition (ΔI_R) is assumed to be generated by every repetition of the response (R), whether reinforced or not, and these increments are assumed to accumulate except as they spontaneously disintegrate with the passage of time.

The second part of the hypothesis deals with the problem of individual differences adumbrated by Pavlov but almost completely neglected by Hull. A statement of this part of the hypothesis might be as follows:

B. Human beings differ with respect to the speed with which reactive inhibition is produced, the strength of reactive inhibition, and the speed with which reactive inhibition is dissipated. These differences themselves are properties of the physical structures involved in the evocation of responses.

The third part of the hypothesis relates A and B to the results of taxonomic work summarized above and states:

CORTICAL INHIBITION, FIGURAL AFTEREFFECT, AND PERSONALITY

C. Individuals in whom reactive inhibition is generated quickly, in whom strong reactive inhibitions are generated, and in whom reactive inhibition is dissipated slowly are thereby predisposed to develop extraverted patterns of behavior and to develop hysterical disorders in cases of neurotic breakdown; conversely, individuals in whom reactive inhibition is generated slowly, in whom weak reactive inhibitions are generated, and in whom reactive inhibition is dissipated quickly, are thereby predisposed to develop introverted patterns of behavior and to develop dysthymic disorders in cases of neurotic breakdown.

Comparatively little work has been done in this field since Pavlov's original fragmentary hypotheses were formulated. The experiments by Welsh and Kubis (45, 46) have lent some support to hypotheses of this type. In one experiment these investigators used PGR conditioning on 82 control subjects and 51 neurotic patients. They found, as could be predicted from the inhibition theory, that their patients, most of whom were of the dysthymic type, conditioned very much more quickly than did the controls (average number of repetitions required for the production of a conditioned response was 8.6 ± 3.1 in the patients and 23.9 ± 8.2 in the controls). Among the patients an attempt was made to rate the degree of anxiety from which they were suffering; it was found that the average number of repetitions required to produce a conditioned response in those with great and moderate anxiety was 7.1 and 8.4 respectively; in those with mild or no anxiety the number of repetitions required was 22.2 and 26.3. (Correlations between conditionability and age and intelligence were quite insignificant; test-retest reliability was .88 in the normal group.)

In another experiment 24 dysthymic patients were contrasted with 22 controls. Again the mean number of repetitions required was significantly different for the two groups, being 7.5 ± 2.31 for the dysthymic patients, and 21.86 ± 7.97 for the controls. Some hysterics were also tested and were found difficult to condition.

The only investigation, however, to put the hypothesis to a proper test by including a matched group of hysterics as well as normal and dysthymic groups was carried out at the Maudsley Hospital by Franks (7). Using the eyewink reflex to a puff of air as the response, and a tone as the conditioned stimulus, he obtained unequivocal evidence that dysthymics condition more quickly than normals, and normals more quickly than hysterics. (The normal group, being a random sample of the population, would include extraverts and introverts in roughly equal proportions and would therefore be ambivert on the average, and consequently intermediate between the extravert-hysteric and the introvert-dysthymic groups.)

Among several other investigators who have succeeded in relating speed of conditioning to dysthymia, the work of Taylor (42) and Taylor and Spence (43) is of particular interest, as these investigators advance an explanation of the phenomenon which is somewhat different from our own.

Making use of Hull's formula $sE_R = sH_R \times D$, where sE_R represents excitatory potential, sH_R = habit strength, and D = drive strength, they argue that anxiety is related to drive level, and that consequently higher states of anxiety should lead to quicker conditioning (sE_R) because of increases in drive strength (D). Their experiments do not provide crucial evidence with respect to the two theories involved as the same prediction would be made in terms of both hypotheses.[2] It seemed necessary, therefore, to choose a prediction which would produce positive effects in terms of our hypothesis, but where no such prediction could reasonably be made in terms of the Taylor-Spence hypothesis. An attempt to formulate such a deduction will be made in the next section.

[2] Spence and Taylor (43) use the Taylor Scale of Manifest Anxiety as a measure of anxiety in spite of the fact that little evidence is brought forward to support any assumption that it correlates with clinical estimates of anxiety. The work of Holtzman (2), as well as that of Sampson and Bindra (35), in which an attempt is made to link up scores on this scale and independent criteria, fails to support Taylor's hypothesis. Franks (7) has shown that contrary to the Spence and Taylor hypothesis hysterics, whose scores on the Taylor scale are about as high as those of dysthymics, are more difficult to condition than members of a normal group, whose scores on the Taylor Scale are very much lower. He also failed, as have other investigators (2, 14), to obtain a significant correlation between conditioning and score on the Taylor Scale. These findings throw considerable doubt on the Spence-Taylor hypothesis.

H. J. Eysenck

Cortical Inhibition and Figural Aftereffect

In searching for a phenomenon which would avoid the ambiguity of results encountered in the work of conditioning, it was found necessary to go back from Hull's development of learning theory to Pavlov's somewhat more fundamental position. Pavlov regarded the conditioned reflex as a tool for investigating the dynamics of cortical action rather than as a paradigm of learning. He considered that the laws discovered by him had perfectly general validity and were not restricted to the very special circumstances of the conditioning experiment; indeed, he suggested explicitly that perceptual and other phenomena could find an explanation in terms of inhibition, excitation, disinhibition, etc. It seems possible, therefore, that we may be successful in our search if we look for perceptual phenomena to which our general theory may be found applicable.

The phenomenon chosen for this purpose was the figural aftereffect discussed by Köhler and Wallach (20), Gibson (9), Luchins (23), and others, in a series of articles. Essentially, the effects observed showed beyond doubt that constant stimulation of parts of certain sensory surfaces, such as the retina, sets up states of inhibition in corresponding areas in the cortex which have measurable effects on the perception of stimuli later presented in the same region. If, for instance, a circle is fixated for a period of one or two minutes, and is then withdrawn, other stimulus objects, such as a small square, appearing within that part of the retina and the cortex which had previously been surrounded by the circle, will appear smaller than a square of precisely the same size appearing elsewhere on the retina and the cortex.

Effects of this kind appear to be exactly in line with the statement quoted in explanation of Part A of our hypothesis to the effect that "all responses leave behind in the physical structures involved in the evocation, a state or substance which acts directly to inhibit the evocation of the activity in question" (17). It should be noted that in accepting the fact of the occurrence of figural aftereffects, we need not necessarily accept Köhler's theory regarding the origin of these aftereffects, just as in accepting the fact of Pavlovian inhibition

we need not accept his theory of cortical inhibition. There is, indeed, a curious resemblance between the arch-atomist Pavlov, on the one hand, and the arch-Gestaltist Köhler, on the other, in that both have proposed what are strictly physiological, molecular theories of brain action to account for their findings, and that both theories are well outside orthodox neurology. Konorski (21) has discussed the relationship between Pavlov's physiological and neurological theories and those of Sherrington and other orthodox workers in some detail and has attempted to account for Pavlov's experimental results in more acceptable terms; Osgood and Heyer (25) have attempted to do a similar service for Köhler's figural aftereffects.

While we need not deal in detail with Köhler's theories, we must note the terminology used by him, which is in part at least bound up with his theory. The reader will find a more extensive discussion in a recent paper by Luchins and Luchins (23). Briefly, then, Köhler assumes that every visual figure is associated with currents in the visual sector of the nervous system, the currents being the results of a difference in density and brightness between figure and ground. (For ease of discussion we are presenting an example from the visual field, but the same arguments apply to all other sensory fields, and the experiment to be described shortly was, indeed, done in the kinaesthetic field rather than in the visual.) The visual sector is considered as a volume conductor, and figure currents are assumed to polarize all surfaces through which they pass. This polarization and certain aftereffects in the affected cells are called *electrotonus*, and it is known that this condition of electrotonus may proceed for some time after the polarizing current has ceased to flow. Köhler uses the term *satiation* to describe electrotonic effect of figure currents on the cortical sector; the term *figural aftereffects* is used to denote the alterations which test objects may show when their figure currents pass through a satiated region.

Satiation has as its main effect a localized inhibition in the sense that polarization of the affected cells increases their resistance to the passage of an electric current, thereby making the appearance of figure currents in that region more difficult, i.e., acting as an inhibiting agent. The main observable fact mediated in this way is the *displacement* of test objects from the affected region. This displacement is measurable, shows pronounced individual differences, and may be used both as a measure and as an operational definition of cortical inhibition in the perceptual field.

The importance of these satiation phenomena in their own right will be obvious to anyone familiar with Köhler's highly original and brilliant work in this field. From the point of view of general psychology, they are of particular interest in that they form a bridge between two large fields of study which have hitherto remained either out of touch or else frankly antagonistic to each other. One of these is the field of conditioning and learning theory; the other is that of perception. In this work on figural aftereffects we find at long last a *rapprochement* between these large groups of workers and the sets of facts unearthed quite independently by them, and it is encouraging to note that the general law of inhibition enunciated by Pavlov, and more explicitly by Hull, appears to be formally identical with that advanced by Köhler in terms of perceptual satiation.[3] As long as we regard only the speculative brain theories of these writers, we will tend to miss the essential similarity of their formulations; once we concentrate on the molar rather than on the molecular parts of their theories the similarity will be striking.

The main aim of this section, however, is not to point to similarities between Pavlovian and Gestalt theories, but rather to link both of these with personality theory. From what has been said above it follows immediately that if our argument is sound and if the "reactive inhibition" of Pavlov and Hull is indeed essentially identical with the factors involved in Köhler's "satiation," then it would follow directly from Parts B and C of our theory that hysterics should show satiation effects more markedly than dysthymics. In fact, three quite specific predictions can be made. In the first place, satiation effects should appear *earlier* in the hysteric group; in the second place, they should appear more *strongly* in the hysteric group; and in the third place, they should disappear more *slowly* in the hysteric group. These are quite specific

[3] Several workers in Great Britain (1, 3) have recently shown interest in attempts to bring together into one framework these two great fields.

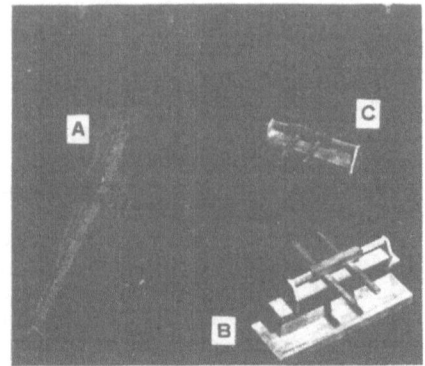

Fig. 2. Photograph of Apparatus used for the Investigation of the Kinaesthetic Figural Aftereffect

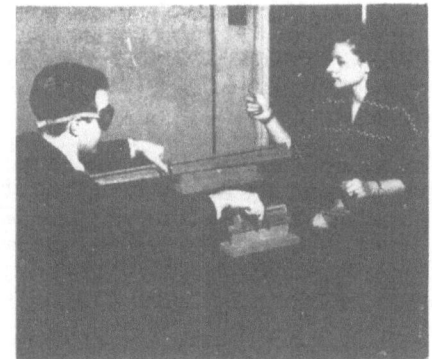

Fig. 3. Subject Undergoing Test to Determine the Extent of Kinaesthetic Figural Aftereffect

predictions which can be tested experimentally, and it is only through such experimental verification that the theory can show its acceptability and usefulness. Our next section will, therefore, be concerned with certain empirical results obtained in comparing a group of hysterics and a group of dysthymics with respect to figural aftereffects.

An Experimental Test of the Cortical Inhibition Hypothesis: Method

Apparatus

The apparatus used in this experiment is an adaptation of that described by Köhler and Dinnerstein (19); the exact form of apparatus and procedure was taken from Klein and Krech (18), who used it in their work on cortical conductivity in the brain injured. As a full description and rationale are given by these authors, our own will be brief; Figs. 2 and 3 show the apparatus set out on a table, and the test in progress, and may serve to facilitate comprehension.

The apparatus consists of a comparison scale (marked "A" in Fig. 2), a test object (marked "B" in Fig. 2), and a stimulus object (marked "C" in Fig. 2). Movable riders are affixed to all three objects in such a way that the position of thumb and forefinger is fixed as the subject moves these two fingers up and down along the sides of the object. All objects are made of unpainted, smoothed hardwood. The apparatus is so arranged as to present the comparison scale to the left of the seated subject, and either the test or stimulus object to his right (see Fig. 3).

Procedure

The subject (*S*) is blindfolded before he has an opportunity of viewing any part of the equipment. Having taken his seat in front of the apparatus, his task is explained in detail and a demonstration given. Then the experiment proper commences. Putting thumb and forefinger of his right hand into the rider on the test object, and thumb and forefinger of his left hand into the rider on the comparison scale, *S* is required to adjust the position of the rider on the comparison scale until the distance between the fingers of his left hand feels equal to the distance between the fingers of his right hand. This is the point of subjective equality, and all changes are measured from this point as the baseline. Four separate determinations are carried out, and the results averaged, to make this baseline more reliable.

The next step in the experiment consists in providing *S* with varying periods of constant tactile stimulation. For this purpose he is instructed to put his fingers into the rider on the stimulus object, which is slightly broader than the test object ($2\frac{1}{2}$ in. as compared with $1\frac{1}{2}$ in.), and to rub the sides of the stimulus object at an even rate for periods of 30 sec., 60 sec., 90 sec., and 120 sec., respectively. Four determinations of subjective equality are made after each period of rubbing, in order to obtain more reliable measures. In this way the effect of rubbing the stimulus object on the perception of the test object is ascertained. Finally, after a five-minutes rest and again after another ten-minutes rest, the subjective width of the test object is again ascertained in order to establish the perseverative effects of the stimulation periods. These two sets of judgments are again obtained four times each in order to increase reliability.

Scoring

The predicted aftereffect consequent upon the rubbing of a stimulus object *broader* than the test object is an apparent shrinking of the test object, which should manifest itself in terms of a decrement in the width on the comparison scale judged equal to the test object. For each subject this decrement is expressed in terms of his own original baseline, so that individual differences in perceived equality are taken into account in the score, which thus is essentially a percentage decre-

ment score, i.e., an estimate of the shrinkage that has occurred as a percentage of the original width of the object as perceived by each subject.

The following scores will be reported in this paper: 1. average percentage decrement after 30 sec.; 2. average percentage decrement after 60 sec.; 3. average percentage decrement after 90 sec.; 4. average percentage decrement after 120 sec.; 5. sum of the above four scores; 6. maximum single percentage decrement obtained from any subject. In addition to these poststimulation aftereffects, the following recovery period scores were obtained: (*a*) average percentage decrement after 5-min rest; (*b*) average percentage decrement after (10 min. + 5 min. =) 15 min. rest; (*c*) sum of these two scores.

Subjects

The *S*s used in this investigation were selected on the basis of two criteria. The first of these was that they should fall into the diagnostic groups of hysterics and dysthymics respectively. Diagnoses of conversion hysteria, hysteria, and psychopathy were accepted as falling into the former group; diagnoses of anxiety state, reactive depression, obsessional and compulsive disorders were accepted as falling into the latter group.

In view of the known unreliability of psychiatric diagnosis, which has been demonstrated, for instance, in *The Scientific Study of Personality* (4), it was considered advisable to have a second criterion which was independent of diagnosis. For this purpose a questionnaire was used which had been shown by Hildebrand (13) to be a good measure of extraversion. This questionnaire is Guilford's Rathymia scale (12), and the reader will find evidence regarding the adequacy of this scale as a measure of extraversion discussed elsewhere (6). The procedure followed was that no one with a score below 31 was accepted as extraverted, and no one with a score above 39 was accepted as introverted.[4] While it would have been desirable to have no overlap at all in the questionnaire scores of the two groups, it proved impossible to find a large enough group of subjects in the time available to

[4] Hysterics were found by Hildebrand (13) to have an average score of 37 ± 12, dysthymics one of 28 ± 10. In our sample the means were 40 ± 12 and 25 ± 10 respectively.

CORTICAL INHIBITION, FIGURAL AFTEREFFECT, AND PERSONALITY

TABLE 1

POSTSTIMULATION FIGURAL AFTEREFFECTS—
DYSTHYMICS

Source	df	MS	F
Between times	3	116.0082	0.7752
Between people	13	2050.0241	13.7010
Residual	39	149.6416	
Total	55		

$r_{11} = 0.9270$

TABLE 3

POSTSTIMULATION FIGURAL AFTEREFFECTS—
HYSTERICS

Source	df	MS	F
Between times	3	38.5519	0.3895
Between people	13	443.9761	4.4860
Residual	39	98.9703	
Total	55		

$r_{11} = 0.7771$

TABLE 2

RECOVERY PERIOD AFTEREFFECTS—DYSTHYMICS

Source	df	MS	F
Between times	1	1.9137	0.0541
Between people	13	642.1574	18.1429
Residual	13	35.3945	
Total	27		

$r_{11} = 0.9449$

TABLE 4

RECOVERY PERIOD AFTEREFFECTS—HYSTERICS

Source	df	MS	F
Between times	1	53.8013	1.1749
Between people	13	319.8050	6.9837
Residual	13	45.7933	
Total	27		

$r_{11} = 0.8568$

reach this ideal. We can only suggest that the results found with the present groups would probably have been improved somewhat if a stricter criterion could have been employed.

There were fourteen subjects in each group, all of them males. The average ages of the two groups were 29.14 (hysterics) and 34.23 (dysthymics), an insignificant difference. Matrix IQ's were 100.86 and 104.92, Mill Hill Vocabulary IQ's 102.79 and 110.25; these differences also were insignificant.

Reliability of Scores

Granted that our methods of scoring, which we have taken over from Klein and Krech (18), are the most obvious ones, we must first of all ask ourselves questions regarding their reliability and consistency. To our knowledge, there are no reports in the literature dealing with this question, which is of crucial importance whenever test results are to be used as psychometric scores. Consequently, two analyses of variance were carried out for each of the two groups with whom we are concerned, i.e., the hysterics and the dysthymics. The first analysis deals with the scores which we have called average poststimulation figural aftereffects; the second analysis deals with the scores from the two recovery periods. With the formula suggested by Hoyt (16), reliabili-

ties of .93 and .94 were found for the dysthymics; both of these were significant at the .001 level. For the hysterics the reliabilities are somewhat lower, being .78 and .86 respectively. Both of these, however, are significant at the .01 level. Full details are given in Tables 1, 2, 3, and 4.[5]

Having found dysthymics to be more consistent in their test performances than hysterics, we would expect to find the correlations among the six scores (four poststimulation scores and two recovery period scores) to be higher for the dysthymics than for the hysterics; this is indeed so. On comparison of the two sets of 15 correlations pair by pair, it was found that in 13 cases the dysthymic correla-

[5] This consistency in itself poses certain problems for the theoretical analysis of the figural aftereffect phenomenon. Some subjects consistently over-rate rather than under-rate the size of the test object after stimulation. This is very difficult to account for in terms of either the Gestalt or the statistical type of hypothesis. A survey of the literature, on other types of inhibition phenomena (massed and spaced learning, reminiscence, etc.) indicates that while most people act in conformity with prediction, some consistently go counter to prediction, i.e., learn better with massed rather than with spaced practice, etc. Theorists usually deal with averages rather than with individual cases and traditionally disregard aberrations of this kind. It seems reasonable to ask that any adequate theory should be able to account for discordant cases as well as for the admittedly large number of concordant ones.

H. J. EYSENCK

TABLE 5

	Poststimulation Figural Aftereffects						Recovery Period		
	30 sec.	60 sec.	90 sec.	120 sec.	ϵ	Max.	5 min.	10 min.	ϵ
	Hysterics								
Means	9.68	10.58	13.09	12.78	46.13	20.74	4.35	8.00	12.35
Variances	9.48	13.57	14.22	16.30	1775.90	97.58	14.65	12.94	645.70
	Dysthymics								
Means	1.70	6.21	2.98	7.96	18.85	15.32	0.89	0.36	1.52
Variances	12.97	21.95	32.83	27.77	8200.10	190.12	15.77	20.59	1284.31

tion was higher; in one case the two were equal; in one case the hysteric correlation was higher. Thus, our expectation is borne out that dysthymics would be more consistent than hysterics.

RESULTS

We must next turn to the main differences between the groups. Means and variances for hysterics and dysthymics respectively are given in Table 5 for the four poststimulation aftereffects, the sum of the poststimulation aftereffects, the maximum poststimulation aftereffect, the five- and ten-minute recovery period aftereffects, and the sum of the rest period aftereffects. Four poststimulation aftereffects and the two rest periods are plotted in Fig. 4. All the results will be seen to be in line with prediction. Figural aftereffects in the

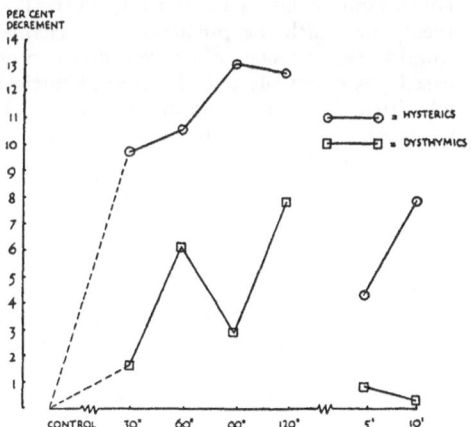

FIG. 4. AMOUNT OF FIGURAL AFTEREFFECT SHOWN AS PERCENTAGE DECREMENT AFTER FOUR DIFFERENT PERIODS OF STIMULATION AND TWO DIFFERENT PERIODS OF REST

hysteric group appear more quickly, are more strongly marked, and disappear more slowly than in the dysthymics.

The significance of the differences between the two groups was tested by means of Hotelling's T test (15). This over-all test invalidated the null hypothesis at between the .01 and .05 levels of significance. Individual one-tail t tests applied to the nine separate scores disclosed that only the 30-sec. period gave results significant at below the .05 level of significance; the other scores were significant at approximately the .10 level only. It is suggested that in future work more attention be paid to short periods of stimulation (between 10 sec. and 30 sec.) as longer periods of stimulation appear to increase variability without increasing differentiation. It might also prove useful to make use of more prolonged rest pauses; times of 15 min., 20 min. and 30 min. might give improved differentiation.

The calculation of differences between groups gives little idea of the strength of the relationship discovered. Accordingly product-moment correlations were calculated between scores on the figural aftereffect test and the R scale. In addition to the 28 hysterics and dysthymics used for the group comparison, an additional seven neurotics were included in this calculation. These Ss had shown a discrepancy between diagnosis and score on the R scale, and had therefore not been included in the group comparisons. Correlations for this group of altogether 35 neurotic subjects were as follows: .374 (30 sec.); .252 (60 sec.); .236 (90 sec.); .218 (120 sec.); .321 (5 min.); .237 (10 min). It will be noted that with increasing periods of stimulation, correlations tend to fall off in a regular progression. As regards significance, the correlation for the 30-sec. period almost reaches the .01 level; of the others only the correlation for the 5-min. rest period passes the .05 level of significance. The remaining correlations just fall short of the .05 level. Significance levels were of course calculated by using one-tailed tests, as follows from the logic of the experimental design.

It is interesting to note the fate of the seven individuals in whom diagnosis and R score disagreed. In each case where a patient was diagnosed hysteric but had an R score which put him on the introverted side, relatively small aftereffects were found. In each case where a patient was diagnosed dysthymic but had an R score which put him on the extraverted side, relatively large aftereffects were found. In other words, when diagnosis and questionnaire disagree, agreement of the experimental test is much closer with the questionnaire than with diagnosis. In view of the widespread habit of heaping contumely upon questionnaires, this fact may deserve stressing.

DISCUSSION

It will not require much discussion to establish the relevance of the results of our experiment to a theory of neurotic disorder. Psychoanalytic theories have usually played down differences between the various types of neurotic symptomatology as accidental, unimportant, and variable; usually the implication has been that hysteria and the dysthymic disorders both lie close to each other along one single dimension of *regression*, and that hysterical symptoms are in a sense merely a defense against the overt anxiety shown by the dysthymic. On the basis of this type of theory, no fundamental differences would be expected on psychophysiological measures of conditioning or of figural aftereffects. The fact that such differences are observed considerably weakens the Freudian theory, and supports the dimensional theory outlined at the beginning of this paper. Another advantage of the dimensional theory appears to be that it can account for the similarities observed in the behavior and the symptomatology of hysterics, brain-injured, and leucotomized patients, a task not even attempted by psychoanalytic writers. A discussion of such an extension of our theory may be in order.

The experimental procedure adopted in section four was taken over directly from Klein and Krech, and a comparison of our results with theirs may be of some interest. They were concerned with differences between brain-injured patients and normals, and found that figural aftereffect was much more strongly marked among the former than in the normal control group. The average size of the over-all figural aftereffect was 12.08 per cent for the brain-injured and 6.25 per cent for the controls. The maximum degree of effect for the brain-injured averaged 19.50 per cent, for controls, 13.00 per cent. Corresponding figures for hysterics and dysthymics are: 11.53 per cent and 4.71 per cent for average over-all effect, 20.74 per cent and 15.32 per cent for maximum effect. There is thus a distinct similarity in the behavior of the brain-injured in Klein and Krech's study and the hysterics in our own. The normal controls tested by Klein and Krech give results intermediate between our hysteric and dysthymic groups, though somewhat closer to the dysthymics.

These figures would seem to indicate similarities between hysteria and brain injury which are important from a theoretical point of view. In a series of studies (28, 29, 30, 31), A. Petrie has shown that one of the psychological aftereffects of leucotomy is an increase in extraversion, as measured by objective tests of personality similar to those used by Hildebrand in his factorial study (13). The theory on which the prediction of a change toward extraversion after leucotomy was based was essentially one of increased cortical inhibition following brain injury.[6] Such an hypothesis is much too broad and general to account for all the known facts and will presumably require a good deal of detailed modification, particularly with respect to the differential activity of various parts of the brain, and the effect of specific incisions and ablations. Thus, recent unpublished work by A. Petrie has shown that a change in the direction of increased extraversion is produced by all prefrontal operations involving the convexity (standard leucotomy, Rostral leucotomy, and

---

[6] Here again Pavlov's theory of negative induction has also been used to account for some of the observed effects (36, 37, 38, 39, 40); it is not clear to what extent negative induction and reactive inhibition can be identified with each other at the phenomenal level.

selective surgery of areas 9 and/or 10). On the other hand, cingulectomy and orbital undercutting, i.e., operations not involving the convexity, do not have aftereffects involving a shift toward extraversion on the tests used. If these results were to be confirmed, they would clearly indicate the need to make this general hypothesis much more specific.

Nevertheless, as a first approximation, this general hypothesis has led to the prediction of the phenomena observed by Petrie (28) and it does account similarly for the results of the Klein and Krech experiment. It would appear worthy of further investigation, particularly as it gives rise to very clear-cut predictions. Thus, we may predict that the formation of conditioned reflexes would be more difficult in the brain-injured than in the intact individual. Some evidence supporting this prediction has just been published by Reese, Doss, and Gantt (33). After leucotomy, we would predict that inhibitory effects would be more strongly marked than before, and we would also be able to make a number of predictions regarding the reactions of leucotomized patients on certain perceptual tests similar to those made in the concluding section of this paper with respect to hysterics.

Klein and Krech, in their paper, advance a somewhat different theory which, however, in most essentials appears to deviate but little from that used in our own work. They assume that

... transmission rate of excitation patterns varies from individual to individual, from time to time within the same individual, and from area to area within a single cortical field at any time. With this assumption it is possible to appeal to *differential* cortical conductivity as a parameter which will help us understand inter- and intra-individual differences in cortical integration and therefore in behavior (18, p. 118).

It may be worth-while to indicate in just one sentence the essential difference between the conductivity hypothesis and the one advocated here. Klein and Krech postulate neural conductivity as a basic personality dimension, assuming that it may be high or low *prior to any stimulation*. We assume that individuals differ not with respect to conductivity, but with respect to the rate at which inhibition is aroused along cortical pathways by the passage of a neural impulse. The latter hypothesis seems to be more securely based on experimental findings, less

subject to unprovable assumptions, and more easily testable. It is for these reasons that it has been preferred in this paper. It should be added, however, that both the conductivity and the inhibition hypothesis give rise to similar predictions in the case of the degree of satiation to be expected in the brain-injured and hysterical patients, and that the data reported here do not in any way disprove the conductivity hypothesis, any more than they prove the inhibition hypothesis.

It may be worth while, however, to indicate very briefly the type of prediction which our theory makes possible, and to suggest lines along which it could be disproved.

1. If we accept Köhler's demonstration that the rate of disappearance with time of the Müller-Lyer and other illusions is a consequence of figural aftereffects, it can be predicted that the rate of disappearance of the illusion should be more rapid with hysterics than with dysthymics, and in the brain-injured as compared with the normal.

2. If we accept Klein's interpretation of the phenomenon, it can be predicted that when the persistence of an afterimage is measured as a function of the duration of stimulus exposure, the duration of the afterimage in hysterics should fall off significantly as compared with dysthymics. Klein has already shown that this is so when the brain-injured are compared with normal subjects (18).

3. Phenomena of apparent motion may be reformulated in terms of the inhibition theory and it may be predicted that the optimal time interval for the perception of apparent movement would be decreased more in hysterics than in dysthymics after the introduction of some form of continuous stimulation in the path of the apparent movement. Shapiro (40) has shown, in experiments using continuous stimulation in order to produce experimental inhibition effects in the occurrence of apparent movement, that under conditions of inhibition the time-interval threshold was 140 sigma, as compared with 250 sigma under noninhibition conditions.

4. If a theory of satiation or inhibition be acceptable as accounting for reversal of perspective, then one would predict not only that the rate of reversal would increase in time as it is known to do, but also that this increase in

rate of reversal should be more marked among hysterics than among dysthymics. Our prediction here, as in the case of the experiment described in this paper, would relate more to a change of rate than to the initial rate of reversal, although the latter also should show differences in favor of the hysterics and the brain-injured.

5. Perceptual disinhibition phenomena of the type studied by Rawdon-Smith (32) and others might be presumed also to show differences between hysterics and dysthymics. On the hypothesis that we are dealing with the inhibition of an inhibition in these cases, it might be predicted that disinhibition should be more pronounced among hysterics than among dysthymics.

6. Critical flicker fusion would be expected to be observed at different frequencies in hysterics and brain-injured, as compared with dysthymics and non-brain-injured. This follows directly from our interpretation of the law of reactive inhibition. Some empirical data are available to support one of these predictions at least (22).

7. Rotation phenomena, such as have been described by Shapiro (40), have been explained by him in terms of inhibition (negative induction). If this hypothesis, which has led to important discoveries in the field of brain injury, should prove acceptable, then we would expect a greater degree of rotation among hysterics than among dysthymics.

In making these predictions, we have purposely kept within the perceptual field, but it is clear that many other predictions could be made in the fields of learning, memory, and motor behavior. Phenomena of reminiscence, of massed and spaced learning, of vigilance, of blocking, and many others have been interpreted in terms of inhibition. While it remains possible, of course, that in each separate case we must have recourse to a different type of inhibition, this does not seem a likely contingency, and the hypothesis certainly appears worth testing that it is the same type of cortical inhibition which causes all these phenomena, as well as the perceptual ones discussed above. The obvious method of testing this hypothesis appears to be in terms of individual differences, i.e., in postulating that a person found to show a high degree of inhibition with respect to any one of these phenomena should also show a high degree of inhibition with respect to all the others. It is hoped to provide evidence with respect to this generalized inhibition hypothesis in the near future.

SUMMARY AND CONCLUSIONS

An attempt has been made in this paper to work out a dynamic theory to account for a number of experimental findings in the field of personality related to the concept of extraversion-introversion. Following Pavlov and Hull, a theory of cortical inhibition was developed to account for observed differences in behavior and a deduction from this principle was made by extending it to the perceptual field. It was predicted that hysterics (as a prototype of the extraverted personality type) would be differentiated from dysthymics (as a prototype of the introverted personality type) in the *speed of arousal, strength,* and *length of persistance* of figural aftereffects. A comparison of two groups of carefully selected subjects showed that (a) hysterics developed satiation and figural aftereffects more quickly than did dysthymics; (b) that hysterics developed stronger satiation and figural aftereffects than did dysthymics; and (c) that hysterics developed more persistent satiation and figural aftereffects than did dysthymics. The differences are statistically significant and are in complete accord with prediction. In the discussion, certain parallels were drawn between hysteria and brain injury in terms of the theory outlined, with particular reference to the aftereffects of leucotomy. Lastly, a number of predictions were made from the theory which should permit of an experimental decision as to its worth-whileness.

REFERENCES

1. BERLYNE, D. E. Attention, perception, and behavior theory. *Psychol. Rev.*, 1951, **58**, 137–146.
2. BITTERMAN, M. E., & HOLTZMAN, W. H. Conditoning and extinction of the galvanic skin response as a function of anxiety. *J. abnorm. soc. Psychol.*, 1952, **47**, 615–623.
3. BROADBENT, D. E. Classical conditioning and human watch-keeping. *Psychol. Rev.*, 1953, **60**, 331–339.
4. EYSENCK, H. J. *The scientific study of personality.* London: Routledge & Kegan Paul, 1952.
5. EYSENCK, H. J. The logical basis of factor analysis. *Amer. Psychol.*, 1953, **8**, 105–114.

H. J. EYSENCK

6. EYSENCK, H. J. *The structure of human personality.* London: Methuen, 1953.
7. FRANKS, C. An experimental study of conditioning as related to mental abnormality. Unpublished doctor's dissertation, Univer. of London, 1954.
8. FRASER, R. *The incidence of neurosis among factory workers.* London: H.M.S.O., 1947.
9. GIBSON, J. J. Adaptation, after-effect and contrast in the perception of curved lines. *J. exp. Psychol.*, 1933, **16**, 1–51.
10. GROSS, O. *Die cerebrale Sekundärfunction.* Leipzig, 1902.
11. GROSS, O. *Über psychopathologische Minderwertig-Keiten.* Leipzig, 1909.
12. GUILFORD, J. P. *An inventory of factors STDCR.* Sheridan Supply Company, 1942.
13. HILDEBRAND, H. P. A factorial study of introversion-extraversion by means of objective tests. Unpublished doctor's dissertation, Univer. of London, 1953.
14. HILGARD, E. R., JONES, L. V., & KAPLAN, S. J. Conditioned discrimination as related to anxiety. *J. exp. Psychol.*, 1951, **42**, 94–99.
15. HOTELLING, H. The generalization of "student's" ratio. *Ann. math. Statist.*, 1931, **2**, 360–368.
16. HOYT, C. Test reliability obtained by analysis of variance. *Psychometrika*, 1941, **6**, 153–160.
17. HULL, C. L. *Principles of behavior.* New York: D. Appleton-Century, 1943.
18. KLEIN, G. S., & KRECH, D. Cortical conductivity in the brain-injured. *J. Pers.*, 1952, **21**, 118–148.
19. KÖHLER, W., & DINNERSTEIN, D. Figural after-effects in kinesthesia. In: *Miscellanea psychologica* (Albert Michotte). Louvain: Institut Supérieur de Philosophie, 1947.
20. KÖHLER, W., & WALLACH, H. Figural after-effects: an investigation of visual processes. *Proc. Amer. phil. Soc.*, 1944, **88**, 269–357.
21. KONORSKI, J. *Conditioned reflexes and neuron organization.* Cambridge: University Press, 1948.
22. LANDIS, C. *An annotated bibliography of flicker fusion phenomena.* Michigan: Michigan Armed Forces—National Research Council, 1953.
23. LUCHINS, A. S., & LUCHINS, E. H. The satiation theory of figural after-effects and Gestalt principles of perception. *J. gen. Psychol.* 1953, **49**, 3–29.
24. McLEOD, H. An experimental study of the inheritance of introversion-extraversion. Unpublished doctor's dissertation, Univer. of London, 1954.
25. OSGOOD, C. E., & HEYER, A. W. A new interpretation of figural after-effects. *Psychol. Rev.*, 1952, **59**, 98–118.
26. PAVLOV, I. P. *Lectures on conditioned reflexes.* Vol. II. London: Lawrence & Wishart, 1941.
27. PAVLOV, I. P. *Conditioned reflexes.* London: Oxford Univer. Press, 1927.
28. PETRIE, A. *Personality and the frontal lobes.* London: Routledge & Kegan Paul, 1952.
29. PETRIE, A., & LE BEAU, J. A comparison of the personality changes after (1) prefrontal selective surgery for the relief of intractable pain and for the treatment of mental cases; (2) cingulectomy and topectomy. *J. ment. Sci.*, 1953a, **99**, 53–61.
30. PETRIE, A., & LE BEAU, J. Études psychologiques des changements de la personnalité produits par certaines opérations préfrontales sélectives. *Rev. de Centre de Psychol. appl.*, 1953b, **4**, No. 1, 1–16.
31. PETRIE, A., & LE BEAU, J. Psychological effects of selective frontal surgery including cingulectomy. *Proc. Vth Int. Congr. Neurol.*, Lisbon, 1953, **4**, 392–395.
32. RAWDON-SMITH, A. R. R. Experimental deafness. Further data upon the phenomenon of so-called auditory fatigue. *Brit. J. Psychol.*, 1936, **26**, 233–244.
33. REESE, W. G., DOSS, R., & GANTT, W. H. Autonomic responses in differential diagnoses of organic and psychogenic psychoses. *AMA Arch. neurol. Psychiat.*, 1953, **70**, 778–793.
34. RIM, Y. S. Perseveration and fluency as measures of extraversion-introversion in abnormal subjects. Unpublished doctoral dissertation, Univer. of London, 1953.
35. SAMPSON, H., & BINDRA, D. "Manifest" anxiety, neurotic anxiety, and the rate of conditioning. *J. abnorm. soc. Psychol.*, 1954, **49**, 256–259.
36. SHAPIRO, M. B. Experimental studies of a perceptual anomaly. *J. ment. Sci.*, 1951, **97**, 90–110.
37. SHAPIRO, M. B. Experimental studies of a perceptual anomaly. II. Confirmatory and explanatory experiments. *J. ment. Sci.*, 1952, **98**, 605–617.
38. SHAPIRO, M. B. Experimental studies of a perceptual anomaly. III. The testing of an explanatory theory. *J. ment. Sci.*, 1953, **99**, 393–410.
39. SHAPIRO, M. B. An experimental investigation of the block design rotation effect. An analysis of psychological effect of brain damage. *Brit. J. med. Psychol.*, 1954a, **27**, 84–88.
40. SHAPIRO, M. B. A preliminary investigation of the effects of continuous stimulation on the perception of "apparent motion." *Brit. J. gen. Psychol.* 1954b, **45**, 58–67.
41. SPEARMAN, C. *The abilities of man.* London: Macmillan, 1927.
42. TAYLOR, J. A. The relationship of anxiety to the conditioned eyelid response. *J. exp. Psychol.*, 1951, **41**, 81–92.
43. TAYLOR, J. A., & SPENCE, K. W. The relationship of anxiety level to performance in serial learning. *J. exp. Psychol.*, 1952, **44**, 61–64.
44. Thurstone, L. L. *Multiple factor analysis: a development and expansion of the vectors of the mind.* Chicago: Univer. of Chicago Press, 1947.
45. WELCH, L., & KUBIS, J. The effect of anxiety on the conditioning rate and stability of the PGR. *J. Psychol.*, 1947a, **23**, 83–91.
46. WELCH, L., & KUBIS, J. Conditioned PGR (psychogalvanic response) in states of pathological anxiety. *J. nerv. ment. Dis.*, 1947b, **105**, 372–381.

Received May 10, 1954.

From *C. Shagass and A. B. Kerenyi* (1958). Journal of Nervous and Mental Disease, *126*, 141-147, *by kind permission of the authors and the Williams and Wilkins Co.*

NEUROPHYSIOLOGIC STUDIES OF PERSONALITY[1]

CHARLES SHAGASS, M.D.[2] AND ALBERT B. KERENYI, M.D.[2]

In the field of personality, the identification and measurement of pertinent dimensions are one of the major problems. MacKinnon (10) has listed a number of dichotomous typologies, or bipolar factors, which have been proposed as fundamental dimensions of personality. Examples are the hysterical and obsessional types of Janet, the cycloid and schizoid types of Kretschmer, and the extraverted and introverted types of Jung. Although the typologies have been subject to a great deal of criticism, many of the terms engendered by them, such as "extravert," have found wide acceptance, suggesting a basis in everyday clinical observation. Over the past decade, the investigations of Eysenck and his group have indicated that some dichotomous typologies may represent the extremes of valid and measureable dimensions of personality. By applying factorial analysis to data obtained with a variety of test procedures, Eysenck isolated three personality factors, which he called: neuroticism, introversion-extraversion and psychoticism (3, 5). The investigations to be reported in this paper bear on a possible neurophysiologic basis for the introversion-extraversion dimension.

The present research arose from a previous study of the sedation threshold in psychoneurosis (16). The sedation threshold, which is an objective neurophysiologic determination of the amount of sodium Amytal required to produce certain EEG changes, was found to differentiate between various types of neurosis. Thresholds were low in patients with hysteria, intermediate in patients with mixed neurosis, and high in patients with anxiety states and neurotic depressions. These findings supported the hypothesis that the threshold was correlated with degree of manifest anxiety. However, they could also be taken to indicate a relationship between the threshold and the position of the patient on a personality continuum ranging from hysterical to obsessional. It was then noted that the order in which the sedation threshold arranged the psychoneuroses corresponded closely to the order in which Hildebrand (8) found them to be arranged by a battery of Eysenck's tests of introversion-extraversion. Furthermore, as Eysenck has recently pointed out (4), the sedation threshold results in psychoneurosis appeared to confirm, in every detail, predictions made from his theory that reactive inhibition is greater in hysterics than in dysthymics (obsessive-compulsives, neurotic depressions, anxiety states) (2).

From the parallels between Eysenck's results on introversion-extraversion and those obtained with the sedation threshold, it seemed reasonable to suggest that the sedation threshold might reflect the state of neural mechanisms involved in this dimension of personality. However, more direct studies of these relationships seemed desirable, as they had so far been inferred mainly from differences between diagnostic groups. Two investigative approaches were employed for this purpose in the present study. In the first, clinical ratings of hysterical-obsessional trend were compared with the sedation threshold. In the second, introversion-extraversion was measured by questionnaires and by determining the ease of formation of the conditioned eyeblink response; these measures were then compared with the sedation threshold. The question-

[1] Read before the Annual Meeting of the Society of Biological Psychiatry, Atlantic City, June, 1957. This study was assisted by grants from the Department of National Health and Welfare and the Defense Research Board (Grant No. DRB 9345-04, Project No. D50-45-04) of Canada.

[2] Allan Memorial Institute of Psychiatry, McGill University, Montreal.

naires used had contributed the greatest weight to Hildebrand's battery (8). The eyeblink conditioning measure was based on the work of Franks (6), who found that conditionability was correlated with questionnaire measures of introversion-extraversion, and differed in hysterics and dysthymics in the direction expected from Eysenck's reactive inhibition theory.

MATERIALS AND METHODS

Rating Study. Subjects were 308 patients, including all those classified as psychoneurotic in a consecutive series of 750; diagnoses and other details have been described elsewhere (14). There were 104 men and 204 women, aged from 16 to 71.

Questionnaire Study. Data-taking for this study had not been completed at time of writing. Results for the first 36 patients will be presented. The only factors influencing selection of these patients were availability for testing and absence of any clinical evidence to suggest the possibility of psychosis. There were 13 men and 23 women, ranging in age from 15 to 57, with a mean of 35 years. The group contained most types of psychoneurosis.

Sedation Threshold Procedure. The procedure has been described in detail in previous publications (13, 16). Sodium Amytal is injected intravenously at the rate of 0.5 mg. per kg. every 40 seconds until well after slurred speech is noted, while the frontal EEG is continuously recorded. The amplitude of the fast (15 to 30 c.p.s.) waves elicited by the drug is measured. Measurements in the earlier cases were done by a hand method (13); an electronic integrator (1) was used in about the last one-third of the "rating" series and in all of the "questionnaire" cases. The amplitude measurements are plotted against the amount of drug to yield a curve, which is usually of sigmoid shape and contains an inflexion point, preceding which the amplitude rises sharply and following which it tends to plateau. This point corresponds roughly to the onset

of slurred speech. The sedation threshold is the amount of sodium Amytal, in mg. per kg. required to produce this inflexion point.

Ratings of Hysterical-Obsessional Trend. Ratings were based on case records, which usually consisted of assistant resident's admission note, intern's case history, and attending psychiatrist's discharge summary. As none of the histories was taken specifically for the purpose of assessing hysterical-obsessional trend, it was anticipated that some cases could not be rated. Two psychiatrists, who had not seen any of the patients, independently rated the case records without knowledge of the sedation threshold. The rating scale consisted of the following points: H3, H2, H1, M1, M2, O1, O2, O3. "H" referred to hysterical, "M" to mixed, and "O" to obsessional personality traits. Patients with clear hysterical conversion symptoms were to be rated H3 and patients with clear obsessive-compulsive symptoms were to be rated O3. The intermediate categories were intended to reflect varying degrees of intensity of one or other personality trend. Following are some illustrative descriptive phrases from the case records, which were used as a basis for rating: under *hysterical*, histrionic, manipulative, usually outgoing, immature, eager to communicate, exhibitionistic; under *obsessional*, meticulous, perfectionistic, conscientious, rigid, hard driving with guilt over failure, preoccupied with detail, afraid of losing control.

Introversion-Extraversion Scales. The Rhathymia (R) and Social-Introversion (S) Scales of the Guilford inventory of factors S, T, D, C and R (7) were used to measure introversion-extraversion. Individual questions were typed on cards; the subject answered them as yes, no or uncertain, by sorting them into three appropriately labeled compartments of a box. The cards were presented in a random order. A French translation was used for French-speaking patients; the French version seemed to give approximately the same results as the English one when both were given to a few bilingual persons. For convenience in presenting the statistics, the raw scores for each of the scales were converted into standard C scores, according to tables supplied in the test manual. The C score statistics did not differ to any extent from those based on the individual raw scores, which were also worked out. As the C scores in the manual were arranged in such a way that they increased with increasing extraversion, they were reversed in order to avoid negative correlations. Also the C scores for R and S were added to provide a combined C score with a possible range from 0 to 20; the higher the combined C score, the greater the degree of introversion.

Conditioning Procedure. In the main, Frank's procedure was followed (6). The conditioned stimulus was a tone of 1100 cycles, produced by an Ediswan oscillator, Type R666, at an output of 22.5 volts, and delivered through S. C. Brown Type K moving coil headphones. The unconditioned stimulus was an air puff to the cornea. The air source was a compressed air supply, with the valve at the main outlet set so that the pressure was 2 ± 0.5 lb. Overall timing was controlled by a R. W. Cramer switch, Type M8 120S with a 0.5 r.p.m. motor, which was set so that 8 interstimulus intervals varying from 11 to 19 seconds would be repeated serially. The tone lasted 650 milliseconds, and, in reinforced trials, it was followed immediately by an air puff, lasting 275 milliseconds. Release of the air was effected by means of an Asco air valve, with relay activated by an electronic timing circuit. The air tube was held in place by a plastic frame attached to the headphones. There were 48 stimuli in the conditioning series; 30 included both tone and air puff and 18 consisted of tone alone. Before the first stimulus of the conditioning series, there was a preliminary series of stimuli; the first 3 were tone alone, then there were 3 air puffs alone, and finally 3 tones alone. Following the conditioning series, there was an extinction series consisting of 10 unreinforced tones.

The retinocorneal potential from two electrodes near the eye provided a recording of eyeblink on one channel of a Grass EEG. The subject was seated during the conditioning procedure; some degree of eye fixation was obtained by having the subject look at a coat hook on the wall in front of him. The experimenter could observe the subject through a window. The subject's room was semidark. In evaluating the conditioning records, all eyeblink deflections of at least 3 mm. amplitude, beginning from 500 to 1000 μseconds after the onset of the tone, were scored as a response. Subjects with 3 or more out of a possible 6 responses to the tones preceding the conditioning series were rejected.

RESULTS

Hysterical-Obsessional Rating. One or the other psychiatrist was unable to rate 84 of the 308 cases. To obtain some estimate of the degree of agreement between raters in the remaining 224 cases, the H3 to O3 scale was treated as an eight point rating scale and the product-moment correlation between the two ratings was determined. The correlation coefficient was 0.78, indicating reasonably good agreement.

Again with the ratings determined as an eight point scale, the correlation between the mean of the two ratings and the sedation threshold was determined. The correlation coefficient was 0.53, which is highly significant statistically and indicates that the sedation threshold was positively correlated with hysterical-obsessional trend. Figure 1 shows the mean hysterical-obsessional rating for each sedation threshold. The graph shows that thresholds of 3.0 or less were obtained in patients generally rated as hysterical, and thresholds of 4.5 or more were obtained in patients generally rated obsessional. Figure 1 also suggests that the sedation threshold discriminates only three, or

CHARLES SHAGASS AND ALBERT B. KERENYI

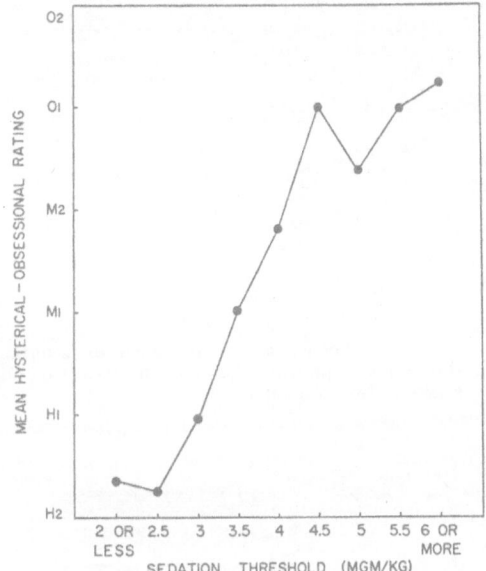

FIG. 1. Mean hysterical-obsessional rating by sedation threshold, 224 patients. Rating for each patient was the mean of two psychiatrists' ratings.

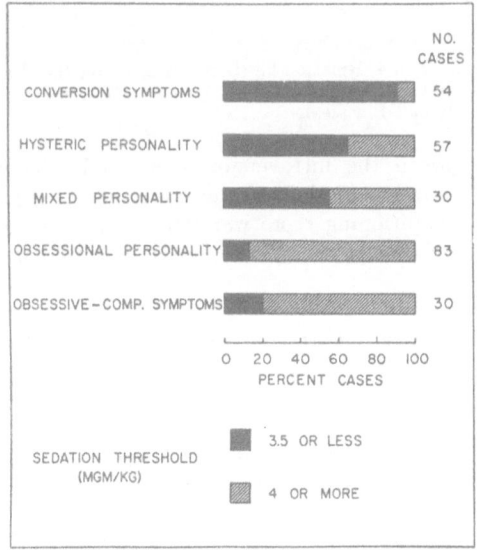

FIG. 2. Relationship between sedation threshold and main reason for hysterical-obsessional ratings made by one psychiatrist. Note that differences between ratings made because of symptoms are greater than differences between ratings based on personality characteristics.

at the most four, points on a hysterical-obsessional continuum.

It was of some interest to determine whether the correlation between hysterical-obsessional trend and the sedation threshold was based more upon symptoms or upon assessments of behavior characteristics. One of the raters was asked to indicate the basis for his ratings in these terms. The reasons could be classified into five categories: conversion symptoms, obsessive-compulsive symptoms, and either hysterical, mixed, or obsessional personality characteristics. Figure 2 shows the proportion of above and below average sedation thresholds for each of these categories in the 254 patients assigned ratings by this psychiatrist. Sedation threshold differences were greatest between patients with frank conversion and obsessive-compulsive symptoms. The differences were less marked between the groups classified on personality characteristics alone, but the trend was statistically significant at better than the 1 per cent level of confidence. Thus, although it appeared that symptoms provided a firmer basis for discrimination with respect to the sedation threshold, there was also a definite relationship between the threshold and personality evaluations based on behavioral characteristics.

As the ratings were based on heterogeneous case materials gathered in a nonstandard fashion, it seemed reasonable to assume that those subjects to whom both psychiatrists assigned the same ratings might offer some approximation of the true relationship between the sedation threshold and hysterical-obsessional trend. Figure 3 shows the distributions of sedation thresholds for all those cases assigned either an H or O rating by both psychiatrists. There was relatively little overlapping between these groups with concordant ratings. The biserial correlation coefficient for the data in Figure 3 was 0.84; this coefficient is spuriously high because the mixed group was omitted, but it gives some indication of the possible relationship.

Guilford Introversion Score. The 36 patients for whom questionnaire scores and sedation thresholds were available contained a somewhat greater than usual number of patients with high thresholds, thus restricting the possible range of variation. Even with a restricted range, the coefficient for the correlation between the threshold and the introversion C score, which was 0.60, was highly significant statistically. The S scale contributed more to the correlation than the R scale. Figure 4 illustrates the relationship between the sedation threshold and the introversion score. These data confirm the hypothesis that the sedation threshold is positively correlated with degree of introversion.

Conditioning. Acceptable conditioning results were available for only 22 of the 36 patients. It was necessary to reject 7 patients because of apparatus breakdown during the conditioning experiments, and 7 more because they gave three or more blink responses during the six preconditioning presentations of the tone alone. Taking the total number of conditioned responses during the unreinforced trials of the conditioning and extinction series as a total conditioning score, the correlations between this score and the introversion C score and sedation threshold were determined. The coefficient for conditioning score *versus* introversion was 0.45, and for conditioning *versus* sedation threshold was 0.23. The former was significant at the 5 per cent level of confidence, while the latter was not significant.

The absence of a significant correlation between conditioning and sedation threshold suggests that these two procedures measure factors which are not similar. If one takes conditioning as another measure of central nervous system function, it is a matter of interest to determine how well introversion-extraversion could be predicted by a combination of the sedation threshold and the conditioning tests. In the 22 subjects for whom all three sets of data were available, the coefficient of multiple correlation be-

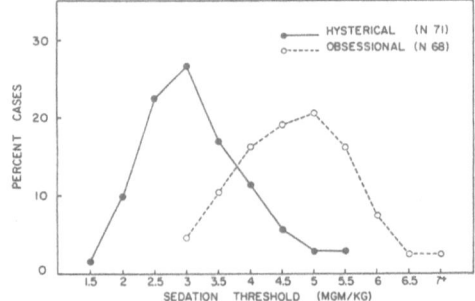

FIG. 3. Percentage distributions of sedation thresholds in patients classed as hysterical or obsessional by both raters.

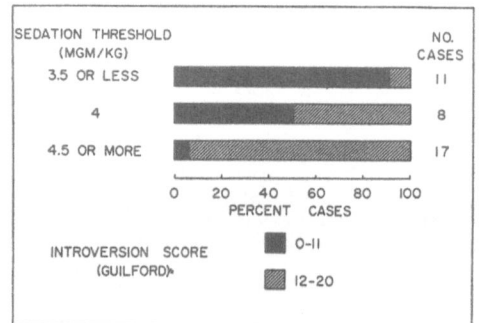

FIG. 4. Relationship between sedation threshold and introversion (Guilford combined C score for R and S scales).

tween the introversion score and a combination of the sedation threshold and the conditioning score was 0.67. This was significant at the 1 per cent level of confidence.

DISCUSSION

Present data support the conclusion that the sedation threshold is correlated with degree of hysterical-obsessional trend or introversion-extraversion. The results are in agreement with Jung's (9) view that the characteristic neurosis of the extrovert is hysteria, whereas that of the introvert is psychasthenia, and they confirm Hildebrand's (8) results showing that hysterics and dysthymics differ on measures of introversion-extraversion. Franks' (6) findings with respect to conditionability and introversion-extraversion are also confirmed, although the hypothesis that the sedation threshold would be correlated with conditionability was not supported by the data.

It is possible that our failure to demonstrate a relationship between conditionability and the sedation threshold may be due to undiscovered technical faults in the conditioning procedure, or that a larger series will yield more positive results. However, these possibilities seem dubious in view of the fact that the present correlation of 0.45 between the conditioning and introversion scores was almost identical with the correlation which Franks found. The present negative conditioning data are not critical for the theory that the dimension of introversion-extraversion is associated with a dimension of central nervous excitation-inhibition, insofar as the sedation threshold, which is a more direct measure of central excitability, was definitely correlated with introversion-extraversion.

In previous studies of the sedation threshold in nonpsychotic subjects, it seemed appropriate to stress the positive correlation between the threshold and degree of manifest anxiety (16, 17). The relationship between the threshold and hysterical-obsessional trend, which present results confirmed, was also noted. As it would be desirable to avoid the problems raised by multiple concepts, one might attempt to bring these two correlates of the sedation threshold together, if it could be demonstrated that manifest anxiety is really dependent upon introversive tendencies. This is a possibility which agrees with much clinical experience, but one cannot ignore the fact that hysterics manifesting apparent anxiety reactions are by no means uncommon. Another reason for retaining the anxiety correlate comes from data showing that, when patients with anxiety states and high sedation thresholds responded to therapy with reduction of anxiety, the sedation threshold decreased (15). To account for these facts, it was suggested that there are several neurophysiologic mechanisms of

anxiety, that the "choice" of mechanism is linked with personality structure, and that the sedation threshold reflects the activity of that anxiety mechanism predominating in obsessional or introverted persons (15). However, if retest studies were to show that a decrease in sedation threshold is accompanied by a corresponding decrease in both anxiety and introversion, it would be possible to regard the personality factor as the primary correlate of the threshold. It should be possible to carry out the research necessary to clarify this issue.

Eysenck (4) has drawn attention to a pharmacologic implication of the sedation threshold; it suggests that the position of a person on the introversion-extraversion continuum may be perhaps the most important factor influencing his therapeutic dosage requirements for a stimulant or depressant drug. Impressions gained by one of us from clinical experience with sedatives seem to substantiate this view. In hysterical patients, small doses of sedatives are often adequate, whereas the larger doses, which are required by dysthymics, tend to produce disturbing side effects. These side effects are often reported in the form of exaggerated complaints, which may sometimes be interpreted by the physician as a need for more sedation; if more is given, this may lead to further side effects, and so on. This differential effect of sedatives in hysterics and dysthymics is allied to Pavlov's observations on the quantitative therapeutic requirements of bromides in dogs with experimental neuroses (11, p. 92). A practical clinical application would be to use personality assessment as a guide to sedative dosage.

Although the exact neurophysiologic function reflected by the sedation threshold is not certain, it most probably measures a time characteristic of neuronal excitability (12). In demonstrating that introversion-extraversion is correlated with a neurophysiologic factor of this order, the present study provides strong support for a theoretical approach to personality which is orientated along neurophysiologic lines.

SUMMARY

The purpose of this study was to test the hypothesis that the sedation threshold is correlated with a personality factor, similar to Eysenck's introversion-extraversion dimension or, in neurotics, a hysterical-obsessional continuum. In one part of the study, two psychiatrists independently rated 308 case records for hysterical-obsessional tendency. Their ratings were significantly correlated with the sedation threshold, a high threshold being associated with obsessional tendencies and a low one with hysterical tendencies. Another investigative method used was to correlate the sedation threshold with questionnaire scores of introversion-extraversion (Guilford R and S scales) in 36 neurotic patients and with ease of conditioned eyeblink formation. The threshold was significantly correlated with the questionnaire scores in the predicted direction, high thresholds being associated with introversion. The threshold was not significantly correlated with conditionability, although high introversion on the questionnaire was associated with greater conditionability. The main conclusion reached from the findings was that there is an objectively demonstrable neurophysiologic basis for the introversion-extraversion dimension.

Acknowledgments. Thanks are due to Dr. J. F. Davis for designing the aparatus used in this study, to Dr. A. L. Jones for rating the case records, to Dr. J. L. Lapointe for translating the Guilford scales into French, and to Herbert Lorenz and Genevieve Servin for technical assistance.

REFERENCES

1. DAVIS, J. F. Low frequency analyzers in electroencephalography. Paper (No. 56–24–1) presented at the Instrument Society of America Meeting, September, 1956.
2. EYSENCK, H. J. A dynamic theory of anxiety and hysteria. J. Ment. Sc., **101**: 28, 1955.
3. EYSENCK, H. J. *Dimensions of Personality.* Routledge & Kegan Paul, Ltd., London, 1947.
4. EYSENCK, H. J. Drugs and personality. I. Theory and methodology. J. Ment. Sc., **103**: 119, 1957.
5. EYSENCK, H. J. *The Scientific Study of Personality.* Routledge & Kegan Paul, Ltd., London, 1952.
6. FRANKS, C. M. Conditioning and personality. A study of normal and neurotic subjects. J. Abnorm. & Social Psychol., **52**: 143, 1956.
7. GUILFORD, J. P. An inventory of factors S, T, D, C, R. *Manual of Directions and Norms,* Sheridan Supply Co., California, 1940.
8. HILDEBRAND, H. P. A factorial study of introversion-extraversion by means of objective tests. Ph.D. Thesis, University of London Library, 1953.
9. JUNG, C. G. *Psychological Types.* Routledge & Kegan Paul, Ltd., London, 1924.
10. MacKINNON, D. W. Personality and the behavior disorders. In *The Structure of Personality* (J. McV. Hunt, editor). Ronald Press Co., New York, 1944, Ch. 1.
11. PAVLOV, I. P. *Conditioned Reflexes and Psychiatry* (Transl. by W. H. Gantt). International Publishers, New York, 1941.
12. SHAGASS, C. A measurable neurophysiological factor of psychiatric significance. Electroencephalog. & Clin. Neurophysiol., **9**: 101, 1957.
13. SHAGASS, C. The sedation threshold. A method for estimating tension in psychiatric patients. Electroencephalog. & Clin. Neurophysiol., **6**: 211, 1954.
14. SHAGASS, C. AND JONES, A. L. A Neurophysiological Test for Psychiatric Diagnosis. Results in 750 patients. Amer. J. Psychiat. (in press).
15. SHAGASS, C., MIHALIK, J. AND JONES, A. L. Clinical psychiatric studies using the sedation threshold. J. Psychosom. Res., **2**: 45, 1957.
16. SHAGASS, C. AND NAIMAN, J. The sedation threshold as an objective index of manifest anxiety in psychoneurosis. J. Psychosom. Res., **1**: 49, 1956.
17. SHAGASS, C. AND NAIMAN, J. The sedation threshold, manifest anxiety and some aspects of ego function. A. M. A. Arch. Neurol. & Psychiat., **74**: 379, 1955.

From R. Lynn (1960). British Journal of Psychology, *51,* 319-324, *by kind permission of the author and the British Psychological Society*

EXTRAVERSION, REMINISCENCE AND SATIATION EFFECTS

By R. LYNN

Exeter University

Eysenck's theory that extraverts accumulate reactive inhibition quickly and that it dissipates in them slowly and his application of this theory to after-effects and reminiscence is made the basis of six predictions: using the spiral after-effect, there should be (1) a negative correlation between extraversion and duration of the after-effect; (2) a tendency for extraverts to see progressively less of the after-effect with repeated massed trials; (3) a tendency for extraverts to recover more in their perception of the after-effect after a period of rest; (4) a negative correlation between the duration of the after-effect and a measure of reminiscence using the inverted alphabet printing task; (5) a positive correlation between extraversion and reminiscence; (6) a tendency for extraverts to show more work decrement with massed practice on the inverted alphabet printing task. Using forty male university students as subjects, predictions 1, 2, 4 and 5 are confirmed at a statistically significant level, and predictions 3 and 6 show non-significant results in the predicted direction.

I. INTRODUCTION

In view of the recent criticisms of Eysenck's (1957) theory linking introversion-extraversion with reactive inhibition, figural after-effects and satiation effects, this paper presents the results of an independent investigation of some predictions from the theory. Essentially, the Eysenck theory postulates that extraverts accumulate reactive inhibition quickly and dissipate it slowly. This theory mediates a large number of predictions, e.g. that extraverts should show greater work decrement and more reminiscence, for which there is confirmatory evidence (Eysenck, 1957). Eysenck has also postulated that figural after-effects and satiation effects are affected by reactive inhibition and hence related to introversion-extraversion and evidence in support of this postulate has been published for the kinaesthetic after-effect and the Archimedes spiral satiation effect (Eysenck, 1957).

The experiment reported here concerns the relation between extraversion, reminiscence and the spiral satiation effect. Eysenck's theory of the spiral satiation effect is as follows: as the subject fixates the spiral reactive inhibition is generated and this interferes with the after-effect according to its strength. Further, the processes underlying the reversal phenomenon must themselves generate satiation and therefore curtail the after-effect. Both processes would tend to make extraverts experience the after-effect less than introverts. Although little direct evidence is available, two additional hypotheses of Eysenck provide deductions about which there is evidence relevant to this theory. First, it is postulated that depressant drugs increase reactive inhibition and hence curtail the after-effect, while stimulant drugs decrease inhibition and hence increase the duration of the after-effect; this deduction has been partially confirmed by Eysenck, Holland & Trouton (1957). Secondly, it is postulated that brain injury increases the tendency to generate reactive inhibition and hence brain injured subjects should have smaller satiation effects. This deduction has been confirmed by Price & Deabler (1955), although some doubt has been thrown on this finding as a result of the findings of Spivack & Levine (1959) and what would appear to be the important question of the site of the injury remains uninvestigated. As far as reminiscence is concerned, Eysenck accepts Hull's theory that reminiscence is due to the dissipation of reactive inhibition; when Eysenck's own postulate that extraverts generate reactive inhibition quickly and dissipate it slowly is added to Hull's theory, the prediction is that extraverts should show greater reminiscence.

This theory has not been without its critics, notably Hamilton (1959) and Rechtschaffen (1958), who maintain that there is insufficient evidence in its support. Rechtschaffen presents evidence showing some positive association between extraversion, figural after-effects and reminiscence using inverted alphabet printing, but the correlations were too low for statistical significance. However, since Rechtschaffen used an unusually short rest interval in his reminiscence test, it is arguable that his experiment cannot be regarded as an adequate test of the theory.

The present paper reports an investigation of six predictions from the Eysenck theory, namely: (1) under certain conditions of administration the inverted alphabet printing task should yield reminiscence scores which correlate positively with extraversion; (2) extraverts should show more work decrement in inverted alphabet printing under conditions of massed practice; (3) there should be a negative correlation between extraversion and duration of the spiral after-effect; (4) with repeated presentation, extraverts should show a greater fall off in the spiral after-effect as a result of their tendency to generate reactive inhibition more quickly; (5) after a period of rest extraverts should show a greater recovery in seeing the spiral after-effect as a result of the dissipation of reactive inhibition; (6) the duration of the spiral after-effect and reminiscence should be negatively correlated.

II. THE INVESTIGATION

Subjects. The sample consisted of forty male university students living in a university hall of residence; volunteers for the experiment were asked for and the first forty to volunteer were taken as the subjects. All subjects fell in the age range 18–23 with the exception of one who was slightly older. On the Maudsley Personality Inventory the mean score for extraversion was 23·5, S.D. 8·42, compared with the norm for the general population of 24·9, S.D. 9·71; and for neuroticism 27·6, S.D. 9·27, compared with the norm for the general population of 19·9, S.D. 11·02. It is evident therefore that the sample was representative of the normal population on the introversion-extraversion dimension but on neuroticism it scored somewhat more neurotic. However, it has been shown that English university students as a whole score more neurotic than the general population by something like $\frac{1}{2}$ S.D. (Lynn, 1959) and it may therefore be concluded that the present sample was representative of English university students though not representative of the general population on the neuroticism dimension.

Procedure. The spiral used in this experiment was a 4-throw spiral of 180° similar to the one illustrated by Eysenck (1957) except that it was 10 in. in diameter; it rotated at 78 rev./min., and subjects were tested in daylight conditions. Subjects were seated 6 ft. from the spiral and instructed to fixate the central point. The after-effect was explained to the subjects, and they were asked to report when the apparent movement ceased. Subjects were given a practice trial of 40 sec. They were then given ten trials of 30 sec. each in 'massed' conditions, i.e. the spiral was rotated as

Extraversion, reminiscence and satiation effects

soon as the subject had made his judgement of the cessation of the after-effect. Following this a 2 min. rest was allowed, after which subjects underwent one more trial. The reliability of this test, calculated by the split-half method, was 0·86.

Subjects were then asked to answer the Maudsley Personality Inventory which gives a measure of introversion-extraversion and neuroticism.

Finally, subjects were asked to do the inverted alphabet printing task. Subjects were instructed to print the alphabet upside down as fast as they could for fourteen trials with massed practice. They were then given a 2 min. rest, and asked to print the alphabet once more.

III. Results

The variables about which predictions were made were scored in the following way: (1) reminiscence: a score was obtained by subtracting the speed on trial 15 of the inverted alphabet printing from the mean of the speeds on the trials 8–14; (2) work decrement: speed on trial 14 of alphabet printing; (3) duration of spiral after-effect: the reported duration on the first trial; (4) decline of the spiral after-effect; a score was obtained by subtracting the time of the after-effect on trial 10 from that on trial 1; (5) recovery of the after-effect with rest: duration of after-effect on the eleventh (post-rest) trial minus duration of the after-effect on trial 10. The product-moment correlations between these variables and extraversion are shown in Table 1. To afford comparison with other studies, the product-moment correlations of neuroticism with some of these measures are also shown in Table 1.

Table 1. *Product moment correlations of measures of*
inhibition with extraversion and neuroticism

Measure	E	N	Measure 3
1. Reminiscence	+0·42*	+0·29	−0·34*
2. Work decrement	+0·21	—	—
3. Duration of spiral after-effect	−0·43*	−0·13	—
4. Decline of spiral after-effect	+0·42*	—	—
5. Recovery of after-effect after rest	+0·18	—	—
Speed of alphabet printing, trial 1	—	+0·29	—

* Significant at 0·05 probability level.

Two extreme groups of 12 extraverts and 11 introverts were obtained by considering only the subjects whose scores fell 7 or more points away from the mean. Fig. 1 shows the mean scores for the two groups over the 11 trials on the spiral after-effect and illustrates the greater decrement of the extraverts with repeated presentation. Fig. 2 shows the mean scores for the two groups on the inverted alphabet printing task and illustrates the tendency of extraverts to slow down and to show greater reminiscence. The means and S.D.'s of these two extreme groups on the measures calculated are shown in Table 2.

R. LYNN

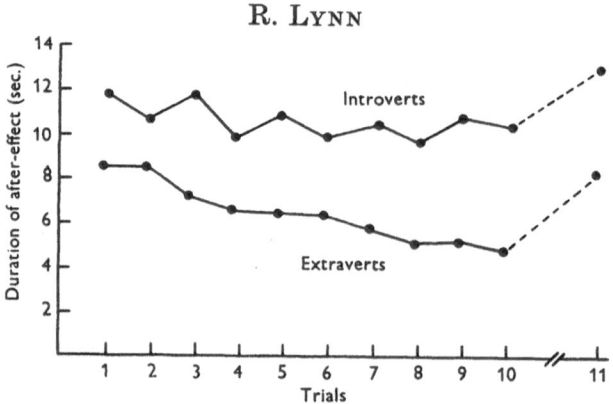

Fig. 1. Duration of spiral after-effects of introverts and extraverts

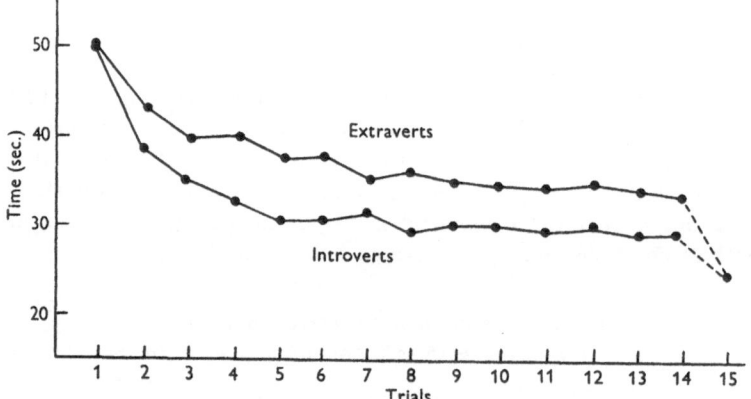

Fig. 2. Mean times and reminiscence of introverts and extraverts
on the inverted alphabet printing task.

Table 2. *Means and* S.D.*'s of introvert and extravert
groups on measures of reactive inhibition*

	Introverts		Extraverts	
	Mean	S.D.	Mean	S.D.
Inverted alphabet printing				
1. Reminiscence	5·10	2·28	10·42	4·98
2. Speed on trial 14	29·18	6·32	33·00	6·00
Spiral after-effect				
3. Duration on trial 1	12·09	8·50	7·52	5·31
4. Decline of after-effect	1·18	5·33	3·65	4·36
5. Recovery of after-effect	2·55	2·62	3·17	4·32

DISCUSSION

It is evident that the correlations tend to support Eysenck's theory. The two that do not reach statistical significance are in the predicted direction and the lowest, that of $+0\cdot18$ between extraversion and recovery of the spiral, is probably reduced by the method of scoring, since the extraverts show a greater proportional post-rest

Extraversion, reminiscence and satiation effects

increase in after-effect which is to some extent masked by considering the absolute increase. On the other hand, it should be noted that the correlation between extraversion and the decline of the after-effect might have been increased by the experimental procedure used, since extraverts experienced more 'massing' as a result of their shorter after-effects.

The difference between the present results and those obtained by Rechtschaffen (1958) deserves some discussion. Rechtschaffen used Guilford's R scale for assessing extraversion, and this correlates only about 0·5 with the extraversion scale of the M.P.I. (Eysenck, 1959). But it is likely that the differences in methods of assessing reactive inhibition are also important. The method employed by Rechtschaffen was to give subjects five trials of distributed practice followed by five trials of massed practice and to obtain an estimate of reactive inhibition by subtracting the number of letters printed under massed practice from the number printed under distributed practice. Using this measure he obtained a correlation of $+0·18$ between extraversion and the amount of reactive inhibition accumulated. He also obtained a score of reminiscence by giving a one minute rest after the five massed trials, followed by two further trials. Reminiscence and extraversion correlated only $+0·08$. The difference between this finding and the present one might be due to at least two factors. First, Rechtschaffen's failure to get large reminiscence scores for his extraverts could be due to an insufficiently long rest pause; the rest given was only 1 min., which is considerably less than most investigators have used with the inverted alphabet printing task, e.g. Archer (1954) gave a 5 min. rest, and Kimble (1949) a 10 min. rest; and Eysenck obtained his correlation between extraversion and reminiscence with a 10 min. rest pause. It is likely that the 1 min. rest is insufficient for reactive inhibition to dissipate fully in extraverted subjects. Hence they would not show the full reminiscence effect obtained with a longer rest interval. Rechtschaffen argues that since it is postulated that extraverts generate reactive inhibition more quickly and dissipate it more slowly, conflicting predictions about reminiscence scores can be made from the Eysenck theory: either extraverts should dissipate more I_R because they have more and hence show more reminiscence; or because they dissipate I_R more slowly they should show less reminiscence; or the two effects might cancel each other out. This argument could easily explain Rechtschaffen's finding using his particular experimental conditions, but it cannot be accepted as a valid criticism of the Eysenck theory; for, once the time interval for reactive inhibition to dissipate in extraverts has been established by the standard method of plotting reminiscence scores with different rest intervals, the theory yields the quite unequivocal prediction that if this time interval is allowed extraverts will show more reminiscence.

A second factor which could explain Rechtschaffen's low correlation between extraversion and reminiscence arises from the part played by conditioned inhibition. Reminiscence scores are most satisfactorily obtained either very quickly, before $_sI_R$ has had time to develop, or after a number of trials, when $_sI_R$ has reached its asymptote. Rechtschaffen's choice of ten trials may be unsatisfactory from this point of view. Since reactive inhibition develops more quickly in extraverts, it is possible that by the eleventh trial they will have greater conditioned inhibition and this would obscure the recovery from reactive inhibition in the measurement of reminiscence. Since in the present study extraverts and introverts both work at the same

R. Lynn

speed on the fifteenth trial, it appears that $_sI_R$ has reached its asymptote and the greater reminiscence of extraverts emerges.

The small correlation of neuroticism with duration of the spiral after-effect confirms previous reports that there is no association between the spiral after-effect and affective states (Price & Deabler, 1955). The correlation between neuroticism and time on trial 1 of the inverted alphabet printing task would be predicted on the basis of the Yerkes–Dodson law, i.e. the task is one in which the dominant habits are incorrect and are made more dominant by high drive, with the result that high drive impairs performance. Although the correlation falls short of significance, it is in the predicted direction and may be regarded as giving some support to the findings of Taylor & Rechtschaffen (1959) of a significant correlation between anxiety and time on inverted alphabet printing. On the other hand, the independence of neuroticism and reminiscence is inconsistent both with Eysenck's (1956) finding of a positive correlation between neuroticism and reminiscence on the pursuit rotor, and Kimble's (1950) finding of a correlation between drive and reminiscence in inverted alphabet printing. The discrepancy adds one more finding to the many reviewed by Jensen (1958) showing that experiments using questionnaire measures of drive give extremely conflicting results, probably determined in part by the degree to which drive is mobilized by the experimental situation.

The writer is indebted to Mr Ian Gordon of Exeter University for help in carrying out part of the experiment.

References

Archer, E. J. (1954). Post-rest performance in motor learning as a function of pre-rest degree of distribution of practice. *J. Exp. Psychol.* 47, 47–51.

Eysenck, H. J. (1956). Reminiscence, drive and personality theory. *J. Abnorm. (Soc.) Psychol.* 53, 328–33.

Eysenck, H. J. (1957). *The Dynamics of Anxiety and Hysteria.* London: Routledge and Kegan Paul.

Eysenck, H. J. (1959). Comments on a test of the personality-satiation-inhibition theory. *Psychol. Rep.* 5, 395–69.

Eysenck, H. J., Holland, H. & Trouton, D. S. (1957). Drugs and personality. III. The effects of stimulant and depressant drugs on visual after-effects. *J. Ment. Sci.* 103, 650–5.

Hamilton, V. (1959). Eysenck's theories of anxiety and hysteria—a methodological critique. *Brit. J. Psychol.* 50, 48–63.

Jensen, A. R. (1958). Personality. *Ann. Rev. Psychol.* 9, 295–322.

Kimble, G. A. (1949). An experimental test of a two factor theory of inhibition. *J. Exp. Psychol.* 39, 15–23.

Kimble, G. A. (1950). Evidence for the role of motivation in determining the amount of reminiscence in pursuit rotor learning. *J. exp. Psychol.* 40, 248–53.

Lynn, R. (1959). Two personality characteristics related to educational attainment. *Brit. J. Educ. Psychol.* 29, 213–6.

Price, A. G. & Deabler, H. L. (1955). Diagnosis of organicity by means of the spiral after-effect. *J. Cons. Psychol.* 19, 299–302.

Rechtschaffen, A. (1958). Neural satiation, reactive inhibition and introversion-extraversion. *J. Abnorm. Soc. Psychol.* 57, 283–91.

Spivack, G. & Levine, M. (1959). Spiral after-effect and measures of satiation in brain injured and normal subjects. *J. Personality,* 27, 211–27.

Taylor, J. A. & Rechtschaffen, A. (1959). Manifest anxiety and reversed alphabet printing. *J. Soc. Abnorm. Psychol.* 58, 221–4.

(*Manuscript received* 26 *May* 1959)

From D. S. Holmes (1967). Journal of Personality and Social Psychology, *5,* 98-103, *by kind permission of the author and the American Psychological Association*

PUPILLARY RESPONSE, CONDITIONING, AND PERSONALITY

DAVID S. HOLMES [1]

Northwestern University

This research tested the relationship of levels of acetylcholine and norepinephrine (as inferred from speed of pupillary constriction and dilation) to awareness of an environmental contingency, performance on a verbal conditioning task, and personality. High levels of acetylcholine, inferred from rapid constriction, were found to be significantly related to greater awareness of an environmental contingency, superior performance in verbal conditioning, and to introverted personality traits as measured by self-report and peer ratings. Relationships between levels of norepinephrine, inferred from speed of dilation, awareness, conditioning, and personality were for the most part inconsistent and nonsignificant. The conclusion was that speed or efficiency of neural transmission at cholinergic synapses, where acetylcholine is the transmitter substance, was related to conditioning and personality. The lack of significant findings regarding norepinephrine was attributed to the probable limitation of this mediator to synapses of the autonomic system.

In the past few years a number of important findings have been reported relating brain chemistry to learning. Rosenzweig, Krech, and Bennett (1958, 1961) have shown that rats which performed better in three different types of situations had greater amounts of cholinesterase (ChE) in the cerebral cortex. It has been known for some time that acetylcholine (ACh) is important in facilitating neural transmission at the synapses (Eccles, 1957), and since ChE breaks up or hydrolyzes ACh after the transmission of the impulse, ChE was used as an indicator of the amount of ACh available; that is, better learning was accompanied by higher levels of ChE and, inferentially, higher levels of ACh. In another approach to the study of neural transmission and learning, Russell, Watson, and Frankenhaeuser (1961) have shown that animals fed a ChE inhibitor, Systox, which consequently reduced the hydrolysis of ACh, showed slower extinction than normal animals. All of these data suggest that there is an important relationship between speed or efficiency of neural transmission and learning.

The application of this work to humans was retarded by the lack of appropriate techniques for measuring ACh or ChE levels. Recently, however, Rubin (1960) proposed that speed of pupillary constriction may be taken as an indicator of the amount of the cholinergic mediator

[1] Now at the University of Texas.

The author wishes to express his appreciation to Lee Sechrest for his assistance in the design of the research and to E. Femme for her assistance throughout the project.

(ACh) present. It should be recalled that synapses employing ACh as a transmitter are called cholinergic, while those employing norepinephrine are called adrenergic (Von Euler, 1959). The pupillary response provided a good measure of cholinergic mediator, because, as Rubin pointed out, "the magnitude of constriction is an increasing monotonic function of the amount of the cholinergic mediator liberated [p. 567]"; that is, faster constriction is indicative of greater amounts of ACh at cholinergic synapses. In like manner, Rubin suggested that speed of pupillary dilation be used as a measure of the amount of the adrenergic mediator (norepinephrine) present at the synapses, for again it seemed justified to assume a monotonic relationship (Rubin, 1964). The introduction of these measures has thus provided what seems to be simple and reliable measures of the transmitter substances and, consequently, predictors of learning.

If pupillary response is a predictor of learning in the human, then the application of this predictor might be carried one step further, into the area of personality. It has been theorized that an individual who learns or conditions rapidly tends to be highly sensitive to his environment, anxious, inhibited, compulsive, introspective, and often ill at ease. Conversely, the individual who conditions slowly would tend to be impulsive, irresponsible, unreliable, and insensitive to the environment and to the feelings of others. A considerable amount of research has been accumulated which supports the relationship between this dimension of personality and speed of conditioning (Eysenck, 1960; Franks, 1956; Johns & Quay, 1962; Quay & Hunt, 1965). Eysenck (1947) has referred to easily conditioned individuals as introverts, and to less easily conditioned individuals as extraverts; he has subsequently developed a scale to measure these characteristics (Eysenck, 1956).

The present study was an attempt to test the relationships between speed of neural transmission, conditionability, and personality. On the basis of earlier work with animals and the theoretical extrapolation to personality, it was predicted that subjects with inferred higher levels of the transmitter substances, as measured by the pupillary responses, would (a) be more aware of an environmental contingency, (b) evidence superior performance in verbal conditioning, and (c) rate themselves and be rated by peers as generally more introverted in personality.

METHOD

The subjects were 49 women in an introductory psychology class at Northwestern University. The first part of the experiment consisted of a verbal conditioning procedure similar to the one reported by Taffel (1955). Each subject was given 80 3 × 5 cards. On each card was typed a different past-tense verb. Below the verb were the pronouns I, we, you, he, she, and they. The pronouns appeared in a different order on each card. The subject's task was to make up a sentence using the verb and the pronoun of her choice. The experimenter sat behind a screen which separated him from the subject and recorded the pronouns used. The experimenter did not reinforce any of the subject's responses on trials 1 through 20. For trials 21 through 80, the experimenter responded with the word "good" in a flat, unemotional tone at the end of any sentence starting with the pronouns I or we. After completing the conditioning procedure, each subject was questioned concerning her awareness of the reinforcement contingency, according to a modified form of the inquiry schedule developed by DeNike and Spielberger (1963). In addition to assessing awareness, two items of the inquiry were used to determine the subject's behavioral intentions; that is, if the subject was aware of the reinforcement contingency, did the knowledge have a conscious effect on her behavior.

Following the verbal conditioning procedure, photographic measurements were taken of pupillary dilation and constriction. During the photographic procedure, the subject sat in a chair with her head held firmly in a Bausch and Lomb chin rest and forehead brace. The photographs of the eyes were taken with an Asahi Pentax single-lens reflex camera which was fitted with an extension bellows and an ƒ4.5, 105 millimeter lens. The lens was 16 inches from the subject's eyes. The adapting light used to constrict the pupils was placed 9 inches from the subject's eyes, at a point 5 inches below the plane between the subject's eyes and the camera lens. This light source consisted of a 3.5-inch square of white frosted glass which was illuminated from behind by a 100-watt white bulb. The lens of this light source was tilted so that the light was aimed directly at the subject's eyes. Eight and one-half inches to either side of the camera lens, and 14 inches from the subject's eyes were the infrared light sources, which were 2.75-inch squares. The illumination for these lights was provided by 200-watt bulbs which were housed in 10-inch photoflood reflectors. The light exposed to the subject was filtered through a Kodak Wratten filter No. 87. Consequently, the only light visible to the subject during the photographing of the dilating pupils was a dull red glow on either side of her field of vision. The intensity of the visible light was less than .5 footcandle.

All subjects were given the following explanation of the apparatus and procedure:

This apparatus will be used for taking photographic measurements of your eye. During the time the photographs are being taken, I will want you to keep your chin firmly in the chin rest and your forehead against the metal brace. While in this position, look straight forward at the lens of the camera. If you cannot see the lens because it is too dark, look straight forward at the point at which you think the lens should be. A series of photographs will be taken with this white light on and a series of photographs will be taken with this light off. When the light is off, you may notice a very dim red glow on each side of the side panels. Ignore these and continue to look straight ahead.

After the subject had her head positioned in the head rest, the room light was extinguished. Ten seconds later the adapting light and the infrared lights were turned on for 15 seconds to maximally constrict the pupil. At the end of this interval, the adapting light was turned off. Photographs of the dilating pupils were taken after intervals of 5, 10, 15, 30, 45, and 60 seconds. Prior to photographing the constricting pupils, the pupils were dark adapted for 1 minute. After 1 minute of complete darkness the adapting light and the infrared lights were turned on. The constricting pupils were photographed after intervals of 1, 2, 3, 4, and 5 seconds with a different trial being used for each measurement. The time intervals were controlled by a Hunter interval timer. Pupillary size after the various intervals of time was determined by projecting the developed negatives on a screen and measuring the diameter of the pupil with a millimeter ruler. The negatives were projected from a distance of 17 feet with a 5-inch lens. Since the photographs of the pupil carried only an identification number and the measurements were recorded on numbered data sheets, the experimenter did not know the identity of the subject who was being measured.

After completion of the photographic procedures, the subjects filled out a questionnaire which contained the Extraversion (E) and Neuroticism (N) scales from the Maudsley Personal Inventory, and the A, R, and MA scales from the MMPI.

Before leaving the laboratory, each subject was given three peer-rating forms and three envelopes. She was instructed to give one form and envelope to each of the three girls whom she felt knew her best and ask them to rate her on the various items. The form consisted of 16 descriptive statements about personality characteristics. All of the items were worded in the positive direction. Eight items described introverted characteristics and eight, extraverted characteristics. Within each set of eight items, half were socially desirable and half less desirable, though none were completely undesirable. Rating of a subject on this form was done by placing an X on a 9-inch graphic scale beneath each item. The scale had end points labeled "Very Descriptive" and "Not Descriptive." All rating forms were returned to the experimenter in sealed, self-addressed envelopes. The scoring key was constructed so that extraverted descriptions received higher scores. The final score on the peer-rating form was the sum of the ratings given by all three judges.

RESULTS

Speed of Pupillary Constriction

The mean and SD of the proportion of constriction after each interval are presented in Table 1. It should be pointed out that 100% constriction was not reported in this table because of what might be called a "bounce effect"; this is, some subjects reached maximal constriction in 3 or 4 seconds and then dilated slightly, which caused a drop in the constriction curve for these subjects and lowered the overall mean proportion of constriction after 4 and 5 seconds. Because of this bounce, the measurement after 4 and 5 seconds for some subjects was not an accurate measure of the speed of constriction, and therefore the measures taken after 1, 2, and 3 seconds were judged to be most accurate for comparing rates of constriction.

Extreme subjects (fast and slow) were identified as those whose proportion of constriction after at least two of the three intervals was plus or minus one SD from the mean of the distribution for each respective interval. Intermediate subjects were identified as those whose

TABLE 1

PROPORTION OF CONSTRICTION AFTER INTERVALS OF TIME

Sec.	M	SD
1.0	63.69	10.15
2.0	82.73	8.07
3.0	92.76	5.35
4.0	98.10	2.57
5.0	98.10	4.78

Note.—$N = 49$.

proportion of constriction was within plus or minus one SD of the mean of each respective distribution. Eight subjects were identified as fast constrictors, 17 as intermediate speed constrictors, and eight as slow constrictors.

Speed of pupillary constriction and awareness. On the basis of their responses to the awareness inquiry, the subjects were classified as either aware or not aware of the reinforcement contingency. (It should be noted that there was 98% agreement between two independent judges with regard to classifying the subjects on awareness or behavioral intentions.) To test the hypotheses relating increased awareness and high ACh levels, the proportions of aware and not aware subjects within the fast and slow constricting groups were compared. A Fisher test of exact probability indicated that there was a significant (.05) relationship between fast constriction and awareness. Of the fast constrictors, 62.5% were aware, while 12.5% of the slow constrictors were aware.

Speed of pupillary constriction and verbal conditioning. Before discussing the relationship between speed of constriction and performance curves in verbal conditioning, some comment should be made concerning the subjects' conscious attitude toward performance on this task. When the postconditioning inquiries were scored for behavioral intentions, it was found that some of the aware subjects had consciously fought against giving conditioned responses. This tendency on the part of some subjects and the effect it had on the data has been noted and reported earlier (Farber, 1963; Holmes, 1966). Since the use of subjects who reported consciously resisting the giving of conditioned responses would distort any relationship between performance and speed of constriction, in Figure 1 where performance curves for fast, intermediate, and slow constrictors are plotted, only those subjects who did not resist conditioning were used.

Analysis of variance for repeated measures (Edwards, 1960) indicated that there were significant differences between the groups ($F = 53.54$, $df = 2,23$, $p < .01$) across blocks of trials ($F = 5.11$, $df = 3,69$, $p < .01$), and the Groups $\times$ Trials interaction was significant ($F = 3.57$, $df = 6,69$, $p < .01$). The correlations between the total number of conditioned responses given on trials 21–80 and the proportion of constriction after intervals of 1, 2, and 3 seconds were .33 ($p < .05$), .44 ($p < .005$), and .52 ($p < .005$), respectively. All of these results clearly indicated that there was a significant relationship between fast pupillary constriction, which was indicative of an inferred high ACh level, and performance on a verbal conditioning task. (It should be noted that since awareness is related to verbal conditioning performance—Farber, 1963; Holmes, 1966; Spielberger, 1965—the findings relating the pupillary response to awareness and to verbal conditioning performance are not completely independent. They were presented separately in this paper because, while related, they represented different types of functioning and behavior which have been of interest to psychologists.)

Speed of pupillary constriction and personality measures. When the fast and slow constrictors were compared over the personality measures, the slow constrictors were found to be more extraverted than fast constrictors, as measured both by the E scale ($t = 3.09$, $df = 14$, $p < .01$) and by the peer-rating form ($t = 1.78$, $df = 14$, $p < .10$). Fast and slow constrictors did not differ significantly on the measures of general maladjustment, that is, the *A*, *MA*, and N scales ($t = .41$, .83, .43, respectively; $df = 14$).

In summary, fast pupillary constriction which is indicative of high levels of ACh was significantly related (*a*) to the development of awareness of a reinforcement contingency, (*b*) to superior performance on a verbal conditioning task, and (*c*) to the personality characteristics of introversion.

Speed of Pupillary Dilation

The mean and *SD* of the proportion of dilation after each of six intervals are presented in

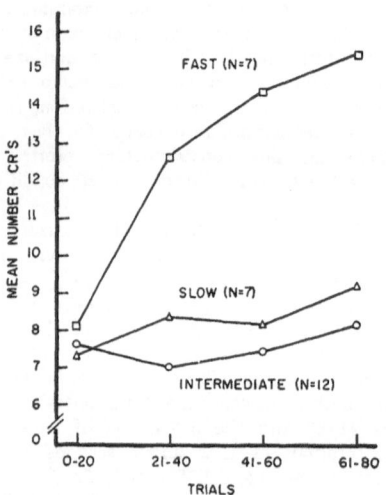

FIG. 1. Verbal conditioning performance curves for subjects with fast, intermediate, and slow pupillary constriction.

TABLE 2

PROPORTION OF DILATION AFTER
SIX INTERVALS OF TIME

Sec.	M	SD
5	77.55	8.74
10	87.86	6.99
15	92.45	5.85
30	95.94	4.43
45	97.59	3.97
60	98.86	1.81

Note.—$N = 49$.

Table 2. Because there was only limited variability in the subjects' responses after the intervals of 30, 45, and 60 seconds, extreme subjects were selected on the basis of their dilation after 5, 10, and 15 seconds. Fast ($N = 8$), intermediate ($N = 19$), and slow ($N = 6$) dilators were then selected in the same way as extreme constrictors.

Speed of pupillary dilation and awareness. A Fisher test of exact probabilities comparing the frequencies of aware and not aware subjects within the fast and slow dilating groups indicated that the distribution was well within the limits of chance occurrence.

Speed of pupillary dilation and verbal conditioning. When comparing the performance curves of the fast, intermediate, and slow dilators, the data from aware subjects who consciously resisted conditioning were not used. Analysis of variance indicated that there was a significant increase in conditioned responses over trials ($F = 5.56$, $df = 3,63$, $p < .01$), but that there were no significant differences between the groups ($F = .06$, $df = 2,21$).

Speed of pupillary dilation and personality measures. When the fast and slow dilators were compared over the personality measures, the fast dilators evidenced significantly higher E-scale scores ($t = 2.70$, $df = 12$, $p < .05$), but the groups did not differ on the peer-rating form measure of extraversion ($t = .51$, $df = 12$). As was the case with subjects differing in speed of constriction, the fast and slow dilators did not differ on the *A*, N, or *MA* scales ($t = 1.4$, 1.62, 1.54, respectively; $df = 14$).

DISCUSSION

The results of the present study clearly related the speed of pupillary constriction to awareness of an environmental contingency, susceptibility to verbal conditioning, and to personality in terms of the introversion-extraversion dimension. Since more rapid constriction is supposedly indicative of greater amounts of ACh at the cholinergic synapses, the results of this study were in agreement with earlier findings on animals where subjects with an inferred higher level of ACh evidenced better performance. The results of the present study, however, extended the findings to the area of personality, and offered support for the hypothesis relating high levels of ACh to environmental awareness, rapid conditioning, and consequently to introverted personality characteristics. That is, subjects with inferred high ACh levels who are more aware and more easily conditioned by environmental contingencies would be more likely to learn, or introject, the rules, restraints, and anxieties of the environment than would their low ACh counterparts. The differences in neural conductivity, and the concomitant differences in reactions and conditioning, would therefore play a major role in their personality characteristics with regard to the dimension of introversion and extraversion.

Some comments might be made in regard to the personality differences which the present author found to be associated with fast and slow constriction. Rubin (1964) recently reported differences in constriction between normals and neurotics. The points on his Figure 2 (p. 564) indicated that after each interval the neurotics had evidenced *more* constriction than had the normals; that is, the neurotics were faster constrictors. Though consistent, the differences were not significant. When the diagnoses of the neurotic subjects were checked (p. 563), it was found that all of these subjects could be classified as suffering from *introverted* disorders. In the present study fast constrictors were significantly more introverted. The independent-dependent variables have been reversed in the two studies, but when Rubin's neurotics are seen as introverted, the results of the two studies are consistent. The fact that Rubin's findings were not significant could be attributed to the fact that his introverted neurotics were compared to an unselected sample of normals, a sample which, it is fairly certain, would have included introverted normals who would thus have decreased the differences between the groups.

The results using speed of dilation, the measure of the adrenergic mediator, were for the most part inconsistent and nonsignificant. This probably stemmed from the fact that "only the cholinergic transmitters have been proved to be transmitters within the brain," while the adrenergic transmitters may be limited to the autonomic system (Morgan, 1965, p. 554); that is, adrenergic synapses may not have played a role in the responses measured in this study.

The consistency of the findings within this study, as well as the agreement between the results of this project and earlier research on animals, was very encouraging. It seems clear that if the pupillary response is in fact a function of ACh, the level of this transmitter substance is an important determinant of psychological functioning.

REFERENCES

DeNike, L., & Spielberger, C. Induced mediating states in verbal conditioning. *Journal of Verbal Learning and Verbal Behavior*, 1963, 1, 339–345.

Eccles, J. *The physiology of nerve cells.* Baltimore: Johns Hopkins Press, 1957.

Edwards, A. *Experimental design in psychological research.* New York: Holt, Rinehart & Winston, 1960.

Euler, U. von. Autonomic neuroeffector transmission. In J. Field, H. Magoun, & V. Hall (Eds.), *Handbook of physiology.* Vol. 1. Washington, D. C.: American Physiological Society, 1959. Pp. 215–237.

Eysenck, H. *Dimensions of personality.* London: Kegan, Paul, 1947.

Eysenck, H. The questionnaire measurement of neuroticism and extraversion. *Revista di psicología*, 1956, 50, 113–140.

Eysenck, H. *Experiments in personality.* London: Routledge & Kegan Paul, 1960.

Farber, I. The things people say to themselves. *American Psychologist*, 1963, 18, 185–197.

Franks, C. Conditioning and personality: A study of normal and neurotic subjects. *Journal of Abnormal and Social Psychology*, 1956, 52, 143–150.

Holmes, D. Awareness, intentions, and verbal conditioning performance. Paper read at Midwestern Psychological Association, Chicago, May 1966.

Johns, J., & Quay, H. The effect of social reward on verbal conditioning in psychopathic neurotic military offenders. *Journal of Consulting Psychology*, 1962, 26, 217–220.

Morgan, C. *Physiological psychology.* New York: McGraw-Hill, 1965.

Quay, H. C., & Hunt, W. A. Psychopathy, neuroticism, and verbal conditioning: A replication and extension. *Journal of Consulting Psychology*, 1965, 29, 283.

Rosenzweig, M., Krech, D., & Bennett E. Brain chemistry and adaptive behavior. In H. Harlow and C. Woolsey (Eds.), *Biological and biochemical bases of behavior.* Madison: University of Wisconsin Press, 1958. Pp. 367–400.

Rosenzweig, M., Krech, D., & Bennett, E. Heredity, environment, brain chemistry, and learning. In R. Patton (Ed.), *Current trends in psychological theory: A bicentennial program.* Pittsburgh: University of Pittsburgh Press, 1961. Pp. 87–110.

Rubin, L. Pupillary reactivity as a measure of adrenergic-cholinergic mechanisms in the study of psychotic behavior. *Journal of Nervous and Mental Disease*, 1960, 130, 386–400.

BRIEF ARTICLES

RUBIN, L. Autonomic dysfunction as a concomitant of neurotic behavior. *Journal of Nervous and Mental Disease,* 1964, **138,** 558–574.

RUSSELL, R., WATSON, R., & FRANKENHAEUSER, M. Effects of chronic reductions in brain cholinesterase activity on acquisition and extinction of a conditioned avoidance response. *Scandinavian Journal of Psychology,* 1961, **2,** 21–29.

SPIELBERGER, C. Theoretical and epistemological issues in verbal conditioning. In S. Rosenberg (Ed.), *Directions in psycholinguistics.* New York: Macmillan, 1965. Pp. 149–200.

TAFFEL, C. Anxiety and the conditioning of verbal behavior. *Journal of Abnormal and Social Psychology,* 1955, **51,** 496–501.

(Received October 6, 1965)

From G. S. Claridge and H. J. Chappa (1973). British Journal of Social and Clinical Psychology, *12*, 175-187, *by kind permission of the authors and the British Psychological Society*

Psychoticism: A Study of its Biological Basis in Normal Subjects

By GORDON S. CLARIDGE and HERBERT J. CHAPPA*

Department of Psychological Medicine, University of Glasgow

Starting from the viewpoint that the psychoses represent extreme forms of personality deviation, a study of the psychophysiological correlates of psychoticism in normal subjects was undertaken, using Eysenck's new PEN scale to select three groups of individuals: high P scorers, high N scorers and low N scorers. The research strategy used was to examine, in each of these three groups, the covariation between the two-flash threshold and skin conductance. This method was derived from previous work showing that what is uniquely different about psychotic patients is that they differ not on any single psychophysiological parameter but in the way in which different measures, including those studied here, covary. A specific comparison was made with a previous study showing that, in normal subjects given LSD-25, two-flash threshold and electrodermal level were related in a U-shaped fashion, compared with the conventional inverted-U function found in the same subjects under placebo. In the present study a U-function, similar to that observed under LSD-25, was evident in high P subjects, this contrasting markedly with the performance found in high N subjects. The difference between high N and high P subjects was particularly obvious in the low range of autonomic arousal, where the groups showed correlations between two-flash threshold and skin conductance which were significant but opposite in sign. Surprisingly, over this low range, low N subjects closely resembled high P individuals. This latter finding was considered to support the view that, in some people, low reported neuroticism may reflect the emotional blunting associated with certain forms of psychotic personality not measured by the Eysenck P scale, which seems mainly concerned with paranoid characteristics. In general, it was concluded that the results provide evidence for psychoticism as a normal personality dimension having, as its biological basis, a particular kind of nervous typological organization seen, in its extreme form, in the psychotic disorders.

In a recent review of the genetic, psychological and psychophysiological evidence Claridge (1972) has argued the case for a nervous typological view of the functional psychoses. According to that view the psychotic disorders would be extreme forms of personality deviation, occupying the end-point of a dimension of psychoticism. Their nervous typological basis would represent an exaggeration of the psychophysiological organization underlying psychoticism as seen in individuals who are psychiatrically well but predisposed to psychotic breakdown. Looked at in this way, psychosis and psychoticism would stand in the same relation to each other as do neurosis and neuroticism.

Apart from the fact that, until recently, the climate of opinion has more strongly favoured disease models, there are two difficulties that have prevented such an approach to the psychoses making the same progress as in the study of the neurotic disorders. First, it has proved particularly difficult to find suitable research strategies and theoretical models with which to investigate psychotic behaviour, which psychophysiologically is certainly more complex than neurosis. Secondly, the study

* Present address: Psychological Medicine, Facultad de Ciencias Medicas, Universidad de La Plata, Argentina.

of psychoticism in normal individuals has received little attention, both in psycho-physiology and in the personality field.

With regard to the first problem it is true of course that a considerable amount of research on the psychophysiology of schizophrenia has been carried out, mainly under the general heading of what Venables (1964) has termed 'input dysfunction'. Explanatory models have made use of the full gamut of psychophysiological concepts, including 'arousal' (Fish, 1961), 'attention' (McGhie, 1969) and, in a short-lived incursion into the field by Eysenck (1961), 'reactive inhibition'. It has become increasingly apparent that none of these concepts is by itself sufficient to account for psychosis, since psychotic patients have never been shown to differ consistently from other individuals when examined on single psychophysiological parameters. This has suggested the need to consider psychosis as involving a more complex type of central nervous organization—or disorganization—in which several psycho-physiological processes interact in a particular way (Claridge, 1967).

The empirical evidence for that conclusion comes from a number of studies showing that psychotic patients differ, not so much in their absolute levels or the range they cover on given measures, but rather in the way in which different measures covary. Thus both Herrington & Claridge (1965) and Krishnamoorti & Shagass (1964) reported that two such measures—the sedation threshold and Archimedes spiral after-effect—were correlated in opposite directions when neurotics and psychotics were compared; yet the range of scores on each measure taken individually was the same in both groups. Around the same time Venables (1963) compared normals and chronic schizophrenics and described a similar reversal of correlation using two quite different measures: skin potential and the fusion threshold for paired light flashes (two-flash threshold).

Subsequent investigation of this unusual feature of psychotic psychophysiology has concentrated on the two measures studied by Venables: the two-flash threshold and skin potential or its alternative, skin conductance (Lykken et al., 1966; Lykken & Maley, 1968; Hume & Claridge, 1965; Hume, 1970). None of these studies has confirmed Venables' original finding in all respects because the actual signs, and sometimes the magnitude, of the correlations found in various groups have differed from those described by him. Indeed, in one experiment, that by Lykken & Maley (1968), the pattern of correlations in psychotics and non-psychotics was diametri-cally opposite to that reported by Venables. However, a recent joint study with Venables and Lykken suggests that these apparent contradictions may arise because of differences in the range of arousal over which subjects in various experiments have been tested (Gruzelier et al., 1972).

Some results recently reported by Claridge (1972) would strongly support their conclusion and in general have helped to elucidate the nature of the relationship between two-flash threshold and electrodermal response in different psychological states. The results in question come from a study, originally carried out by Claridge & Hume (1966), concerned with the effects of LSD-25 on normal subjects. The aim of the experiment was to set up a drug model of Venables' comparison of schizo-phrenic and normal subjects; the prediction being that the effect of LSD-25, compared with a placebo, would be to alter the covariation between two-flash threshold and skin potential. Recent re-examination of the data from that experiment has revealed that the two variables did indeed covary in opposite directions under the two conditions but that in both cases the relationships were strongly curvilinear. Under placebo the relationship between two-flash threshold and skin potential formed a conventional inverted-U; that is to say, perceptual discrimination improved up to a moderate level of autonomic arousal and then deteriorated. Under LSD, however, a curious U-function was found, heightened perceptual sensitivity occurring when the concurrent level of arousal was either very high or very low and being poorest at a moderate arousal level. The actual signs of the correlations between two-flash threshold and skin potential, under both conditions, therefore depended critically on the range of arousal sampled.

Although the picture that begins to emerge is more complex than was once thought, the results just described do suggest that one consistent, if unexplained, characteristic of psychosis, whether naturally occurring or induced pharmacologically, is a peculiar inversion of the covariation between autonomic and perceptual function. The question that remains is whether the psychophysiological state underlying these empirical data is a qualitatively distinct one or whether it actually forms the nervous typological basis of a continuously variable personality characteristic of psychoticism. In other words, is it a discrete result of 'illness' or does it represent one kind of nervous typological organization, perhaps predisposing the individual to psychotic breakdown?

A direct attack on this problem has hitherto been difficult because of the unavailability of suitable instruments for investigating psychoticism as a normal personality characteristic—the second reason, referred to earlier, why the dimensional/nervous typological approach to psychosis has so far made little progress. Of the personality questionnaires the MMPI certainly contains scales aimed at the measurement of psychotic behaviour: and indeed Gottesman & Shields (1968), who have also argued from the genetic evidence for the continuity model of schizophrenia, have suggested that the Sc scale of that inventory may be useful for detecting individuals prone to psychotic breakdown. However, the MMPI may be considered of doubtful value on several counts: its theoretical derivation, factorial purity, and validity as an instrument for measuring personality traits in normal individuals (Griffiths, 1970).

A more promising development has been Eysenck's recent attempt to construct a questionnaire which will measure psychotic traits in psychiatrically well individuals. Of course, it has always been an implicit assumption in Eysenck's theory that psychoticism forms a dimension of personality additional to neuroticism and extraversion (Eysenck, 1955; Eysenck, 1956). However, the P (psychoticism) scale of his new PEN inventory represents his first published questionnaire instrument for measuring that dimension (Eysenck & Eysenck, 1968). Even the PEN inventory is apparently still in a transitional stage of development, the P scale in particular being regarded essentially as an exploratory research tool.

Despite this, the ready availability of appropriate psychophysiological and PEN inventory data on a group of normal subjects seemed to provide a sufficient rationale for carrying out the present study, the general aim of which will already be clear. That was to examine the psychophysiological correlates of the P scale in normal

individuals using the experimental strategy described earlier, namely the investigation of the covariation between two-flash threshold and electrodermal response,
in this case skin conductance. The expectation was that in individuals with high
scores on the P scale the relationship between these two measures would be opposite
in direction to that found in other subjects tested over the same range of autonomic
arousal. As a basis for comparison, two other types of subject were studied, both
selected in terms of their scores on the N (neuroticism) scale of the PEN inventory.
One, those with low N (and low P) scores, were individuals who, according to
Eysenck, would be regarded as extremely stable and lacking in personality abnormality. The second comparison group consisted of individuals who had *high* N
scores, but low P scores, and who would therefore be considered to be extreme in
neurotic, but not psychotic, tendency.

The data reported on below actually form only one part of a larger set of results
obtained in an investigation of the effects of chlorpromazine on a variety of psychophysiological and performance variables and only those aspects of the procedure
and results relevant to the present discussion will be considered here. Because high
scorers on the P scale tend to be rather rare it proved necessary to combine data
from two separate experiments in order to obtain a sample of reasonable size.
However, apart from some minor procedural differences mentioned below, the
experimental conditions for these two experiments were identical. A final point to be
noted is that only readings taken under the placebo conditions of the two experiments were utilized, since it was clearly necessary to avoid the complicating influence
which it was anticipated chlorpromazine would have on the psychophysiological
variables being considered. Analyses of the complete data from a pharmacological
viewpoint will be reported on in later papers.

METHOD

Subjects

The total sample available consisted of 61 subjects forming the combined placebo groups
of the two drug experiments referred to earlier. These subjects were allocated to subgroups
according to their scores on the P and N scales of the PEN inventory. This was done in the
following way. The sample was first divided into low and high P subjects, using as a lower
cut-off point for high P a score of 3 on the psychoticism scale. The low P part of the sample
was then further subdivided into high and low N individuals, the former being subjects with
a neuroticism score of 12 or more and the latter subjects with a neuroticism score of 8 or less.
This procedure resulted in three groups: a high P group (11 subjects), a high N (low P) group
(14 subjects) and a low N (low P) group (21 subjects).

Measures

Two-flash threshold. This was determined by presenting paired light flashes, 1 msec.
in length, via a Ferranti type CL-64 cathode tube, reduced in intensity with a 1·5 Kodak
neutral density filter, and situated at eye-level 2·2 m from the subject. All measurements
were taken in dim illumination in an air-conditioned, sound-proofed room. After the ingestion of two (placebo) pills incorporated in the design of both drug experiments a series of
estimations of the two-flash threshold were made at regular intervals. Each estimation
represented the mean of an upper and a lower threshold determined from ascending and
descending series. In the ascending series, starting from a point below the subject's approximate threshold, the inter-flash interval of the light pairs was increased in 2 msec. steps until
the subject changed his judgement from 'one' to 'flicker' on four consecutive presentations.

Psychoticism: A Study of its Biological Basis in Normal Subjects

The reverse procedure was used for descending series. In one of the experiments eight estimations of the two-flash threshold were made at 15, 30, 45, 60, 75, 135, 150 and 165 min. after ingestion of the placebo. In the other experiment five estimations were made at 0, 20, 60, 80 and 100 min. A single overall measure of each subject's two-flash threshold was obtained by averaging the eight, or five, estimations as appropriate.

Skin conductance level. Throughout each experiment the subject's skin resistance was monitored continuously on a Grass Model 5 polygraph, using silver/silver chloride electrodes with a KCl electrolytic jelly attached to the palmar surface of the distal phalanx of the left index finger (active site) and to the ventral surface of the forearm, approximately 10 cm above the wrist. The records were analysed by taking readings of skin resistance level coinciding with each estimation of the two-flash threshold. On each occasion two such readings were actually taken, one for the ascending and one for the descending threshold, these then being averaged. The mean of the eight (or five) resistance levels so obtained, converted to conductance units, was used as the overall measure of the subject's skin conductance level.

PEN Inventory. This questionnaire was administered to each subject during the rest intervals between two-flash threshold estimations.

RESULTS

The main comparisons between the three groups studied are clearly brought out in Figs. 1–3, where it should be noted that the two-flash threshold readings have been plotted so that changes in an upward direction indicate *improved* perceptual discrimination. In the case of high P subjects (Fig. 1) it can be seen that, although there

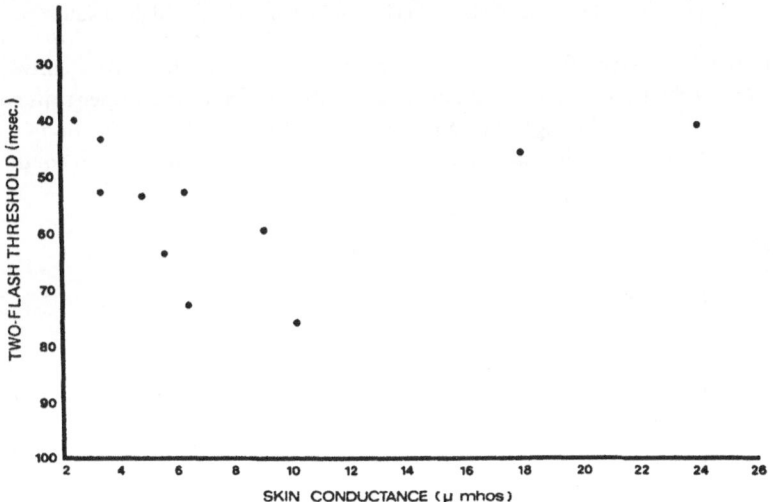

Fig. 1. Two-flash threshold and skin conductance level in high P subjects. On this and later figures the scale for two-flash threshold is arranged so that changes in the upper direction indicate improved perceptual discrimination.

were few subjects in the upper range of skin conductance, the overall relationship between that measure and two-flash threshold was generally U-shaped. In this respect it was very reminiscent of that found under LSD as described earlier. Certainly, over the *low* range of autonomic arousal there was a clear tendency, as

GORDON S. CLARIDGE AND HERBERT J. CHAPPA

under LSD, for increasing skin conductance to be accompanied by a progressive impairment of perceptual discrimination.

Contrasting markedly with the finding for high P subjects was the kind of covariation observed in high N subjects whose results are shown in Fig. 2. It can be seen

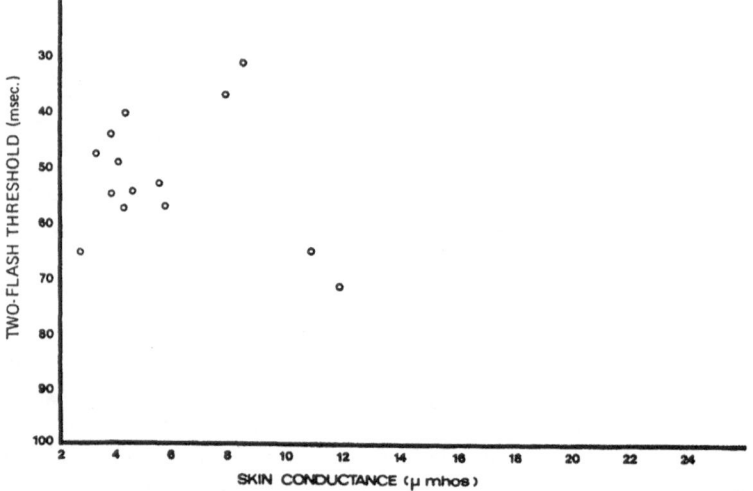

Fig. 2. Two-flash threshold and skin conductance level in high N subjects.

there that the overall function in that group tended rather towards a conventional *inverted*-U relationship, although again few subjects fell in the upper skin conductance range. As in the high P group the relationship was clearest in the low range, where perceptual discrimination improved in an orderly fashion as skin conductance increased.

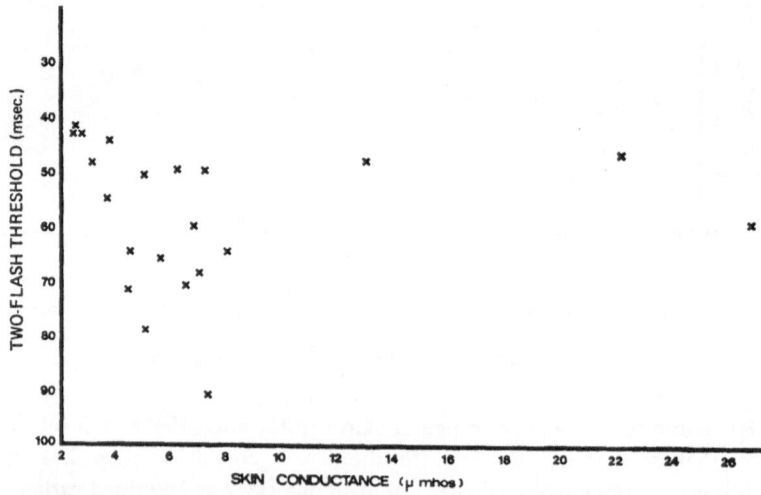

Fig. 3. Two-flash threshold and skin conductance level in low N subjects.

Psychoticism: A Study of its Biological Basis in Normal Subjects

Finally, the results for low N subjects are shown in Fig. 3. The overall picture here is less clear than in the other two groups, at least over the upper range of skin conductance. However, over its lower range low N individuals closely resembled high P subjects, perceptual discrimination worsening as autonomic arousal increased.

In all three groups it is evident that, although of different shape, the functions relating two-flash threshold and skin conductance were suggestive of curvilinearity, in that respect being entirely consistent with our LSD experiment. However, because of the small number of subjects with very high levels of skin conductance statistical analysis of the results was confined to data falling in the lower range of autonomic arousal. Observation of the plotted scores indicated that a skin conductance of 10·25 μmhos provided a suitable cut-off point which, for the three groups, included all two-flash threshold readings occurring before the various points of inflexion.

In each group product moment correlations were calculated between two-flash threshold and skin conductance over this low range of autonomic arousal, as just

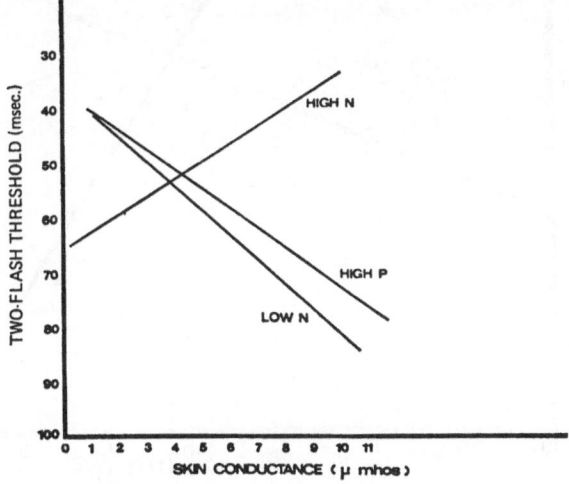

Fig. 4. Regression lines relating skin conductance level and two-flash threshold in high P, low N and high N subjects in skin conductance range up to 10·25 micromhos.

defined. In this respect it should be noted that the convention is used here of presenting the signs of correlation from the point of view of their interpretation in terms of 'arousal'. That is to say, a positive correlation indicates that a high level of skin conductance is associated with *improved* perceptual discrimination. Negative correlations indicate that perceptual discrimination is *poorer* at high skin conductance levels.

As expected from the graphical representation of the results, high correlations between two-flash threshold and skin conductance were found in all three groups, though of course the signs differed in the various samples. In the nine high P subjects falling in the low range of skin conductance the value for r was -0.78 ($P < 0.05$). In the 12 comparable high N subjects the correlation was also significant but positive in direction ($r = +0.64$, $P < 0.05$); while low N subjects resembled high P individuals, r being -0.58 ($P < 0.05$, $n = 18$). This close similarity between high P and low N subjects, and the difference between both of those groups and high N subjects, is brought out clearly in Fig. 4, where the regression lines relating the two measures together over the low skin conductance range have been drawn for each of the three groups.

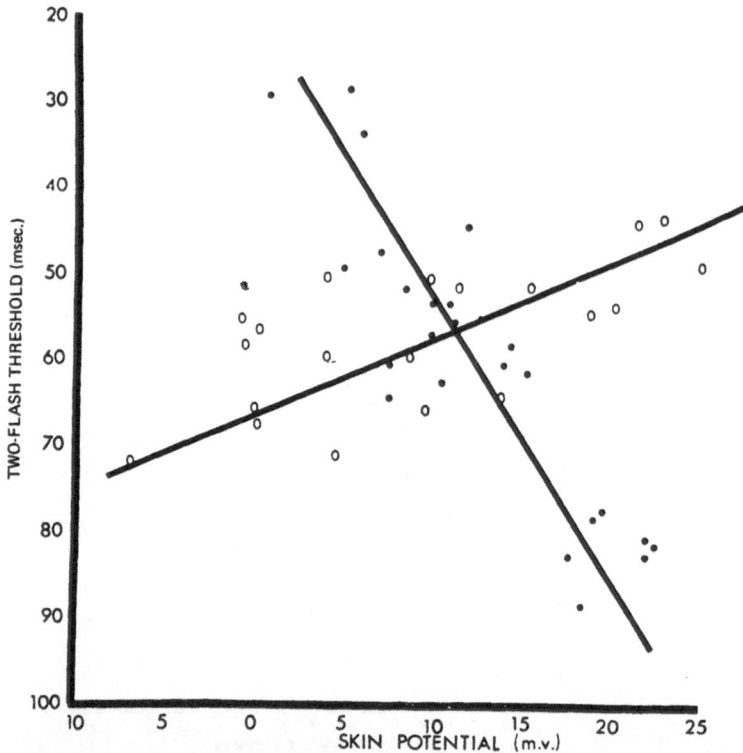

Fig. 5. Relationship between two-flash threshold and skin potential under LSD-25 and placebo conditions in skin potential range up to 25 mV. Compare similarity with equivalent data for high P and low N subjects and for high N subjects, shown in Fig. 4. The signs of skin potential readings have been reversed. ●, LSD-25, rho = -0.82; ○, placebo, rho = $+0.74$.

Finally, it is of interest to compare directly the findings of the present study with those of the LSD experiment referred to earlier. Fig. 5 shows the two-flash threshold and skin potential readings under LSD-25 and placebo measured over a low range of autonomic arousal equivalent to that covered for skin conductance in Fig. 4. Comparing the two diagrams it can be seen that there is a remarkable coincidence between the two sets of data, the direction and extent of covariation between the perceptual and autonomic measure being identical for the high N group and the placebo condition, on the one hand, and for the high P/low N subjects and the LSD condition, on the other.

Psychoticism: A Study of its Biological Basis in Normal Subjects

DISCUSSION

The theoretical position adopted here has contained two assumptions. One is that psychoticism represents a continuously variable dimension of personality. The other is that this dimension has definable psychophysiological correlates; or, put another way, is, because of the obvious involvement of biological processes in psychotic disorder, most appropriately investigated from a nervous typological viewpoint. The research strategy necessary to test both of these assumptions is obvious: that of examining the psychophysiological status of psychiatrically well individuals judged to be high in psychoticism using techniques derived from the study of psychotic patients. When these two areas of research are brought together, as they have been here, the results seem to be extremely promising and to add one further set of proofs to the mounting evidence, from many different sources, that the functional psychoses are not qualitatively distinct illnesses, but extreme forms of personality deviation.

Another, more specific, assumption made at the beginning of this paper was that the biological basis of psychoticism (and psychosis) lies in a particular kind of nervous typological organization, as reflected empirically in the covariation between different psychophysiological measures. This assumption, too, seems to have found strong support here. Even using a lenient cut-off point on a personality questionnaire still under development it has been possible to show that individuals relatively high on its psychoticism scale show a distinctive kind of covariation between the two measures chosen for investigation. However, perhaps what is more important, the *direction* of this covariation is identical with that found in normal subjects in whom a psychotic state was induced pharmacologically and in whom, incidentally, electrodermal activity was monitored differently, i.e. with skin potential rather than skin conductance.

As observed here, the covariation between two-flash threshold and electrodermal response associated with psychoticism seems to take on a curious U-shape. Whether this is in line, as would be expected, with that found in psychosis itself can, at the moment, only be determined by extrapolation from existing results obtained on patient samples. This is because no investigator has yet reported the crucial experiment, namely a comparison of the two-flash threshold and electrodermal activity in a group of *drug-free* acute psychotics covering the *whole range* of autonomic arousal. So far, as we have seen, various authors have reported correlations which differ in sign and magnitude; the measures almost certainly sampling different parts of the arousal scale. It is also difficult to build up a composite picture by piecing together the results of various studies, since the experimental procedures adopted by different investigators have rarely been comparable. In one case, however, identical techniques *were* used for measuring both skin potential and two-flash threshold. Thus, the recording techniques described by Venables (1963) in his original study of two-flash threshold and skin potential were replicated exactly in the LSD experiment from which the data described here were taken (Claridge & Hume, 1966). It is therefore possible to compare, across the two experiments, the direction of covariation between two-flash threshold and skin potential for equivalent ranges of electrodermal response. When this is done it emerges that most of

Venables' subjects—both psychotic and normal—had a skin potential level of more than 25 mV, that is beyond the upper cut-off point used to define the high range in our LSD experiment. In other words, Venables seems mainly to have tested subjects in a state of *high* autonomic arousal. The direction of correlations he reports for normal and non-paranoid schizophrenics is therefore directly in line with those that would be predicted from our data for LSD and high P subjects.

In his original paper reporting the inversion of correlation between two-flash threshold and skin potential in psychotics, Venables interpreted his findings by suggesting that it may be due to a failure of some feedback mechanism that normally intervenes between cortical and autonomic arousal. Claridge (1967), attempting to explain his comparable finding on the sedation threshold and spiral after-effect, reached a not dissimilar conclusion, though he adopted a rather different model of central nervous activity. He suggested that psychosis may involve the dissociation between two important psychophysiological systems: one concerned with arousal as such, the other with attention and the regulation of sensory input. He also argued at that time, incidentally, that the 'dissociated' state found in psychotic patients may represent in an extreme form a particular kind of central nervous organization found to a lesser degree in normal subjects highly loaded on psychoticism.

In a general sense it may be supposed that the results reported here are consistent with some kind of model of nervous activity which incorporates the notion of feedback between different psychophysiological systems, whether these are visualized anatomically as 'cortical' and 'autonomic' or in terms of their respective functions in controlling arousal, on the one hand, and attention or perceptual sensitivity, on the other. It seems feasible to suppose that different kinds of interaction between these systems give rise to the different varieties of nervous typological organization underlying the major personality dimensions. In that case it may be significant that the particular organization apparently associated with psychoticism and psychosis is, according to the present results, a very unusual one. Thus the U-shaped function relating two-flash threshold to electrodermal response could be said to represent a highly unstable physiological state, since changes in arousal in either direction from the optimum would result in quite disproportionate increases in perceptual sensitivity. In an extreme form such changes might disrupt mental function drastically and could account for some of the major symptoms of psychotic disorder, particularly those involving perception and attention. By comparison, the conventional inverted-U function would seem, intuitively at least, to represent a more regulated condition for the nervous system to be in, since it implies the operation of some protective mechanism at high levels of arousal.

A startling feature of the present results, and one which requires further comment, is the close similarity found here between high P subjects and individuals with very low neuroticism scores. Taken at face value the finding might seem to negate much of the foregoing discussion, since according to Eysenck low scores on his N scales are intended to reflect normality of personality. Statistically, of course, this is not so and we would suggest that individuals reporting low neuroticism scores could be regarded as having the lack of anxiety and emotional responsiveness appropriate to certain forms of psychoticism which are not tapped by Eysenck's P scale. Inspec-

Psychoticism: A Study of its Biological Basis in Normal Subjects

tion of the latter's item content, for example, reveals that many of its questions reflect paranoid tendencies. A similar conclusion was reached by Teasdale *et al.* (1971), who considered that seven of the P scale items are paranoid in nature. In addition, several other items could be construed in a similar way, namely those referring to excessive concern with ill-luck and with contagion from disease. What seems most obvious is an almost complete absence of questions concerned with other prominent signs of psychosis, namely withdrawal, flatness of affect, lack of interest and drive, and the inability to express emotion. It is these characteristics which could be reflected in abnormally low levels of neuroticism and, while it seems unlikely that all low N scores can be interpreted in that way, the tendency in the present sample may have been sufficiently strong to bring out the psychophysiological relationships observed.

Such an interpretation of the questionnaire findings would be consistent with a number of other facts about psychosis, in general, and about the P scale, in particular. Elsewhere Claridge (1967) has provided evidence for a dimension of psychoticism running from active (paranoid) to retarded (non-paranoid) psychosis. From what has been said it seems reasonable to suppose that low N scoring provides some measure of the latter, the Eysenck P scale reflecting only that group of personality traits clustering at the 'active' end of Claridge's dimension.

In this respect it is interesting to note that in a recent study Birchall (1971) found that the P scale correlated positively with those characteristics which Claridge considered to be associated with 'active' psychosis, namely impulsivity and self-control as measured by the CPI and hypomania derived from the MMPI.

A further feature of the P scale would support the view that it is measuring only one aspect of psychoticism. This concerns the statistical distribution of scores obtained on the scale. The findings of Teasdale *et al.* (1971), Birchall (1971) and the present authors all agree with the original sampling data reported by the Eysencks in showing a score distribution which is quite asymmetric, with the modal frequency falling at zero. In all cases the distribution is smoothly J-shaped, apparently forming exactly half a normal one.

Clearly, some of the findings reported here strongly challenge Eysenck's assumption of independence between the major personality dimensions, at least when studied with the biological or 'causal' procedures he himself so favours. On the other hand, our results obtained with the P scale provide some validity for his questionnaire measure of psychoticism and help to carry the nervous typological approach into this relatively unexplored area of personality. Here, as the possible biological basis of psychoticism and psychosis, we have stressed the *organization* of central nervous processes, rather than the simple deviation along some single psychophysiological continuum such as 'arousal'. That this organization should be uniquely different in the clinically recognizable psychotic disorders is not too surprising. That it should form the basis of a dimension of normal personality is, to say the least, fascinating and must lead one to speculate particularly about the biological adaptiveness of a set of characteristics which in extreme form are associated with gross mental disturbance.

Finally, one further general point is worth making. If the view that the psychoses represent gross variations of normal personality characteristics continues to find support, then there could be important implications for the methodology of research into the nature of those disorders. The difficulty of obtaining reliable experimental data on acutely disturbed patients is well known—a difficulty not unconnected, perhaps, with the peculiar nervous typology which may underlie psychotic behaviour. An even greater practical problem is that of collecting samples of non-institutionalized drug-free patients in whom the processes that need to be studied can be seen in pure form. It is feasible that a more complete understanding of the psychoses may come through a shift of emphasis in research, away from the study of the psychiatric patient, and towards the investigation of similar, but less deviant, forms of personality abnormality found in the general population.

The work of Dr Chappa was carried out while he was a British Council Scholar at the University of Glasgow. The authors wish to thank the Council for their financial assistance in this respect and for the provision of funds to pay the expenses of the subjects taking part in one of the experiments reported here. The remaining subjects were paid from Grant ACMR 689 from the Advisory Committee on Medical Research, to whom thanks are also due.

REFERENCES

BIRCHALL, P. M. A. (1971). Some measures of personality and their relation to psychiatric illness. (M.Sc. thesis, University of Glasgow.)

CLARIDGE, G. S. (1967). *Personality and Arousal*. Oxford: Pergamon Press.

CLARIDGE, G. S. (1972). The schizophrenias as nervous types. *Br. J. Psychiat.* **121**, 1–17.

CLARIDGE, G. S. & HUME, W. I. (1966). Comparison of effects of dexamphetamine and LSD-25 on perceptual and autonomic function. *Percept. mot. Skills* **23**, 456–458.

EYSENCK, H. J. (1955). Psychiatric diagnosis as a psychological and statistical problem. *Psychol. Rep.* **1**, 3–17.

EYSENCK, H. J. (1961). Psychosis, drive and inhibition: a theoretical and experimental account. *Am. J. Psychiat.* **118**, 198–204.

EYSENCK, S. B. G. (1956). Neurosis and psychosis: an experimental analysis. *J. ment. Sci.* **102**, 517–529.

EYSENCK, S. B. G. & EYSENCK, H. J. (1968). The measurement of psychoticism: a study of factor stability and reliability. *Br. J. soc. clin. Psychol.* **7**, 286–294.

FISH, F. J. (1961). A neurophysiological theory of schizophrenia. *J. ment. Sci.* **107**, 828–838.

GOTTESMAN, I. I. & SHIELDS, J. (1968). In pursuit of the schizophrenic genotype. In S. G. Vandenberg (ed.), *Progress in Human Behaviour Genetics*. Baltimore: Johns Hopkins Press.

GRIFFITHS, R. D. (1970). Personality assessment. In P. Mittler (ed.), *The Psychological Assessment of Mental and Physical Handicap*. London: Methuen.

GRUZELIER, J. H., LYKKEN, D. T. & VENABLES, P. (1972). Schizophrenia and arousal revisited: two-flash thresholds and electrodermal activity in activated and nonactivated conditions. *Archs gen. Psychiat.* **26**, 427–432.

HERRINGTON, R. N. & CLARIDGE, G. S. (1965). Sedation threshold and Archimedes' spiral after-effect in early psychosis. *J. psychiat. Res.* **3**, 159–170.

HUME, W. I. (1970). An experimental analysis of arousal. (PhD. thesis, University of Bristol.)

HUME, W. I. & CLARIDGE, G. S. (1965). A comparison of two measures of 'arousal' in normal subjects. *Life Sci.* **4**, 545–553.

KRISHNAMOORTI, S. R. & SHAGASS, C. (1964). Some psychological test correlates of sedation threshold. In J. Wortis (ed.), *Recent Advances in Biological Psychiatry*. New York: Plenum Press.

LYKKEN, D. T. & MALEY, M. (1968). Autonomic versus cortical arousal in schizophrenics and non-psychotics. *J. psychiat. Res.* **6**, 21–32.

LYKKEN, D. T., ROSE, R., LUTHER, B. & MALEY, M. (1966). Correcting psychophysiological measures for individual differences in range. *Psychol. Bull.* **66**, 481–484.

Psychoticism: A Study of its Biological Basis in Normal Subjects

McGHIE, A. (1969). *Pathology of Attention.* Harmondsworth: Penguin Books.

TEASDALE, J. D., SEGRAVES, R. T. & ZACUNE, J. (1971). 'Psychoticism' in drug-users. *Br. J. soc. clin. Psychol.* 10, 160–171.

VENABLES, P. H. (1963). The relationship between level of skin potential and fusion of paired light flashes in schizophrenic and normal subjects. *J. psychiat. Res.* 1, 279–287.

VENABLES, P. H. (1964). Input dysfunction in schizophrenia. In B. A. Maher (ed.), *Progress in Experimental Personality Research.* New York: Academic Press.

Section Four

Cortical Substrates of Behaviour

Editorial Commentary

on

Cortical Substrates of Behaviour

It is the unfortunate state of affairs that our present understanding of cortical neuro-anatomy is sufficiently puerile to preclude statements relating personality traits to specific mechanisms in the brain. This presumes, of course, that enduring traits of personality do indeed have some origin in the brain. For the sake of argument, let us assume some contribution exists and see if we can augur what it might be.

Professor John Fulton, in delivering the Sir Charles Scott Sherrington Lectures at the University of Liverpool in 1952, related the following anecdote. A Roman physican by the name of Scribonius Largus writing in the first century A.D. described his mode of treatment for patients suffering from a headache. He placed a large Mediterranean 'torpedo' across the patient's brow and induced a discharge 'until the patient's senses were benumbed'. The efficacy of this treatment is not surprising when one realizes that the Mediterranean torpedo electricus develops electrical potentials of 100–150 volts at high amperage. Who would have a mere headache after that! Dr. Largus' writings were first published in 1529, and within 70 years the use of torpedos to relieve labour pains had become common practice. It took almost another 300 years before the implications of the 'torpedo technique' were realized. Professor Friedrich Leopold Goltz of Strassburg found that his dogs exhibited dramatic behavioural changes after he ablated large sections of their central hemispheres. He reported his results in 1874,

catalyzing a chain of experiments that ended up in the first prefrontal lobotomy, performed by Egas Moniz in 1935. The following year, Cerletti (appropriately from Rome) first introduced to the modern world electroshock as a therapeutic technique (or should I say 'reintroduced'). Thus, almost 1900 years after Dr. Largus, we replaced the fish with electrodes.

Between the time that Professor Moniz and his colleague Almeida Lima introduced the leucotomy in 1935 and 1950 there were about 20 000 humans lobotomized. It took a sizable surgical "N" before it became apparent to neurosurgeons that an essential distinction had to be made between the neo-cortex and the so-called visceral brain. This distinction was made quite elegantly some years later by Paul Maclean (1973) in describing the 'triune brain', consisting of the midbrain (olfactostriatum, corpus striatum and globus pallidus), the limbic system and the neocortex. Lesioning in the visceral brain alone produced no impairment in learning capacity, whereas neocortical lesions (particularly Brodmann's areas 9, 10, 11, 12) produced severe learning impairment. Thus, the optimum 'cut', from the standpoint of leaving intact the maximum number of functions while eliminating the unwanted behaviour, was localized in the medial ventral quadrant of the frontal lobe. A second important consequence of lobotomy was reported by Freeman and Watts (1946), namely the relief of intractable pain. As Professor Fulton has described, sectioning the

medial ventral quadrant transects a large
ascending visceral sensory system projecting
to the hypothalamus and medial thalamic
nuclei and eventually to the orbito-frontal
cortex and posterior orbital gyrus. Thus, the
pain messages are never delivered, something
akin to snipping the telephone line.

So how far have we come? Granted we can
interrupt the pathways that conduct pain
messages and even lesion tissue that seems to
be responsible for delusional thought, but what
can we say about the relatively stable and
idiosyncratic profile of behaviours that define
our personality? To begin with I will finesse
the question of personality by addressing
myself to *low intensity* emotional response,
such as introversion–extraversion, assertive–
submissive, gregarious–shy, cheerful–sombre,
calm–frenetic, active–lazy, secure–insecure,
pleasant–irascible, and the like. Most would
agree that these dimensions fall under the
rubric of personality. Many of the dimensions,
however, are probably inappropriate for our
present inquiry, being subject to the greater
forces of social learning (assertive–submissive,
secure–insecure, altruistic–selfish, trust-
worthy–untrustworthy, etc.). We are left
then with a cluster of dimensions of emotional
response (most seeming to involve activity
level) that may be exhibited enough of the time
to fetch a label.

Let me digress for one minute. The past 10
years has ushered in a frontier of research in
brain stimulation, mostly infrahuman. The
results of this research have forcibly
demonstrated the ability to reliably produce
high intensity emotional reactions with electrical stimulation (fear, aversion, pain and
rage are principal examples). The question
then is to what extent are invariant patterns of
low intensity emotional response attributable
to brain mechanisms. Is an introverted,
retiring, sombre sort of chap responding to
hyperactivity of his RAS, which in turn
initiates septo-hippocampal inhibition? Does
heightened *cortical* arousal lead to increased
behavioural inhibition? If so, is this negative
feedback loop of the kind described by Gray,
involving the orbito-frontal cortex, the medial
septal area and the hippocampus? At the
cortical level, there is little question but that
the limbic system is involved in emotional
behaviour (Papez, 1937; Maclean, 1955). At
the *subcortical* level, behavioural arousal

seems to result from adreneric stimulation or
serotonergic blocking (ergotropic dominance
to use W. R. Hess' term). With grave regard
to the abuse of parsimony, a subcortical
(probably midbrain) imbalance results in
central limbic adrenergic stimulation or
depression. What is missing is the elaborate,
heterogeneous biochemical formula that turns
hypothetics into an advanceable theory.

This section is devoted to research on the
role of cortical and subcortical structures in
influencing, initiating or regulating behaviour.
While the question of 'personality' in this
regard is a very difficult one, hopefully some
light will be shed in this area as well.

An important point to keep 'in mind' is that
structural function in the brain is heterogeneous, nothing happens in isolation without
impact on neighbouring tissue or structures.
The brain is the most intricate labyrinth of
neuronal pathways. The cortex alone contains
about fifteen *billion* neurons. One example will
hopefully suffice to imprint this message.

One system that has been mentioned a
number of times is the limbic system or 'limbic
lobe', a term coined by Broca 100 years ago.
The limbic system has profuse connections
with the olfactory system (rhinencephalon),
the diencephalon (thalamus, hypothalamus
and epithalamus) and certain areas of the
neocortex. Perhaps the most important pathway is the medial forebrain bundle, the major
telegraph line between the limbic system, the
hypothalamus and the subcortex (midbrain).
In brief, the limbic system consists of the
amygdala, septal area, hippocampal formation, fornix, stria terminalis, stria
habenularis, cingulate and parihippocampal
gyri, piriform lobe, olfactory bulb, nerves and
tract and medial and lateral olfactory striae
and gyri. Just defining the boundary of this
system has been a matter of controversy. So
many structures within the system are
functionally interconnected with regions outside the system, it has not been clear 'where
to draw the line'. Let's consider the complexity
of isolating just one structure within the sytem.
The hippocampal formation alone includes the
prehippocampal rudiment, indusium griseum,
dentate gyrus, subiculum, Ammon's horn and
gyrus fasciolaris. Each of these structures has
its own connectivity pattern. As you might
guess, we can break it down still farther. The
subiculum, for example, is divided into four

areas: the parasubiculum, presubiculum, subiculum and prosubiculum. In sum, when we speak about the relationship of the limbic system to personality let us not forget what our conjecture involves.

References

Freeman, W., and Watts, J. W. (1946). Pain of organic disease relieved by prefrontal lobotomy. *Lancet,* **1,** 953–955

Fulton, J. F. (1972). *The Frontal Lobos and Human Behaviour.* (Liverpool: University of Liverpool Press)

MacLean, P. D. (1955). Limbic sytem ("visceral brain") in relation to central gray and reticulum of brain stem: Evidence of interdependence in emotional process. *Psychosomat. Med.,* **17,** 355–366

MacLean, P. D. (1973). *A Triune Concept of the Brain and Behaviour.* (Toronto: University of Toronto Press)

Papez, J. W. (1937). A proposed mechanism of emotion. *Arch. Neurol. Psychiatry,* **38,** 725–743

From A. A. Ward Jr. (1948). Proceedings of the Association for Research in Nervous and Mental Disease, *27,* 438-445, *by kind permission of the author and Raven Press, New York*

THE ANTERIOR CINGULATE GYRUS AND PERSONALITY

ARTHUR A. WARD JR., M.D.

LONG ago, sometime prior to 1670, Felix Plater, the Professor of Medicine at Basle, recorded the unusual case of the good knight, Caspar Bonecurtius, who gradually became mentally deranged over the course of two years, until he was utterly incapable of any reasoning. He spent most of the time sitting with arms on the table, supporting his head in his hands. He did not respond to events in his environment, occasionally uttered a few words but they were rarely relevant. This state of altered personality continued for six months when he suddenly died. At autopsy a globular tumor was found over the anterior portion of the corpus callosum which must certainly have partially destroyed the anterior portion of the cingulate gyrus.

Until relatively recently, little definite information was available as to the function of this region—also known as the anterior limbic area, Brodmann's area 24 or LA of Economo. Because of certain early anatomical studies, the anterior limbic area was supposed to be a part of the rhinencephalon and thus to be olfactory. However, it is now clear that this region is a powerful autonomic effector region and has no particular relation to olfactory processes. It is also known to be one of the most powerful of the cortical suppressor regions.

Anatomy

The cytoarchitecture of this region has been described by von Bonin (4) and Bailey (3) for the various primates. The only known subcortical afferents to this region are from the anteromedial nucleus of the thalamus (5, 16). It is well known that the anteromedial nucleus receives the termination of the mammillothalamic tract and this nucleus is also said to be connected with the other anterior thalamic nuclei as well as with the nuclei of the midline. Probably few other afferents to the anterior limbic area exist in view of the statement by von Bonin (4) that "in the inner main layer of LA (area 24) there are relatively few oblique fibers, from which one could conclude that there is a dearth of specific afferents." This area is also very poorly connected with the rest of the cerebral cortex.

No cortical afferents to area 24 have been demonstrated by physiological neuronography (9). It, in turn, projects only to areas 32 and
31 and locally into 6a and 4s (2, 20). The main efferent pathway from
this region passes down the internal capsule into the ventral and
medial portions of the cerebral peduncles, giving off no myelinated
collaterals to the basal ganglia, thalamus or hypothalamus. At the
upper end of the pons, fibers leave the peduncles and pass dorsally
into the medial reticular formation, from just below the superior
olive to just above the pyramidal decussations (21). This medial
portion of the bulbar reticular system has been shown by Magoun
and Rhines (11) to suppress all muscular action. In common with
other suppressor regions, strychninization of the anterior limbic
cortex demonstrates that the axons from area 24 en route to the
reticular formation send collaterals to the nucleus caudatus which
are presumably unmyelinated (7). Physiological neuronography has
recently confirmed a projection from this area back to the anterior
thalamic nuclei (4), thereby making this a closed circuit.

Effects of stimulation

The effects of electrical stimulation of the rostral cingular cortex
in the monkey (18, 21) can be divided into three groups.

1. *Autonomic responses.* These include both sympathetic and
parasympathetic responses. The pupillary dilatation which may be
obtained from the dorsal portion of this area is probably primarily a
sympathetic response since it is readily obtained following section
of the 3rd nerve. Piloerection follows stimulation of the more caudal
portions of area 24. Marked respiratory slowing and arrest up to 25
seconds may be obtained from the more rostral and deeper portions
of this region, being most marked anteriorly. Marked cardiovascular
effects are also obtained, consisting of vagal slowing of the heart,
cardiac arrest and a marked fall as well as the occasional rise in
blood pressure.

2. *Motor effects.* Stimulation of the deeper and more caudal portions of this region under deep anesthesia (21) elicits tonic, bilateral
movements which may start in either both arms or both legs and
spread to involve the whole body in slow, postural movements
somewhat similar to the adversive movements obtained from stimulation of area 8 on the lateral surface of the hemisphere. Under
different conditions of anesthesia, stimulation of the rostral cingular
cortex causes prompt vocalization and complex facial movements
(18).

3. *Suppressor action.* Electrical stimulation of this region (9) causes a relaxation of existing muscular contractions and a holding in abeyance of motor after-discharge, both these effects appearing and disappearing promptly. There is also suppression of the motor response to stimulation of the sensorimotor cortex. Local strychninization of this area (2) causes a widespread and profound suppression of the electrical activity of the remainder of the cortex which appears after a variable latency. It has been established by McCulloch (9) that this suppression of cortical activity is mediated via the caudate nucleus while the powerful suppression of motor response is mediated through the bulbar reticular formation in the pons (10). During the period of stimulation, there is not only a complete loss of normal muscle tone, but also an abolition of all the deep reflexes (18, 21).

Effects of ablation

Immediately following either unilateral or bilateral subpial resection of the rostral cingular gyrus in the monkey (21) there is an obvious change in personality. The monkey loses its preoperative shyness and is less fearful of man. It appears more inquisitive than the normal monkey of the same age. In a large cage with other monkeys of the same size, such an animal shows no grooming behavior or acts of affection toward its companions. In fact, it treats them as it treats inanimate objects and will walk on them, bump into them if they happen to be in the way and will even sit on them. It will openly eat food in the hand of a companion without being prepared to do battle and appears surprised when it is rebuffed. Such an animal never shows actual hostility to its fellows. It neither fights nor tries to escape when removed from a cage. It acts under all circumstances as though it had lost its "social conscience." This is probably what Smith (17) saw and called "tameness." It is thus evident that following removal of the anterior limbic area, such monkeys lose some of the social fear and anxiety which normally governs their activity and thus lose the ability to forecast accurately the social repercussions of their own actions.

Function of area 24

Although the superstition still persists that the whole cingular gyrus is olfactory, Economo and Koskinas in 1925, on anatomical grounds, had conjectured that it contained the cortical representation of the vegetative nervous system. One might have guessed this because a well-developed gyrus cinguli is present in certain aquatic mammals that have no olfactory bulbs and is disproportionately well-developed in man whose sense of smell is vestigial.

It is now clear that area 24 has two powerful functions. It suppresses cortical activity and motor performance and it dominates the autonomic nervous system. The cortical suppressor areas on the lateral surface of the hemisphere are so distributed that each is associated with a major functional subdivision of the cortex: area 19 with vision, area 2 with somaesthesia, area 4s with motor control and area 8 with the associative activity of the frontal pole. Thus area 24 is similarly related to the rest of the limbic lobe. All the suppressor areas are known to have descending axons with collaterals to the nucleus caudatus. From the nucleus caudatus, by an indirect path, they can prevent impulses, ascending into the thalamus, from being relayed to the cortex and so can block the interplay of cortex and thalamus. This circuit, which has the properties of negative feed-back, operates as an automatic volume control to keep afferent excitation within normal bounds and to prevent the activity of one cortical system from overpowering the rest. In contrast to all the other cortical suppressor areas, however, the anterior limbic area is, in addition, the main motor outflow of its own system—the autonomic. It is thus perhaps not surprising that its removal should cause a profound change in cerebral function which is manifested as an alteration of personality. Papez (15) has long contended that "the hypothalamus, the anterior thalamic nuclei, the gyrus cinguli, the hippocampus and their interconnections constitute a harmonious mechanism which may elaborate the functions of central emotion as well as participate in emotional expression." Although portions of this circuit are now known to exist, it is probable that the phenomenon of emotion is mediated over far more complex circuits.

Area 24 in man

Little is known of this area in man. The cytoarchitecture of this region shows a remarkable constancy from mouse to man and the same may hold for its connections. The only evidence of these connections in man suggests it to be the cortical field of the anteromedial nucleus of the thalamus (14). It is not known that this region is either a powerful suppressor area or that it is the main cortical autonomic effector region in man.

However, there is some circumstantial evidence that it is concerned with mental processes. It is well known that tumors in the region of the corpus callosum often produce mental symptoms, and

Ironside and Guttmacher (8) noted that mental signs were more prominent with tumors of the anterior callosum. In the vast majority of these cases the anterior limbic area was partially or completely destroyed. It is now definite that mental symptoms are not due to interruption of the corpus callosum since they are absent following its surgical section (1) and congenital defects of the callosum in man are present without mental impairment (13). Thus changes in personality in such patients may well be due to damage to area 24. Furthermore, Vonderahe (19) has described one patient in which destruction of the gyrus cinguli was followed by total lack of affect with development of indifference and finally complete apathy.

The question arises as to whether this area or its projections may be injured by the operation of frontal lobotomy which is currently widely used in the treatment of many psychoses. Although anatomicopathological reports are scanty, it is probable that the cingulum or other projections of area 24 are only infrequently destroyed (12). However, Freeman and Watts (6) have noted that, during section of the white matter in the frontal lobe, flattening and disorientation do not occur until certain stab incisions are made in the depths of the quadrantic sweeping incisions. In some cases it seemed as though a relatively small bundle of fibers was preserving the patient's contact with reality. When this was sectioned, the patient drifted off into confusion and unresponsiveness. As nearly as they could tell, the bundle was close to the midline at about the level of the genu of the corpus callosum. The fasciculus cinguli lies in this location.

It is obviously of great importance to know more of the function of the anterior limbic area in man. Because of the dramatic results of anterior cingulate gyrectomy in the monkey, the fibers entering and leaving the anterior limbic area have been sectioned in one patient which may be briefly mentioned at this time. This was a girl, about 25 years old, who for nine years had been institutionalized with the diagnosis of hebephrenic schizophrenia. She had deteriorated so far as to be mute or to answer at random, never responded with any signs of feeling and talked in a monotone. Her actions were stereotyped and there were frequent outbursts of ill-directed activity. Under general anesthesia, bilateral trepanations were made in the coronal suture, leaving a bridge of bone 1 cm. wide over the longitudinal sinus in the midline. Through vertical holes which permitted direct vision down to the artery that lies in the bottom of the cingulate sulcus, the white matter underlying area 24 was bilaterally sectioned in a parasaggital plane, thus completely undermining the anterior limbic area. After operation the patient slept and could not be fully roused for 62 hours. She remained apathetic for about a week. By the end of this time she would smile at me and respond appropriately to simple questions. On return to the psychiatric ward, she drifted back toward her original state but remained more manageable. To make certain that the patient could not be further helped, the usual type of bilateral frontal lobotomy was then performed. Upon recovering from the anesthetic, she was as before operation. I can only conclude that lobotomy does no more for such a case than section of the connections of area 24.

From the removal of area 24 in monkeys, one would expect greatest improvement not in schizophrenics, but in those anankastic cases whose obsessions or compulsions are charged with fear somehow referable to their fellows. They are too busy with these anxious preoccupations to attend and adjust to the world about them. One has only a certain number of cells and connections in his brain. And Wiener (22) has already pointed out that this sort of trouble increases disproportionately with increase in size of brain. In his words:

"The human brain is one of the largest of all, and of the large brains it has by far the thickest cortex. Now if we double the size of a brain keeping all gross tissues in proportion, we shall multiply the number of cells by 8 and the number of connecting fibers only by 4 since their length is also doubled. In other words, we have a relative deficiency of direct remote connectors between different parts of the brain, and if we have effective connections at all, it is at the cost of a larger number of intermediate stages.

"Thus the crowding problem of the brain is of importance, very much as the traffic problem is of importance in every large city. Combined with the absence of a complete clearing process, we see that concomitant mental processes in the same brain are likely to compete for internuncial space and memory space and that this competition is likely to increase the traffic-jam still more. It may be in the future that we can do something better with situations where circulating memories have led to bad traffic jams than to destroy a part of the connections of the brain by a frontal lobotomy or to intervene brutally in all synaptic connections by one or the other varieties of shock therapy."

The only conclusion I would draw is that at present the best we can do is to limit our destruction to the fewest streams of traffic which will relieve the jam.

DISCUSSION

Dr. John F. Fulton (New Haven, Conn.): One of the purposes of this meeting has been to find out more concerning functional localization in the frontal lobe and more particularly

THE FRONTAL LOBES

with regard to the operation of frontal lobotomy. It is clearly suggestive. Dr. Ward just pointed out that this profound change in behavior occurs when a lesion is limited to the cingular gyrus, and I am hoping that Dr. Freeman and others will comment on the possibility which Dr. Ward has just mentioned, that perhaps the major results seen following the larger operation are due to encroaching upon this part of the rhinencephalon.

DR. WALTER FREEMAN (Washington, D. C.): Dr. Ward, I have a specimen here in which an operation was performed from above and destroyed the anterior cingulate area as well as the superior frontal convolution, done by a different surgeon after we had failed in an original operation. That was ten years ago, and the patient spent most of those ten years in an institution. He was utterly fearless and completely indifferent to the social obligations that were required of him. We have intentionally aimed at this particular area, and have, for the most part, seen nothing comparable to what Dr. Ward has told us about.

Our other experience in regard to the limbic lobe was an instance in which the anterior cerebral artery was lacerated on one side, leading to massive thrombosis and infarction on the whole inner aspect of one hemisphere. This patient, who was also operated on nearly ten years ago, was completely helpless and paralyzed and ate enormously. At one sitting she consumed 4000 calories of food, and followed it by three-quarters of a pound (excuse my mixing of the apothecary and the metric system, but that is what the nurse said) of chocolate candy, vomited, and was ready to start again.

We tried in a couple of pain cases to interrupt the distressing visceral sensations by means of an operation aimed strictly at the anterior cingulate area, and failed.

Actually, our present ideas on this subject are that we can't demonstrate any definite effects from this particular localized operation, and the effects that we have seen from it have been mostly disagreeable.

PRESIDENT FULTON: I don't think the patient whom Dr. Freeman has just mentioned in which the anterior cerebral artery got loose could be used as a real argument against the point of view which Dr. Ward has adopted, but the case does emphasize that the region is difficult to get at surgically, and unless some simple means of isolated destruction of the area is devised, it will be something of a surgical problem, but I have intimate confidence in the ingenuity of our neurological colleagues when it comes to making localized lesions of this character.

DR. FRED A. METTLER (New York, N. Y.): The only question I had was, was Dr. Ward careful to preserve the venous drainage to the superior sagittal sinus of these cases?

DR. WARREN S. McCULLOCH (Chicago, Ill.): I would be grateful if you would contrast the effects of stimulation of 24 with that of any of the other suppressor areas.

DR. ARTHUR A. WARD, JR. (Seattle, Wash.) [Closing discussion]: In answer to Dr. Mettler's question, an occasional small vein to the longitudinal sinus had to be clipped in the monkey experiments. Histological studies demonstrated a minimal amount of superficial damage at the edge of the hemisphere due to retraction, but no damage to the cortex of the lateral surface. Of course, in the human cases, the veins to the sinus were not interfered with as the approach was transcortical and lateral to the sinus.

To answer Dr. McCulloch's question, area 24 has two functions. It is the main autonomic effector region and also is a powerful suppressor region. In what way is it different from the other suppressor regions of the cortex? You all remember that the cortical suppressor areas of the lateral surface of the hemisphere are all so distributed that each is associated with a major functional subdivision of the cortex. Thus area 8 is associated with the associative activity of the frontal pole, area 4-s with the motor system, area 2 with somesthesia and area 19 with vision. In a similar manner area 24 is associated with the limbic lobe.

CINGULATE AND PERSONALITY

In contrast to all the other cortical suppressor areas, however, this area 24 is not only the suppressor area for its own system, but it is also that system's main motor outflow—namely, the autonomic. So, therefore, it is perhaps not surprising that ablation of such an area which has two such powerful functions localized in the same place should cause fairly marked changes in the general activity of the brain.

In response to Dr. Freeman's comments, I was very interested to hear of his experience with lesions in this vicinity. In the two cases which he just described, massive lesions were present and for that reason I think that no clear conclusions can be drawn. Furthermore, I I do not believe we can say anything definite about the function of this área in the human until it is studied by careful, direct stimulation and also by observing the effects of minute lesions confined to area 24 alone.

PRESIDENT FULTON: Is it not also true, Dr. Ward, that area 24 projects directly to the supra-optic nuclei?

DR. WARD: There is no evidence on that.

REFERENCES

1. AKELAITIS, A. J. E. *Amer. J. Psychiat.*, 1941, *97:* 1147–1157.
2. BAILEY, P., BONIN, G. VON, DAVIS, E. W., GAROL, H. W., McCULLOCH, W. S., ROSEMAN, E. AND SILVEIRA, A. *J. Neurophysiol.*, 1944, *7:* 51–56.
3. BAILEY, P. *Res Publ. Ass. nerv. ment. Dis.*, 1948, *27:* 67–83.
4. BONIN, G. VON. *Res. Publ. Ass. nerv. ment. Dis.*, 1948, *27:* 84–94.
5. CLARK, W. E. LE GROS AND BOGGON, R. H. *J. Anat., Lond.*, 1933, *67:* 216–226.
6. FREEMAN, W. AND WATTS, J. W. *Ann. Rev. Physiol.*, 1944, *6:* 517–542.
7. GLEES, P. *J. Anat., Lond.*, 1944, *78:* 47–51.
8. IRONSIDE, R. AND GUTTMACHER, M. *Brain*, 1929, *52:* 442–483.
9. McCULLOCH, W. S. Pp. 212–242 in *The precentral motor cortex*. P. C. Bucy, ed. University of Illinois Press, 1944.
10. McCULLOCH, W. S., WARD, A. A. Jr., AND MAGOUN, H. W. Unpublished observations.
11. MAGOUN, H. W. AND RHINES, R. *J. Neurophysiol.*, 1946, *9:* 165–171.
12. MEYER, A. AND BECK, E. *J. ment. Sci.*, 1945, *91:* 411–425.
13. MINGAZZINI, G. *Der Balken: Eine Anatomische, Physio-pathologische und Klinische Studie.* Berlin, J. Springer, 1922.
14. NORMAN, R. M. *J. Neurol. Neurosurg., Psychiat.*, 1945, *8:* 52–56.
15. PAPEZ, J. W. *Arch. Neurol. Psychiat., Chicago*, 1937, *38:* 725–743.
16. ROSE, J. E., WOOLSEY, C. N., AND JARCHO, L. W. *Fed. Proc.*, 1947, *6:* 193.
17. SMITH, W. K. *Fed Proc.*, 1944, *3:* 42.
18. SMITH, W. K. *J. Neurophysiol.*, 1945, *8:* 241–255.
19. VONDERAHE, A. R. *Ohio State med. J.*, 1943, *39:* 325–330.
20. WARD, A. A. JR., PEDEN, J. K., AND SUGAR, O. *J. Neurophysiol.*, 1946, *9:* 453–462.
21. WARD, A. A. JR. *J. Neurophysiol.*, 1948, *11:* 13–23.
22. WIENER, N. Time, communication and the nervous system. [In preparation]

From G. Rylander (1948). Proceedings of the Association for Research in Nervous and Mental Disease, *27*, 691-705, *by kind permission of Raven Press, New York*

PERSONALITY ANALYSIS BEFORE AND AFTER FRONTAL LOBOTOMY

GÖSTA RYLANDER, M.D.

TO START with, I want to thank you for the great honor you have shown me by the invitation to address this meeting. I think I should tell you in advance that my series of lobotomized cases is not large. It consists of only 32 patients: melancholics, schizophrenics, obsessives and some psychopaths. The number of my cases suitable for closer psychiatric studies before and after the operation is still smaller, amounting to only one-fourth of the series.

The therapeutic effects of lobotomy on the symptoms from which my patients have suffered are quite in accordance with the findings of other authors. The psychotics have improved, some of them very much. Of the eight nonpsychotics, seven have been released from their compulsive phenomena totally or partially and their hypersensitiveness and anxiety have disappeared. One patient with phantom limb pains did not improve. I shall pass over all the details of their recovery—as well as the histories of the patients—with a few exceptions.

That lobotomy lessens the symptoms of certain mental diseases is beyond any doubt. But is anything of the original personality destroyed; at the same time, do any nondesirable mental changes occur after the operation? That is a question of paramount importance both from a theoretical and practical point of view. I shall limit my discussion to this difficult subject. It has interested me ever since I took up the problem of frontal lobotomy as a consequence of my earlier studies of excisions of cerebral tissue, and Freeman and Watts' painstaking investigation was the initial stimulus to my work with the psychic sequels of lobotomy.

That personality changes follow lobotomy is well known, but what are those changes in detail? And is there any intellectual deterioration after lobotomy? Very little is known about these questions. It has been shown by considerable evidence that excisions of parts of the frontal lobes cause special emotional and intellectual changes. Is is possible, then, to cut many thousands of the pathways to and from the frontal lobes without provoking similar changes? That emotional changes of the frontal lobe type do occur goes without saying. In fact, the operation is performed in order to change the depressed, introverted self-occupied patients into slightly euphoric, extroverted, easygoing persons.

Most authors agree that emotional phenomena are the main factors that cause the alteration of the patient's behavior, but opinions differ very much as to the amount of alteration. Some investigators claim that the behavior changes are slight. The pattern of the original personality is not much altered, as an American

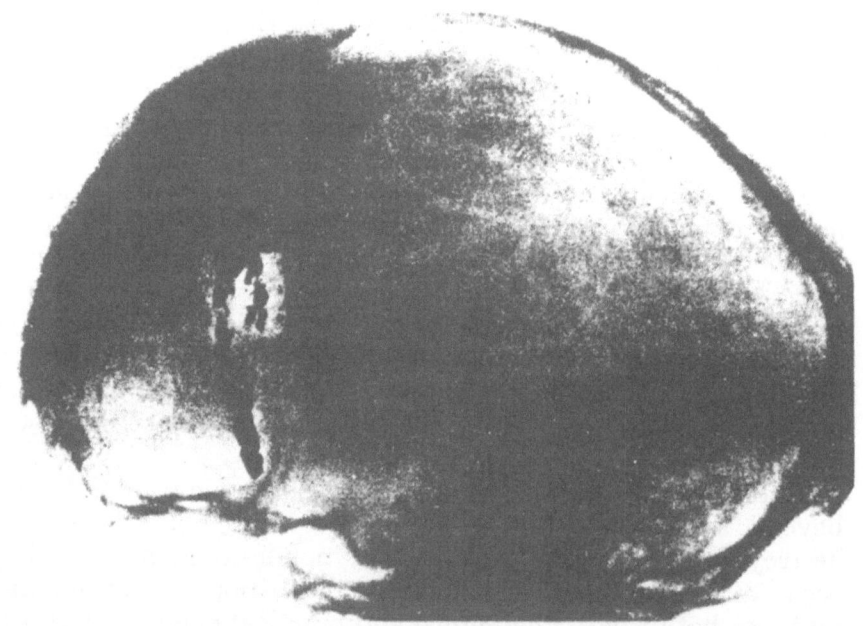

Fig. 199. X-ray showing line of lobotomy incision.

psychologist recently asserted. But others—and I belong to that group—consider the changes rather grave.

The disagreement is still greater concerning the intellectual sequels of lobotomy. Most authors declare that they have found no intellectual deterioration. Cases have also been published which show better results in intelligence tests after lobotomy than before. Isn't that a rather marvelous result of a mutilating brain operation! Of course it cannot depend on a real increase in intelligence. Non-intellectual factors—to use a concept of Wechsler—factors which have disturbed the testing, have been reduced by the operation.

The pioneers in this field, Freeman and Watts, stated in *Psychosurgery* (9) that there was no impairment of intelligence in 50 patients—most of them tested before and after the operation. Even later Freeman and Watts have indicated that no intellectual deficits are produced, measurable by tests, although some reduction in planning capacity may occur.

The literature indicates that most investigators are of the same opinion: Frank, Strecker, Fleming, McGregor, Eng, Hutton in England, Lyerly and Worchel in the United States. Some others seem to be rather uncertain whether lobotomy is followed by intellectual impairment—for example, Kisker, Carmichael and Cobb. A few observers have found slight intellectual changes. Mary Robinson (36) in a thorough study with the suggestive title, "What price lobotomy," found that what she called prolonged attention or deliberativeness was reduced by the operation. Reitman (35), using the pin-man test, found that lobotomized patients did not describe the meanings of the attitudes but only the position of the figures. Porteus and Kepner (34) found a slight drop in mental age after lobotomy in five of their patients, but in six others a slight gain was noted. They tested their patients a few weeks to several months after the operation. Goldstein (12), with his extensive knowledge of frontal lobe functions, is sure that intellectual deficits occur.

Thus, opinions differ greatly as to the sequels of lobotomy. But this is not astonishing, considering the different abnormalities for which the operation has been used, and the very heterogeneous anatomical results of the cuts in the white matter, as has been shown so dramatically by Alfred Meyer in his recent paper published in *Brain*. In addition, all authors have tested psychotic patients with the exception of Halstead, Carmichael and Bucy (17), who analyzed eight neurotics. They found that what they call biological intelligence is not impaired by lobotomy, but the biological intelligence of these patients was already impaired before the operation, although they were not chronic cases. The impairment index indicated a frontal lobe lesion before the operation.

If a schizophrenic or melancholic person, on the other hand, is examined before operation, the results of the tests usually are greatly lowered by splitting or inhibition, faulty concentration, etc. After the operation, when these handicaps are reduced or removed, the patient can use his intellectual tools to greater advantage. The results may be better than the preoperative ones, even when the intellectual faculties have become impaired. Too little regard has been paid to these facts in most of the studies published hitherto.

Halstead's statement a year ago in the *American Journal of*

Psychiatry (17) still holds good; he says: "Not a single patient has been adequately studied....There has been phenomenal array of case statistics. Unfortunately, the pyramid of unknowns is scarcely a pathway to knowledge."

To my mind, when comparing results of testing on different occasions, it is of outstanding importance to select individuals who are test-reliable, who really can make use of their maximal intellectual capacity when tested. Such persons are rare and like precious stones in the great mass of psychotics, whom we can help but not use for scientific studies of intellectual changes after lobotomy. Certain persons with obsessive ideas are probably the best subjects for comparative preoperative and postoperative

TABLE 24

1. Nurse	35 yrs.	Obsessive-compulsive	I.Q. 134	Postop. Obs. 22 mos.
2. Skilled mechanic	45 yrs.	Obsessive-compulsive	I.Q. 114	Postop. Obs. 27 mos.
3. Housekeeper	39 yrs.	Hysterical psychopath with anxiety periods	I.Q. 110	Postop. Obs. 23 mos.
4. Wife of electrician	28 yrs.	Anxiety periods with compulsive and hysterical fits	I.Q. 118	Postop. Obs. 16 mos.
5. Clerk	49 yrs.	Sensitive psychopath with periods of depression	I.Q. 118	Postop. Obs. 19 mos.
6. Widow of civil servant	51 yrs.	Hypochondriac-paranoid state	—	Postop. Obs. 7 wks.
7. Detonation foreman	58 yrs.	Phantom limb pains	—	Postop. Obs. 12 mos.
8. School teacher	48 yrs.	Hypochondriacal state	I.Q. 105	Postop. Obs. 5 mos.

examinations. They are conscientious, often introspective and highly cooperative.

In Table 24 is given a résumé of my most closely studied, suitable patients. Patient 6 was observed only six weeks after the operation. Cases 7 and 8 I was not able to examine preoperatively.[1] Figure 196 illustrates the type of cut made by Dr. Olof Sjöqvist, the brain surgeon who was my coworker. All the cases have been operated upon with the same technique by Sjöquist, who has followed Freeman and Watts' instructions but using another instrument. Immediately after the cut in all cases lipiodol was injected and Roentgenphotos were taken.

---

[1] I wish to thank Dr. F. Wiesel and Dr. B. Cronholm in Stockholm for permitting me to use their patients for my study.

PERSONALITY ANALYSIS

All of the patients on the list have shown changes in behavior of the well-known type, namely, tactlessness, emotional lability with tendencies to outbursts, extrovertness and slight euphoric traits. I shall pick out some features which seem to me to be more interesting, and then base my statements also on patients of my series other than those in the table.

The wife of Patient 2 says: "Doctor, you have given me a new husband. He isn't the same man." The mother of Patient 4 declares, "She is my daughter but yet a different person. She is with me in body but her soul is in some way lost. Those deep feelings, the

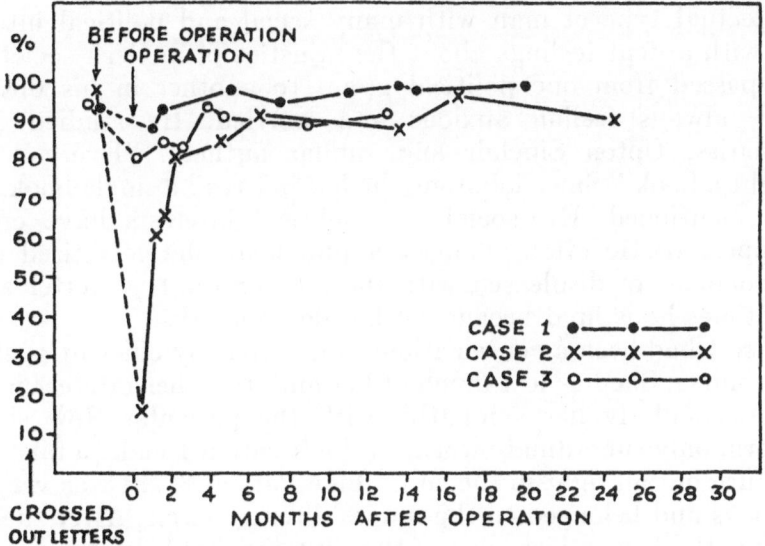

Fig. 200. Bourdon's test. (Crossing out of 202 N's and E's in a text of 224 words.)

tendernesses are gone. She is hard, somehow." The brother, a clergyman, of Patient 3 states that her personality has altered; her interests, her outlook on life, her behavior, are different. "I have lost my husband. I'm alone. I must take over all responsibilities now," says the wife of a schoolteacher. "I'm living now with another person," says the friend of Patient 7. "She is shallow in some way."

The similarity with Hutton's report (22), published in January this year, is striking. The wife of one of Hutton's patients said, "His soul appears to be destroyed."[2] Another observation is that my patients have partially lost the sense of the value of money. They

---

[2] The expression of the relatives, quoted in this paper, should not be identified with the religious idea of soul.

do not waste money on a large scale, but buy things they would not have bought before and are not concerned about the prices. Some of my patients have lost the ability to dream.

The patients themselves behave in the most perfect way at the examinations. They are smiling, polite, answer the questions rapidly and openly, and say that they are very pleased with the results, that everything is all right and that they have not altered. But questioned in detail, they will explain that they forget things and that they have lost many of their interests. The more introspective of them may allege that they are unable to feel as before. They can feel neither real happiness nor deep sorrow. Something has died within them.

The skilled mechanic, Case 2, before the operation was a rather intellectual type of man with many social and political interests, and with ardent feelings about the injustice of modern society. He had passed from one political group to another in his obsessive state, always feeling anxious and worried. He studied Marx, Buchariss, Upton Sinclair and similar authors. "Every week I bought a book." Since lobotomy he has not read a single book of the type mentioned. His social and political interests have entirely disappeared. He often changes employment—he gets tired of the environment or displeased with the boss or wants a better salary; sometimes he is fired because of heedless remarks.

Case 1 had been a conscientious and extremely efficient operating room nurse. She has lost much of her ambition, her interest in work and particularly her sympathy with the patients. Now she can perform only subordinate work. "I don't care if I make a mistake, it will turn out all right in the end." Like Patient 3, she was very fond of books and belonged to the nurses' literary circle. After the operation both of them lost most of their interest in books.

Patient 4 loved classical music. Now she cares only for dance tunes. Earlier she was religiously inclined, attending church now and then, especially when her brother preached. Now she thinks religion is humbug and often teases her brother because of his vocation. She had suffered from periods of anxiety with hysterical outbursts and had tried to commit suicide several times. She was a rather dangerous patient, smashing things and fighting the nurses in her temper tantrums. After lobotomy I engaged her as a cook in my household, thus getting excellent opportunities to study her at work and in daily life. She bought Christmas presents for me and my father, quite above her resources. Originally she was a clever cook, but now she had difficulty in using new recipes and made ridiculous mistakes. But her old cooking methods she usually applied faultlessly. Going out to buy food she might disappear for half a day.

She had met a friend, had coffee with her, and chatted, forgetting time and duties. In her acts and reasoning she often had difficulties in seeing the possibility of more than one solution to a problem. I think she lacked the normal individual's fund of associations.

The clerk, Case 5, was a hypersensitive man who started brooding. and got depressed over trifles. This led him to alcoholism. He suffered from asthma and the specialists could not help him. His sensitiveness disappeared and so did the asthmatic troubles, but he became rather aggressive, developing a slightly paranoid attitude.

Unfortunately there is not time for further details. The rest of the patients on the list show more or less the same symptoms mentioned above. I must now pass on to the test findings. Generally I have done the testing myself, but occasionally a psychologist has taken over the job in order to check the personal factor. Our results have always corresponded. Attention is quickly restored, the curve having reached the pre-operative level after 4–6 months. The curve is probably of logarithmical type, which from the psychological point of view is of interest.

The power of concentration measured in the 100–3 and 100–7 test was generally restored after one month, but for a fairly long time the calculations were done more slowly.

I have examined the rate of intellectual work, using the old Kraepelin addition test. The rate does not quite reach the pre-operative standard (Fig. 201). The curve is of the same type as in the Bourdon test. Memory, tested in different ways, showed no impairment after the lapse of a couple of months. Nevertheless, four or five patients complained of forgetfulness. I shall discuss that contradiction later. A rather striking change was revealed in the word enumeration test. The subject must name as many nouns as possible during three minutes with eyes closed to exclude visual stimulation. A definite and considerable reduction followed the operation (Fig. 203).

Patients start enumerating the words, then suddenly stop, complaining, "My brain becomes a blank, I run completely out of words. I can't think any more." The nurse when tested 20 months after the operation said, "This is the most difficult test you have. I have practiced it many times at home. I know there are masses of words but it is impossible to get at them." Sometimes patients change over too often from one category of nouns to another, sometimes they stick to the same category in absurdum. The availabilities of association seem to be restricted or, according to Thurstone, a diminishing of the fluency factor must have occurred.

Figure 204 shows in detail the course of development during the

256

first seven weeks after the operation. The curves are, on the whole, of the same type as in the figures above. Two remarks ought to be

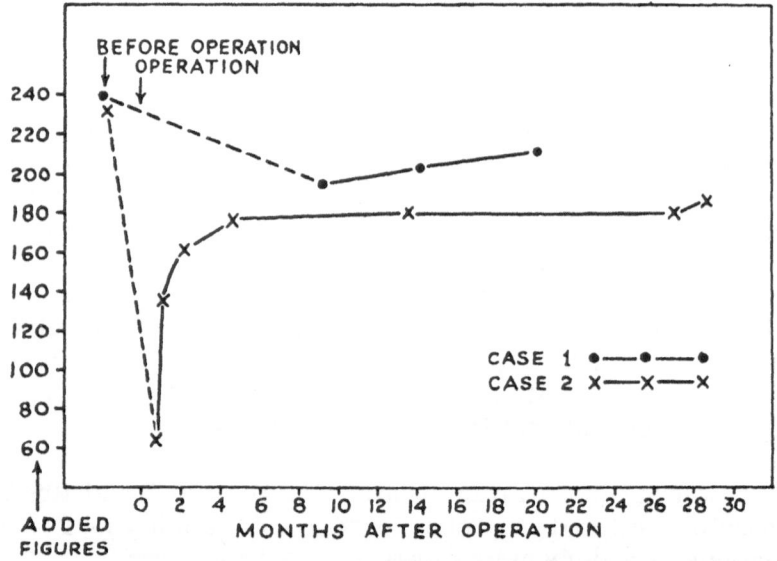

Fig. 201. Kraepelin's test. (Addition of one-place figures in two's for five minutes)

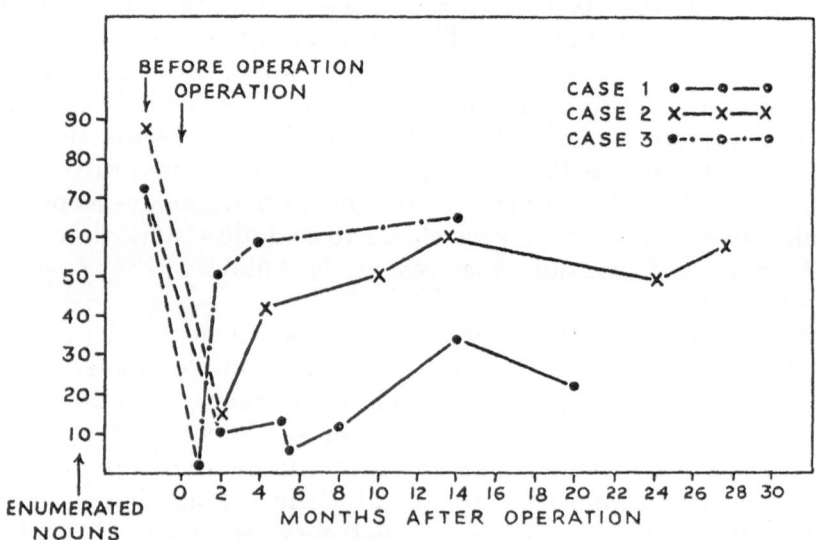

Fig. 202. Enumeration of nouns.

made. The result in Bourdon's test seven days after the operation is lower than the result four days after the operation. The explanation is that on the seventh day the patient (some time before I tested her) had been shown to medical students during a lecture. She became somewhat tired and upset by this, and her scores were lower than they had been several days before. That observation illustrates

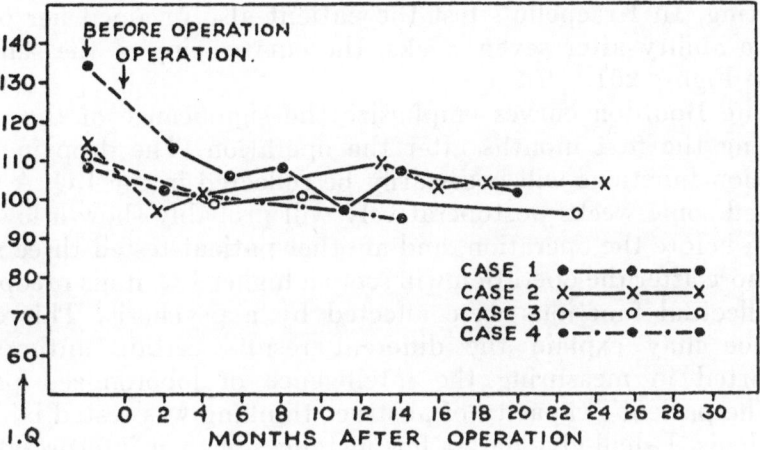

Fig. 203. Intelligence quotients.

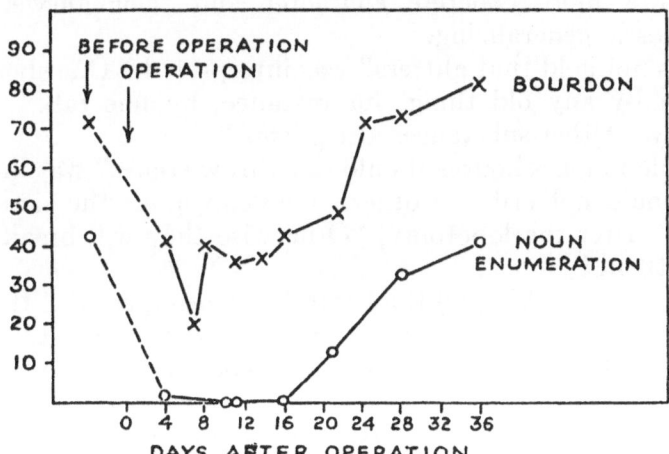

Fig. 204. Results in the Bourdon test and the noun enumeration test during the first five weeks post lobotomy (Case 6).

how sensitive to disturbances are lobotomized patients shortly after operation. The results in experimental psychology must be interpreted with great caution.

The patient's ability to recite words preoperatively was not as good as might have been anticipated from her I.Q. of 105. She was somewhat hampered by her paranoid state and performed the test in a rather unusual way. She started enumerating nouns which began with A, and having gone through as many as she could find, she went on with the letter B, losing time thereby. After the operation she did not follow that pattern and soon regained her preoperative level of reciting. In Kraepelin's test the patient also regained her preoperative ability after seven weeks, the curve being of the same type as in Figure 201.

The Bourdon curves emphasize the significance of the changes during the first months after the operation. The drop in the attention functions will necessarily be reflected in the I.Q. A patient tested some weeks postoperatively will probably show a lower I.Q. than before the operation, and another patient tested three months or more after the operation will score a higher I.Q. if his preoperative intellectual functions were affected by a psychosis. This circumstance may explain the different results certain authors have reported in measuring the intelligence of lobotomized patients.

The patient's capacity of abstract thinking was tested by several methods. I shall give only a few instances of their interpretations of proverbs and fables. After the lobotomy their interpretations acquired a more concrete character and their answers showed difficulties in generalizing.

"All is not gold that glitters" was interpreted, "One should not be taken in by any old thing; for instance, by fine talk." After the lobotomy, "Other substances also glitter."

"People in glass houses should not throw stones" was interpreted, "One should not criticize others. One can make the same mistake oneself." After the lobotomy, "Otherwise they will break the walls around them."

"Too many cooks spoil the broth" was interpreted, "If too many people are working with something it won't be good." After the lobotomy, "If too many people do the cooking, the food will not be so good."

The fables of the Stanford Revision were interpreted in the same concrete way. "The Farmer, His Son and The Donkey" was explained, "One should not act only on the advice of others." After the operation, "They should not both have ridden on the donkey."

The answers I have picked out are typical but extreme. I want to stress particularly that in other cases the interpretations are not as restricted. One of the patients (No. 5) did show very little or no change in his interpretation of fables and proverbs. I do not know why. In his general behavior and judgment, however, there were obvious signs of defects just as in the other patients. The defects in abstract thinking probably have their background in the reduced association power. In Rothman's sorting test the patients showed difficulties in finding the sorting principles. They also showed a tendency to repeat their mistakes.

The intelligence quotients were lowered after the operation. The differences between the preoperative and the postoperative I.Q. were not large, but there was a reduction in every case (Fig. 202). In the fifth case, not seen on the curve, the I.Q. fell from 115 to 107. From Figure 203 it can be noted that two patients were tested seven times. I have used the Stanford Revision and Terman-Merrill, Forms L and M. I have used the same method several times. A training effect must appear, but in spite of that, the curves of the I.Q.'s do not reach the preoperative level.

Detailed analysis reveals that tests which require familiarity with abstract concepts were not answered as well. Certain abstract words were less clearly defined and sometimes confused with words of a similar form. The same unclearness was sometimes observed as regards the definitions of similarities and differences between pairs of abstract words. Tests requiring a high degree of combination ability, e.g., the code test, showed a slight reduction in systematic thinking.

The consequences of lobotomy in some of our patients with high intellectual level have forced us in Stockholm to be very reluctant to operate on nonpsychotic patients. That is why my series of more closely analyzed cases is not large. However, there is no reason to regret the operation on the patients mentioned here. As has already been said, they were, with one exception, released from their severe mental pain. All of them had been crippled by their diseases. The task is to evaluate the suffering of the patient with the sequels of lobotomy as regards his personality.

I know that definite conclusions cannot be drawn from the cases described here. The human brain is constructed in different ways, and some people can mentally endure brain lesions better than others, but my findings are at least a warning that intellectual damage may follow lobotomy. I should like to mention that Dr. Bingley-Wennstroem at Olivecrona's Clinic in Stockholm has found similar changes in five nonpsychotic patients, studied with the same methods. The observation time, however, does not exceed six months. It seems to me somewhat risky to perform lobotomy in patients with periodic psychosis, true melancholia and periodic schizophrenia, as has been proposed recently by certain English and American authors. The periods may disappear in many cases, but the great danger is that something is taken away from the mind of the patient, something that is more valuable than the therapeutic effects of the operation.

Finally, I want to point out that my observations were made on patients operated upon after the technique of Freeman and Watts. Most of the white matter was cut through, as can be seen in Figure 196. I do not know anything of the intellectual sequels of partial lobotomy; no one knows at present. A less extensive operation should be worked out, and several brain surgeons have already tried to accomplish this. Perhaps such an operation could be used in cases of periodic psychosis and obsessive states without any intellectual deficit.

I shall refrain from starting further theories on association phenomena beyond those meager ones already mentioned. I think that in regard to frontal lobe functions skyscrapers of theories have already been built upon a rather unstable foundation of insufficient facts.

DISCUSSION

PRESIDENT FULTON: Dr. Rylander, I don't think I need add anything to this expression of warm appreciation on the part of the Association and its guests. We are very, very happy to have you here, and we thank you for this most stimulating address.

DR. RICHARD M. BRICKNER (New York, N. Y.): Without going into theory, particularly at this point following Dr. Rylander's note of caution, the manner in which he made his observations deserves emphatic comment. The studies were not limited entirely to psychological tests; they included living, working and dealing in every way with his patients. In this way it is possible to get vastly more important information about a patient and about his deficits than it is if you limit your observations entirely to tests. There is a flavor and a knowledge that cannot be derived from tests alone, a point that should be particularly stressed in days when formal tests are getting to dominate the scene more and more.

I want to congratulate Dr. Rylander upon having done his work in this way.

PRESIDENT FULTON: I had rather hoped that Dr. Rylander might tell of still another case of a Salvation Army worker who had certain troubles of a religious nature. The case seems to me of very great significance.

DR. RYLANDER: I think you can do it better than I.

PRESIDENT FULTON: I think you must tell it.

DR. RYLANDER: This patient was a Salvation Army worker, a very high ranking officer. She married a clergyman. For years she lay in the hospital, constantly saying that she had committed sins against the Holy Ghost. She complained of it for weeks and months, and her poor husband did his best to distract her, but without success. Then we decided to operate upon her. Sjöqvist performed the operation in the usual way. She complained of committing a sin. When the operation was finished, she was quite silent. After the dressing had been taken

PERSONALITY ANALYSIS

off, I asked her, "How are you now? What about the Holy Ghost?" Smiling, she answered, "Oh, the Holy Ghost; there is no Holy Ghost." (Laughter)

DR. WALTER FREEMAN (Washington, D. C.): If I understood correctly one of Dr. Rylander's conclusions, it was that something is taken away from the mind of the patient which is more important than the relief afforded. Is that a correct quotation from Dr. Rylander?

DR. RYLANDER: That is right.

DR. FREEMAN: I think that has to be very clearly understood and interpreted, because in the case of the Salvation Army worker who for seven years was in torment because of ruminations on her sins against the Holy Ghost, she could apparently rather easily adjust to the absence of the Holy Ghost.

It is a serious matter. Will Dr. Rylander agree that there is something in the frontal lobe function that determines and prolongs the activity of these useless parasitic ideas which are so distressing and disabling to the patient? This chart that Dr. Rylander didn't have time to throw on the screen shows a reduction at the 28th day in the Bourdon test from the level of 82 to 74 in the level of noun enumeration, which is an awfully good test, from 40 to 34. To me, these are relatively inconsiderable reductions in comparison with the behavior of character-istics and general adaptability of the patients. He has selected as jewels in his jewel casket, one might say, nonpsychotic individuals who have been perplexed and obsessed by painful ideas over long periods of time, and he has shown that there is a reduction in their intelligence quotient from an average, we will say, of 115 down to an average of 104. This does not reflect, it seems to me, the adaptability of the patient in his surroundings, and if he were to test a number of psychotic individuals whose I.Q. was in the neighborhood of 60 or 50 or 40, de-pending upon the disturbance and behavior and inability of a patient to comprehend and to cooperate in the tests, I think he would find that their postoperative I.Q. leveled off about the level of 100 to 105, which means, maybe, that the lobotomy operation is a great leveler of the intellectual capacity.

It seems to me that this capacity has a good deal of significance in connection with these studies. We will grant, I think, that patients who have previously manifested superior abilities in the matter of nursing, mechanics, cooking, Salvation Army work and liberal radical ideas are no longer capable of maintaining the same interest in those features.

We find quite often in our studies that patients who have reached a high level of intellectual achievement are no longer intrigued or interested in those activities. Nevertheless, following operation they are relieved of their harassing doubts, fears and distress and can adjust in the social medium at a better level than they could during the period of their illness. So it seems to me that Dr. Rylander's conclusion that lobotomy takes away something from an individual should be judged in the light of what lobotomy gives back to the individual in relation to his prepsychotic adjustability in his social surroundings.

PRESIDENT FULTON: Thank you, Dr. Freeman.

I think the Chair would like to rise in Dr. Rylander's defense. At least as I understood Dr. Rylander, he merely posed the question of whether the operation did not in certain instances remove something that was more valuable than the therapeutic effect. I don't think it was his conclusion, but he raised the question, as I understood him.

DR. DAVID M. RIOCH (Rockville, Md.): It is interesting that at the present period of social development excision of large parts of patients' brains is socially acceptable. The significance of this social attitude we probably won't know for some time, but while we are engaged in such ablation experiments on humans, I think we are to be congratulated that there are men like Dr. Rylander and Dr. Halstead who are really interested in what happens—in the results—and that we are not completely concerned with the prestige values of percentage "cures."

THE FRONTAL LOBES

These studies, I think, will always be of use and will, I hope, establish landmarks in the field of neurophysiology. I hope, however, that it may not be necessary for us to continue using this type of clinical procedure. We may be able to learn how to let the brain do what it can do, namely, to modify and improve its own form of functioning in terms of appropriate responses from the environment. There are definite indications that such is possible in the work of Dr. John N. Rosen of this city. He has treated functionally over forty consecutive patients, of the category sometimes designated as "backward schizophrenics," with the result of their returning to life as normal as most of us neurotics are. This is genuinely dealing with the function of the brain. We have to stop and consider whether destroying function is really a scientific way of studying function. However, while we are destroying function, I think we are to be congratulated that a few people are exerting extra effort to find out precisely what the results are.

Dr. Roy R. Grinker (Chicago): I should like to voice my appreication for this frank and honest statement of the lobotomy problem. I would like to point out that the observer has not only used laboratory tests and observations on the ward isolated from the patients' real life, but he has also utilized the comments and observations of families and associates of the patients in their real life situations. These procedures may well have been done in this country also, but there seems to be something different in the attitudes of the observers in the real life situations which color their reports. Here, with our extremely materialistic culture, there is an intense wish for rapid and magical recovery from all illness by means of nostrums and operations, and less patience with time-consuming and slowly moving therapies. The public is not so much concerned with the kind of deficit that is expressed by the Swedish families when they state, "After lobotomy he has lost his soul."

It is this simple observation that I think is one of the most valuable that we have heard, for it indicates a great deal of deficit after lobotomy which laboratory tests and examinations in hospital wards completely miss.

Dr. Johannes M. Nielsen (Los Angeles, Cal.): I should like to ask Dr. Rylander to pass on a little epigrammatic statement of the function of the frontal lobe which has seemed to me quite apropos, that from the area 6 backward we have our concepts. That is, that is the part of the brain that we really test in determining the intelligence quotient. This is one kind of knowledge, the ability to gather facts and have them in your brain. Another kind of knowledge is the knowledge of what to do with those facts, and it seems to me that resides in the area anterior to 6. I would like to ask Dr. Rylander what he thinks of that, that there are two kinds of knowledge—one of facts, the other of what to do with facts. The latter is wisdom, and that resides anterior to area 6.

Dr. Gösta Rylander (Stockholm, Sweden) [Closing discussion]: I agree partially with Dr. Freeman. One should choose between the extent of troubles of the patient before lobotomy and balance them against any unpleasant side-effects of the operation. If the patient is crippled by his symptoms and suffers a great deal and is relieved by operation, it doesn't matter if he loses something of his abstract thinking. It seems to me very important to make a thorough analysis of the heredity, personality and environment of the patient—not merely to see him in the reception room and then decide upon operation. In Stockholm we don't operate upon a patient until after at least several weeks' observation in a hospital.

I agree with Dr. Grinker; life itself is the best test, of course. I am rather skeptical of using too much apparatus in test work. The situation seems unfamiliar and artificial to the patients. They feel uneasy and sometimes they approach the type of behavior which Goldstein has called catastrophic reactions. As a consequence, test results may vary and are not reliable.

Dr. Nielsen's question I cannot answer. I dare not go into details concerning the functions of different areas of the frontal lobes. I know too little about those very tangled problems.

PERSONALITY ANALYSIS

REFERENCES

1. ACKERLY, S. *Amer. J. Psychiat.*, 1935, *92:* 717–792.
2. BERLINER, F., MAYER-GROSS, W., *et al. Lancet*, 1945, *2:* 325–328.
3. COBB, S. *Borderland of psychiatry.* Harvard University Press, 1943.
4. DAX, E. C. AND RADLEY SMITH, E. *J. J. ment. Sci.*, 1943, *89:* 182–185.
5. FALCON, J. *Ann. méd.-psychol.*, 1946, *104:* 301–305.
6. FRANK, J. *Proc. R. Soc. Med.*, 1945, *38:* 317–320.
7. FRANK, J. *J. ment. Sci.*, 1946, *92:* 497–508.
8. FREEMAN, W. AND WATTS, J. W. *Amer. J. med. Sci.*, 1946, *211:* 1–8.
9. FREEMAN, W. AND WATTS, J. W. *Psychosurgery.* Springfield, Ill., Charles C Thomas, 1942.
10. FREEMAN, W. AND WATTS, J. W. *J. ment. Sci.*, 1944, *90:* 532–537.
11. FULTON, J. F. *Physiology of the nervous system.* Oxford University Press, 1938.
12. GOLDSTEIN, K. *J. Psychol.*, *Provincetown*, 1944, *17:* 187–208.
13. GOLDSTEIN, K. AND SCHEERER, M. *Psychol. Monogr.*, 1945, *53:* 1–149.
14. GOLLA, F. *J. ment. Sci.*, 1943, *89:* 189–191.
15. HALSTEAD, W. C. *Amer. J. Psychiat.*, 1940, *96:* 1263–1291.
16. HALSTEAD, W. C. *Arch. Neurol. Psychiat.*, *Chicago*, 1940, *44:* 1140–1142.
17. HALSTEAD, W. C., CARMICHAEL, H. T., AND BUCY, P. C. *Amer. J. Psychiat.*, 1946, *103:* 217–228.
18. HANFMANN, E. AND KASANIN, J. *J. Psychol.*, *Provincetown*, 1937, *3:* 521.
19. HOFSTATTER, L., SMOLIK, E. A., AND BUSCH, A. K. *Arch. Neurol. Psychiat.*, *Chicago*, 1945, *53:* 125–130.
20. HUTTON, E. L. *J. ment. Sci.*, 1942, *88:* 275–281.
21. HUTTON, E. L. *J. ment. Sci.*, 1945, *91:* 153–165.
22. HUTTON, E. L. *J. ment. Sci.*, 1947, *93:* 31–42.
23. HUTTON, E. L. *J. ment. Sci.*, 1947, *93:* 333–341.
24. HUTTON, E. L., FLEMING, G. W. T. H., AND FOX, F. E. *Lancet*, 1941, *2:* 3–7.
25. KISKER, G. W. *Psychosom. Med.*, 1944, *6:* 146–150.
26. KISKER, G. W. *Arch. Neurol. Psychiat.*, *Chicago*, 1945, *50:* 691–696.
27. KISKER, G. W. *Ohio St. med. J.*, 1943, *39:* 913–916.
28. KISKER, G. W. *Amer. J. Psychiat.*, 1943, *100:* 180–184.
29. KISKER, G. W. *Psychiat. Quart.*, 1944, *18:* 43–52.
30. MACGREGOR, J. S. AND CRUMBIE, J. R. *J. ment. Sci.*, 1942, *88:* 534–540.
31. MEYER, A. AND BECK, E. *J. ment. Sci.*, 1945, *91:* 411–425.
31a. MEYER, A., BECK, E., AND MCLARDY, T. *Brain*, 1947, *70:* 18–49.
32. PARKER, C. S. *J. ment. Sci.*, 1946, *92:* 719–733.
33. PETERSEN, M. C. AND BUCHSTEIN, H. F. *Amer. J. Psychiat.*, 1942, *99:* 426–430.
34. PORTEUS, S. D. AND KEPNER, R. D. *Genet. Psychol. Monogr.*, 1944, *29:* 3–115.
35. REITMAN, F. *J. ment. Sci.*, 1947, *93:* 55–61.
36. ROBINSON, M. *J. abnorm. (soc.) Psychol.*, 1946, *41:* 421–434.
37. RYLANDER, G. *Acta psychiat.*, *Kbh.*, 1939, *Suppl. 30:* 3–327.
38. RYLANDER, G. *Acta psychiat.*, *Kbh.*, 1943, *Suppl. 25:* 5–81.
39. RYLANDER, G. AND SJÖQVIST, O. *Nord. Med.*, 1946, *29:* 557–602.
40. STRECKER, E. A., PALMER, H. D., AND GRANT, F. C. *Amer. J. Psychiat.*, 1942, *98:* 524–532.

From K. Goldstein (1952). Psychiatry, *15*, 245-260, *by kind permission of the William Alanson White Psychiatric Foundation*

The Effect of Brain Damage on the Personality[†]

Kurt Goldstein[*]

WHEN I WAS ASKED to speak before the Psychoanalytic Association about the changes of the personality in brain damage, I was somewhat hesitant because I was not quite sure that I would be able to make myself understood by an audience which thinks mainly in such different categories and speaks in such a different terminology from my own. I finally accepted the invitation, because I thought that members of the Association apparently wanted to hear what I think and because it brought me the opportunity to express an old idea of mine—the idea that it is faulty in principle to try to make a distinction between so-called organic and functional diseases, as far as symptomatology and therapy are concerned.[1] In both conditions, one is dealing with abnormal functioning of the same psychophysical apparatus and with the attempts of the organism to come to terms with that. If the disturbances—whether they are due to damage to the brain or to psychological conflicts—do not disappear spontaneously or cannot be eliminated by therapy, the organism has to make a new adjustment to life in spite of them. Our task is to help the patients in this adjustment by physical and psychological means; the procedure and goal of the therapy in both conditions is, in principle, the same.

This was the basic idea which induced a group of neurologists, psychiatrists, and psychotherapists—including myself—many years ago, in 1927, to organize the Internationale Gesellschaft für Psychotherapie in Germany and to invite all physicians interested in psychotherapy to meet at the First Congress of the Society. Psychotherapists of all different schools responded to our invitation, and the result of the discussions was surprisingly fruitful. At the second meeting in 1927, I spoke about the relation between psychoanalysis and biology.[2] During the last twenty years, in which I have occupied myself intensively with psychotherapy, I have become more and more aware of the similarity of the phenomena of organic and psychogenic conditions.

It is not my intention to consider the similarities in this paper. I want to restrict myself to the description of the symptomatology and the interpretation of the behavior changes in patients with damage to the brain cortex, particularly in respect to their personality, and would like to leave it to you to make comparisons.

The symptomatology which these patients present is very complex.[3] It is the effect of various factors of which the change of personality is only one. Therefore, when we want to characterize the

[2] K. Goldstein, "Die Beziehungen der Psychoanalyse zur Biologie"; in *Verhandlungen d. Congresses für Psychotherapie in Nauheim;* Leipzig, Hirzel, 1927.

[3] See K. Goldstein, *Aftereffects of Brain Injuries in War;* New York, Grune & Stratton, 1942.

[*] M.D. Univ. of Breslau, Germany 03; Prof. of Neurol. & Psychiat., Med. School, Univ. of Frankfurt am Main; Director, Neurol. Inst., Frankfort am Main 14-30; Director, Hosp. for Brain-Injured Soldiers 19-30; Rockefeller Rsc. Fellow (in Holland) 33-34; New York Med. License 36; Chief, Neurophysiol. Lab., and Attend. Neurologist, Montefiore Hosp., New York City 36-40; Clin. Prof. of Neurol. & Psychiat., Columbia Univ. 36-40; Lecturer in Psychopathol., Harvard Univ. 38; Clin. Prof. of Neurol., Tufts Med. College, Boston 40-45; Director, Neurol. Lab., Boston Dispens. 40-45; Visiting Prof. in Psychol., City College, New York City 45-. Member, Amer. Neurol. Soc.; fellow, Amer. Psychiatric Assn.; member, Assn. for Rsc. in Nerv. & Mental Disease of the Eastern Psychol. Assn.; fellow, New York Acad. of Sci.; diplomate, Amer. Board of Neurol. & Psychiat.; co-editor, *Journal of Nervous and Mental Disease.* For bibliography, see Reference Lists section of this issue.

[†] This paper was presented, by invitation, at the Annual Meeting of the American Psychoanalytic Association, Atlantic City, May 1952.

[1] See K. Goldstein, "Ueber die gleichartige functionelle Bedingtheit der Symptome in organischen und psychischen Krankheiten," *Monatschr. f. Psychiat. u. Neurol.* (1924) 57:191.

change of personality, we have to separate it from the symptoms due to other factors: (1) from those which are the effect of *disturbance of inborn or learned patterns* of performances in special performance fields—such as motor and sensory patterns; (2) from those which are the *expression of the so-called catastrophic conditions;* and (3) from those which are the *expression of the protective mechanisms* which originate from the attempt of the organism to avoid catastrophies.

In order to avoid terminological misunderstandings, I want to state what I mean by personality: Personality shows itself in behavior. Personality is the mode of behavior of a person in terms of the capacities of human beings in general and in the specific appearance of these capacities in a particular person. Behavior is always an entity and concerns the whole personality. Only abstractively can we separate behavior into parts—as for instance, bodily processes, conscious phenomena, states of feelings, attitudes, and so on.[4]

According to my observation, all the phenomena of behavior become understandable if one assumes that all the behavior of the organism is determined by one trend,[5] the *trend to actualize itself*—that is, its nature and all its capacities. This takes place normally in such harmony that the realization of all capacities in the best way possible in the particular environment is permitted. The capacities are experienced by a person as various *needs* which he is driven to fulfill with the cooperation of some parts of the environment and in spite of the hindrance by other parts of it.

Each stimulation brings about some disorder in the organism. But after a certain time—which is determined by the particular performance—the organism comes back, by a process of *equalization*, to its normal condition. This process guarantees the constancy of the organism.

A person's specific personality corresponds to this constancy. Because realization has to take place in terms of different needs and different tasks, the behavior of the organism is soon directed more by one than by another need. This does not mean that organismic behavior is determined by separate needs or drives. All such concepts need the assumption of a controlling agency. I have tried to show in my book, *The Organism*, that the different agencies which have been assumed for this purpose have only made for new difficulties in the attempt to understand organismic behavior; they are not necessary if one gives up the concept of separate drives, as my theory of the organism does. All of a person's capacities are always in action in each of his activities. The capacity that is particularly important for the task is in the foreground; the others are in the background. All of these capacities are organized in a way which facilitates the self-realization of the total organism in the particular situation. For each performance there is a definite figure-ground organization of capacities; the change in the behavior of a patient corresponds to the change in the total organism in the form of an alteration of the normal pattern of figure-ground organization.[6]

Among patients with brain damage we can distinguish between alterations which occur when an area belonging to a special performance field—such as a motor or sensory area—is damaged somewhat isolatedly, and alterations which occur when the personality organization itself is altered. In lesions of these areas—according to a dedifferentiation of the function of the brain cortex[7]—qualities and patterns of behavior (both those developing as a result of maturation and those acquired by learning) are disturbed. Indeed, these patterns never occur isolatedly. They are always embedded in that kind of behavior which we call personality. The personality structure is disturbed particularly by lesions of the frontal lobes, the parietal lobes, and the

[4] See K. Goldstein, *The Organism: A Holistic Approach to Biology;* New York, Amer. Book Co., 1939; pp. 310 ff.
[5] See K. Goldstein, *Human Nature in the Light of Psychopathology;* Cambridge, Harvard Univ. Press, 1940; p. 194.
[6] Reference footnote 4; p. 109.
[7] Reference footnote 4; p. 131.

insula Reili; but it is also disturbed by diffuse damage to the cortex—for instance, in paralysis, alcoholism, and trauma, and in metabolic disturbances such as hypoglycemia. The effect of diffuse damage is understandable when we consider that what we call personality structure apparently is not related to a definite locality of the cortex [8] but to a particular complex function of the brain which is the same for all its parts. This function can be damaged especially by lesions in any of the areas I have mentioned. The damage of the patterns certainly modifies the personality too. Although for full understanding of the personality changes, we should discuss the organization of the patterns and their destruction in damaged patients, that would carry us too far and is not absolutely necessary for our discussion. I shall therefore restrict my presentation to consideration of the symptoms due to damage of the personality structure itself. [9]

There would be no better way of getting to the heart of the problem than by demonstrating a patient. Unfortunately I have to substitute for this a description of the behavior of patients with severe damage of the brain cortex. Let us consider a man with an extensive lesion of the frontal lobes. [10] His customary way of living does not seem to be very much disturbed. He is a little slow; his face is rather immobile, rather rigid; his attention is directed very strictly to what he is doing at the moment—say, writing a letter, or speaking to someone. Confronted with tasks in various fields, he gives seemingly normal responses under certain conditions; but under other conditions he fails completely in tasks that seem to be very similar to those he has performed quite well.

This change of behavior becomes apparent particularly in the following simple test: We place before him a small wooden stick in a definite position, pointing, for example, diagonally from left to right. He is asked to note the position of the stick carefully. After a half minute's exposure, the stick is removed; then it is handed to the patient, and he is asked to put it back in the position in which it was before. He grasps the stick and tries to replace it, but he fumbles; he is all confusion; he looks at the examiner, shakes his head, tries this way and that, plainly uncertain. The upshot is that he cannot place the stick in the required position. He is likewise unable to imitate other simple figures built of sticks. Next we show the patient a little house made of many sticks—a house with a roof, a door, a window, and a chimney. After we remove it, we ask the patient to reproduce the model. He succeeds very well.

IMPAIRMENT OF ABSTRACT CAPACITY

If we ask ourselves what is the cause of the difference in his behavior in the two tasks, we can at once exclude defects in the field of perception, action, and memory. For there is no doubt that copying the house with many details demands a much greater capacity in all these faculties, especially in memory, than putting a single stick into a position which the patient has been shown shortly before. A further experiment clarifies the situation. We put before the patient two sticks placed together so as to form an angle with the opening pointing upward (V). The patient is unable to reproduce this model. Then we confront him with the same angle, the opening downward this time (Λ), and now he reproduces the figure very well on the first trial. When we ask the patient how it is that he can reproduce the second figure but not the first one, he says, "This one has nothing to do with the other one." Pointing to the second one, he says, "That is a roof"; pointing to the first, "That is nothing."

These two replies lead us to an understanding of the patient's behavior. His first reply makes it clear that, to him, the two objects with which he has to deal are totally different from one another. The second answer shows that he appre-

[8] Reference footnote 4; pp. 249 ff.
[9] See K. Goldstein, *Handbuch der normalen und pathologischen Physiologie;* Berlin, J. S. Springer, 1927; vol. 10, pp. 600 ff. and 813.
[10] K. Goldstein, "The Significance of the Frontal Lobes for Mental Performances," *J. Neurol. and Psychopathol.* (1936) 17:27-40; and "The Modifications of Behavior Consequent to Cerebral Lesions," *Psychiatric Quart.* (1936) 10:586.

hends the angle with the opening downward as a concrete object out of his own experience, and he constructs a concrete thing with the two sticks. The two sticks that formed an angle with the opening upward apparently did not arouse an impression of a concrete thing. He had to regard the sticks as representations indicating directions in abstract space. Furthermore, he had to keep these directions in mind and rearrange the sticks from memory as representatives of these abstract directions. To solve the problem he must give an account to himself of relations in space and must act on the basis of abstract ideas. Thus we may conclude that the failure of the patient in the first test lies in the fact that he is unable to perform a task which can be executed only by means of a grasp of the abstract. The test in which the opening of the angle is downwards does not demand this, since the patient is able to grasp it as a concrete object and therefore to execute it perfectly. It is for the same reason that he is able to copy the little house, which seems to us to be so much more complicated. From the result of his behavior in this and similar tasks we come to the assumption that these *patients are impaired in their abstract capacity*.

The term "abstract attitude," which I shall use in describing this capacity, will be more comprehensible in the light of the following explanation.[11] We can distinguish two different kinds of attitudes, the concrete and the abstract. In the concrete attitude we are given over passively and bound to the immediate experience of unique objects or situations. Our thinking and acting are determined by the immediate claims made by the particular aspect of the object or situation. For instance, we act concretely when we enter a room in darkness and push the button for light. If, however, we reflect that by pushing the button we might awaken someone asleep in the room, and desist from pushing the button, then we are acting abstractively. We transcend

[11] See K. Goldstein and M. Scheerer, *Abstract and Concrete Behavior;* Psychol. Monogr. No. 239, 1941.

the immediately given specific aspect of sense impressions; we detach ourselves from these impressions, consider the situation from a conceptual point of view, and react accordingly. Our actions are determined not so much by the objects before us as by the way we think about them: the individual thing becomes a mere accidental representative of a category to which it belongs.

The impairment of the attitude toward the abstract shows in every performance of the brain-damaged patient who is impaired in this capacity. He always fails when the solution of a task presupposes this attitude; he performs well when the appropriate activity is determined directly by the stimuli and when the task can be fulfilled by concrete behavior. He may have no difficulty in using known objects in a situation that requires them; but he is totally at a loss if he is asked to demonstrate the use of such an object outside the concrete situation, and still more so if he is asked to do it without the real object. A few examples will illustrate this:

The patient is asked to blow away a slip of paper. He does this very well. If the paper is taken away and he is asked to think that there is a slip of paper and to blow it away, he is unable to do so. Here the situation is not realistically complete. In order to perform the task the patient would have to imagine the piece of paper there. He is not capable of this.

The patient is asked to throw a ball into open boxes situated respectively at distances of three, nine, and fifteen feet. He does that correctly. When he is asked how far the several boxes are from him, he is not only unable to answer this question but unable even to say which box is nearest to him and which is farthest.

In the first action, the patient has only to deal with objects in a behavioral fashion. It is unnecessary for him to be conscious of this behavior and of objects in a world separated from himself. In the second, however, he must separate himself from objects in the outer world and give himself an account of his actions and of the space relations in the world facing him. Since he is unable to do this, he fails. We could describe this failure also by saying that the patient is unable to deal with a situation which is only possible.

A simple story is read to a patient. He may repeat some single words, but he does not understand their meaning and is unable to grasp the essential point. Now we read him another story, which would seem to a normal person to be more difficult to understand. This time he understands the meaning very well and recounts the chief points. The first story deals with a simple situation, but a situation which has no connection with the actual situation of the patient. The second story recounts a situation he is familiar with. Hence one could say the patient is able to grasp and handle only something which is related to himself.

Such a patient almost always recognizes pictures of single objects, even if the picture contains many details. In pictures which represent a composition of a number of things and persons, he may pick out some details; but he is unable to understand the picture as a whole and is unable to respond to the whole. The patient's real understanding does not depend on the greater or smaller number of components in a picture but on whether the components, whatever their number, hang together concretely and are familiar to him, or whether an understanding of their connection requires a more abstract synthesis on his part. He may lack understanding of a picture even if there are only a few details. If the picture does not reveal its essence directly, by bringing the patient into the situation which it represents, he is not able to understand it. Thus one may characterize the deficiency as an inability to discover the essence of a situation which is not related to his own personality.

Memory and Attention

This change in behavior finds its expression in characteristic changes in memory and attention. Under certain circumstances the faculty for reproduction of facts acquired previously may be about normal. For example, things learned in school may be recalled very well, but only in some situations. The situation must be suited to reawakening old impressions. If the required answer demands an abstract attitude on the part of a patient or if it demands that he give an account of the matter in question, the patient is unable to remember. Therefore he fails in many intelligence tests which may seem very simple for a normal person, and he is amazingly successful in others which appear complicated to us. He is able to learn new facts and to keep them in mind; but he can learn them only in a concrete situation and can reproduce them only in the same situation in which he has learned them. Because the intentional recollection of experiences acquired in infancy requires an abstract attitude toward the situation at that time, the patient is unable to recall infancy experiences in a voluntary way; but we can observe that the aftereffect of such experiences sometimes appears passively in his behavior. Such a patient has the greatest difficulty in associating freely; he cannot assume the attitude of mind to make that possible. He is incapable of recollection when he is asked to recall things which have nothing to do with the given situation. The patient must be able to regard the present situation in such a way that facts from the past belong to it. If this is not the case, he is completely unable to recall facts which he has recalled very well in another situation. Repeated observation in many different situations demonstrates clearly that such memory failures are not caused by an impairment of memory content. The patient has the material in his memory, but he is unable to use it freely; he can use it only in connection with a definite concrete situation.

We arrive at the same result in testing attention. At one time the patient appears inattentive and distracted; at another time, he is attentive, even abnormally so. The patient's attention is usually weak in special examinations, particularly at the beginning before he has become aware of the real approach to the whole situation. In such a situation he ordinarily seems much distracted. If he is able to enter into the situation, however, his attention may be satisfactory; sometimes his reactions are even abnormally keen. Under these circumstances he may be totally untouched by other stimuli from the environment to which normal persons will unfailingly react. In some tests he will always seem distracted; for example, in those situations which demand a change of approach (a choice), he always seems distracted because he is incapable of making a choice. Consequently, it is not correct to speak of a change of attention in these patients in terms of plus or minus. The state of the patient's attention is but part of his total behavior and is to be understood only in connection with it.

Emotional Responses

The same holds true if we observe the emotions of the patients. Usually they are considered emotionally dull and often they appear so, but it would not be correct to say simply that they are suffering from a diminution of emotions. The same patients can be dull under some conditions and very excited under others. This can be explained when we consider the patient's emotional behavior in relation to his entire behavior in a given situation. When he does not react emotionally in an adequate way, investigation reveals that he has not grasped the situation in such a way that emotion could arise. In fact, we might experience a similar lack of emotion through failing to grasp a situation. The patient may have grasped only one part of the situation—the part which can be grasped concretely—and this part may not give any reason for an emotional reaction. The lack of emotion appears to us inappropriate because we grasp with the abstract attitude the whole situation to which the emotional character is attached. This connection between the emotions and the total behavior becomes understandable when we consider that emotions are not simply related to particular experiences but are, as I have

shown on another occasion,[12] inherent aspects of behavior—part and parcel of behavior. No behavior is without emotion and what we call lack of emotion is a deviation from normal emotions corresponding to the deviation of behavior in general. From this point of view, one modification of reactions that is of particular interest in respect to the problem of emotions in general, becomes understandable. Often we see that a patient reacts either not at all or in an *abnormally quick manner*. The latter occurs particularly when the patient believes he has the correct answer to a problem. Although this behavior might seem to be the effect of a change in the time factor of his reactivity, it is rather the *effect of an emotional factor*—that is, it is the modification of his emotional feelings because of the impairment of his ability for abstraction—which in turn modifies the time reaction.

Pleasure and Joy

These patients are always somewhat in danger of being in a catastrophic condition—which I shall discuss later—as a result of not being able to find the right solution to a problem put before them. They are often afraid that they may not be able to react correctly, and that they will be in a catastrophic condition. Therefore, when they believe they have the right answer, they answer as quickly as possible. Because of impairment of abstraction, they are not able to deliberate; they try to do what they can do as quickly as possible because every retardation increases the tension which they experience when they are not able to answer. The quick response is an effect of their *strong necessity to release tension;* they are forced to release tension because they cannot handle it any other way. They cannot bear anything that presupposes deliberation, considering the future, and so on, all of which are related to abstraction.

This difference in behavior between these patients and more normal people

[12] See K. Goldstein, "On Emotions: Considerations from the Organismic Point of View," *J. Psychol.* (1951) 31:37-49.

throws light on the nature of the *trend to release tension.* These patients must, so to speak, follow the "pleasure principle." This phenomenon is one *expression of the abnormal concreteness* which is a counterpart to the impairment of abstraction. The *trend to release tension appears to be an expression of pathology* —the effect of a protective mechanism to prevent catastrophic condition. To normal behavior belong deliberation and retardation; but in addition there is the ability to speed up an activity or a part of it to correspond to the requirements of the task, or at least part of the requirements, so that its performance guarantees self-realization. Sometimes the ability to bear tension and even to enjoy it are also a part of this normal behavior. In contrast, the patients that I am talking about are only able to experience the pleasure of release of tension; they never appear to enjoy anything—a fact which is often clearly revealed by the expression on their faces. This becomes understandable if we consider that immediate reality is transcended in any kind of joy and that joy is a capacity we owe to the abstract attitude, especially that part of it concerned with possibility. Thus brain-injured patients who are impaired in this attitude cannot experience joy. Experience with brain-injured patients teaches us that we have to distinguish between *pleasure by release of tension,* and the active *feeling of enjoyment* and freedom so characteristic of joy. Pleasure through release of tension is the agreeable feeling which we experience on returning to a state of equilibrium after it has been disturbed—the passive feeling of being freed from distress. Pleasure lasts only a short time till a new situation stimulates new activity; we then try to get rid of the tension of the new situation which acts to shorten the span of pleasure. In contrast, we try to extend joy. This explains the different speeds of joy and pleasure. Because of the capacity for joy, we can experience the possibility of the indefinite continuation of a situation. The two emotions of joy and pleasure play essentially different roles in regard to self-realiza-

tion; they belong to different performances or different parts of a performance; they belong to different moods. Pleasure may be a necessary state of respite. But it is a phenomenon of standstill; it is akin to death. It separates us from the world and the other individuals in it; it is equilibrium, quietness. In joy there is disequilibrium. But it is a productive disequilibrium, leading toward fruitful activity and a particular kind of self-realization. This difference in approach between the normal person and the brain-injured patient is mirrored in the essentially different behavior of the latter and the different world in which he lives. The different significance of the two emotional states in his total behavior is related to their time difference.

Edith Jacobson,[13] in the outline of her paper presented to the Psychoanalytic Association, speaks about the speed factor in psychic discharge processes and comes to the conclusion that discharge is not the only process which produces pleasure—that we have to distinguish between different qualities of pleasure in terms of the slow rising and the quick falling of tension. That is very much in accordance with my conclusions derived from experience with brain-injured patients. If one distinguishes two forms of pleasure, one should, for clarity's sake, use different names for them; I think that my use of pleasure and joy fits the two experiences. But I would not like to call them both discharge processes: the one is a discharge process; the other one a very active phenomenon related to the highest form of mental activity—abstraction. From this it becomes clear why they have such an essentially different significance in the totality of performance: the one is an equalization process which prepares the organism for new activity; the other one is an activity of highest value for self-realization. They belong together just as in general equalization process and activity belong together. Therefore

[13] Edith Jacobson, "The Speed Pace in Psychic Discharge Processes and Its Influence on the Pleasure-Unpleasure Qualities of Affects," paper read before the Amer. Psychoanal. Assn., Atlantic City, May, 1952.

they cannot be understood as isolated phenomena.

The Phenomenon of Witticism

From this viewpoint of the emotions of brain-injured patients, the phenomenon of witticism appears in a new aspect. We can see that even though a patient makes witty remarks, he is not able to grasp the character of situations which produce humor in an average normal individual. Whether or not some situation appears humorous depends upon whether it can be grasped in a concrete way which is suited to producing the emotion of humor. In accordance with the impairment of his ability for abstraction, such a patient perceives many humorous pictures in a realistic way, which does not evoke the expected humor. But of course any of us who might at a given time perceive a humorous picture in a realistic way would respond similarly. On the other hand a patient may make a witty remark in relation to a situation which is not considered humorous by us, because he has experienced the situation in another way. Thus we should not speak of witticism as a special characteristic of these patients. It is but one expression of the change in their personality structure in the same way that their inability to understand jokes under other conditions expresses this change. Indeed, these patients are in general dull because of their limited experience, and their witticisms are superficial and shallow in comparison with those of normal people.

Friendship and Love

The drive towards the release of tension, which I have already mentioned, is one of the causes of the strange behavior of these patients in friendship and love situations. They need close relationships to other people and they try to maintain such relationships at all cost; at the same time such relationships are easily terminated suddenly if the bearing of tension is necessary for the maintenance of the relationship.

The following example is illustrative: A patient of mine, Mr. A, was for years a close friend of another patient, Mr. X. One day Mr. X went to a movie with a third man. Mr. X did not take Mr. A along because Mr. A had seen the picture before and did not want to see it a second time. When Mr. X came back, my patient was in a state of great excitement and refused to speak to him. Mr. A could not be quieted by any explanations; he was told that his friend had not meant to offend him, and that the friendship had not changed, but these explanations made no impression. From that time on, Mr. A was the enemy of his old friend, Mr. X. He was only aware that his friend was the companion of another man, and he felt himself slighted. This experience produced a great tension in him. He regarded his friend as the cause of this bad condition and reacted to him in a way that is readily understandable in terms of his inability to bear tension and to put himself in the place of somebody else.

Another patient never seemed to be concerned about his family. He never spoke of his wife or children and was unresponsive when we questioned him about them. When we suggested to him that he should write to his family, he was utterly indifferent. He appeared to lack all feeling in this respect. At times he visited his home in another town, according to an established practice, and stayed there several days. We learned that while he was at home, he conducted himself in the same way that any man would in the bosom of his family. He was kind and affectionate to his wife and children and interested in their affairs insofar as his abilities would permit. Upon his return to the hospital from such a visit, he would smile in an embarrassed way and give evasive answers when he was asked about his family; he seemed utterly estranged from his home situation. Unquestionably the peculiar behavior of this man was not really the effect of deterioration of his character on the emotional and moral side; rather, his behavior was the result of the fact that he could not summon up the home situation when he was not actually there.

Lack of imagination, which is so apparent in this example, makes such patients incapable of experiencing any expectation of the future. This lack is apparent, for instance, in the behavior of a male patient toward a woman whom he later married.[14] When he was with the girl, he seemed to behave in a friendly, affectionate way and to be very fond of the girl. But when he was separated from her, he did not care about her at all; he would not seek her out and certainly did not desire to have a love relationship with her. When he was questioned, his answers indicated that he did not even understand what sexual desire meant. But in addition he had forgotten about the girl. When he met her again and she spoke to him, he was able immediately to enter into the previous relation. He was as affectionate as before. When she induced him to go to bed with her and embraced him, he performed an apparently normal act of sexual intercourse with satisfaction for both. She had the feeling that he loved her. She became pregnant, and they were married.

Change in Language

Of particular significance in these patients is the change in their language because of their lack of abstract attitude.[15] Their words lose the character of meaning. Words are not usable in those situations in which they must represent a concept. Therefore the patients are not able to find the proper words in such situations. Thus, for instance, patients are not able to name concrete objects, since as shown by investigation, naming presupposes an abstract attitude and the abstract use of words. These patients have not lost the sound complex; but they cannot use it as a sign for a concept. On other occasions, the sound complex may be uttered; but it is only used at those times as a simple association to a given object, as a property of the object, such as color and form, and not as representative of a concept. If a patient has been particularly gifted in language before his brain is damaged and has retained many such associations or can acquire associations as a substitute for naming something, then he may utter the right word through association, so that an observer is not able to distinguish between his uttering the sound complex and giving a name to something; only through analysis can one make this distinction.[16] Thus we can easily overlook the patient's defect by arriving at a conclusion only on the basis of this capacity for a positive effect. In the same way we can be deceived by a negative effect which may only be an expression, for instance, of the patient's fear that he will use the wrong word. I have used the term *fallacy of effect* to describe the uncertain and ambiguous character of a conclusion which is based only upon a patient's effective performance. This term applies not only to language but to all performances of the patients. It is the source of one of the most fatal mistakes which can be made in interpretation of phenomena observed in organic patients; incidentally, it is a mistake which can be made also in functional cases.

Frontal Lobotomy

In reference to the fallacy of effect, I want to stress how easily one can be deceived about the mental condition of patients who have undergone frontal lobotomy. The results of the usual intelligence test, evaluated statistically, may not reveal any definite deviation from the norm; yet the patient can have an impairment of abstraction that will become obvious through tests which take into consideration the fallacy of effect.[17] My experience with frontal lobotomy patients and my evaluation of the literature on frontal lobotomy leave no doubt in my mind that at least many of these patients

---

[14] K. Goldstein and J. I. Steinfeld, "The Conditioning of Sexual Behavior by Visual Agnosia," *Bull. Forest Sanit.* (1942) vol. 1, no. 2, pp. 37-45.

[15] See K. Goldstein, *Language and Language Disturbances;* New York, Grune & Stratton, 1948; p. 56.

[16] Reference footnote 15; p. 61.

[17] Thirty years ago we constructed special tests when we were faced with the problem of re-educating brain-injured soldiers. (See K. Goldstein and A. Gelb, "Ueber Farbennamenamnesie," *Psychol. Forsch.* [1924] 6:127.) These tests, which were introduced in America by Scheerer and myself (reference footnote 11), proved to be particularly useful not only for studying the problem of abstraction in patients, but also for the correct organization of treatment.

show impairment of abstract capacity, although perhaps not to such a degree as do patients with gross damage of the brain. Because of the fallacy of effect, which tends to overlook the defect in abstraction, the reports of the relatives that the lobotomized patient behaves well in everyday life are often evaluated incorrectly by the doctor.[18] In the sheltered, simple life that these patients have with their families, the patients are not often confronted with tasks which require abstract reasoning; thus the family is likely to overlook their more subtle deviations from the norm. Sometimes peculiarities of the patient are reported which definitely point to a defect in abstraction, which is more serious than it is often evaluated: for instance, a patient who in general seems to live in a normal way does not have any relationship with even the closest members of his family and manifests no interest in his children; another patient exists in a vacuum so that no friendship is possible with him.

A woman patient after lobotomy still knows how to set a table for guests, and how to act as a perfect hostess. Before lobotomy, she was always a careful housewife, deciding everything down to the last detail; but now she does not care how the house is run, she never enters the kitchen, and the housekeeper does all the managing, even the shopping. She still reads a great number of books, but she does not understand the contents as well as before.

A skilled mechanic, who is still considered an excellent craftsman, is able to work in a routine way; but he has lost the ability to undertake complicated jobs, has stopped studying, and seems to have resigned himself to being a routine worker; apparently all this is an effect of the loss of his capacity for abstraction, which is so necessary for all initiative and for creative endeavor. Thus we see that even when the behavior of the patients appears not to be overtly disturbed, it differs essentially from normal behavior—in the particular way which is characteristic of impairment in abstract attitude. Freeman,[19] who was originally so enthusiastically in favor of the operation, has become more cautious about its damage to the higher mental functions. He writes:

The patients with frontal lobotomy show always some lack of personality depth; impulse, intelligence, temperament are disturbed; the creative capacity undergoes reduction—the spiritual life in general was affected. They are largely indifferent to the opinions and feelings of others.

He apparently discovered the same personality changes in his patients as those which we have described as characteristic of the behavior of patients with impaired capacity for abstraction. Thus we should be very careful in judging personality change following frontal lobotomy. Although I would not deny the usefulness of the operation in some cases, I would like to say, as I have before, that the possibility of an impairment of abstraction should always be taken into consideration before the operation is undertaken.

I would now like to present a survey of the various situations in which the patient is unable to perform. He fails when he has: (1) to assume a mental set voluntarily or to take initiative (for instance, he may even be able to perform well in giving a series of numbers, once someone else has presented the first number, but he cannot begin the activity); (2) to shift voluntarily from one aspect of a situation to another, making a choice; (3) to account to himself for his actions or to verbalize the account; (4) to keep in mind simultaneously various aspects of a situation or to react to two stimuli which do not belong intrinsically together; (5) to grasp the essence of a given whole, or to break up a given whole into parts, isolating the parts voluntarily and combining them into wholes; (6) to abstract common properties, to plan ahead ideationally, to assume an attitude toward a situation which is only possible, and to think or perform symbolically; (7) to do

[18] See K. Goldstein, "Frontal Lobotomy and Impairment of Abstract Attitude," *J. N. and M. Disease* (1949) 110:93-111.

[19] W. Freeman and J. Watts, *Psychosurgery*, second edition; Springfield, Ill., Thomas, 1950.

something which necessitates detaching the ego from the outer word or from inner experiences.

All these and other terms which one may use to describe the behavior of the patients basically mean the same. We speak usually, in brief, of an *impairment of abstract attitude.* I hope that it has become clear that the use of this term does not refer to a theoretical interpretation but to the real behavior of the human being and that it is suitable for describing both normal and pathological personality.

In brief, the patients are changed with respect to the most characteristic properties of the human being. They have lost initiative and the capacity to look forward to something and to make plans and decisions; they lack phantasy and inspiration; their perceptions, thoughts, and ideas are reduced; they have lost the capacity for real contact with others, and they are therefore incapable of real friendship, love, and social relations. One could say they have no real ego and no real world. That they behave in an abnormally concrete way and that they are driven to get rid of tensions are only expressions of the same defect. When such patients are able to complete a task in a concrete way, they may—with regard to the effect of their activity—not appear very abnormal. But closer examination shows that they are abnormally rigid, stereotyped, and compulsive, and abnormally bound to stimuli from without and within.

To avoid any misunderstanding, I would like to stress that the defect in patients with brain damage does not always have to manifest itself in the same way—not even in all frontal lobe lesions. To what degree impairment of abstraction appears depends upon the extensiveness, the intensity, and the nature of the lesion. To evaluate the relationship between a patient's behavior and his defect, we have to consider further that personal experience plays a role in determining whether a patient can solve a problem or not. One patient reacts well—at least at face value—when he is given a task, al-

though another patient has failed the same task; to the first patient the task represents a concrete situation; for the second patient it is an abstract situation. But in both cases, the defect will always be revealed by further examination.

CATASTROPHIC CONDITIONS

Impairment of abstraction is not the only factor which produces deviations in the behavior of patients, as I have stated before. Another very important factor is the occurrence of a catastrophic condition.[20] When a patient is not able to fulfill a task set before him, this condition is a frequent occurrence. A patient may look animated, calm, in a good mood, well-poised, collected, and cooperative when he is confronted with tasks he can fulfill; the same patient may appear dazed, become agitated, change color, start to fumble, become unfriendly, evasive, and even aggressive when he is not able to fulfill the task. His overt behavior appears very much the same as a person in a state of anxiety. I have called the state of the patient in the situation of success, *ordered condition;* the state in the situation of failure, *disordered or catastrophic condition.*

In the catastrophic condition the patient not only is incapable of performing a task which exceeds his impaired capacity, but he also fails, for a longer or shorter period, in performances which he is able to carry out in the ordered state. For a varying period of time, the organism's reactions are in great disorder or are impeded altogether. We are able to study this condition particularly well in these patients, since we can produce it experimentally by demanding from the patient something which we know he will not be able to do, because of his defect. Now, as we have said, impairment of abstraction makes it impossible for a patient to account to himself for his acts. He is quite unable to realize his failure and why he fails. Thus we can assume that catastrophic condition is not a reaction of the patient to failure, but rather belongs intrinsically to the situation of

[20] Reference footnote 4; pp. 35 ff.

the organism in failing. For the normal person, failure in the performance of a nonimportant task would be merely something disagreeable; for the brain-injured person, however, as observation shows, any failure means the impossibility of self-realization and of existence. The occurrence of catastrophic condition is not limited therefore to special tasks; any task can place the patient in this situation, since the patient's self-realization is endangered so easily. Thus the same task produces anxiety at one time, and not at another.

Anxiety

The conditions under which anxiety occurs in brain-injured patients correspond to the conditions for its occurrence in normal people in that what produces anxiety is not the failure itself, but the resultant danger to the person's existence. I would like to add that the danger need not always be real; it is sufficient if the person imagines that the condition is such that he will not be able to realize himself. For instance, a person may be in distress because he is not able to answer questions in an examination. If the outcome of the examination is not particularly important, then the normal person will take it calmly even though he may feel somewhat upset; because it is not a dangerous situation for him, he will face the situation and try to come to terms with it as well as he can by using his wits, and in this way he will bring it to a more or less successful solution. The situation becomes totally different, however, if passing the examination is of great consequence in the person's life; not passing the examination may, for instance, endanger his professional career or the possibility of marrying the person he loves. When self-realization is seriously in danger, catastrophe may occur together with severe anxiety; when this occurs, it is impossible for the person to answer even those questions which, under other circumstances, he could solve without difficulty.

I would like to clarify one point here—namely, that anxiety represents an emo-

tional state which does not refer to any object. Certainly the occurrence of anxiety is connected with an outer or inner event. The organism, shaken by a catastrophic shock, exists in relation to a definitive reality; and the basic phenomenon of anxiety, which is the occurrence of disordered behavior, is understandable only in terms of this relationship to reality. But anxiety does not originate from the experiencing of this relationship. The brain-injured patient could not experience anxiety, if it were necessary for him to experience this relationship to reality. He is certainly not aware of this objective reality; he experiences only the shock, only anxiety. And this, of course holds true for anxiety in general. Observations of many patients confirm the interpretation of anxiety by philosophers, such as Pascal and Kierkegaard, and by psychologists who have dealt with anxiety—namely, that the source of anxiety is the inner experience of not being confronted with anything or of being confronted with nothingness.

In making such a statement, one must distinguish sharply between *anxiety* and *fear*—another emotional state which is very often confused with anxiety.[21] Superficially, fear may have many of the characteristics of anxiety, but intrinsically it is different. In the state of fear we have an object before us, we can meet that object, we can attempt to remove it, or we can flee from it. We are conscious of ourselves, as well as of the object; we can deliberate as to how we shall behave toward it, and we can look at the cause of the fear, which actually lies before us. Anxiety, on the other hand, gets at us from the back, so to speak. The only thing we can do is to attempt to flee from it, but without knowing what direction to take, since we experience it as coming from no particular place. We are dealing, as I have shown explicitly elsewhere, with qualitative differences, with different attitudes toward the world. Fear is related, in our experience, to an

[21] See K. Goldstein, "Zum Problem der Angst," *Allg. ärztl. Ztschr. f. Psychotherap. u. psych. Hygiene* (1929) 2:409-437. Also, reference footnote 4; p. 293.

object; anxiety is not—it is only an inner state.

What is characteristic of the object of fear? Is it something inherent in the object itself, at all times? Of course not. At one time an object may arouse only interest, or be met with indifference; but at another time it may evoke the greatest fear. In other words, fear must be the result of a specific relationship between organism and object. What leads to fear is nothing but the experience of the possibility of the onset of anxiety. What we fear is the impending anxiety, which we experience in relation to some objects. Since a person in a state of fear is not yet in a state of anxiety but only envisions it —that is, he only fears that anxiety may befall him—he is not so disturbed in his judgment of the outer world as the person in a state of anxiety. Rather, driven as he is by the tendency to avoid the onset of anxiety, he attempts to establish special contact with the outer world. He tries to recognize the situation as clearly as possible and to react to it in an appropriate manner. Fear is conditioned by, and directed against, very definite aspects of the environment. These have to be recognized and, if possible, removed. Fear sharpens the senses, whereas anxiety renders them unusable. Fear drives to action; anxiety paralyzes.

From these explanations it is obvious that in order to feel anxiety it is not necessary to be able to give oneself an account of one's acts; to feel fear, however, presupposes that capacity. From this it becomes clear that our patients do not behave like people in a state of fear— that is, they do not intentionally try to avoid situations from which anxiety may arise. They cannot do that because of the defect of abstraction. Also from our observation of the patients we can assume that they do not experience fear and that they only have the experience of anxiety.

Anxiety, a catastrophic condition in which self-realization is not possible, may be produced by a variety of events, all of which have in common the following: There is a discrepancy between the individual's capacities and the demands made on him, and this discrepancy makes self-realization impossible. This may be due to external or internal conditions, physical or psychological. It is this discrepancy to which we are referring when we speak of "conflicts." Thus we can observe anxiety in infants, in whom such a discrepancy must occur frequently, particularly since their abstract attitude is not yet developed or not fully. We also see anxiety in brain-injured people, in whom impairment of abstraction produces the same discrepancy. In normal people, anxiety appears when the demands of the world are too much above the capacity of the individual, when social and economic situations are too stressful, or when religious conflicts arise. Finally we see anxiety in people with neuroses and psychoses which are based on unsolvable and unbearable inner conflicts.

THE PROTECTIVE MECHANISMS

The last group of symptoms to be observed in brain-injured patients are the behavior changes which make it possible for the patient to get rid of the catastrophic condition—of anxiety.[22] The observation of this phenomenon in these patients is of special interest since it can teach us how an organism can get rid of anxiety without being aware of its origin and without being able to avoid the anxiety voluntarily. After a certain time these patients show a diminution of disorder and of catastrophic reactions (anxiety) even though the defect caused by the damage to the brain still exists. This, of course, can occur only if the patient is no longer exposed to tasks he cannot cope with. This diminution is achieved by definite changes in the behavior of the patients: They are withdrawn, so that a number of stimuli, including dangerous ones, do not reach them. They usually stay alone; either they do not like company or they want to be only with people whom they know well. They like to be in a familiar room in which everything is organized in a definite way. They show extreme orderliness in every respect;

---

[22] Reference footnote 4; p. 40 ff.

everything has to be done exactly at an appointed time—whether it is breakfast, dinner, or a walk. They show excessive and fanatical orderliness in arranging their belongings; each item of their wardrobe must be in a definite place—that is, in a place where it can be gotten hold of quickly, without the necessity of a choice, which they are unable to make. Although it is a very primitive order indeed, they stick fanatically to it; it is the only way to exist. Any change results in a state of very great excitement. They themselves cannot voluntarily arrange things in a definite way. The orderliness is maintained simply because the patients try to stick to those arrangements which they can handle. This sticking to that which they can cope with is characteristic for their behavior; thus any behavior change can be understood only in terms of this characteristic behavior.

An illustration of this characteristic behavior is the fact that they always try to keep themselves busy with things that they are able to do as a protection against things that they cannot cope with. The activities which engross them need not be of great value in themselves. Their usefulness consists apparently in the fact that they protect the patient. Thus a patient does not like to be interrupted in an activity. For instance, although a patient may behave well in a conversation with someone he knows and likes, he does not like to be suddenly addressed by someone else.

We very often observe that a patient is totally unaware of his defect—such as hemiplegia or hemianopsia—and of the difference between his state prior to the development of the symptoms and his present state. This is strikingly illustrated by the fact that the disturbances of these patients play a very small part in their complaints. We are not dealing simply with a subjective lack of awareness, for the defects are effectively excluded from awareness, one might say. This is shown by the fact that they produce very little disturbance—apparently as the result of compensation. This exclusion from awareness seems to occur particularly when the degree of functional defect in performance is extreme. We can say that defects are shut out from the life of the organism when they would seriously impair any of its essential functions and when a defect can be compensated for by other activities at least to the extent that self-realization is not essentially disturbed.

One can easily get the impression that a patient tries to deny the experience of the functional disturbance because he is afraid that he will get into a catastrophic condition if he becomes aware of his defect. As a matter of fact, a patient may get into a catastrophic condition when we make him aware of his defect, or when the particular situation does not make possible an adequate compensation. Sometimes this happens—and this is especially interesting—when the underlying pathological condition improves and with that the function.

A patient of mine who became totally blind by a suicidal gunshot through the chiasma opticum behaved as if he were not aware of his blindness; the defect was compensated for very well by his use of his other senses, his motor skill, and his knowledge and intelligence. He was usually in a good mood; he never spoke of his defect, and he resisted all attempts to draw his attention to it. After a certain time, the condition improved; but at the same time he realized that he could not recognize objects through his vision. He was shocked and became deeply depressed. When he was asked why he was depressed, he said, "I cannot see." We might assume that in the beginning the patient denied the defect intentionally because he could not bear it. But why then did he not deny it when he began to see? Or we might assume that in the beginning he did not deny his blindness, but that in total blindness an adjustment occurred in terms of a change of behavior for which vision was not necessary; and because of this it was not necessary for him to realize his blindness. The moment he was able to see, he became aware of his defect and was no longer able to eliminate it. The exclusion of the blindness defect from awareness could thus be considered a secondary effect of the adjustment. But in this patient who was mentally undisturbed a more voluntary denial cannot be overlooked. A voluntary denial is not possible in patients with impairment of abstraction as in brain-injured patients. Here the unawareness of the defect can only be a secondary effect—an effect of the same behavior, which we have described before, by which the brain-injured person is protected against catastrophes which may occur because of his defect. As we have said, the patient, driven by the trend to realize himself as well as possible, sticks to what he is able to do; this shows in his whole behavior. From this point of view, the patient's lack of awareness of his defect, as well as his peculiarities in general, becomes understandable. For instance, in these terms, it is understandable why an aphasic patient utters a word which is only on the normal fringe of the word that he needs; for the word that he needs to use is a word that he cannot say at all or can say only in such a way that he could not be understood and would as a result be in distress.[23] Thus a patient may repeat "church" instead of "God," "father" instead of "mother," and so on; he considers his reaction correct, at least as long as no one makes him aware of the fact that his reaction is wrong. This same kind of reaction occurs in disturbances of recognition, of feelings, and so on.

One is inclined to consider the use of wrong words or disturbances of recognition, actions, and feelings as due to a special pathology; but that is not their origin. Since these disturbances are reactions which represent all that the individual is able to execute, he recognizes them as fulfillment of the task; in this way, these reactions fulfill this need to such a degree that no catastrophe occurs. Thus the protection appears as a passive effect of an active 'correct' procedure and could not be correctly termed denial, which refers to a more intentional activity, 'conscious' or 'unconscious.'

This theory on the origin of the protective behavior in organic patients deserves consideration, particularly because the phenomena observed in organic patients shows such a similarity to that observed in neurotics. One could even use psychoanalytic terms for the different forms of behavior in organic patients. For instance, one might use the same terms that Anna Freud [24] uses to characterize various defense mechanisms against anxiety. Both neurotic and organic patients show a definite similarity in behavior structure and in the purpose served by that structure. In organic patients, however, I prefer to speak of protective mechanisms instead of defense mechanisms; the latter refers to a more voluntary act, which organic patients certainly cannot perform, as we have discussed earlier. In neurotics, the development of defense mechanisms generally does not occur so passively through organismic adjustment, as does the development of protective mechanisms in the organic patients; this is in general the distinction between the two. It seems to me that this distinction is not true in the case of neurotic children, however; some of these children seem to develop protective mechanisms in a passive way, similar to organic patients. Such mechanisms can perhaps be found in other neurotics. Thus, in interpreting these mechanisms, one should take into account the possibility of confusing the neurotic patient with the organic patient.

I would like to add a last word with regard to the restrictions of the personality and of the world of these patients which is brought about by this protective behavior. The restrictions are not as disturbing in the brain-injured patients as is the effect of defense mechanisms in neuroses. In a neurotic, defense mechanisms represent a characteristic part of the disturbances he is suffering from; but the organic patient does not become aware of the restriction since his protective mechanisms allow for some ordered form of behavior and for the experience of some kind of self-realization—which

---

[23] Reference footnote 15; p. 226.

[24] A. Freud, *The Ego and the Mechanisms of Defense;* New York, Internat. Univ. Press, 1946.

is true, of course, only as long as the environment is so organized by the people around him that no tasks arise that he cannot fulfill and as long as the protecting behavior changes are not hindered. This is the only way the brain-damaged person can exist. The patient cannot bear conflict—that is, anxiety, restriction, or suffering. In this respect he differs essentially from the neurotic who is more or less able to bear conflict. This is the main difference which demands a different procedure in treatment; in many respects, however, treatment can be set up in much the same way for both.[25] In treating these patients, it is more important to deal with the possible occurrence of catastrophe rather than with the impairment of abstraction, for my observations of a great many patients for over ten years indicate that the impairment of abstraction cannot be alleviated unless the brain damage from which it originated is eliminated. There is no functional restitution of this capacity by compensation through other parts of the brain. Improvement of performances can be achieved only by the building up of substitute performances by the use of the part of concrete behavior which is preserved; but this is only possible by a definite arrangement of the environment.

I am well aware that my description of the personality change in brain damage is somewhat sketchy. The immense material and the problems involved, so manifold and complex, make a more satisfactory presentation in such a brief time impossible. I hope that I have been successful in outlining, to the best of my ability, the essential phenomena and problems of these patients. In addition, I trust that I have shown how much we can learn from these observations for our concept of the structure of the personality, both normal and pathological, and for the treatment of brain-damaged patients and also, I hope, of patients with so-called psychogenic disorders.

1148 FIFTH AVE.
NEW YORK 28, N. Y.

---

[25] See K. Goldstein, "The Idea of Disease and Therapy," *Rev. Religion* (1949) 14:229-240.

From R. G. Heath (1975). Journal of Nervous and Mental Disease, *160*, 159-175, *by kind permission of the author and the Williams and Wilkins Co.*

BRAIN FUNCTION AND BEHAVIOR

I. Emotion and Sensory Phenomena in Psychotic Patients and in Experimental Animals

ROBERT G. HEATH, M.D., D.M.Sci.[1]

For the past 25 years, the research program of the Tulane University Department of Psychiatry and Neurology has been directed primarily to the development of treatment for patients with certain psychiatric and neurological disorders that have been resistant to commonly used therapy. In the course of investigations, using a variety of approaches, new techniques have evolved which have permitted simultaneous exploration of brain activity and behavior. The data reported substantiate an anatomical localization in the brain for the syndrome of psychotic behavior. Further, observations in patients, coupled with animal investigations, have led to the demonstration of brain pathways and previously undisclosed anatomical connections which provide a physical substrate for the clinically observed relation between perception and emotionality. These findings provide a basis for the development of specific biological methods for the treatment of behavioral disorders.

Since 1949, the extensive experimental and clinical research program of the Tulane University Department of Psychiatry and Neurology has been directed primarily to the development of treatment for patients with certain psychiatric and neurological disorders that have been resistant to commonly used therapy. In the course of these physiological and anatomical studies, new techniques have evolved which have permitted us to explore brain activity and behavior simultaneously. Correlations established between brain function and certain behavioral characteristics are the subject of this report.

Emotion has subjective, as well as objective components. The subjective components, which are accessible only through human subjects capable of reporting their feelings, are essential for a comprehensive study of emotion. In our treatment program for intractably ill patients with use of physiological techniques, we have had the opportunity to gain a better understanding of the activity and organization of the human brain. Much of the data concerning brain mechanisms in emotionality presented herein were gathered from patients who were psychotic and displaying characteristic profound pathological changes in emotionality. Our findings suggested new, heretofore unidentified brain pathways, which we were later able to demonstrate by anatomical methods. By and large, they refute the concept that the limbic brain constitutes the physical-anatomical substrate for emotional expression (1, 17, 44).

In the classification of disorders of behavior, the traditional concept prevails that cellular abnormality demonstrable under the light microscope must underlie all clinical signs and symptoms if the pathogenesis is to be considered organic or physical. In the absence of demonstrable cellular pathology, the cause of the disorder is sought in the social-environmental sphere. In the organic psychoses, varied lesions have been described at many different brain sites and of various etiological origins. Although cellular lesions have

[1] Professor and Chairman, Department of Psychiatry and Neurology, Tulane University School of Medicine, 1430 Tulane Avenue, New Orleans, Louisiana 70112.

been histopathologically identified at widely disparate sites, correlations between the site of the cytopathological lesion and clinical manifestations have been inconsistent. In some psychotic patients (with schizophrenia and manic-depressive illness), no cellular abnormalities have been disclosed and, by default, their diseases have been termed "functional" (16, 34). On the other hand, certain other states (dyskinesia and many types of epilepsy) are consensually classified as organic neurological disorders despite absence of demonstrable cellular pathology. It is evident, therefore, that new procedures are required to identify the pathological sites in the brains of persons suffering from psychotic signs and symptoms and ultimately to delineate the nature of the "functional" pathological problem. In our investigations we have followed the traditional two-step neurological approach—localization of the physiological change producing the signs and symptoms, followed by delineation of its causative pathological process. The resulting data provide the basis for development of specific treatment.

The psychotic state, a disorder of thinking, feeling, and perceiving, is a mental disease. Man is the only species capable of reporting his thoughts and feelings, thereby providing access to mental function, a necessary source of data for correlation of aberrant mental function with brain disturbances. It is these data which provide the most specific leads for the application of physiological methods to the study of the brain. And it is in cross-relating the data gathered by the two approaches that one gains understanding of the "mind-brain" association. It is therefore incongruous that psychiatrists have so widely resisted use of physiological techniques and that brain-behavior physiologists and neurologists have almost universally rejected psychodynamic data (16).

In the Tulane laboratories, therapeutic use of depth electrode techniques for human psychiatric and neurological disor-ders (preceded by and always augmented by numerous animal studies) has yielded data that have permitted us to move toward localization of pathological sites underlying psychotic behavior. By implantation of electrodes into various predetermined specific brain sites of patients capable of reporting thoughts and feelings, we have been able to make long term observations of functional changes while simultaneously monitoring mental activity (23, 28, 32). From the data gathered by these techniques in patients, together with supplemental information from animal experiments suggested by the human data, we believe that we have identified a consistent correlation between brain function and psychotic signs and symptoms (9, 20). The septal region of the brain, as defined in the early 1950s (10), has unfailingly shown aberrant electrical activity, in the form of spikes and slow waves, during psychotic episodes, regardless of cause. Our observations during 25 years of investigations are summarized here. During this period, the only published report of independent studies in which the researchers used our techniques was confirmatory (43).

The data reported herein substantiate an anatomical localization in the brain for the syndrome of psychotic behavior. Validation of our findings in psychotic patients required control studies of nervous system activity in nonpsychotic, conscious human subjects and in experimental animals. During the course of these studies, data were also collected which identified brain pathways for emotional expression. It became evident that the anatomical bases for the relation between brain structures for emotional expression and levels of awareness, on the one hand, and brain nuclei for sensory perception on the other, were pathophysiological components of the psychotic state.

THE PSYCHOTIC STATE

The psychotic state is a syndrome, or a group of signs and symptoms. A variety of causes, of which schizophrenia is probably the most common, can generate it. While some of its features are constant, others differ with the underlying etiology. The psychotic state is characterized by gross impairment of feelings and emotional expression, a fluctuating level of (sometimes profound reduction in) psychological awareness, and disturbances in sensory perception. When the cause is schizophrenia, the altered emotionality is manifested by defective integration of pleasurable feelings, often associated with excessively painful (emergency) emotional behavior (42). In certain drug-induced psychoses, on the other hand, the affect may even be one of pleasure. Lowered thought level is characterized by primary process thinking, in which ego defenses are weakened and the normally hidden unconscious thought processes, manifested in gross disorders of thought (delusions), become conscious reality. Self-image, which also vacillates with fluctuating level of awareness, is correspondingly fuzzy. Perceptive disturbances usually take the form of distorted bodily image (sometimes characterized as a proprioceptive disorder) and hallucinations—auditory more often than visual. Altered perception of stereognosis, resembling mild parietal cortical dysfunction, often also occurs.

Since many of these symptoms characteristic of the psychotic state are primarily subjective, their correlation with brain mechanisms required synchronization of brain physiological studies with the subjective data disclosed through the "reporting" of conscious human subjects. Before moving to studies in patients, however, we studied the objective components of the basic clinical manifestations in animals to establish whatever objective correlates were possible. And the animal studies were pursued to the point where findings suggested possibilities for effective therapeutic intervention.

In using the objective components to construct bridges between activity of the mind and of the brain, we have tried to identify brain sites and pathways where activity correlates with emotional expression and levels of awareness, and to determine, by physiological and anatomical techniques, how they interrelate with brain sites involved in sensory perception. Such data, in addition to allowing greater precision in physiological treatment, also provide a foundation for development of specific pharmacological therapy.

BACKGROUND AND HYPOTHESIS

Our earliest studies, initiated in animals and later extended to patients, were prompted by observations of the limited desirable effects of frontal lobe operation (including cingulectomy) in the treatment of psychotic schizophrenic patients (38). Such intervention is effective in altering emotions associated with memory and is somewhat beneficial in treating patients handicapped by painful affect due to anticipatory thoughts (the intractable obsessive-compulsive, borderline psychotic patient) or by intractable depression, with associated feelings of rejection, anguish, gloom, despair, and suicidal ideation. Frontal lobe operation, however, fails to correct the defective mechanism of emotional expression of the psychotic (impaired pleasure or anhedonia, flat affect) or the impaired level of awareness. This ineffectuality suggested that the brain mechanism for these phenomena was principally elsewhere than in the cortex. Extensive animal experiments in our laboratory had pointed to a certain rostral medial forebrain site, which we termed the "septal region" (10), as a key neural site for emotional expression and level of awareness. Whereas destruction of the septal region of animals reduced awareness and profoundly impaired emotional expression, electrical stimulation of that region heightened awareness (alerting) and induced what appeared to be a pleasurable state (25, 26). Beginning in 1950, when stimulation techniques were applied to patients, the subjective reports of these patients confirmed the impressions from animal experiments that septal region stimulation elicited pleasurable feelings (27).

Since impaired affect (specifically, the inability to integrate pleasure) and reduced awareness are recognized clinical features of psychotic behavior, we postulated that function of the septal region of the psychotic was impaired, either by direct cellular damage (organic psychoses with septal lesions) or as a functional abnormality (physiological abnormality due to local chemical changes), in the absence of cellular damage (functional psychoses and organic psychoses with cellular pathology elsewhere in the brain). The pathological behavior of patients with organic psychoses who had lesions elsewhere than in the septal region, we speculated, might be due to changes in the function of the septal region as a consequence of the effect of lesions at distal, but connected, brain sites. A further, and critical, assumption was also made that pathological activity, in the absence of cellular damage at a given brain site, would induce essentially the same effects as a destructive lesion.[2]

ELECTRODE IMPLANTATION

The therapeutic rationale for the investigation of these hypotheses in patients was based on studies in animals with electrodes implanted into the brains. Our findings in animals suggested that activation of an "impaired" septal region might correct faulty emotional responsivity by activation of pleasure responsivity and elevation of the level of psychological awareness (20, 27). This animal evidence was sufficient for us to adapt the procedure to patients with certain psychotic disorders with reasonable confidence that it would be more effective than existing modes of therapy. Over the years, rigid criteria have been applied in selection of patients for this procedure; foremost has been the failure of the patient to respond to all conventional forms of treatment.

For correlation of brain activity with behavior to be meaningful, certain other criteria had to be met. Electrodes had to

[2] Heath, R. G. Destructive brain lesions—effects on muscle. In preparation.

be implanted into numerous deep and surface brain sites, since recordings from a single site were of little value in identifying sites of origin of brain changes responsible for clinical phenomena. Further, such multiple implantations would permit evaluation of nonspecific effects from the trauma of implantation and would allow localization of recording abnormalities. Because all parts of the brain are so richly interconnected, it is impossible to localize the site from which aberrant activity originates unless activity from numerous sites is viewed simultaneously. Altered activity at one site, as well as clinical signs and symptoms, can originate either from a cellular lesion at that site or from propagation of abnormal activity at a distal site. Similarly, one could not be certain that focal recordings around the electrode induced symptoms; clinical effects might just as well have been the result of propagated distal effects from focally damaged cells. In many instances, recordings from a single site proved misleading in localization of brain lesions. For example, "epileptic foci" localized by electroencephalographic (EEG) recordings and extirpated surgically as treatment for seizures sometimes proved to be "mirror" or distal reflections of the primary focus. Abnormal recordings from the amygdala, which sometimes correlate with pathological behavior, may also be only distal reflections of primary disturbances at another site.

Since behavior continually fluctuates, it was also essential, in order to correlate brain activity and behavior, to leave the electrodes in exact position for long periods. Techniques were therefore developed which permitted long term study and treatment with electrical stimulation for months to several years in a few instances (29). Later, when a cannula was developed that could be accurately implanted, fixed into position to remain as long as the electrodes, and used repeatedly, chemical stimulation, by introduction of putative synaptic transmitter chemicals, was also possible (21, 22). Although primarily therapeutic, these procedures also permitted collection of data concerning brain activity in association with widely variable behavior, that is, during normal psychological fluctuations (sleep, wakefulness), as well as during changes occurring during psychotic behavior.

Most of our early patients, particularly those in the first reported group of 26 studied between 1950 and 1952, were schizophrenic (27). It became evident, however, that meaningful evaluation of the data from schizophrenic patients required comparative data from nonpsychotic subjects suffering from other previously intractable illnesses which might be alleviated by our procedures. Over the years, therefore, increasing numbers of patients who participated in our studies have had diseases other than schizophrenia. In fact, our last schizophrenic patient was operated on in 1962, the effects of electrical and chemical stimulation having proved to be not much better than the effects of the antipsychotic drugs which were then coming into wide use. Further, the focus of our studies of schizophrenia shifted more to identification of the nature of the basic pathological process affecting the brain to produce the consistent recording changes.[3]

Our continuing studies in human subjects with other intractable illnesses than schizophrenia, many without significant behavioral pathological changes, were prompted by the need to characterize the impaired emotional responsivity of the schizophrenic patient by acquiring comparative data that could be obtained only from such patients.

[3] Some of the refocusing has involved approaches centered in isolation of taraxein (8, 20, 30, 31, 35, 37). But it was the data from our depth electrode studies in schizophrenic patients, indicating a physiological abnormality in recordings from the septal region in association with psychotic behavior, that provided the appropriate assay (the rhesus monkey with similarly implanted electrodes) for these other approaches. Investigations to determine the pathological process responsible for changes in function and in the biochemical substrate for the physiological activity will be the subject of another review article.

CORRELATION OF BRAIN ACTIVITY WITH SPECIFIC EMOTION

As data from the treatment of patients have continued to accumulate, it has become possible to identify those brain sites and pathways in man that are associated with specific emotional states, such as pleasurable emotion and adversive emotion. Our findings do not coincide with conventional textbook presentations. Further, extensions of these studies, to elucidate relations between perception and emotion, have shown that the physical substrate for emotion involves the sensory systems in a manner not formerly described. A summary of previously reported data, based on physiological studies in conscious, reporting patients, identifying brain sites for pleasurable and for painful feelings, will suffice as background for our newer data, which show the anatomical relations of these sites for emotional expression and levels of awareness with sites in pathways for sensory perception.

Sites and pathways for pleasurable emotional expression include the septal region and the medial forebrain bundle to, and including, the interpeduncular nuclei in the mesencephalon. Sites for adversive emotional expression, on the other hand, are the hippocampi and parts of the amygdalae, periaqueductal sites in the mesencephalon, and sites in the medial hypothalamus near the third ventricle. Activity of other brain sites into which electrodes were implanted could not be related to either pleasurable or painful emotional states.

The pleasure system of the brain, as we have demarcated it, is substantiated by data demonstrating how it is activated:

1. Passive electrical stimulation of sites in the pleasure system induced intense pleasure (19, 27, 29). Moreover, when a patient was given the opportunity selectively to self-stimulate various deep brain regions, he repeatedly and exclusively stimulated these sites (12, 19, 29).

2. Introduction of putative synaptic

chemical transmitter agents (most effective of which was acetylcholine) directly into this pleasure system induced a similar response (18, 19).

3. Feelings of pleasure, spontaneous or induced by an action (notably, sexual orgasm) or by association through psychiatric interview, similarly activated the septal region and occasionally other directly connected sites, as evidenced by EEGs (18, 23). Septal recordings were characterized predominantly by bursts of slow, high amplitude activity when the pleasurable state was one of relaxation, such as the behavior induced by pleasant memories (23, 28). On the other hand, electrical activity of the septal region was characterized by faster frequencies of high amplitude and sharp spiking, often coupled with a slow wave, resembling activity we have recorded throughout the brain during an epileptic seizure, when pleasure was intense and explosive (18) (Figure 1). When patients were alerted by anticipation of pleasure, spindling recordings were obtained from the same sites of similar frequency and amplitude as those recorded during adversive states (19, 23).

4. Administration of certain pleasure-inducing agents (marijuana) similarly activated the pleasure system, as reflected in the patient's EEGs (15) (Figure 2).

Further substantiation of this pleasure system of the brain is the fact that human ability to experience pleasure is reduced if function of the system is impaired by:

1. The psychotic state with associated abnormal recordings (spikes and slow waves) from the septal region (Figure 3). Particularly when the etiology of the psy-

PLEASURABLE EMOTION

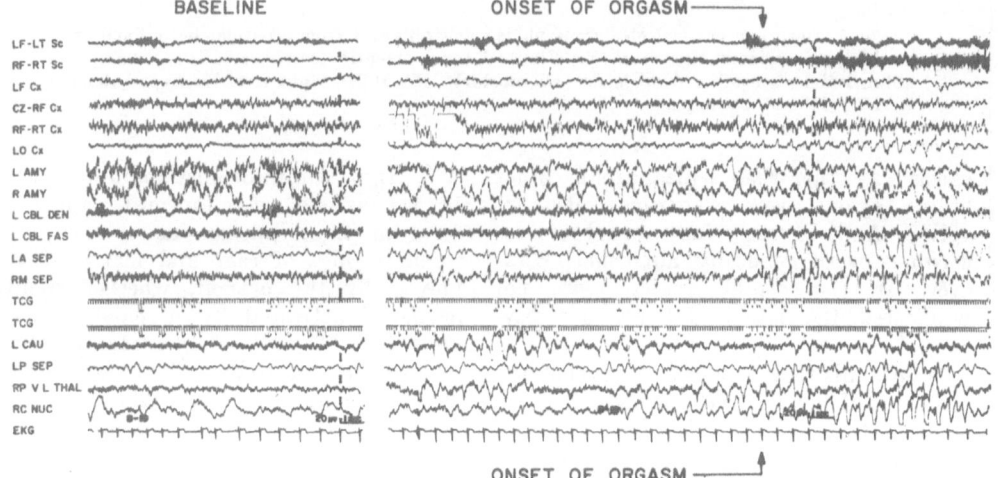

FIG. 1. Deep, cortical, and scalp electroencephalograms obtained from a patient while he was alert (baseline) and later, with onset of orgasm. Cortical leads: LF-LT Sc, left frontal to left temporal scalp; RF-RT Sc, right frontal to right temporal scalp; LF Cx, left frontal cortex (bipolar); CZ-RF Cx, central zero to right frontal cortex; RF-RT Cx, right frontal to right temporal cortex; LO Cx, left occipital cortex (bipolar). Deep leads (all bipolar): L AMY, left amygdala; R AMY, right amygdala; L CBL DEN, left cerebellar dentate; L CBL FAS, left cerebellar fastigius; LA SEP, left anterior septal region; RM SEP, right midseptal region; TCG, time code generator; L CAU, left caudate nucleus; LP SEP, left posterior septal region; RP V L THAL, right posterior ventral lateral thalamus; RC NUC, right central nucleus thalamus; EKG, electrocardiogram.

BRAIN FUNCTION AND BEHAVIOR

PLEASURABLE EMOTION

MARIHUANA

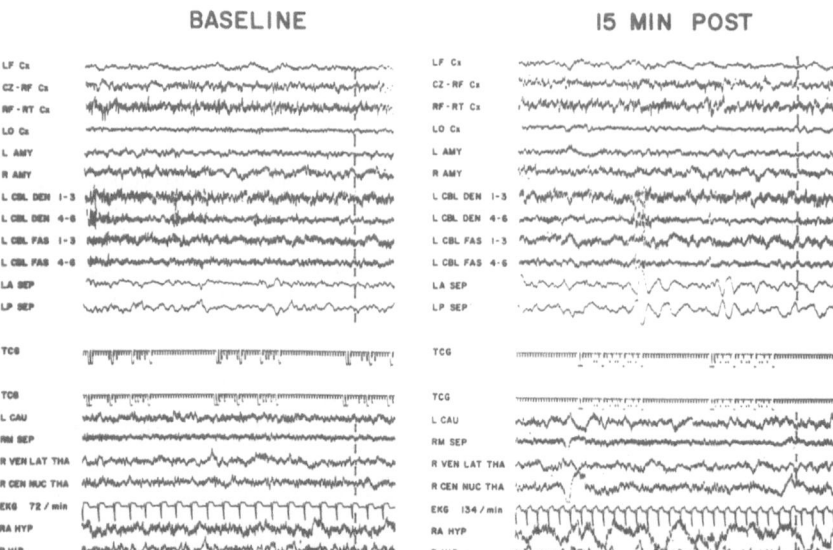

FIG. 2. Deep and cortical electroencephalograms obtained from a patient before and after smoking a marijuana cigarette. (See Figure 1 for explanation of abbreviations.) Additional abbreviations are other deep leads (all bipolar): RA HYP, right anterior hypothalamus; R HIP, right hippocampus.

chosis was other than schizophrenia, other brain regions were sometimes also involved. And, in many instances, brain recordings were generally abnormal. However, if the septal region was not implicated, the patient did not show psychotic behavior.

2. Administration of some psychotomimetics or of taraxein (the protein fraction obtained from schizophrenic sera) (30, 35, 37). These agents, when given to monkeys with implanted electrodes, have consistently induced septal spiking (Figure 4).

3. Induction of spiking in the septal region by electrical stimulation of remote brain sites which, by direct connection, influence the septal region (12).

Correlation of adverse emotional responses and brain activity was also established by several methods.

1. High amplitude fast spindling (12 to 14 per second) spontaneously appeared, focal in the hippocampus or amygdala, when feelings of rage and fear were displayed by the patient, whether spontaneous or activated by psychiatric interview (23) (Figure 5). In a recent patient in whom electrodes had also been implanted into the cerebellum and cingulate gyrus because animal data had indicated their direct connections to deep temporal lobe nuclei, similar activity was recorded from these regions concomitant with her display of emergency emotion (Figure 6).

2. Focal epileptiform activity, presumably a consequence of the basic pathological disturbance in epilepsy, invariably appeared in these same nuclear sites (hippocampus or amygdala) deep in the

ROBERT G. HEATH

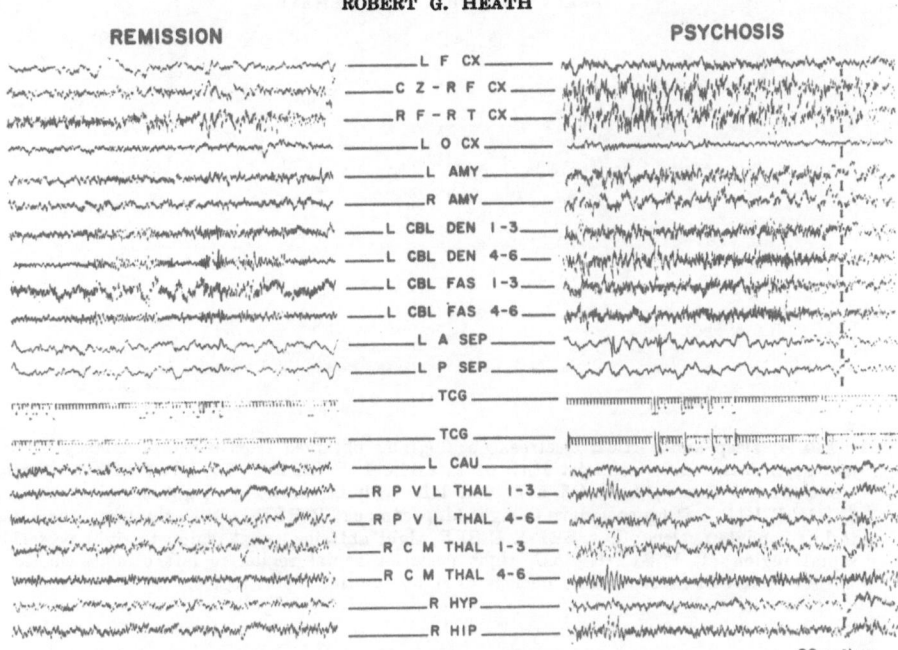

FIG. 3. Deep and cortical electroencephalograms obtained from a patient during states of remission and psychosis. (See Figure 1 for explanation of abbreviations.) Note sharp spike in anterior septal leads, appearing also in cerebellar leads.

temporal lobe of epileptic patients when they had aura characterized by intense fear or rageful outbursts (11, 19).

3. Electrical stimulation to the hippocampus, to many sites within the amygdala, and to numerous medial hypothalamic and mesencephalic periaqueductal sites induced an emergency state dominated by fear or rage. When patients were given the opportunity to self-stimulate in this system, they always abstained. Indeed, they inactivated the self-stimulation device (12, 19).

4. Introduction of levarterenol into the hippocampus induced epileptiform activity and associated emergency emotion (19).

Whereas these correlations of activity at specific brain sites with painful emotion are consistent, strong emotional arousal, not particularly adversive and sometimes in anticipation of pleasure, has been accompanied in several instances by similar changes at these sites, suggesting that the cerebellar-cingulate-hippocampal-amygdala spindling may be a correlate of intense arousal of emotion, not necessarily painful.

Each system of the brain (pleasure and pain) is seemingly capable of overwhelming or inhibiting the other. Activation of the pleasure system by electrical stimulation or by administration of drugs eliminates signs and symptoms of emotional or physical pain, or both, and obliterates changes in recordings associated with the painful state. Similarly, activation of brain sites for adversive emotional response replaces pleasurable feelings with painful feelings, and obliterates recording correlates of the pleasure state.

These studies in patients have provided a physiological basis for clinical observations of the apparent relation between states of painful and pleasurable emotion. It is clinically assumed that a deficient pleasure mechanism in patients with schizophrenia and some borderline states causes an unpleasant or painful emotional state.

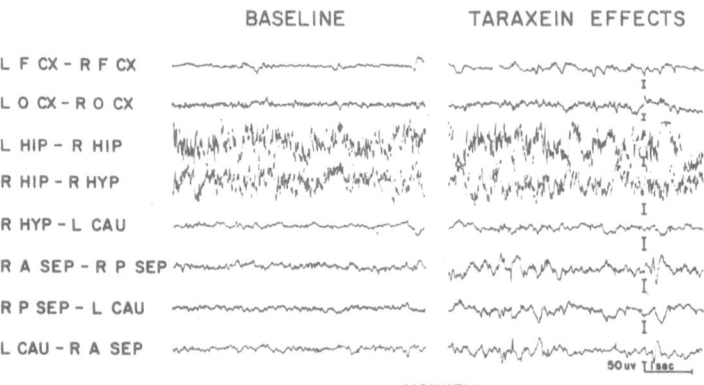

BRAIN FUNCTION AND BEHAVIOR

FIG. 4. Deep and cortical electroencephalograms obtained from a rhesus monkey before and after intravenous administration of taraxein. L F CX-R F CX, left frontal cortex to right frontal cortex; L O CX-R O CX, left occipital cortex to right occipital cortex; L HIP-R HIP, left hippocampus to right hippocampus; R HYP-L CAU, right hypothalamus to left caudate nucleus; R A SEP-R P SEP, right anterior septal region to right posterior septal region; R P SEP-L CAU, right posterior septal region to left caudate nucleus; L CAU-R A SEP, left caudate nucleus to right anterior septal region.

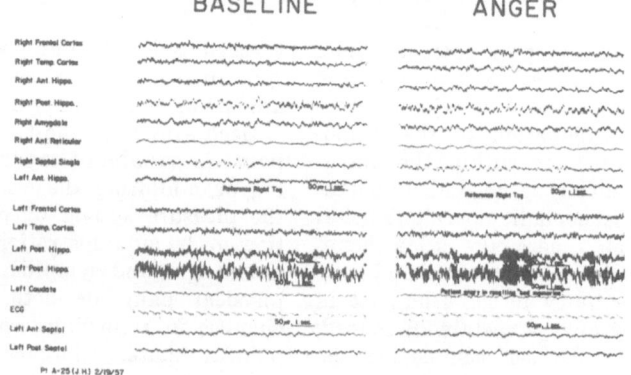

FIG. 5. Deep and cortical electroencephalograms obtained from a patient when he was alert and calm (baseline) and, on another occasion, when he became angry in "recalling bad memories."

A physiological correlate for this state has now been demonstrated in our large series of schizophrenic patients. Further, overwhelming emergency emotion (adversive emotion) in both schizophrenic and non-schizophrenic patients has been shown to correlate with excessive activity of deep temporal lobe nuclei and related brain sites.

RELATION OF EMOTIONAL RESPONSIVITY AND PERCEPTION

Beginning with the earliest concepts of emotion advanced by James and Lange

ROBERT G. HEATH

PAINFUL EMOTION
PSYCHIATRIC INTERVIEW

BASELINE   FEAR

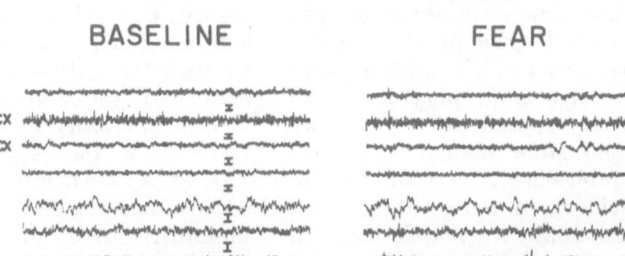

FIG. 6. Deep and cortical electroencephalograms obtained from a patient when she was alert and calm (baseline) and later, when psychiatric interview prompted a state of anxiety-fear. (See Figure 1 for explanation of abbreviations.) Additional deep leads (bipolar): L CIN, left cingulate gyrus; L CBL, left cerebellum subcortex.

(33) and by Cannon (3), sensory input has been considered of primary importance. Sensory stimuli can induce emotion, as can memory experiences. It is usually the subject's interpretation of the sensory stimulus against the background of memory experiences that determines the intensity of the emotional response. It is apparent, therefore, that the effector mechanism for emotionality is activated both through sensory receptor mechanisms and from higher neural centers. The correlative studies described heretofore have demarcated those brain sites where function relates to qualitatively specific emotional states. Other researchers (1, 39, 41, 44) have described neural pathways between cortical sites and these subcortical sites for specific emotions. In this discussion, the focus will be on those subcortical sites at which activity has been correlated with emotion. (Back-and-forth connections to the higher cortical levels will not be considered in the present report.)

There is abundant clinical evidence of the effect of sensory stimuli on emotion and, reciprocally, the effect of an emotional state on perception. An obvious relation similarly exists among level of awareness (alertness), emotional state, and sensory receptivity. Interrelations of impaired emotionality with the altered level of awareness of the psychotic state and perception have also been extensively documented. On the other hand, and in contrast to the abundant clinical evidence, there is sparse evidence of the anatomical-physiological tie-in of structures involved in perception with those involved in emotion and levels of awareness. Data from recent studies in our laboratories indicate that these systems, usually considered separate, are so functionally interrelated as to constitute one system.

It is consistent clinical observations in our reporting patients that have permitted identification of brain sites where activity is correlated with emotion. These observations, in turn, have pointed the way for our physiological studies in animals, which

BRAIN FUNCTION AND BEHAVIOR

have provided direction for anatomical studies. Data derived from these continuing animal investigations have, in turn, prompted additional studies in human subjects. And these newer studies in patients have substantiated some of the observations of the structural-functional interrelation between sensory phenomena and emotion. Sensory stimuli can move a person's emotional state toward heightened pleasure or intensified adversion. This influence is evident in our everyday life. Movement stimulation (muscle-joint-tendon) can be very pleasant: children like to be picked up, rocked, and swung; merry-go-round and roller coaster rides are fun; deep muscle massage and various forms of vibration can be exceedingly pleasant; physical exercise, particularly that of contact sports, is exhilarating. Other sensory stimuli, such as the warm temperature of a bath, can induce relaxation and a feeling of well-being, but perhaps less profoundly than proprioceptive stimuli. The emotional effects of sound vary widely—from the soothing symphonies of Beethoven to the stirring marches of John Phillip Sousa, from the soft lapping of water against a shore to the shrill blaring of horns on a traffic-congested street; from dulcet murmurs to piercing screams. A wide range of visual, olfactory, and tactile stimuli similarly affect one's emotional state. Reciprocally, acumen for specific sensory stimuli is influenced by one's prevailing emotional state. A frightened person responds to sights, sounds, and somatosensory stimuli differently from one who is in an amorous mood. Emotional state, level of awareness, and sensory perception are seemingly inter-related phenomena; a change in one affects the others.

During psychotic states, the inter-relations of these phenomena are perhaps more evident. The psychotic person's disturbances in feeling and emotional expression are inevitably associated with changes in sensory perception and levels of awareness. Textbooks describe these classical symptoms (2, 34). Further, certain programmed manipulation of one of these basic phenomena can predictably alter the others. Numerous studies show that sensory isolation or prolonged sleep deprivation (altering level of awareness) induces transient psychotic behavior in human subjects (36). When primates, from birth through the critical first 6 months of life, are raised in isolation and thereby deprived of certain sensory stimuli, basic behavioral features of the psychotic state develop (5). In all such instances, deprivation of somatosensory stimuli, particularly of the kinesthetic-vestibular type, is proving to be the primary cause for the syndrome.

Data from the isolation-rearing studies of primates prompted our initial investigations of anatomical relations between sensory systems and brain sites for emotional response. In these seriously disturbed monkeys, recording abnormalities from brain sites where activity was correlated with emotionality were similar to those we had obtained from the same brain sites in psychotic patients (13). In the monkeys, however, because sensory deprivation, particularly of proprioceptive and somatosensory stimuli, had induced the emotional disturbance, we had also implanted electrodes into the somatosensory thalamus and into deep cerebellar nuclei known to be part of the vestibular proprioceptive system. When recordings from the septal region and hippocampus of these monkeys were abnormal, gross abnormalities were also recorded from the implanted sensory relay nuclei (13). Furthermore, computer analyses, showing frequent and almost simultaneous spiking in sensory relay nuclei and in sites for emotional expression, offered the first suggestion of direct connections between these sites, that is, an anatomical substrate for the relationship suggested by clinical observations (14, 17).

These leads prompted us to undertake anatomical and physiological studies in animals (rhesus monkeys and cats), which revealed a number of heretofore undescribed neural connections between brain sites involved in emotional expression and sensory relay nuclei. These observations thus substantiated the clinical leads. Additional studies in animals demonstrated the functional inter-relations among these sites (14, 17, 24). When we applied these findings to a few patients in our depth electrode series, the recording changes from related brain sites coupled with the reporting of these human subjects confirmed that the functional physiological relations among these interconnected brain sites are indeed basic to emotional expression in man as well as in the animals (15, 18, 28).

EVOKED POTENTIAL STUDIES IN ANIMALS

The evoked potential technique used in cats and monkeys, in which bipolar electrodes had been chronically implanted into specific brain sites, consisted in the delivery of a brief stimulus to one nuclear site under study while recordings were obtained from other sites suspected of being interconnected. Delay time from stimulus to onset of response (speed of conduction) provided an indication of the kind of pathway involved, that is, the degree to which it was myelinated and whether or not the connection was direct (monosynap-

tic) or indirect (polysynaptic). Our data from these studies have previously been reported in detail (6, 7, 14, 17, 24). Findings important to the present thesis were the demonstrations of: 1) monosynaptic connections within nuclear sites involved in emotional expression, that is, among the hippocampus, amygdala, and septal region; 2) direct monosynaptic connections within pertinent sensory relay nuclei: the posterior ventral lateral nucleus of the thalamus for somatosensory sensation, the fastigial nuclei of the cerebellum for proprioception, the medial geniculate bodies for audition, and the lateral geniculate bodies for vision; and 3) direct back-and-forth monosynaptic connections between these sensory relay nuclei and the sites for emotional expression, both for pleasurable and adversive states. Figure 7 illustrates the evoked potential technique for demonstrating these anatomical connections. A richly interconnected network demonstrating an integral relation between brain sites for emotional expression and those for sensory perception was thus established physiologically in animals.

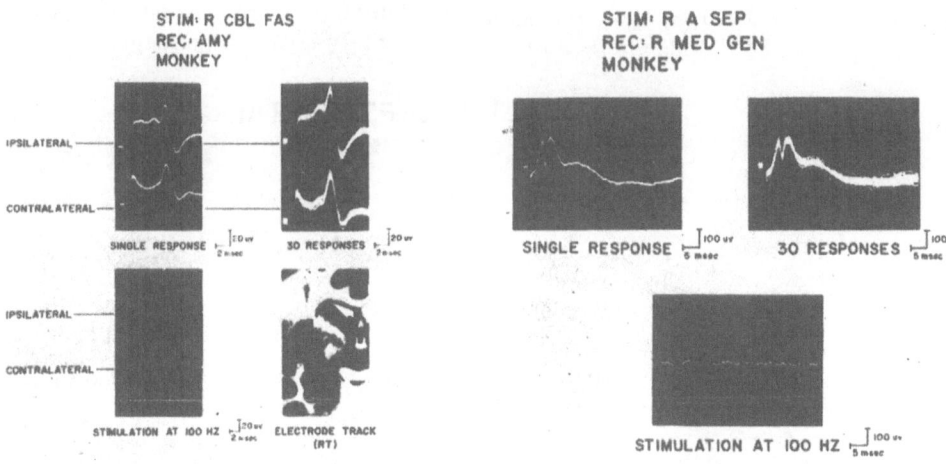

FIG. 7. Evoked potentials demonstrating direct (indicated by short latency) connections between sensory relay nuclei and some sites in the pathways for emotional expression. The response is validated by the fact that high frequency stimulation eliminates it and, further, that it is consistent, as shown by the 30 superimposed responses. The anatomical section shows the site of the recording electrode. (See Figure 1 for explanation of abbreviations.)

BRAIN FUNCTION AND BEHAVIOR

ANATOMICAL TECHNIQUES

Most of the pathways demonstrated by evoked potential techniques have now been verified by use of anatomical techniques (6, 7, 24).[4] A lesion-producing electrode was implanted stereotaxically into a selected nuclear site of monkeys and cats, and fulgerating, continuous, unidirectional current was applied at two sites within the nucleus. The animals were killed on different days after the surgical procedure, and the brains were fixed, sectioned, and stained by three methods: the Nauta-Gygax (40) method for degenerating axons, the Fink-Heimer (4) procedure I for degenerating axoplasm and synaptic terminals, and cresylechtviolet for clarification of cytoarchitectural details. With these methods, we have verified monosynaptic (direct) connections from the fastigial nucleus to the somatosensory thalamus, to the medial and lateral geniculates, and to the septal region, hippocampus, and amygdala. Many other ascending and descending connections between sites for emotional expression and the sensory relay nuclei that were demonstrated by use of evoked potentials were also substantiated by this technique (6, 7, 24).[4]

[4] Heath, R. G., and Harper, J. W. Descending projections of the septal region. In preparation.

IRRITANT DISTAL FOCUS STUDIES

Another technique, involving stereotaxic implantation of cobalt into a selected brain site, has demonstrated the functional inter-relations among these directly connected brain sites. In cats and monkeys prepared with deep and surface electrodes and implanted with an irritant, cobalt or alumina, a primary epileptiform focus developed at the implantation site and was later propagated over efferent pathways to activate secondary epileptiform activity in nuclei directly connected with the primary site.

Figure 8 shows how a primary epileptiform focus induced in the septal region, on one side, by cobalt implantation induced secondary epileptiform activity in the posteroventral lateral thalamus and in the fastigial nucleus of the cerebellum. This demonstration illustrates how function of the septal region, involved in pleasurable emotion, can alter function of the cerebellum, which is involved in movement and proprioception. The reverse relation between these nuclei has also been demonstrated. The primary epileptiform discharge from the fastigial nucleus of the cerebellum, induced by cobalt implantation there, spread to encompass the septal region, hippocampus, and amyg-

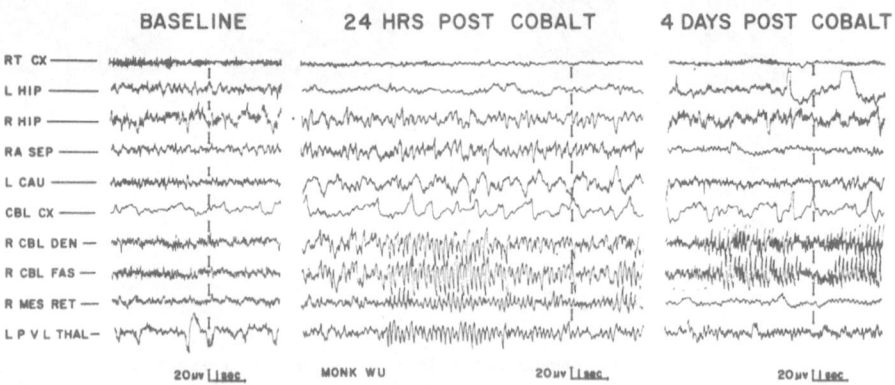

FIG. 8. Recordings obtained from a monkey before and after (24 hours and 4 days) implantation of cobalt into the septal region. (See Figure 1 for explanation of abbreviations.)

dala, and then involved the temporal cortex, this activity coinciding with onset of a generalized epileptic seizure (17).

With this technique, functional relations have also been shown between nuclear sites for emotional expression and those for perception of sensory stimuli. These demonstrations lend further support to data of other studies which indicated integral functional relations among these sites.

CORROBORATIVE FINDINGS IN HUMAN SUBJECTS

Although the demonstrations in animals of many new brain pathways were provocative, the only conclusive proof of the importance of this anatomical substrate to behavioral and neurological phenomena was the demonstration that neural activity at these specific brain sites occurred concomitantly with specific mental phenomena. During the past few years, to assist in diagnosis and treatment, we have implanted electrodes into some sensory relay nuclei of a few intractably ill patients. In one patient (B-19), during orgasmic climax, striking changes in electrical activity were recorded from the somatosensory thalamus (RP V L THAL, Figure 1), as well as from the septal region and part of the amygdala, anatomical sites where activity has been correlated consistently with feelings of pleasure (in other patients in our depth electrode series as well) (18, 27, 29). In another patient (B-22), intermittent high amplitude spindle bursts were recorded not only in the hippocampus and amygdala at frequencies of 10 to 14 cycles per second (typical of recordings we had obtained previously in other patients in our series) in association with intense emergency emotion, but also in deep cerebellar structures for proprioception and in the cingulate gyrus when the patient reported profound anxiety (28). The single patient (B-16) in our series who has had electrodes in the medial geniculate body, the auditory relay station, was an epileptic with an occasional aura of auditory hallucinations. Activity in the geniculate of this patient was unusual only

occasionally. On one occasion pertinent to this discussion, the relation between the medial geniculate body and brain sites where activity was correlated with specific emotional states was demonstrated when the patient was drowsy, but not asleep. High amplitude delta activity, first recorded in the septal region (pleasure site), spread to involve the medial geniculate body (Figure 9). Upon being questioned by the interviewing psychiatrist, the patient reported erotic fantasies associated with recall of provocative music.

The animal studies not only demonstrated direct connections among nuclei for emotional expression and among those for sensory perception, but also direct connections between the two groups of nuclei. A functional relation among these sites was also shown. The few studies in patients demonstrated that physiological relations between these key sites did indeed correlate with the subjective phenomenon of emotion. Taken together, these findings provide evidence that sensory relay nuclei and the rostral septal region, along with the deep temporal nuclei (more commonly identified with emotion), are functionally related and are involved in the substrate for emotional expression. Figure 10, a schematic diagram of a monkey brain against the background of stereotaxic coordinates summarizes principal direct connections among the nuclear sites for sensory perception and emotional expression.

COMMENT

By the techniques described herein, we have observed correlations between emotional states and brain activity at specific sites. Our studies in patients have permitted the identification of an anatomical substrate for emotion and awareness. These findings have been followed by precise anatomical studies in animals. The pathways that we have demonstrated are different from those based solely on animal experiments that have been described in textbooks and in earlier reports. Further, the approaches described have led to the dem-

BRAIN FUNCTION AND BEHAVIOR

EMOTION – PERCEPTION

BASELINE

SEP – HIP – AMY AND M GEN

RELATIONSHIP

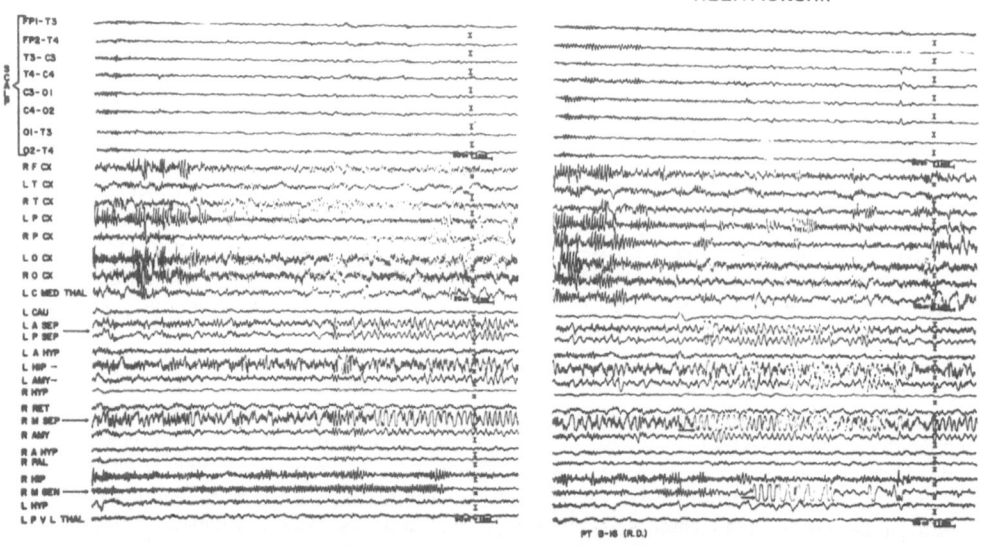

FIG. 9. Deep, cortical, and scalp electroencephalograms obtained from a patient who had electrodes implanted into the medial geniculate. (See Figure 1 for explanation of abbreviations.)

onstration of previously undisclosed anatomical connections, which provide a physical substrate for the clinically observed relation between perception and emotionality. It is generally agreed that there is a chemical, as well as an emotional substrate for emotion. A structural-functional relation between the pathways described herein and the nuclear sites for putative neurotransmitters will be the subject of a related article. And, in a third article in this series, efforts to identify the pathological process affecting function of this physiological substrate for emotional expression will be described.

Healthy (appropriate) emotion is generally accepted to be nuclear to the development of normal behavior, whereas inappropriate emotion is the basic pathognomonic factor in disordered behavior. The demonstrations of the anatomical-functional substrate for emotion provide a basis for the development of specific bio-

logical methods for the treatment of behavioral disorders.

REFERENCES

1. Akert, K., and Hummel, P. The Limbic System—Anatomy and Physiology. Roche Laboratories, Nutley, New Jersey, 1968.
2. Bleuler, E. Dementia Praecox or The Group of Schizophrenias. International Universities Press, New York, 1950.
3. Cannon, W. B. The James-Lange theory of emotions: A critical examination and an alternative theory. Am. J. Psychol., 39: 106–124, 1927.
4. Fink, R. P., and Heimer, L. Two methods for selective silver impregnation of degenerating axons and their synaptic endings in the central nervous system. Brain Res., 4: 369–374, 1967.
5. Harlow, H. F., and Harlow, M. Social deprivation in monkeys. Sci. Am., 207: 137–146, 1962.
6. Harper, J. W., and Heath, R. G. Anatomic connections of the fastigial nucleus to the rostral forebrain in the cat. Exp. Neurol., 39: 285–292, 1973.
7. Harper, J. W., and Heath, R. G. Ascending projections of the cerebellar fastigial nu-

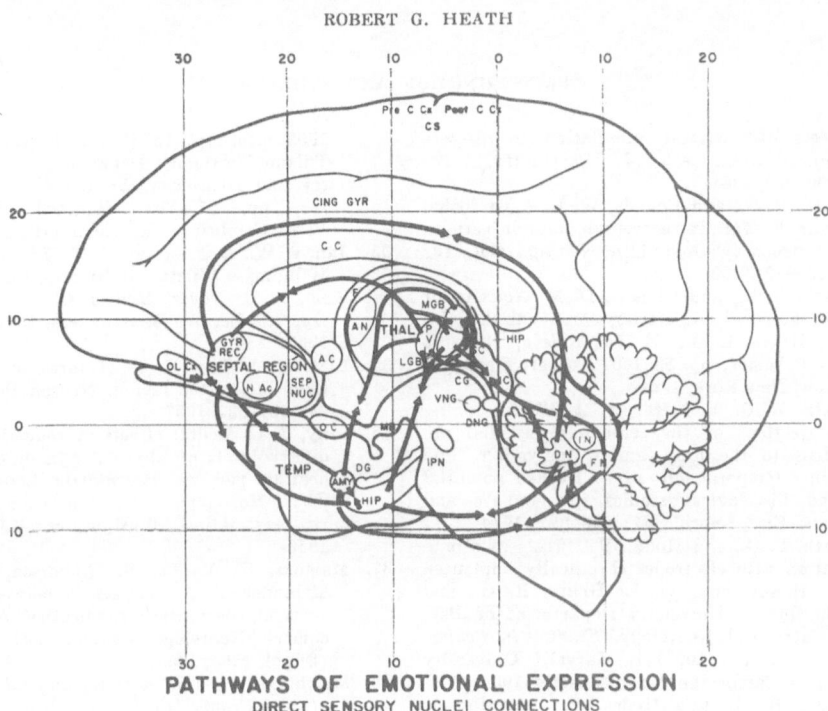

PATHWAYS OF EMOTIONAL EXPRESSION
DIRECT SENSORY NUCLEI CONNECTIONS

FIG. 10. Diagram of a monkey brain against the background of stereotaxic coordinates. (See Figure 1 for explanation of abbreviations.)

clei: Connections to the ectosylvian gyrus. Exp. Neurol., *42:* 241–247, 1974.

8. Heath, R. G. An antibrain globulin in schizophrenia. In Himwich, H. E., Ed. *Biochemistry, Schizophrenias, and Affective Illnesses,* pp. 171–197. Williams & Wilkins, Baltimore, 1970.

9. Heath, R. G. Common characteristics of epilepsy and schizophrenia: Clinical observation and depth electrode studies. Am. J. Psychiatry, *118:* 1013–1026, 1962.

10. Heath, R. G. Definition of the septal region. In Heath, R. G., and the Tulane University Department of Psychiatry and Neurology. *Studies in Schizophrenia,* pp. 3–5. Harvard University Press, Cambridge, Massachusetts, 1954.

11. Heath, R. G. Depth recording and stimulation studies in patients. In Winter, A., Ed. *The Surgical Control of Behavior—A Symposium,* pp. 21–37. Charles C Thomas, Springfield, Illinois, 1971.

12. Heath, R. G. Electrical self-stimulation of the brain in man. Am. J. Psychiatry, *120:* 571–577, 1963.

13. Heath, R. G. Electroencephalographic studies in isolation-raised monkeys with behavioral impairment. Dis. Nerv. Syst., *33:* 157–163, 1972.

14. Heath, R. G. Fastigial nucleus connections to the septal region in monkey and cat: A demonstration with evoked potentials of a bilateral pathway. Biol. Psychiatry, *6:* 193–196, 1973.

15. Heath, R. G. Marihuana: Effects on deep and surface electroencephalograms of man. Arch. Gen. Psychiatry, *26:* 577–584, 1972.

16. Heath, R. G. Perspectives for biological psychiatry: Presidential address. Biol. Psychiatry, *2:* 81–88, 1970.

17. Heath, R. G. Physiologic basis of emotional expression: Evoked potential and mirror focus studies in rhesus monkeys. Biol. Psychiatry, *5:* 15–31, 1972.

18. Heath, R. G. Pleasure and brain activity in man: Deep and surface electroencephalograms during orgasm. J. Nerv. Ment. Dis., *154:* 3–18, 1972.

19. Heath, R. G. Pleasure response of human subjects to direct stimulation of the brain: Physiologic and psychodynamic considerations. In Heath, R. G., Ed. *The Role of Pleasure in Behavior,* pp. 219–243. Hoeber, Harper & Row, New York, 1964.

20. Heath, R. G. Schizophrenia: Biochemical and physiologic aberrations. Int. J. Neuropsychiatry, *2:* 597–610, 1966.

21. Heath, R. G., and deBalbian Verster, F. Ef-

fects of chemical stimulation to discrete brain areas. Am. J. Psychiatry, *117:* 980–990, 1961.

22. Heath, R. G., and Founds, W. L. A perfusion cannula for intracerebral microinjections. Electroencephalogr. Clin. Neurophysiol., *12:* 930–932, 1960.

23. Heath, R. G., and Gallant, D. M. Activity of the human brain during emotional thought. In Heath, R. G., Ed. *The Role of Pleasure in Behavior*, pp. 83–106. Hoeber, Harper & Row, New York, 1964.

24. Heath, R. G., and Harper, J. W. Ascending projections of the cerebellar fastigial nucleus to the hippocampus, amygdala, and other temporal lobe sites: Evoked potential and histological studies in monkeys and cats. Exp. Neurol., *45:* 268–287, 1974.

25. Heath, R. G., and Hodes, R. Effects of stimulation with electrodes chronically implanted in rhesus monkeys. In Heath, R. G., and the Tulane University Department of Psychiatry and Neurology. *Studies in Schizophrenia*, pp. 109–111. Harvard University Press, Cambridge, Massachusetts, 1954.

26. Heath, R. G., and Hodes, R. Induction of sleep by stimulation of the cuadate nucleus in macaqus rhesus and man. Trans. Am. Neurol. Assoc., *77:* 248, 1952.

27. Heath, R. G., and the Tulane University Department of Psychiatry and Neurology. *Studies in Schizophrenia*, Harvard University Press, Cambridge, Massachusetts, 1954.

28. Heath, R. G., Cox, A. W., and Lustick, L. S. Brain activity during emotional states. Am. J. Psychiatry, *131:* 858–862, 1974.

29. Heath, R. G., John, S. B., and Fontana, C. J. The pleasure response: Studies by stereotaxic technics in patients. In Kline, N., and Laska, E., Eds. *Computers and Electronic Devices in Psychiatry*, pp. 178–189. Grune & Stratton, New York, 1968.

30. Heath, R. G., Krupp, I. M., Byers, L. W., and Liljekvist, J. I. Schizophrenia as an immunologic disorder. Arch. Gen. Psychiatry, *16:* 1–33, 1967.

31. Heath, R. G., Martens, S., Leach, B. E., Cohen, M., and Agel, C. A. Effect on behavior in humans with the administration of taraxein. Am. J. Psychiatry, *114:* 14–24, 1957.

32. Heath, R. G., Peacock, S. M., Monroe, R. R., and Miller, W. H. Electroencephalograms and subcorticograms recorded since the June 1952 meetings. In Heath, R. G., and the Tulane University Department of Psychiatry and Neurology. *Studies in Schizophrenia*, pp. 573–608. Harvard University Press, Cambridge, Massachusetts, 1954.

33. James, W., and Lange, G. C. *The Emotions.* Williams & Wilkins, Baltimore, 1922.

34. Kolb, L. C. *Noyes' Modern Clinical Psychiatry*, 7th Ed. W. B. Saunders, Philadelphia, 1968.

35. Lief, H. I. The effects of taraxein on a patient in analysis. Arch. Neurol. Psychiatry, *78:* 624–627, 1957.

36. Lilly, J. C. Mental effects of reduction of ordinary levels of physical stimuli on intact, healthy persons. *Psychiatric Research Reports*, No. 5, pp. 1–28. American Psychiatric Association, Washington, D.C., June, 1956.

37. Martens, S., Vallbo, S., Andersen, K., and Melander, B. A comparison between taraxein and some psychotomimetics. Acta Psychiatr. Neurolog. Scand., *34:* 361–368 (Suppl. 136), 1959.

38. Mettler, F. A., Ed. *Selective Partial Ablation of the Frontal Cortex.* Hoeber, Harper & Bros., New York, 1949.

39. Nauta, W. J. H. Hippocampal projections and related neural pathways to the midbrain in the cat. Brain, *81:* 319–340, 1958.

40. Nauta, W. J. H., and Gygax, P. A. Silver impregnation of degenerating axons in the central nervous system: A modified technique. Stain Technol., *29:* 91–93, 1954.

41. Papez, J. W. A. A proposed mechanism of emotion. Arch. Neurol. Psychiatry, *38:* 725–743, 1937.

42. Rado, S., Buchenholz, B., Dunton, H., Karlen, S. H., and Senescu, R. Schizotypal organization. Preliminary report on a clinical study of schizophrenia. In Rado, S., and Daniels, G. E., Eds. *Changing Concepts of Psychoanalytic Medicine*, pp. 225–235. Grune and Stratton, New York, 1956.

43. UCLA Conference. Clinical neurophysiology: Newer diagnostic and therapeutic methods in neurological disease and behavior disorders. Ann. Intern. Med., *71:* 619–645, 1969.

44. Zanchetti, A. Subcortical and cortical mechanisms in arousal and emotional behavior. In Quarton, G. C., Melnechuk, T., and Schmitt, F. O., Eds. *The Neurosciences*, pp. 602–614. Rockefeller University Press, New York, 1967.

From C. Schooler, T. P. Zahn, D. L. Murphy and M. S. Buchsbaum (1978). Journal of Nervous and Mental Disease, *166,* 177-186, *by kind permission of the authors and the Williams and Wilkins Co.*

PSYCHOLOGICAL CORRELATES OF MONOAMINE OXIDASE ACTIVITY IN NORMALS

CARMI SCHOOLER, PH.D.,[1] THEODORE P. ZAHN, PH.D.,[2] DENNIS L. MURPHY, M.D.,[3] AND MONTE S. BUCHSBAUM, M.D.[4]

This study replicates and extends earlier work by finding that low levels of platelet monoamine oxidase (MAO) activity correlate with sensation seeking, high ego strength, positive affect, and high leisure time activity levels, somewhat similar psychological correlates also being found for plasma amine oxidase activity. Although there are several ways in which a schizophrenia/MAO relationship may exist and still be congruent with the present data, these results pose difficulties for theories which link low MAO activity levels specifically to schizophrenia. Nothing in the present findings, however, is incongruent with the possibility of an association between low platelet MAO activity and bipolar affective disorder.

A recent series of papers (10, 12, 14, 18) empirically link reduced levels of platelet monoamine oxidase (MAO) activity to both chronic schizophrenia and bipolar (manic-depressive) affective disorder. On the basis of these findings, it has been suggested that low platelet MAO activity might represent a genetic, predisposing factor for both disorders (10). As MAO is an enzyme with regulatory effects on biogenic amine metabolism in nerve endings, there are a number of mechanisms whereby a reduction in its activity might be postulated to result in behavioral pathology. For example, MAO inhibition has been found to result in changes in brain dopamine, an increased formation of methylated amine derivatives, and an increased accumulation of other amines with neurotransmitter-modulating properties (*e.g.,* phenylethylamine, octopamine). On a behavioral level, pharmacologically induced MAO inhibition can result in hyperactivity, psychotic behavior, and other psychological changes in medical and psychiatric patients as well as normal individuals (8). Thus, changes in neurotransmitter amines, related to low levels of MAO activity, are quite possibly etiologically relevant in the development of schizophrenic and manic-depressive behavior (10).

There is, however, substantial evidence suggesting that reduced MAO activity is not a sufficient cause of either of these disorders, but rather that MAO activity may interact with other factors to produce overt illness (10). Since low MAO activity by itself may not result directly in psychosis, useful knowledge can be gained by studying nonpsychotic individuals with low MAO activity in order to see whether they show psychological traits which might, in different circumstances, contribute to the development of psychosis. Since in normal volunteers MAO activities are generally relatively stable traits, with test-retest correlations at 8 to 10 weeks of $r = .86$, they are suitable measures for such studies (13). Exploring this possibility, Murphy *et al.* (9) examined the correlations between platelet MAO activity and Zuckerman Sensation-Seeking Scales (20) and the Minnesota Multiphasic Personality Inventory (MMPI) (6) in a nonpsychiatric patient population of college age volunteers. "The MMPI was chosen ... because large differences between patients with bipolar *vs.* unipolar affective disorders have been reported in both MMPI scores and platelet MAO activ-

[1] Laboratory of Socio-environmental Studies, National Institute of Mental Health, Building 10, Room 3D42, Bethesda, Maryland 20014.

The authors would like to thank Peter Fehrenbach, Christine Thompson, and Pearl Slafkes for their help in collecting the data, Anna Nichols for assistance with the enzyme analysis, Mimi Silberman and Ms. Slafkes for their help in the statistical analysis. They are also indebted to Ms. Slafkes for her important and extensive editorial assistance.

[2] Laboratory of Psychology and Psychopathology, NIMH.

[3] Chief, Clinical Neuropharmacology Branch, NIMH.

[4] Biological Psychiatry Branch, NIMH.

ity ... the Zuckerman because ... 'sensation-seeking' seemed related to some impulsive, extroverted behavioral features of bipolar patients" and "because of reported ... similarities in cortical average evoked responses ... between normal individuals scoring high on this scale and bipolar patients" (9, p. 150).

In terms of platelet MAO, Murphy *et al.* (9) found that "low MAO males manifested generalized elevations in their MMPI profile and Zuckerman sensation-seeking scale scores. In addition, negative correlations were found for most of the platelet MAO ... psychological test score relationships in males" (9, p. 155) although the correlation coefficients reached statistical significance for only four of the personality measures (MMPI-F Scale, Zuckerman General, Disinhibition, and Tendency-to-Boredom Scales). No significant relationships emerged for females, although there was a pattern of positive correlations of MMPI Scale scores with platelet MAO activity—a relationship opposite to that found for the males.

Significant correlations were also found between the psychological variables and activities of plasma amine oxidase, an enzyme which, although exhibiting some substrate similarities to platelet MAO, is clearly dissimilar to the platelet enzyme in many other characteristics[5] (10). Although no

[5] The plasma amine oxidase enzyme exhibits some substrate similarities to the platelet enzyme although it is clearly dissimilar to the platelet enzyme in many other characteristics (11). Unlike plasma amine oxidase, the platelet enzyme is extremely sensitive to inhibition by all of the agents used clinically as MAO inhibitors in the treatment of depression (11). This suggests that the level of platelet MAO activity may be more directly linked to psychological functioning than that of plasma amine oxidase. Thus, platelet amine oxidase inhibition by such drugs as phenelzine, isocarboxazid, and iproniazid used in the treatment of unipolar depression regularly leads to accumulation of neurotransmitter amines in brain and other tissues (10). These inhibitors are seen as having their effect through their influence on the regulation of synaptic effects in biogenic amine-mediated neurotransmitter pathways (10). Amine oxidase activity with characteristics of the plasma amine oxidase is found in blood vessels (5), and conceivably could affect vascular perfusion in tissues, including brain. Some possible mechanisms through which plasma amine oxidase activity might be relevant to psychological functioning have been considered elsewhere (9).

pattern emerged among females, among males there were significant negative correlations between plasma amine oxidase and six of the personality measures examined (Hy, Mf, Pa, and Sc Scales of the MMPI, General and Experience-Seeking Scales of the Zuckerman). Eleven of the 12 other correlations, although not significant, were also negative—suggesting the possibility of a general tendency toward impulsive acting-out behavior among men with low MAO activity.

The present study continues to explore the relationship between MAO activity levels and psychological functioning in normal persons in an attempt to clarify further the relationship between MAO activity and mental illness. Since the data employed are part of a larger ongoing study of how autonomic arousal and perceptual task performance relate to each other, the psychological measures used were chosen because of their established relationship with psychophysiological functioning among normals.

Because of the evidence that people who augment on cortical average evoked response tend to be sensation seekers (21), the present study replicates in part the Murphy *et al.* (9) study by using the Zuckerman (20) Sensation-Seeking Scale as one of its measures. The second measure used, the Nowlis Mood Scale (15), is related to psychophysiological functioning; positive moods have been shown to be correlated with high frequency and amplitude of skin conductance responses to stimuli (19). The third psychological measure, the Barron Ego Strength Scale (1), was chosen because it appears to be related to a particular pattern of psychophysiological reactivity. In a wide range of tasks, subjects high on this scale " ... respond 'discriminatively' physiologically, an ability [that] low ego strength subjects lack" (17, p. 319).

Finally, in an attempt to extend the data somewhat beyond the preferences expressed on the Zuckerman Sensation-Seeking Scale, the subjects were asked a series of questions in an attempt to gain some information about the level of activity and stimulus seeking of their social and leisure time pursuits.

Subjects

Ninety-three subjects were tested. All were paid volunteers, students or staff members, from a nearby community college.[6] They were selected randomly from a larger group of 375 who had provided blood samples for MAO determinations.[7] They then participated in a study of relationships between psychophysiological arousal and perceptual task performance, for which the psychological data of the present paper were gathered. Characteristics of the subjects are given in Table 1. Although the subjects tested obviously did not represent a true probability sample, the results would seem to be reasonably generalizable to similar populations. The following measures were used:

PSYCHOLOGICAL SCALES

Zuckerman Sensation-Seeking Scale (20). This was scored according to the author's original instructions, resulting in five measures: the General Sensation-Seeking Scale and the Thrill-Seeking, Experience-Seeking, Disinhibition, and Boredom-Susceptibility Subscales.

Nowlis Mood Scale (15). Subjects filled out the Nowlis checklist on two occasions separated by an interval of at least 24 hours. Separate principal component orthogonal factor analyses were performed for each day's responses. Six factors were extracted from each day's data, four of which were similar on both days (Vigorous-Cheerful Mood, Morose Mood, Paranoid Mood, and Warmhearted Mood).[8] Individual factor

scores were then computed for each subject. In order to create measures that would represent response characteristics generalizable beyond a single occasion, the individual's factor scores for these four factors for day 1 and day 2 were then combined.

Barron Ego Strength Scale (1). This was scored according to original instructions.

AMINE OXIDASE MEASURES

In the assay procedures for platelet and plasma amine activity, platelet-rich plasma obtained from venous blood samples was analyzed for platelet counts and for [^{14}C]-benzylamine deamination in duplicate aliquots with and without the addition of 0.2 mM pargyline HCl (13). The results are reported in units of nmol/10^8 platelets/hour for the platelet enzyme and nmol/ml/hour for the plasma enzyme. In looking for the psychological and behavioral correlates, we evaluated platelet and plasma amine oxidase activity levels in two ways: linearly and categorically.

Linearly. Nanomoles/10^8 platelets/hour for platelet MAO and nmol/ml/hour for plasma amine oxidase.

Categorically. a) For the extreme high enzyme activity analyses (extreme high platelet MAO and extreme high plasma amine oxidase), persons whose enzyme activities were more than one standard deviation above the means for members of their sex were scored 1; all others were scored 0. b) For the extreme low enzyme activity analysis (extreme low platelet MAO and extreme low plasma amine oxidase), persons whose enzyme activities were more than one standard deviation below the means for members of their sex were scored 1; all others were scored 0.

---

[6] All subjects were fully informed as to the nature of their participation and the purposes of the experiments in which they took part, and all agreed in writing to participate fully.

[7] The upper and lower 10 per cent of the 375 were studied separately by Buchsbaum *et al.* (3). Of these individuals, only 10 overlap with the 93 subjects reported here.

[8] Principal component factor analysis with rotation to simple structure was used. The loadings over .40 on the day 1 Vigorous-Cheerful factor were: active .75, energetic .74, vigorous .64, overjoyed .64, sluggish −.58, elated .55, playful .53. The parallel loadings for day 2 were: vigorous .68, energetic .65, elated .58 carefree .57, active .55, playful .53, overjoyed .41, drowsy −.62, tired −.66, sluggish −.73. For Morose, the day 1 factor loadings were: egotistic .74, sad .71, self-sufficient .70, regretful .56, angry .47. The parallel

loadings for day 2 were: sorry .84, sad .80, angry .46. The loadings on day 1 for the Paranoid factor were: suspicious .78, skeptical .68, dubious .62, fearful .59, rebellious .41. The parallel loadings for the Paranoid factor for day 2 were: dubious .80, suspicious .75, defiant .60, fearful .59, skeptical .46, rebellious .42. The loadings for the Warmhearted factor for day 1 were: warmhearted .79, kindly .78, witty .59, affectionate .46, pleased .50, carefree .49, boastful .41. The parallel loadings on day 2 for the Warmhearted factor were: affectionate .76, warmhearted .75, kindly .62, witty .58, overjoyed .49, playful .42, active .40.

SCHOOLER *et al.*

TABLE 1
Characteristics of Sample

	Male	Female	
No. in sample	46	47	
$\bar{X}$ age	21.8	22.0	
$\bar{X}$ platelet MAO (units of nmol/10^8 platelets/hour)	10.01	12.72	
Standard deviation: platelet MAO	3.55	3.89	
t-value			$3.49\ p < .001$
$\bar{X}$ Plasma amine oxidase (units of nmol/ml/hour)	19.49	19.33	
Standard deviation: plasma amine oxidase	4.04	5.63	
t-value			.16 N.S.[a]

[a] N.S., not significant.

LEISURE TIME BEHAVIOR

Questions asked about leisure time activities were: a) "In an average day, how many hours do you spend watching TV?"; "About how many hours of sleep do you get in an average night?"; "During the last 6 months, how many times have you attended a rock concert or festival? Aside from rock concerts, during the last 6 months how many times have you gone to a museum, concert, or play?"

Results

The data revealed no significant correlation between the two enzymes; the correlation between platelet and plasma amine oxidase levels was .01 for the total sample, −.04 for the males, and .07 for the females. The mean platelet MAO and plasma amine oxidase activity levels for males and females are given in Table 1. As has been reported in earlier studies (10), the platelet MAO activity values for women were significantly higher than they were for men. Since there were significant sex differences in MAO activity, the linear correlations are presented in three ways: a) total sample, statistically controlling sex through partial correlations; b) males only; and c) females only. It is not necessary, however, to partial the effects of sex in the extreme group analyses because the activity level needed for placement in the extreme categories was determined separately for each.sex. Unless otherwise noted, all correlations discussed in the text are significant at least at the .05 level using a two-tailed test. Since the number of subjects in the separate sex analysis is halved, a noticeably higher correlation is needed to achieve significance than is the case in analysis of the total sample.

PLATELET MAO ANALYSIS

Zuckerman Sensation-Seeking Scales. Platelet MAO activity was negatively related to sensation seeking. In the total sample partialling sex, the correlation between MAO platelet activity and the Zuckerman General Sensation-Seeking Scale was −.47 (Table 2). For men the correlation was −.52, replicating the findings of Murphy *et al.* (9). A similar significant negative relationship was found among women as well, a finding differing from that of the earlier study. Further results indicated that all of these findings were not merely due to subjects who had extremely high levels of platelet MAO activity; the negative correlation between MAO activity and sensation seeking remained significant even when extreme high platelet MAO subjects were excluded from the analysis ($r = -.32$, $p < .01$). Furthermore, although there was some indication in the earlier study that the negative relationship between platelet MAO activity and sensation-seeking was due to the high sensation-seeking scores of a subgroup with extremely low MAO activity (9), for the present total sample this was not the case; there was no significant correlation between extreme low platelet MAO activity and sensation seeking.

Examining the effects of extreme low platelet MAO activity in each sex separately, we found that although for men there was a positive relationship between extreme low platelet MAO activity and general sensation seeking (Table 2), the linear relationship between sensation seeking and low platelet MAO activity remained negatively significant ($r = -.48$, $p < .001$) even when the subgroup of male subjects with extreme low MAO activity scores was ex-

TABLE 2
Significant Correlations of Platelet MAO Activity with Psychological Variables

Psychological Variables	Linear						Categorical											
							Extreme low MAO individuals = 1, Others = 0						Extreme high MAO individuals = 1, Others = 0					
	Total		Male		Female		Total		Male		Female		Total		Male		Female	
	r	p	r	p	r	p	r	p	r	p	r	p	r	p	r	p	r	p
Zuckerman Sensation-Seeking Scales																		
General Sensation-Seeking	−.47	=.001	−.52	=.001	−.43	=.004			.30	=.05			−.37	=.001			−.41	=.006
Thrill-Seeking	−.25	=.02			−.39	=.009								=.04			−.40	=.008
Experience-Seeking	−.43	=.001	−.43	=.003	−.42	=.004							−.22	=.004	−.32	=.03		
Disinhibition	−.24	=.02											−.30		−.29	=.05		
Boredom-Susceptibility	−.33	=.002	−.41	=.006			.21	=.05					−.22	=.04				
Nowlis Mood Scale																		
Morose mood	.24	=.03	.39	=.008			−.24	=.02	−.31	=.04								
Barron Ego Strength Scale	−.22	=.04					.21	=.05					−.21	=.05			−.30	=.05

cluded from the analysis. Thus, the results strongly suggested that for men the negative relationship between platelet MAO and sensation seeking was a linear one existing throughout the continuum of platelet MAO activity.

When we looked to see whether the negative relationship between MAO activity level and stimulus seeking among women was due to an extreme group, the results were more ambiguous. Although the negative linear relationship between platelet MAO activity and sensation seeking was significant (Table 2), the extreme high platelet MAO women showed a significant decrement in sensation seeking (Table 2), and when this extreme group was omitted, the linear negative relationship between platelet MAO activity and sensation seeking among women was reduced and ceased to be significant ($r = -.13, p = .243$).

In addition to the General Sensation-Seeking Scale, the Zuckerman (20) Scale consists of four subscales. A general pattern in the results suggested negative relationships between all of these subscales and platelet MAO activity (Table 2). Among the subscales, the strongest and most consistent relationships were in the subscale measuring experience seeking (Table 2).

Nowlis Mood Scale. High platelet MAO activity also appeared to be related to negative affect. There was a positive linear correlation between platelet MAO activity and the Morose Mood factor score (Table 2), with high loadings on such negative moods as sad, angry, and sorry both for the total sample partialling sex and for men only. It appears that these overall findings were due, at least in part, to the absence of morose mood among those with extreme low platelet MAO activity (Table 2). Thus, when the extreme low platelet MAO activity group was removed from the analysis and the linear correlations were replicated with the remaining portion of the sample, the correlations between platelet MAO activity and morose mood, although still in the same direction, ceased to be significant (the correlation for the total sample partialling sex being .11, $p = .36$, and for the men .25, $p = .11$).

Barron Ego Strength Scale. In the total

sample there was a small but significant negative correlation between ego strength and platelet MAO activity (see Table 2). Here, too, however, the result appeared to be influenced primarily by the extreme groups: the positive correlation between the Ego Strength Scale and the extreme low score, and the negative correlation between the Ego Strength Scale and the extreme high platelet MAO score being of the same magnitude as the negative linear correlation between the Ego Strength score and platelet MAO activity (Table 2). When the sexes were analyzed separately, a negative relationship between platelet MAO activity and ego strength was found for females only, where the extreme high platelet MAO group (Table 2) showed low ego strength, as measured by the Barron Scale.

In summary then, in this sample of normal individuals platelet MAO activity was negatively correlated with sensation seeking across the whole range of MAO activity levels. Individuals in the extreme low range of MAO activity also showed high ego strength and the absence of negative affect, while those in the extreme high range of MAO activity had relatively low scores on the Ego Strength Scale. Although these results are compatible with the picture of a manic prone person, as suggested by the hypothesis that low platelet MAO is a precursor of an illness with a manic component, they are, on the face of it, difficult to reconcile with the commonly accepted picture of the schizophrenic or preschizophrenic personality.

PLASMA AMINE OXIDASE ANALYSIS

Zuckerman Sensation-Seeking Scale. Low plasma amine oxidase activity also was related to sensation seeking, but much less extensively than was low platelet MAO activity. The findings all involved the extreme low plasma groups. Thus, for the total sample and among men and women separately, persons in the extreme low plasma groups scored high on the Zuckerman Tendency-to-Boredom Subscale; among women only there was a similar relationship with the Zuckerman Experience-Seeking Subscale (Table 3).

Nowlis Mood Scale. In terms of the lin-

TABLE 3

Significant Correlations of Plasma Amine Oxidase Activity with Psychological Variables

	Linear						Categorical											
							Extreme low individuals = 1, Others = 0						Extreme high individuals = 1, Others = 0					
	Total		Male		Female		Total		Male		Female		Total		Male		Female	
Psychological Variables	r	p	r	p	r	p	r	p	r	p	r	p	r	p	r	p	r	p
Zuckerman Sensation-Seeking Scales																		
General Sensation-Seeking											.33	=.03						
Boredom-Susceptibility					.52	=.001	.33	=.001	.32	=.03	.35	=.02						
Nowlis Mood Scale																		
Paranoid	.35	=.001											.28	=.008			.47	=.001
Vigorous					-.29	=.057												

ear analysis, there was a negative relationship between vigorous mood and plasma amine oxidase activity among women (Table 3). A somewhat more general finding was the positive linear correlation of plasma amine oxidase activity with paranoid mood, occurring not only among women but also in the total sample when the effects of sex were partialled (Table 3). This positive correlation between plasma amine oxidase activity and a mood factor highly loaded on suspicious, dubious, and fearful moods seemed to be at least partially the result of the high level of paranoid mood among the extreme high plasma amine oxidase activity group. When the latter group was removed from the analysis, the linear correlations, although still in the same direction, were reduced, the partial correlation for the total sample being .21, $p = .07$, and for women $r = .16, p = .34$.

Barron Ego Strength Scale. As opposed to the findings for platelet MAO activity, no significant relationships were found between plasma amine oxidase activity and the Barron Ego Strength Scale.

Despite the lesser number of significant correlations between psychological characteristics and plasma amine oxidase activity than between such characteristics and platelet MAO activity, the results were similar to those of platelet MAO in suggesting that low amine oxidase activity is related to sensation seeking and comparatively positive affect.[9]

LEISURE TIME ACTIVITIES

MAO activity level was also related to the way in which individuals spend their leisure time and, although these correlations were not as consistent or as significant, they paralleled those of the psycho-

[9] A brief measure of anxiety was also included (7). Only one significant relationship between this measure of anxiety and MAO activity was found, but it was an intriguing one. Those individuals who were within one standard deviation of the mean for their sex in both the level of their plasma and platelet MAO activity showed less anxiety. The correlation for the total sample was $-.32, p = .002$; for the men only $-.43, p = .003$; and for the women $-.25, p = .08$. Thus, those in the midgroup of both MAO measures showed less anxiety than those who did not have such a generally balanced level of amine oxidase activity.

logical variables (Table 4). Thus, for example, in the total sample there was a tendency for those with low platelet MAO activity to seek the stimulation of rock concerts ($p < .07$) and museums, concerts, and plays ($p < .08$). In the separate sex analysis, men in the extreme high platelet MAO activity group tended to go less to rock concerts ($p < .07$) and museums, concerts, and plays ($p < .08$). Among women, those with extreme high platelet MAO activity slept more.

A somewhat similar pattern emerged for plasma amine oxidase activity. In the total sample, low plasma amine oxidase activity was linearly related to more museum going and to less TV watching ($p < .08$) and sleeping ($p < .06$) (Table 4). The latter two findings, however, may have been due to the extreme high amine oxidase activity group since those in this group showed a tendency both to sleep more ($p < .06$) and watch TV more ($p = .10$). In the separate sex analysis, among women there was a positive linear correlation between plasma amine oxidase levels of activity and TV watching and a negative correlation between the plasma amine oxidase activity level and going to museums, concerts, and plays. Among men, there was a significant positive correlation between extreme low plasma amine oxidase activity and going to rock concerts and museums and between extreme high plasma amine oxidase activity and sleep, whereas women in the high plasma amine oxidase group watched TV more (Table 4).

Although somewhat spotty, these relationships between MAO platelet and plasma amine oxidase activity and leisure time behavior gave further support to the picture which emerged of low MAO activity individuals—a picture which, in both its psychological and behavioral aspects, was quite congruent with the mania associated with bipolar illness but was difficult to reconcile with the clinical course of schizophrenia.

Discussion

The most striking result of this study was that we generally replicated and extended earlier findings linking activity dif-

TABLE 4

Correlations of Amine Oxidase Activity with Leisure Time Activities (p ≤ .10)

Activities	Linear						Categorical											
							Extreme low individuals = 1, Others = 0						Extreme high individuals = 1, Others = 0					
	Total		Male		Female		Total		Male		Female		Total		Male		Female	
	r	p	r	p	r	p	r	p	r	p	r	p	r	p	r	p	r	p
Platelet																		
Sleep					.26	=.07											.29	=.05
Attend rock concerts	−.19	=.07																
Go to museums	−.19	=.08																
Plasma																		
Watch TV	.19	=.08											−.18	=.08				
Sleep	.19	=.06											−.19	=.08				
Attend rock concerts			.34	=.02	.43	=.003	.28	=.007	.37	=.01			.17	=.10				
Go to museums	−.23	=.03			−.25	=.01	.24	=.02	.42	=.004			.19	=.06	.31	=.04	.30	=.05

ferences in two biogenic amine-related enzymes to differences in psychological functioning among normal persons. We found that low levels of MAO activity measured in platelets were related to sensation seeking, high ego strength, positive affect, and high activity levels. Interestingly, we found generally similar, although somewhat weaker, psychological correlates for plasma amine oxidase activity even though no intercorrelation between the activities of the two enzymes was found in either the present or previous studies (9, 13). Although similar personality correlates for the plasma enzyme have been previously reported (9), we have no clear understanding of the basis for these correlations between the plasma enzyme and psychological functioning.

Although the pattern of correlations between platelet MAO activity and psychological functioning (9) seems compatible with a previously reported association between reduced MAO activity and the occurrence of bipolar (manic-depressive) affective disorders (12), it does not appear to be compatible with reported associations of low MAO activity and some of the more common conceptions of a preschizophrenic, particularly prechronic schizophrenic, personality. Hence, the findings of this paper pose problems for theories which relate low MAO activity levels specifically to schizophrenia. In recognition of such discrepancies between MAO findings and classical psychiatric diagnostic entities, it has been suggested that rather than being related to a specific psychiatric syndrome, reduced MAO activity may be associated with some general vulnerability factor increasing the risk for psychopathology of various forms (3, 10).

There are, nevertheless, several ways in which a schizophrenia/MAO relationship may exist and still be congruent with the present findings. One possibility is that low MAO activity does not have an effect unless it occurs in conjunction with other biochemical alterations, for example, the presence of another enzymatic defect or of stress-induced changes in catecholamines or other central neuromodulator amines. In such a model, MAO is viewed as a regulatory enzyme, and a reduction in MAO activity as a limiting, less adaptive factor in the biological response to physiological or psychological stressors. Such a possibility is suggested by the finding that the combination of extremely low MAO activity and low dopamine β-hydroxylase is associated with deficits in attentional performance (4). Another possibility suggesting that a schizophrenia/MAO relationship may exist is that the psychological effects of low MAO activity may increase the likelihood of the occurrence of schizophrenia in individuals made susceptible to the disorder by other factors. For example, it is quite possible that the stimulant effects, including increased psychomotor activity, which characterize one of the common forms of behavioral toxicity observed during the administration of MAO-inhibiting drugs to both normals and psychiatric patients (8) might be so stressful to a schizophrenia-prone person as to cause a breakdown or exacerbation of symptoms.

Although these speculations about the relationship between lowered MAO activity and schizophrenia are at best tentative, the present findings are congruent with the possibility of an association between low platelet MAO activity and the manic phase of bipolar disorder.

There is also evidence linking low MAO activity levels to the depressive poles of the illness. Buchsbaum et al. (3) found that low MAO activity levels were related to suicidal behavior. Further research by these workers indicated that suicidal tendencies among low MAO activity individuals are in fact congruent with our general picture, since such psychopathological correlates of low MAO activity appear to occur most frequently among individuals with an augmenting style of stimulus intensity control (2). This suggests that the negative effects of low MAO activity are most likely to occur when a low level of MAO activity interacts with a response style that enhances and magnifies the behavioral activating effects of low MAO activity.

In terms of our understanding of the manic pole of bipolar disorder, our finding of a relationship between low MAO activity and psychological functioning congruent with that of the manic personality is supported by the results of research with rhesus monkeys. Redmond and Murphy (16) found correlations in such monkeys between platelet MAO activity and behaviors similar to those we found among normal human subjects. Monkeys with low MAO activity were more social, more active, more playful, and slept less. If further research continues to indicate that low MAO individuals are characterized by sensation seeking, high activity level, high ego strength, and positive affect, it would suggest that if low MAO activity is a vulnerability factor for manic-depressive illness, it is a genetic factor whose presence may also be of some benefit to the individual, a factor determined by a gene whose positive effect on the likelihood of the individual's reproducing himself insures its own continuation.

REFERENCES

1. Barron, F. An ego-strength scale which predicts response to psychotherapy. In Welsh, G. S., and Dahlstrom, W. G., Eds., *Basic Readings on the MMPI in Psychology and Medicine*, pp. 226–234. University of Minnesota Press, Minneapolis, 1956.
2. Buchsbaum, M. S., Haier, R. J., and Murphy, D. L. Suicide attempts, platelet monoamine oxidase and the average evoked response. Acta Psychiatr. Scand., *56:* 69–79, 1977.
3. Buchsbaum, M. S., Murphy, D. L., and Coursey, R. D. The biochemical high risk paradigm: Behavioral and familial correlates of low platelet monoamine oxidase activity. Science, *194:* 339–341, 1976.
4. Buchsbaum, M. S., Murphy, D. L., Coursey, R. D., Lake, R., *et al.* Platelet monoamine oxidase, plasma dopamine-beta-hydroxylase and attention in a biochemical high-risk sample. J. Psychiatr. Res. In press.
5. Goridis, C., and Neff, N. H. Selective localization of monoamine oxidase forms in rat mesenteric artery. In Usdin, E., and Snyder, S., Eds., *Frontiers in Catecholamine Research*, pp. 157–160. Pergamon Press, Oxford, England, 1973.
6. Hathaway, S. R., and McKinley, J. C. *Minnesota Multiphasic Personality Inventory*. Psychological Corporation, New York, 1943.
7. Kohn, M. L., and Schooler, C. Class, occupation, and orientation. Am. Sociol. Rev., *34:* 659–678, 1969.
8. Murphy, D. L. The behavioral toxicity of monoamine-oxidase inhibiting antidepressants. Adv. Pharmacol. Chemother., *14:* 71–105, 1977.
9. Murphy, D. L., Belmaker, R., Buchsbaum, M. S., *et al.* Biogenic amine-related enzymes and personality variations in normals. Psychol. Med., *7:* 149–157, 1977.

SCHOOLER *et al.*

10. Murphy, D. L., Belmaker, R., and Wyatt, R. J. Monoamine oxidase in schizophrenia and other behavioral disorders. J. Psychiatr. Res., *11:* 221–247, 1974.

11. Murphy, D. L., and Donnelly, C. H. Monoamine oxidase in man: Enzyme characteristics in platelets, plasma, and other human tissues. In Usdin, E., Ed., *Neuropsychopharmacology of Monoamines and Their Regulatory Enzymes,* pp. 71–85. Raven Press, New York, 1974.

12. Murphy, D. L., and Weiss, R. Reduced monoamine oxidase activity in blood platelets from bipolar depressed patients. Am. J. Psychiatry, *128:* 1351–1357, 1972.

13. Murphy, D. L., Wright, C., Buchsbaum, M., *et al.* Platelet and plasma amine oxidase activity in 680 normals: Sex and age differences and stability over time. Biochem. Med., *16:* 254–265, 1976.

14. Nies, A., Robinson, D. S., Lamborn, K. R., *et al.* Genetic control of platelet and plasma monoamine oxidase activity. Arch. Gen. Psychiatry, *28:* 834–838, 1973.

15. Nowlis, V. Research with the mood adjective check list. In Tomkins, S., and Izard, E., Eds., *Affect, Cognition, and Personality,* pp. 353–389.

Springer, New York, 1965.

16. Redmond, D. E., and Murphy, D. L. Behavioral correlates of platelet monoamine oxidase (MAO) activity in rhesus monkeys. Psychosom. Med., *37:* 80, 1975.

17. Roessler, R. Personality, psychophysiology, and performance. Psychophysiology, *10:* 315–327, 1973.

18. Wyatt, R. J., Murphy, D. L., Belmaker, R., *et al.* Reduced monoamine oxidase activity in platelets: A possible genetic marker for vulnerability to schizophrenia. Science, *179:* 916–918, 1973.

19. Zahn, T. P., and Little, B. C. The Psychophysiology of Everyday Life: Autonomic Concomitants of Daily Changes in Mood. Read before the Annual Meeting for the Society for Psychophysiological Research, Salt Lake City, Utah, 1974.

20. Zuckerman, M. The sensation seeking motive. In Maher, B., Ed., *Progress in Experimental Personality Research,* Vol. 7, pp. 79–148. Academic Press, New York, 1974.

21. Zuckerman, M., Murtaugh, T., and Siegel, J. Sensation seeking and cortical augmenting-reducing. Psychopharmacologia, *11:* 535–542, 1974.

Section Five

Behavioural Genetics

Editorial Commentary

on

Behavioural Genetics

Looking to heredity for answers to the origins of personality is a comparatively ancient procedure. Over 100 years ago Galton distinguished between mono- and dizygotic twins. The simple, straightforward hypothesis deriving from Galton's distinction was that any differences between identical (mono-zygotic-MZ) twins must be attributable to the environment (since genetic contribution had presumably been held constant). Differences between fraternal (dizygotic-DZ) twins could be due to either heredity or the environment. At the outset, it should be pointed out that the assumption that MZ twins are genetically identical is less a postulate of the laws of inheritance than a hypothesis (Darlington, 1954). Darlington notes that intra-chromosomal genetic changes (gene mutations or chromosome errors at mitosis) may result in asymmetry. Indeed, it is even possible for two sperms to fertilize the halves of one egg. One additional cogent criticism of this research strategy concerns the evidence that MZ twins have a more homogeneous environment than DZ twins (Scarr, 1965; Smith, 1965). That is, some of the variance in high MZ intragroup correlations may be accounted for by highly similar environments rather than genetics. This criticism obviously does not effect those studies that examined twins raised in separate homes. For the moment, however, we shall accept with candor the dominant research design contrasting sets of twins.

One of the earliest attempts to empirically examine twin sets with regards to mental and physical characteristics was the often cited Newman, Freeman and Holzinger (1937) study. 50 fraternal and 50 identical twins were compared on a battery of tests. The following is the author's widely quoted conclusion: "the physical characteristics are least affected by the environment, that intelligence is affected more; educational achievement still more; and personality or temperament, if our tests can be relied upon, the most," p. 192. Eysenck (1967) points out that not only are there serious questions about the reliability and validity of the personality instruments used by Newman, Freeman and Holzinger but the tests were designed for adults, not children. Despite the obvious drawbacks, which can be made in armchair comfort with the help of retrospect, the early research was certainly foundational and served heuristic purposes. Some 30 years after the Newman study, Gottesman (1965) reported the results of a study using 82 pairs of MZ twins and 68 pairs of DZ twins. According to the MMPI, significant differences in heritability were found, for sexes combined, on the depression, psychopathic deviate, paranoia, schizophrenia, and social introversion scales. Those readers interested in a reasonably comprehensive review of the early research on heritability and personality should consult Eysenck (1967).

A recent, ambitious attempt to examine genetic contributions to personality was made by Claridge, Canter and Hume, published in monograph form in 1973. Their sample consisted of 44 pairs of MZ twins and 51 pairs of DZ twins, selected from the city of Glasgow and controlled for sex, age, SES, IQ and length of separation. Approximately three-quarters of the sample was female. Included in the extensive test battery were four personality questionnaires (EPI, 16PF, Fould's Hostility Scale and the Sociability/Impulsivity Scale), five cognitive instruments to look at divergent thinking (such as word association, Making Objects Test and Gottschaldt Figures), three conceptual thinking tests (such as Chapman's Card Sorting tests) and eight psychophysiological tests (skin potential, finger pulse volume, alpha activity, heart rate, two-flash threshold, spiral aftereffect, habituation to twenty 1 kHz tones of 1 second duration and the cold pressor test). The first four were considered tests of sympathetic responsiveness, the next two perceptual tests and the last two physiological stressors. The results were reported in intraclass correlations and F values looking at within-pair variances. The logic of such analysis dictated that high within-group correlations for MZ twins – relative to the DZ twins – indicated a genetic component on that dependent measure. According to the personality questionnaires, the MZ twins were significantly more alike on sociability, self-criticism and intropunitiveness, the last two traits being attributable to variations in anxiety and extraversion. Four of the five correlations for individual cognitive tests were higher in MZ twins than DZ twins, however, only one difference actually achieved significance. This test, word association, was highly loaded on an intelligence factor in a principle components analysis, suggesting that the MZ/DZ differences may reflect a genetic contribution to IQ. There was a significant difference between the twin groups on Chapman's Card Sorting Test 1, which looks at the effects of distraction. This suggests that genetic factors may be important in those areas of conceptual performance where exclusion of irrelevant stimuli is required. The psychophysiological tests must be viewed from a slightly different perspective. It is assumed that none of the measures reflect invariant patterns of response for an individual. Consequently, the direct question of whether a particular mechanism is affected by genetic factors is misleading. Rather, the appropriate consideration should be whether a situational *reaction,* as monitored by a physiological measure, is affected by genetic factors. Factor analysis of the 27 psychophysiological

components yielded five separate factors: (1) autonomic level, (2) sympathetic response measures, (3) EEG, (4) electrodermal activity, (5) perceptual efficiency. Based on the factor analysis, four physiological systems were described: (1) autonomic balance, (2) sympathetic responsivity, (3) alpha activity, (4) spontaneous skin potential activity. The influence of genetics seems to be most apparent in the first (MZ $r = 0.57$; DZ $R = 0.16$) and last (MZ $R = 0.54$; DZ $r = 0.10$) factors, though it is noteworthy that all four factors combined accounted for *less than half* of the total variance.

Before embarking on a number of past and current considerations on the genetics of personality, it would be worthwhile to address several general points. Assuming that introversion/extraversion was influenced by some genetic component, that influence could be specific or polygenic. Most gene determined human variability derives from polygenic effects. This amounts to the simultaneous occurrence of numerous *minor* aberrations which when all lumped together are not individually detectable. In fact, they blend into a Gaussian distribution for that trait. A polygene is something like a Mendelian major gene; it has a small multiply-mediated effect on trait variation relative to all the variation observed in that trait. The expression of certain traits depends much more on the cumulative pulling power of all genes concerned than on a few unspecific genes. Hence, polygenes tend to be very sensitive to environmental factors (endogenous as well as exogenous). The principle alternative to polygenes are those disorders with specific gene aetiologies. Huntington's chorea, for instance, is caused by *one* dominant gene, though as yet we are unable to trace the pathway from the gene to its behavioural expression. Phenylketonuria (PKU) is caused by two recessive alleles, wherein a specific congenital metabolic error exists. In the case of PKU, heterozygotes can be identified biochemically, whereas in Huntington's disease the biochemical error is unknown and unaffected heterozygotes cannot be identified.

The cases of single-gene substitution are relatively straightforward. However, it sometimes happens that a continuous distribution of genotypes results in discrete phenotypes for certain disorders. The disorder would appear to have a continuously distributed liability, and would only be manifested when some variable exceeds a threshold. The phenotypic discontinuity is not genetic, arising only when the threshold is exceeded. There are many assorted quasicontinuous disorders, such as diabetes mellitus, ulcers and cleft palate. Some theorize that schizophrenia falls in this category.

If we wish to argue that a personality trait, such as introversion/extraversion, has a genetic component we are, in effect, saying that a specific genetically-coded biochemical error exists which results in the behaviour we label introversion or extraversion. The trait itself *cannot* be inherited. There must be some intermediary effect, such as a genetic code, which results in a biochemical error. Such a biochemical error, if we accept the Pavlov–Gray nervous system typology, may result in an imbalance of the autonomic nervous system (i.e. sympathetic or parasympathetic dominance). This effect could derive from blocking or facilitation of the ARAS. Given what we know about the behavioural manifestations of introversion/extraversion, it is highly *un*likely that it could be tied to a specific gene, or for that matter, exclusively to heredity without regard to the environment.

These concluding introductory remarks form an essential backdrop to the readings in this section. It is easy to be lulled into the conclusion that one can literally inherit personality. Rather, our mission is to ask what aspect of the personality, if any, is genetically controlled. The problem we face is precisely that explored by Dobzhansky, namely teasing apart genetic fixity from phenotypic plasticity. Dobzhansky (1960) maintains 'that an essential feature of human evolution which has made our species unique has been the establishment of a genetically controlled plasticity of personality traits.' Were we able to hold

development constant, observed variance in personality traits would reflect genotypic variability. In reality, development is unique for every individual. Hence, variance in personality traits unequivocally reflects environmental factors. Returning then to the 'mission', the question is to what extent we inherit consitutional factors which influence the acquisition of certain personality traits. If something akin to 'sympathetic dominance' is inherited, there is, in effect, a predisposition to behaviour patterns that might be labelled introversion (and the panoply of traits associated with introversion).

References

Claridge, G. S., Hume, W. I., and Canter, S. (1973). *Personality Differences and Biological Variations: A Study of Twins.* (Oxford: Pergamon Press)

Darlington, C. D. (1954). Heredity and environment. Proceedings of the IX International Congress of Genetics. *Caryologia,* 370–381

Dobzhansky, T. (1960). *The Biological Basis of Freedom.* p. 52. (New York: Columbia University Press)

Eyzenck, H. J. (1967). *The Biological Basis of Personality.* (Springfield Charles C. Thomas)

Gottesman, I. I. (1965) Genetic variance in adaptive personality traits. Paper read at the Annual Meeting of the American Psychological Association, Division of Developmental Psychology

Newman, H. H., Freeman, F. N., and Holzinger, K. J. (1937). *Twins.* (Chicago: University of Chicago Press)

Scarr, S. (1965). The inheritance of sociability. Paper read at the Annual Meeting of the American Psychological Association

Smith, R. T. (1965). A comparison of socioenvironmental factors in monozygotic and dyzygotic twins. In S. G. Vandenberg (eds.), *Methods and Goals in Human Behavior Genetics.* (New York: Academic Press)

From H. J. Eysenck (1956). Acta Psychologica, *12*, 95-110, *by kind permission of the author and North-Holland Publishing Company*

THE INHERITANCE OF EXTRAVERSION-INTROVERSION

BY

H. J. EYSENCK

Institute of Psychiatry (Maudsley Hospital), London University

1. INTRODUCTION

The data reported in this paper formed part of an investigation conducted under the writer's direction by Dr. H. McLeod and Dr. D. Blewett from 1951—1953. This investigation was in part made possible by a grant from the Eugenics Society. Some of the results have been reported in Ph. D. theses (2, 16) and in article form (3).

The investigation as a whole was designed to answer a number of different questions, some of which only will be discussed in this paper. In essence we shall be concerned with two closely related problems. The first of these is the factorial definition and measurement of the personality dimension or continuum known as extraversion-introversion; the other is the discovery of the degree to which heredity plays a part in determining a person's position on this continuum. Most of the work on extraversion-introversion has been done with adult subjects; in this study we shall be concerned with school children, mostly of an age between 145 and 185 months.

A number of questions arose in the course of the investigation, or were from the outset considered to determine the design of the experiment. These additional questions, such as, for instance, the relationship between extraversion-introversion and Rorschach's concept of the extratensive/introvertive type of personality, will be discussed as they arise in the course of this paper.

2. THE PROBLEM OF MEASUREMENT

A considerable amount of experimental material relevant to the measurement of extraversion-introversion has been discussed in previous publications by the present writer (5, 6, 10). By and large the results reported there have shown that there is experimental evidence in favour of the existence of some such personality continuum as Jung postulated, at least among adults; that this dimension can be found, both among normal and among neurotic subjects; and that a variety of different tests could be constructed to measure this dimension with different degrees of reliability and validity. It was further found that, as Jung had postulated, extraverted neurotics tended to develop hysterical or psychopathic symptoms, whereas introverted neurotics tended to develop dysthymic symptoms, such as anxiety, reactive depression, or obsessional features. None of the studies carried out in this laboratory, or available in the literature, had concerned themselves with measurement of extraversion-introversion in children. Consequently it appeared worth-while to test the hypothesis that behavioural relationships similar to those found among adults could also be found among children to define an extravert-introvert continuum.

Among the types of measures used with adults had been objective behaviour tests, ratings, and self-ratings, and it seemed desirable to include these divergent types of measures in the children's study also. In addition, however, it was decided to include a rather different type of test, namely, the Rorschach. Although the writer has been somewhat critical of its use as a "global" measure of personality, some attempts made by members of the department had indicated that when socres on this test are used in the usual psychometric manner, meaningful relations can be established, although (or possibly because) the test thus loses its subjective and interpretive character (4). The main reason for introducing the Rorschach into the experiment was, of course, the fact that Rorschach's theory contains the concept of the opposed types of the "extratensive" and the "introvertive" person. Although Rorschach workers often deny that these terms are co-extensive with Jung's typology, nevertheless it seemed a reasonable hypothesis to expect a considerable degree of similarity. Curiously enough no test of this hypothesis had ever been carried out previously to our knowledge, and consequently a number of Rorschach scores were included in our battery.

In addition to the variables discussed so far, we also included a battery of intelligence tests and a battery of autonomic measures. There are two main reasons for the inclusion of the battery of intelligence tests. In the first place, some at least of the tests used for the measurement of extraversion were known to be also measures of intelligence. Without the inclusion of reliable and valid measures of intelligence, therefore, contamination between the effects of extraversion and those of intelligence might easily have taken place. This is particularly obvious in the case of some of the Rorschach variables. Thus, for instance, a high movement score on the

Rorschach, according to Klopfer, indicates high intelligence. It also, however, indicates introversion. Assuming, for the moment, both these hypotheses to be true, before using the $M \%$ score as a measure of extraversion, we would have to partial out that part of the variance assignable to intelligence.

The second reason for including tests of intelligence in our battery was as follows. Most of the work on the inheritance of intelligence has made use of a single test. This does not seem permissible as Eysenck and Prell (11) have argued in a recent paper, because the fact that the score on a given test has a high h^2 when a comparison is made between the scores of identical and fraternal twins, is indeterminate as long as we have no way of assigning the hereditary component indicated in this way to a specific part of the factor variance.[1] Thus, for example, if the Binet test were found to give much higher intra-class correlations for identical than for fraternal twins, we would still not know whether the hereditary influence thus indicated affected the general intellectual ability measured by the test, or the verbal ability also measured, or the numerical ability, or any of the other factors contributing to the total variance. The conclusion reached by Eysenck and Prell was that it is not test scores which should be submitted to such analysis but factor scores, and accordingly a number of intelligence tests were included here to make possible such an analysis of factor scores.

Also included were a number of autonomic measures, such as systolic and diastolic blood pressure, pulse rate in the resting state and under stress, sub-lingual and finger temperature, and dermographic latency. The main reason for the inclusion of these measures was as follows. In "The Structure of Human Personality" (8) a number of studies have been summarized suggesting that autonomic lability may be related to neuroticism. If this were true, then it should follow that autonomic measures of this type should correlate with measures known to be good indicators of neuroticism, such as, for instance, body sway suggestibility. Thus, if autonomic measures and a few known tests of neuroticism were included, and if the theory were to be substantiated by our research, then we would expect, in addition to a factor of extraversion-introversion and a factor of intelligence, also to find a factor of neuroticism containing some, if not all, of these autonomic tests. In this way it was hoped to extend the work begun by Eysenck and Prell in 1951 (11).

---

[1] h^2 is the symbol used by Holzinger to denote a statistic proposed by him as a measure of the degree of hereditary determination of a given trait or ability. For a critical discussion of it, cf. May (17).

The actual tests and measures included in this study will be described briefly in the third section; a much longer description will be found in the theses by McLeod and Blewett (16, 2). In most cases the rationale for including a test has not been given here because considerations of space make this impracticable. A thorough documentation can be found in the writer's previous summaries of work done on these problems. Quite generally it may be said that a test was included as a possible measure of introversion-extraversion when it either had in the past been found in factorial analyses to have significant projections on this factor among adults, or when it had in the past been found to differentiate significantly between hysterics, the neurotic prototype of the extravert, and dysthymics, the neurotic prototype of the introvert. This would, of course, be reasonable only on the assumption that the behaviour of children and their responses to the test situation are similar to those of adults. This assumption appears to be reasonable and, as will be seen in the section on Results, is, in fact, borne out.

3. THE SAMPLE STUDIED

Little need be said here as in all essentials this study is a duplication of the Eysenck–Prell study. We have relied again on the differences found between identical and fraternal twins to give us evidence regarding the hereditary determination of any particular test score or factor score used in the investigation. The general theory is too well-known to be discussed in any detail: it depends on the fact that differences between identical twins must be due to environment; differences between fraternal twins may be due to either environment or heredity. If, therefore, differences between identical twins and differences between fraternal twins are equal in size, the total variance of the particular test under investigation can be ascribed to environmental influences. The greater the similarity of identical twins as compared with fraternal twins, the greater will be the amount of hereditary influence it is necessary to postulate. A convenient formula to assess the amount of hereditary influence has been given by Holzinger. His statistic, which he calls h^2, has frequently been criticized. A general discussion of the twin method, the difficulties which it gives rise to, and possible criticisms of it is given elsewhere (11), and a discussion of Holsinger's h^2 statistic will be found in another paper from this department (17).

The exact details of the population of children used in the present study have been published by Blewett (3). Here it is merely necessary to summarize the main points. Our sample was drawn from four metropolitan boroughs in South London. Our thanks here are due to the co-operation of the London County Council who wrote to headmasters of all the L.C.C. secondary schools in the boroughs of Camberwell, Southwark, Lambeth and Lewisham, requesting a report on any twins on their registers. 102 pairs of twins were located, of whom 56 pairs were subsequently tested. Four of these were later dropped on a random basis to equate numbers of pairs in the four groups: male identical, female identical, male fraternal, and female fraternal, retaining 13 pairs in each group. A thorough check was carried out to avoid various well-known sources of error in the selection of the sample; these are discussed in detail by Blewett.

The criteria used in this study were practically identical with those used by Eysenck and Prell, including rating scales for closeness of similarity of facial features, general habitus, hair colour and distribution, iris pigmentation, shape of ears, and teeth. Height and weight were measured and the ability of the subjects to taste phenyl-thio-carbamide was established. In addition, blood groupings and finger-prints were taken into account. Again, details are given by Blewett (3) and there is little doubt that the final decision regarding the zygoticity of the twin pairs arrived at on the basis of all these criteria is essentially correct. The mean age of the children tested was 166 months, with a standard deviation of 11 months. Age was partialled out from the intercorrelations in the factor analysis as it seemed essential to have data not contaminated by this variable.

4. TESTS USED

The tests used in this investigation will now be briefly described. In connection with each will be given an index which will enable the reader to identify it in the factor analysis. The first two variables included in the factor analysis are zygoticity (index number 1), and sex (index number 2); these are not exactly tests in any sense of the word, but are referred to here, nevertheless, in order to keep all the index numbers together. The scoring in these cases was as follows: zygoticity — $M = 1$, $D = 2$; sex — $M = 1$, $F = 0$.

Next we have the set of intelligence tests included in this investigation. Most of these were taken from Thurstone's tests of primary mental abilities for ages 11—17. These are so widely used that it would serve no useful purpose to describe them in detail. The directions given in the Revised Manual (1949) were followed in the administration, and Thurstone's scoring methods were used throughout. The particular tests used were the verbal scale (index number 8), the numbers scale (index number 9), the space scale (index number 16), the reasoning scale (index number 17), the fluency scale (index number 18) and the total score (index number 19), calculated according to Thurstone's formula:

$V + S + 2N + 2R + W.$

In addition, we used the Furneaux level and speed tests. These are described in some detail by Eysenck (7) and by Blewett (3).

Our next set of scores is derived from the Rorschach test. Standard methods of administration, enquiry, and testing the limits were employed. We followed the method outlined by Klopfer and Kelly (15). The following scores were used: Popular responses (index number 28), average response time (index number 29), D (index number 31), To $\div$ de $(H + A \div Hd + Ad)$ (index number 32), $FM \div M$ (index number 33), $F \%$ (index number 34), $M \%$ (index number 36), $FM + m$ $- Fc + c + C'$ (index number 37), range of response times (index number 13), and lastly a composite score of pathological indicators devised by Blewett and given in detail in his thesis (index number 30). Most of these variables had odd and abnormal distributions and had to be transformed in various ways, usually by a logarithmic transformation.

Also included with the Rorschach group might be another test, the Rosenzweig Picture Frustration test, as this too is often considered as a projective technique. The only score used here was the extrapunitive one (index number 35).

The autonomic tests employed were as follows: Systolic blood pressure (index number 39) and diastolic blood pressure (index number 40). (Room temperature and humidity were measured at the time this and the other autonomic tests were administered, and wherever a significant relationship was found, temperature and humidity were partialled out.) The other measures used were pulse rate after stress (the stress consisted of pulling a hand dynamometer ten times as hard as possible) and pulse rate after resting (index numbers 41 and 42). Sub-lingual temperature (index number 43) and finger temperature (index number 44) were also taken. Lastly, dermographic latency (index number 35) was determined using Wenger's method (23).

The next set of variables consisted of ratings and sociometric measures. Questionnaire scales were used, both in the form of self-assessments and teachers' assessments. The scales used were adaptations of Guilford's C and R scales, which have been shown to be good measures of neuroticism and extraversion respectively (8). The detailed scales employed are given in the theses by Blewett and McLeod respectively (2, 16). Based on these scales, then, we have a teacher's rating of extraversion (index number 4), a teacher's rating of neuroticism (index number 15), self-ratings of extraversion (index number 5), and self-ratings of neuroticism (index number 7). A lie scale based on the well-known M.M.P.I. — but adapted for use with children — was also employed (index number 6).

Two sociability scores were obtained, both derived from a sociometric examination. The subjects were asked simply to write down names of their choice to a series of questions. These questions were of the following kind: "Whom would you like to sit by during class?" "Who do you think would choose you to sit beside them in class?" "Whom would you like to be with after school?" and so forth. The two scores were the total number of names given (index number 53) and the total number of *different* names given (index number 54). The hypothesis underlying this test was, of course, that extraverts, being more sociable, would give a larger number of names in both categories.

The last set of tests to be considered consists of objective behaviour tests. The first of these is the body sway test of suggestibility (index number 11); the second, the finger dexterity test (index number 14). Both these tests are described fully in "The Scientific Study of Personality" (6). Next, we have three tests or rigidity taken from the work of Ferguson and his colleagues (20). These are the opposites test (index number 22), the alphabet test (index number 23), and the arithmetic test (index number 24). These tests are based on the interfering effects of highly habituated culturally induced behaviour patterns in tasks involving largely cognitive processes. Another index of rigidity, called the index of flexibility, is a measure of the amount of change in level of aspiration by actual performance (index number 25). It is taken from a test using the so-called triple tester described in "The Scientific Study of Personality" (6), as is the affective discrepancy score (index number 50) which is the sum of the goal discrepancy and the judgment discrepancy scores. The rationale and meaning of these scores are discussed in "Dimensions of Personality" (5).

Two tests of persistence were included, namely, the leg persistence test (index number 26) and the dynamometer persistence test (index number 27). Both tests have been described in previous publications. As a test of expressive movement two of Mira's (19) tasks were used, namely, the drawing of sagittal lines and the drawing of vertical lines. The score on this test was the total area covered by the lines (index number 38). Two tests of humour were included, one of orectic (index number 46) and one of cognitive (index number 47) humour. The test consisted of 30 cartoons which had to be rated with respect to the amusement derived from them;

the rationale for this test is given in "Dimensions of Personality" (5).

The Porteus Maze test was also given to the children. As Hildebrand (13) and Foulds (12) have shown, certain qualitative performances differentiate hysterics from dysthymics. Included in our study, therefore, were scores "wrong directions" (index number 48) and "lifted pencils" (index number 49). Two scores were also taken from the track tracer described in "Dimensions of Personality" (5). One of these is an accuracy score, the other one a speed score (index numbers 51 and 52).

Last of all, a score was included consisting of the level-speed discrepancy on the Furneaux test (index number 21). Here a high score indicates a lack of such discrepancy; in view of results reported by Eysenck (7), this may be regarded as evidence of normality.

5. RESULTS

Variables indexed in the section above were intercorrelated, the effect of age was partialled out from the intercorrelations, and a factorial analysis undertaken of the resulting matrix. In order to avoid subjective determination of axis rotations by the writer, the rotations were carried out in the statistical section of the writer's department under the direction of Mr. A. E. Maxwell. The results are therefore not influenced by the writer's own conceptions, although this may, of course, intrude in the interpretation of the results given later on. However, the reader will be able to check these interpretations against the figures. Table 1 gives the factor saturations for the 52 variables on the 6 factors extracted, as well as the communalities. The peculiar constitution of the sample, i.e. the fact that it is composed of closely related subjects, makes it impossible to apply any known tests of significance to the residuals, and we have probably erred in taking out more factors than is warranted. However, no interpretation is here attempted of the last three factors, and those with which we shall be concerned are indubitably both significant and meaningful.

The main loadings on factors 1 and 2 have been plotted in Figure 1 and it will be seen that we are dealing essentially with the factors of intelligence and extraversion-introversion. The identification of the intelligence factor leaves very little room for doubt. The Thurstone total score has a loading of .947. All the other Thurstone scores have appropriately high loadings (verbal = .695; number = .569; space = .635; reasoning = .821; frequency = .629). The two Furneaux scores had loadings of .529 and .677. Finger dexterity, as is reasonable with children, has a loading of .389. Two of the rigidity tests have high loadings; the opposites

THE INHERITANCE OF EXTRAVERSION-INTROVERSION

TABLE I

Variable:	I	II	III	IV	V	VI	h^2
22	.579	−.103	−.055	.091	.019	−.034	.359
14	.389	.012	−.215	.037	.099	−.016	.209
8	.695	−.016	.014	−.181	−.050	.062	.523
11	.258	.090	.061	−.162	−.062	−.025	.109
20	.529	−.006	−.041	−.293	−.092	−.042	.378
16	.635	.105	−.066	.106	.037	−.033	.432
19	.947	.075	.124	.036	−.015	.075	.925
10	.677	−.019	.291	.285	.101	−.086	.642
18	.629	−.071	.225	−.057	−.048	.092	.465
9	.569	.096	.200	.047	.025	.162	.402
40	.232	−.230	.452	.015	−.014	−.046	.314
17	.821	.095	.123	.198	.040	−.021	.739
23	.656	.151	.264	.197	−.011	.038	.563
6	.374	.200	.109	−.301	−.046	−.015	.285
34	−.296	.286	.095	.089	−.124	−.067	.206
24	−.161	−.106	.219	−.140	−.010	−.099	.115
48	−.448	.013	.110	−.231	−.021	.071	.272
51	−.389	.162	.041	−.016	.006	−.098	.189
15	−.159	.165	−.177	.084	.021	.005	.091
44	.031	.300	−.181	−.066	.056	−.023	.132
33	−.090	.501	−.292	.137	−.013	−.046	.365
1	.167	.217	−.166	−.226	.057	−.010	.157
46	−.149	.162	−.026	−.358	−.077	−.002	.183
28	.095	.242	.107	−.227	.023	.106	.142
31	.164	.510	.106	−.192	.047	.077	.343
26	−.004	.229	.129	−.087	.050	.167	.107
53	.073	.632	−.017	.061	.011	−.067	.413
54	.121	.574	−.094	.094	.029	−.083	.370
43	−.121	.200	.620	.034	.011	.096	.450
36	.191	−.626	.175	−.084	−.030	.014	.467
52	−.098	−.378	−.047	−.171	.050	.115	.200
30	.013	−.396	−.022	−.272	.096	−.078	.247
32	.112	−.189	−.191	−.264	−.013	.050	.157
38	−.045	.027	.184	−.215	.051	−.087	.088
49	−.148	−.111	.177	−.250	−.092	−.049	.137
42	.076	−.066	.913	.148	.006	−.026	.894
2	.065	−.057	.855	.122	−.054	−.025	.781
29	−.079	.032	.162	.594	−.126	−.016	.402
5	−.104	−.091	−.282	−.030	−.135	.011	.118
27	−.020	.013	−.197	.141	−.037	.127	.077
50	.124	.007	−.447	.123	−.164	.009	.257
21	−.136	−.015	−.240	−.466	−.172	.035	.324
45	.193	−.002	−.216	−.233	.023	−.049	.141
47	−.096	−.056	−.192	−.406	.001	−.096	.223
13	−.006	−.100	.109	.530	−.118	−.024	.317
7	.076	.095	.140	−.350	−.073	−.023	.163
4	.042	.176	−.042	−.326	.073	−.045	.148
35	.096	.119	.103	−.228	.021	.024	.087
25	.032	−.009	.062	−.197	−.048	.082	.053
39	−.019	−.132	.389	.063	.066	.037	.179
41	.108	−.123	.839	.115	−.002	−.013	.744
37	.065	−.121	.290	−.059	−.027	−.011	.107

test .579 and the alphabet test .656. The nature of the material used makes these high correlations intelligible and suggests that these tests cannot properly be used with children. It is not unexpected to find that the Mazes "wrong direction" score has a high negative correlation with intelligence (—.448) or that inaccuracy on the track tracer has a somewhat slighter negative correlation (—.389). It may be surprising and is certainly interesting that the more intelligent apparently give more truthful self-ratings; the correlation between truthfulness on the lie scale and the intelligence factor is .374.

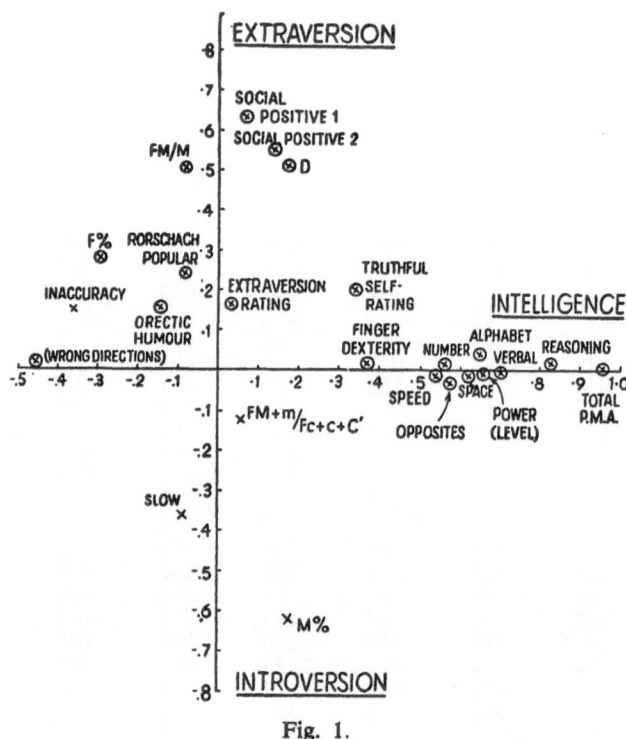

Fig. 1.

An interesting feature of this study is the complete failure of the Rorschach scores to correlate with intelligence. The only one to achieve even the very modest correlation of —.296 is the Rorschach F %. This, in spite of the fact that of all the scores included, the F % score is one of the few that is in general considered *not* to be a measure of intelligence. M, which is usually taken as a good index of intelligence, only achieves a correlation of .191. It is difficult not to conclude that the Rorschach scores which we have used here, and for many of which extravagant claims have been made as measures of ability, fail to measure intelligence to any significant extent.

We now come to the second factor which has been identified as extraversion. Before discussing this interpretation it will be necessary to present some details regarding the method followed in interpreting the Rorschach scores. While there is a good deal of agreement among Rorschach writers in the interpretation of certain scores, this agreement is far from perfect, and it would be possible in *a posteriori* fashion to explain away discordant findings by referring to some obscure authority as having interpreted this particular score in the manner required to substantiate one's own hypothesis. To avoid this danger, the following method was followed. The scores used were communicated to an expert who had been using the Rorschach clinically and teaching it to students for a number of years. He was requested to write down in detail the relevance of each of the scores to the three variables of intelligence, extraversion-introversion, and neuroticism. He was to base himself entirely on the agreed interpretations of the most widely accepted Rorschach authorities, and on independent factual research evidence. His decisions were written down and implicitly followed in our interpretation; wherever necessary they will be quoted in full. This, of course, does not ensure that other Rorschach experts will necessarily agree; it does ensure that our interpretation of the results is not falsified by an attempt to justify observed findings in the manner outlined at the beginning of this paragraph.

Let us now look at the variables defining the two poles of the factor which we have identified as one of extraversion-introversion. The variable having the highest saturation on the introverted side is $M \%$ (—.626). According to the expert "a high M suggests introversion, a low M extraversion". This interpretation has found a good deal of factual support, such as, for instance, a recent study by Barron (1) who has attempted to devise a psychometric measure of M by means of a series of specially constructed blots, and who found considerable correlations between movement scores and introverted personality traits. The other introversion score is indicative of slow and accurate work on the track tracer (—.378); this Himmelweit (14) and Eysenck (5) have found indicative of introversion.

On the extraverted side, the two scores having the highest saturations are the two sociometric scores indicative of social popularity and general social liking (.632 and .574). This relationship between extraversion and positive social relationships is, of course, in line with our hypothesis. Only slightly less highly correlated with extraversion is the Rorschach D score (.510). This is what our authority has to say about a high D score:

"A high D is said to indicate "practical" man, a down to earth extravert; a low D is said to indicate a "theoretical" man, a "theoriser". A high D is associated with hysteria, a low D with dysthymia." The interpretation is thus in accord with our hypothesis. Almost equally high as the D score is the $FM \div M$ score (.501). This score, of course, is not independent of the M score we have already considered, and can therefore not be used to add very much to our interpretation of the latter. However, for what it is worth, our authority summarizes the literature by saying that a high $FM \div M$ ratio "may indicate extraversion", a low $FM \div M$ ratio "may indicate normality, but also introversion and intelligence."

The $F \%$ score has a correlation with the extraversion factor of .286. The interpretation of this score appears excessively difficult. Our authority says that "a high $F \%$ is found in the records of psychopaths"; a high $F \%$ is found in the records of many hysterics ("flat hysterics")". This would suggest that a high $F \%$ is indicative of extraversion. Against this hypothesis speaks the fact that "a high $F \%$ indicates "over-control" which could characterize an introverted neurotic". Altogether, "experts seem in some disagreement" so that we cannot really interpret this particular score. The next Rorschach score, the number of popular replies, has a factor of .242. According to our expert "a large number of popular responses suggests a dull extraverted person or hysteric." Apparently "a small number of popular responses suggests a person out of contact with his environment, or may be due to a perfectionist attitude exhibited by obsessive, compusive neurotics". In all, he concludes that "a high number of popular responses might, therefore, suggest extraversion, a low number introversion".[2]

Three more scores are to be considered and lend weight to this interpretation. Inaccurate work on the track tracer has a loading of .162 which, although low, is in the right direction. Orectic humour also has a loading of .162 which is also low, but again in the right direction. Truthful

---

[2] Score 37, the Rorschach $FM + m \div Fc + c + C'$ has a loading of −.121 and should therefore be a measure of introversion. According to our authority "high $FM + m$ is probably introverted, high $Fc + c + C'$ probably extraverted by majority opinion". This is in line with our hypothesis, but the correlation is much too small to carry any weight. It may, however, serve to counterbalance item 32, the Rorschach To $\div$ de where "a high score is indicative of an uncritical attitude, perhaps suggesting abnormal extraversion". Here also the correlation (−.189) is too small to carry much weight. Ratios, in view of their well-known statistical unreliability, should never be used in work of this kind, particularly when the scores entering into the ratios are themselves not very reliable (18).

self-ratings, with a loading of .200, is slightly higher and also in line with previous work which has shown a slight tendency for extraverts to obtain more truthful scores on the lie scale. With the possible exception of the $F \%$ score, we can therefore say that all the scores considered support the interpretation of this factor as one of extraversion-introversion.

A number of items have moderately high correlations with the factor but have not been considered in this connection because they neither argue for nor against our interpretation and may be chance projections on this factor. Among these scores are, for instance, item 44, high finger temperature, which has a correlation of .300, and item 40, high diastolic blood pressure, which has a correlation of —.230. Our data are not sufficient to make it possible for us to say whether these additional items, which the reader may like to study intensively in Table 1, throw any additional light on either the identification of the factor or its measurement. The work of Theron and of Van der Merwe (21, 22), as summarized in "The Structure of Human Personality", has opened up the possibility that extraversion-introversion may be related to certain autonomic measures, and certainly this line of enquiry is promising and deserves to be followed up. It cannot, however, be maintained that at the present moment our results throw any further light on this problem.

A few words may be said about the third factor. This, quite clearly, is an autonomic one, having very high saturations indeed on pulse rate resting (.913), pulse rate stressed (.839), systolic and diastolic blood pressure (.389 and .452), and on sub-lingual temperature (.620). Finger temperature is rather out of line (—.181), but this may be due to difficulties and inaccuracies of measurement. Dermographic latency has a relatively low loading of —.216. The interpretation of this factor as an autonomic one appears somewhat invalidated, however, by the fact that item 2 (sex) has a very high loading of .855. This suggests that quite possibly the correlations observed are produced very largely by sex differences, and are therefore of less interest than they sight otherwise be. No further analysis or discussion of this factor will be given here as it does not seem relevant to our main purpose. The same may be said of the remaining three factors, which do not lend themselves to any obvious interpretation and will therefore not be considered any further.

Factor scores were estimated for the first three factors. For the Extraversion-Introversion factors, the following items were used: 53, 54, 31, 33, 28, 4, 6, 46, 52, 36. For the Intelligence factor, the following items were used: 17, 10, 16, 18, 8, 9, 20, 14, 48. For the Autonomic factors, the following items were used: 39, 40, 41, 42, 43, 44, 45. Thus, each one of our subjects obtained scores on the three factors of intelligence, extraversion, and autonomic activity.

Intercorrelations of factor scores were calculated for fraternal twins and identical twins separately, and are given in Table 2. It will be seen

TABLE II

	Intelligence	Extraversion	Autonomic
Intelligence	—	.030	−.103
Extraversion	.155	—	−.018
Autonomic	−.074	.001	—

Intercorrelations of factor scores for identical twins (below leading diagonal) and for fraternal twins (above leading diagonal).

that there are no significant relationships between the factors. Next, intra-class correlations were run for the three factors between the identical and also between the fraternal sets of twins. These correlations, as well as the h^2 values calculated from them, are given in Table 3. A test was

TABLE III

	Identical:	Fraternal:	h^2
Intelligence	.820	.376	.712
Extraversion	.499	−.331	(.624)
Autonomic	.929	.718	.748

Intraclass correlations for identical and fraternal twins, on three factor scores.

made of the significance of the differences betwene the intraclass correlations. For the intelligence factor, $t = 2.13$; for the extraversion factor, $t = 2.43$; for the autonomic factor, $t = 2.09$. The t values for the intelligence and autonomic factors are significant at the 5 % level; the t value for extraversion is significant at the 2 % level. We may, therefore, conclude with some statistical justification that the differences observed between identical and fraternal twins are unlikely to have been caused by chance factors and would be found again if the study were duplicated. From this it may be concluded that heredity plays a significant part in the causation of all three factors.

One feature in Table 3 requires discussion. It will be seen that the intra-class correlation for the fraternal twins on the extraversion factor has a negative sign. This is an extremely unlikely occurrence on any reasonable hypothesis, but a thorough checking of the figures failed to reveal any errors in calculation. It seems likely that this value represents a chance deviation from a true correlation of zero, or of some slight positive value, an assumption strengthened by the fact that a correlation of the observed size is not statistically significant. Under the circumstances, however, we cannot regard the h^2 statistic derived for the factor of extraversion as having very much meaning, and it has therefore been put in brackets in Table 3 to indicate its extremely doubtful status. Much more reliance, fortunately, can be placed on the significance of the differences between identical and fraternal twins for this factor which, as has been shown above, is fully significant.

6. SUMMARY AND CONCLUSIONS

In this study an effort has been made to provide evidence for the existence of a factor of extraversion-introversion among children, similar to that found among adults, and to measure this factor. By and large, this attempt has been successful and the factorial analysis reported in this paper gives clear evidence of a strong factor of extraversion-introversion.

It was hypothesized that the concept of extraversion-introversion, as operationally defined in the writer's previous work, would be closely parallel to Rorschach's concept of extratensive-introvertive personality. The inclusion of a number of R scores in the factor analysis made it possible to test this hypothesis, and the results on the whole favoured acceptance of this theory.

Two further factors were isolated in the analysis, namely, one of intelligence and one of autonomic activity. These additional factors were found to be independent of each other and also to be independent of extraversion-introversion. Factor scores were calculated for all three factors for the members of the experimental populations.

As the major aim of the investigation was to study the effects of heredity on extraversion-introversion, the subjects of the investigation were 13 pairs of male identical twins, 13 pairs of female identical twins, 13 pairs of male fraternal twins, and 13 pairs of female fraternal twins. By using standard methods of intra-class correlation for different types of twins, it was shown that for all three factors, identical twins resembled each other significantly more closely than did fraternal twins. This was regarded as proof that heredity played an important part in the determination of intelligence, extraversion, and autonomic reactivity.

REFERENCES

1. Barron, F., An attempt to study the human movement response by constructing a measure of M-threshold. *To appear*.
2. Blewett, D. B., *An experimental study of the inheritance of neuroticism and intelligence*. Ph. D. Thesis, University of London Library, 1953.
3. ———, An experimental study of the inheritance of intelligence. *J. ment. Sci.*, 1954, 100, 922–933.
4. Cox, S. M., A factorial study of the Rorschach responses of normal and maladjusted boys. *J. genet. Psychol.*, 1951, 79, 95–115.
5. Eysenck, H. J., *Dimensions of personality*. London: Kegan Paul, 1947.

H. J. EYSENCK

6. Eysenck, H. J., *The scientific study of personality*. London: Routledge and Kegan Paul, 1952.

7. ————, La rapidité du fonctionnement mental comme mesure de l'anomalie mentale. *Rev. Psychol. Appl.*, 1953, 3, 367–377.

8. ————, *The structure of human personality*. London: Methuen, 1953.

9. ————, *The psychology of politics*. London: Routledge and Kegan Paul, 1954.

10. ————, A dynamic theory of anxiety and hysteria. *J. ment. Sci.*, 1955, 101, 28–51.

11. ———— and Prell, D. B., The inheritance of neuroticism: an experimental study. *J. ment. Sci.*, 1951, 97, 441–465.

12. Foulds, G. A., Temperamental differences in maze performance. Part 1. Characteristic differences among psychoneurotics. *Brit. J. Psychol.*, 1951, 42, 209–218.

13. Hildebrand, H. P., *A factorial study of introversion-extraversion by means of objective tests*. Ph. D. Thesis, University of London, 1953.

14. Himmelweit, H. T., Speed and accuracy of work as related to temperament. *Brit. J. Psychol.*, 1946, 36, 132–144.

15. Klopfer, B. and Kelly, D., *The Rorschach Technique*. London: Harrap, 1952.

16. McLeod, H., *An experimental study of the inheritance of introversion-extraversion*. Ph. D. Thesis, University of London, 1953.

17. May, J., Note on the assumption underlying Holzinger's h^2 statistic. *J. ment. Sci.*, 1951, 97, 466–467.

18. Meadows, A. W., *A factorial study of projection test responses of normal, psychotic and neurotic subjects*. Ph. D. Thesis, University of London, 1951.

19. Mira, E., Myokinetic psychodiagnosis: a new technique of exploring the conative trends of personality. *Proc. Roy. Soc. Med.*, 1940, 33, 9–30.

20. Oliver, J. A. and Ferguson, G. A., A factorial study of tests of rigidity. *Can. J. Psychol.*, 1951, 5, 49–59.

21. Theron, P. A., Peripheral vasomotor reactions as indices of basic emotional tension and lability. *Psychosom. Med.*, 1948, 10, 335–346.

22. Van der Merwe, A. B., The diagnostic value of peripheral vasomotor reactions in the psychoneuroses. *Psychosom. Med.*, 1948, 10, 347–354.

23. Wenger, M. A., Studies of autonomic balance in army air forces personnel. *Comp. Psychol. Monog.*, 1948, 19, 1–111.

From R. B. Cattell, D. B. Blewett and J. R. Beloff (1955). American Journal of Human Genetics, *7*, 122-146, *by kind permission of the authors and the University of Chicago Press*

The Inheritance of Personality

A Multiple Variance Analysis Determination of Approximate Nature-Nurture Ratios for Primary Personality Factors in Q-Data

RAYMOND B. CATTELL, DUNCAN B. BLEWETT AND JOHN R. BELOFF

Laboratory of Personality Assessment and Group Behavior, University of Illinois

I. THE MULTIPLE VARIANCE ANALYSIS DESIGN

WITH INCREASING appreciation in psychology of the importance both for theory and practice of greater functional understanding of the role of heredity in abilities and personality development, including abnormal personality development, the problem of nature-nurture research techniques has recently been attacked with renewed vigor. The research now to be described differs in three significant ways from any previous work in the field.

1. It uses a multiple variance analysis design, recently described and discussed (8), in the place of the usual comparison of identical with fraternal twins. (1) (2) (11) (20) (24) (25) (27) (31) (36).
2. It deals with *dimensions* of personality which have been established by *factor analytic* investigations upon personality responses in rating data, questionnaire data, and objective tests. (6) (9) (19).
3. It estimates the reliability of measurement of the *essential factor* and works out the nature-nurture ratio for this factor rather than for the tests themselves.

To put this research approach in perspective in regard to other studies, it is necessary first to point out that it follows one of the two chief *possible* avenues, the other being the approach by Mendelian ratios, which is not adapted to most normal psychological dimensions, because they are, presumably, multi-gene determined. Within this aim of nature-nurture ratio determination, previous work has examined just three dimensions, namely, general mental capacity, (1) (2) (24), rigidity or perseveration (11) (36), and general neuroticism (18). General ability has been studied extensively (28), but a few names, such as those of Newman, Freeman and Holzinger (24) and Burks (2) stand out in decisive studies. Their work has been judiciously appraised by Schwesinger (28), Thorndike (33) and Woodworth (35) and recently confirmed by Blewett (1). The inheritance of rigidity was examined some years ago by Yule (36) and, along with fluency, by Cattell and Malteno (11), but inconclusively; while an exploratory study of the inheritance of neuroticism has recently been reported by Eysenck and Prell (18). Practically all of these studies used the identical twin-fraternal twin comparison, and did not adequately distinguish between the ratio for the test measurements and the ratio for the implied factor.

The present study is considered still to be at the exploratory level. For, introducing

Received July 7, 1954.

as it does a new method, and entering a factor domain in which less than one-sixth of the dimensions here investigated have been previously studied, it could and does encounter some difficulties. Because of this exploratory nature of the design, we have felt justified in working with the most convenient and brief experimental device, namely the questionnaire. The Q-data thus obtained, however, can be related to behavior ratings and objective personality tests through previous researches (6) (12) (16) integrating factor measures from different media. Accordingly, we regard our findings as initial, approximate statements of these important nature-nurture ratios, which are to be followed by more exact values based on objective test measurements, made with whatever methodological improvements are developed through the present exploratory study. The nature and meaning of the individual personality factor measurements and the nature-nurture ratios will be examined after we have set out the basic design, in the present section, as it applies to the factors generally.

What we have called the Multiple Variance Analysis Design (8) must be clearly distinguished in objectives and design from the typical analysis of variance design, though it is related to it in so far as it deals with analysis-of-variance principles. It differs in that it attempts to determine ratios for hypothetical contributions, and in that it is not concerned primarily with a significance test but with determining a *quantitative value for a ratio*. In the previous article on this design (8), we have pointed out that the hitherto prevalent method of comparing differences between identical twins with differences between fraternal twins has several weaknesses (25). First, it does not give us all the ratios in which we are interested when we are dealing with the practical psychological problems of everyday life. In particular it fails to give the ratio of between-family variance from environmental causes and between-family variance from hereditary causes. This is one of the most important ratios in many clinical and social calculations. Secondly, it is unable to estimate or allow for the correlation between within-family variance due to heredity and within-family variance due to environment. Thirdly, it makes the assumption, which every psychologist knows to be false, that the particular within-family variance due to environment which it determines—namely, that of twins—is the same as the general within-family variance (of sibs) due to environment. Actually, the differences of environment between siblings, born at different periods in the family life and not reacted to as "twins" are, is bound to be greater than this determination would indicate.

Multiple variance analysis was described by the senior author as a new method in the original article (8) but it has since transpired that although it is new to psychology something closely similar has been independently developed in certain agricultural researches (3) (17) (22) (26). However, the latter have commonly been considered as *ad hoc* extensions of analysis of variance and have apparently not explicitly developed the methodological statement that (a) ratios rather than significance tests *per se* are sought (b) hypothetical variances not directly measurable constitute the concepts under consideration (c) these are reached not by experimentally holding constant all but the required variance, but by solving a sufficiency of simultaneous equations. In the present, psychological data the aim is to solve both for variances and correlations, and to test the significance of the magnitudes of the ratios obtained for the hypothetical, contributory, environmental and hereditary, intra- and interfamilial variances.

II. THE ELEVEN OR FIFTEEN POSSIBLE SIMULTANEOUS EQUATIONS

In our original statement of the multiple variance design we restricted ourselves to the use of five or six equations, but in our further explanations of the design it became evident that we could get eleven equations, or fifteen if we gathered data also on half-sibs. For reasons explained later we cannot solve for eleven unknowns by the eleven equations, but since other researchers might find them useful we shall set them all down. The remaining four equations for half-sibs, on which we have no data, will be merely listed, without discussion. In each case the value given on the left is an experimentally obtained variance. In our studies it can be and is corrected for error by subtracting from it the error variance, which is a function of the test reliability (general consistency coefficient, specific to the sample). The values on the right are the hypothetical constituent hereditary and environmental variances.

It has seemed best to us to arrange the equations with the first six dealing with variance among individuals and the later equations with variance among families. However, the reader will notice that another arrangement must also be kept in mind, namely, the supplementary relations between "within" and "between" family variances for the same types of 'family', which would indicate that we adjoin equations 3 and 7, 4 and 8, 5 and 9, 1 and 10, and 2 and 11.

1. $$\sigma^2_{ITT} - (1 - r_{ITT}) \sigma^2_{ITT} = \sigma^2_{we'}$$

This indicates that the differences between identical twins squared, summed and divided by $2n$, (n being the number of pairs), can be considered as due to the within-family environmental difference in the factor being measured, e.g., in intelligence, plus the error of measurement in the test. It will be noticed that the *we* has a prime upon it, indicating that it is different from the more common within-family environmental difference[1]—*we*—where ordinary *siblings* are involved. (ITT = Identical twins raised together.)

2. $$\sigma^2_{FTT} - (1 - r_{FTT}) \sigma^2_{FTT} = \sigma^2_{wh} + \sigma^2_{we'} + 2r_{wh.we'}\sigma_{wh}\sigma_{we'}$$

This states that the variance among fraternal twins reared together (FTT) is equal to the usual inter-sibling hereditary variance, which we shall in general call the within-family hereditary variance, and which is due to the differential segregation of the parental genes, and the within-family environmental variance, in this case again differentiated as that peculiar to fraternal twins. Since the environmental effects may be correlated with the hereditary effects within the family, in that a child showing a certain hereditary endowment may get treatment different from one

---

[1] The environmental variance, within families, among twins, must also include that *among twin pairs* (when more than one pair of twins are considered typical of a "twin family"). When we pair sibs at random the intra-pair differences include the equivalent of this difference. For simplicity of representation we shall assume that we' does also, though we could split it into two terms.

with a different hereditary endowment, we must introduce the term $2r_{wf.we''}\sigma_{wf}\sigma_{we''}$ on the assumption that this r cannot be treated as zero. (However, we are compelled later to treat $r_{wh.we''}$ and $r_{wh.we}$ as identical).

The present equations are, of course, statements of expectation, on theoretical grounds, about the hypothetical variances that will contribute to an observed variance, and about their modes of combination. In both respects there are five shades of difference of possible assumption into which we do not have space to enter here. For example, we have differentiated σ^2_{we}, $\sigma^2_{we'}$ and $\sigma^2_{we''}$ where some investigators might not think it necessary, and in the later half-sib equations we have assumed that mother and father contribute equally to hereditary variations where a finer distinction might take into account the X chromosome. The principle assumptions that the reader might wish to debate, however, are those concerning covariances or correlations that may or may not be considered zero among variances. Our procedure has been to consider all the *mathematically possible* combinations of the variances that enter a given equation and to reject immediately, at this first stage, those which, on analysis of variance principles, could not enter into the final variance. At a second stage, *after* setting out the present equations, we shall argue that some of the correlation terms must be, on general biological and social grounds, absolutely trivial and that there is no reason for retaining them. Thirdly, when we combine these "cleaned up", *scientifically* appropriate equations and find we cannot get an algebraic solution without a further assumption about correlation terms, we shall proceed to *approximate* solutions by dropping some more (or assuming fixed values for them). These three stages in the form of the equations should be realized in the subsequent developments.

3.
$$\sigma^2_{ST} - (1 - r_{ST})\,\sigma^2_{ST} = \sigma^2_{wh} + \sigma^2_{we} + 2r_{wh.we}\sigma_{wh}\sigma_{we}$$

This expression, for siblings reared together (ST), is just the same as the previous one except that it has the full range of intra-familial environmental variance—*we*.

4.
$$\sigma^2_{SA} - (1 - r_{SA})\,\sigma^2_{SA} = \sigma^2_{wh} + \sigma^2_{we} + \sigma^2_{be} + 2r_{wh.we}\sigma_{wh}\sigma_{we}$$

This refers to the formula for siblings reared apart from birth in different families. It should be noted that within-family environmental variance must still be introduced since the brothers are not only in different families but may occupy different positions in the families into which they are adopted. It is conceivable that a prime could be added to *we* and *be* here, on the assumption that foster homes have a slightly different within and between-family environmental range than normal families, but we have approximated and simplified by rejecting this assumption.

5.
$$\sigma^2_{UT} - (1 - r_{UT})\,\sigma^2_{UT} = \sigma^2_{wh} + \sigma^2_{we} + \sigma^2_{bh} + 2r_{wh.we}\sigma_{wh}\sigma_{we} + 2r_{wh.bh}\sigma_{wh}\sigma_{bh} + 2r_{we.bh}\sigma_{we}\sigma_{bh}$$

This is the variance for unrelated children reared together. Again it will be noted that the within-family variance term must enter, (in this case the within-family *hereditary* variance). It enters because although they are from different families they present different possibilities in the hereditary compositions derivable from the

CATTELL, BLEWETT AND BELOFF

parents of that family. Thus, these children possess both the between-family heredity and the within-family heredity variance. Being brought up in the same family they do not have the between-family environmental variance.

Unrelated children could include the situation where all are also unrelated to the acting parents, or where all but one are unrelated, but we have aimed at the first situation. In neither case, however, is there any ground for expecting a relation between bh and wh, so we can say even at this stage that the fifth term on the right would vanish, and it will so be omitted from later equations.

6. $\quad \sigma^2_{UA} - (1 - r_{UA}) \sigma^2_{UA} = \sigma^2_{wh} + \sigma^2_{we} + \sigma^2_{bh} + \sigma^2_{be} + 2r_{we.wh}\sigma_{we}\sigma_{wh} + 2r_{be.bh}\sigma_{be}\sigma_{bh}$

This is the variance for unrelated children reared apart. That is to say, we are dealing with the variance for people taken at random from the general population. Naturally, it includes all four sources of variance, but, as argued in (5), drops $bh.wh$ and $be.we$ terms.

Next we begin a series of five between-family variances corresponding to the within-family variances of equations 1 through 5. The individual measures on which these are based are not, it is true, experimentally independent of those in equations 1 through 5; but, in terms of *sampling*, the within and between variances are independent (have independent distributions and are uncorrelated) and hence are usable, for example, as independent estimates of the total population variance. Strictly, these "variances" are "mean squares" rather than variances. For it is simplest in conception and computation to deal with equations using terms of between family *differences* and the resulting totals are twice the variance of family means and half the variance of family sums. Thus the corresponding "within" and "between" variances mentioned above—equations 3 with 7, 4 with 8, 5 with 9, 1 with 10 and 2 with 11—sum to *twice* the total population variance actually obtained directly— that in equation 6. This follows in accordance with the analysis of variance model, when we take $k - 1$ degrees of freedom for k families in calculating the between variance, and $km - k$, (where m is 2—the two sibs or twins) for the within variance. However, the difficulties we later encounter in the use of these ensuing equations have nothing to do with this trivial "catch", but arise from interaction of the systematic paired relationships of equations just discussed. The result is, that except where some special correlation of variance term breaks the relation, the later equations are obtainable as linear combinations of these earlier ones. They thus fail to be algebraically usable as additional equations permitting solutions for additional terms. However, they will now be stated, because they can nevertheless be used in different combinations and for a least squares solution.

7. $\quad \sigma^2_{BNF} - (1 - r_{BNF}) \sigma^2_{BNF} = 2\sigma^2_{bh} + 2\sigma^2_{be} + 4r_{bh.be}\sigma_{bh}\sigma_{be} + \sigma^2_{we} + \sigma^2_{wh}$
$$+ 2r_{we.wh}\sigma_{we}\sigma_{wh}$$

The expression BNF means "between natural families" and is obtained from the differences of the means of pairs of siblings in different natural families from the mean of all such families. This can be obtained by taking the same experimental data as is used in equations 1, 2, and 3, above.

INHERITANCE OF PERSONALITY

8. $\sigma^2_{BBF} - (1 - r_{BBF})\,\sigma^2_{BBF} = \sigma^2_{we} + \sigma^2_{wh} + \sigma^2_{be} + 2\sigma^2_{bh} + 2r_{we.wh}\sigma_{we}\sigma_{wh} + 4r_{we.bh}\sigma_{we}\sigma_{bh}$

Just as the values in 7 were obtained by taking inter-familial differences from experimental data already used in equation 3, so here we obtain inter-familial differences from the same data that is used in an intra-familial sense in equation 4. Siblings reared apart belong to the same biological hereditary family. Hence the expression *BBF* means "between biological families", i.e., true families which are socially dispersed. It should be noted that the coefficient of the last term would need to be modified from 4 to 2 if we dealt with situations where one child is raised in its own family and one in a foster family. For in the former case there could be no covariance of *we* and *bh*, since *bh* is constant as *we* varies. However, we completely avoided such cases.

9. $\sigma^2_{BSF} - (1 - r_{BSF})\,\sigma^2_{BSF} = \sigma^2_{we} + 2\sigma^2_{be} + \sigma^2_{bh} + \sigma^2_{wh} + 2r_{we.wh}\sigma_{we}\sigma_{wh} + 2r_{we.bh}\sigma_{we}\sigma_{bh}$
$$+ 2r_{wh.bh}\sigma_{wh}\sigma_{bh}$$

Similarly, this takes the inter-familial variance for the data analyzed intra-familially in equation 5. That is, it takes the differences of mean among families that are merely *social families*, consisting of adopted children from hereditarily different families, gathered within the same social families. As in 5 we can decide straightway that $r_{wh.bh}$ is essentially zero and that the last term will therefore disappear from subsequent calculations.

10. $\sigma^2_{BITF} - (1 - r_{BITF})\,\sigma^2_{BITF} = \sigma^2_{we'} + 2\sigma^2_{wh} + 2\sigma^2_{be} + 2\sigma^2_{bh} + 4r_{be.bh}\sigma_{be}\sigma_{bh}$

This is the variance among the means of identical twin families. It uses a specific within-family environmental variance but assumes nothing specific about the between-family heredity of twin families.

11. $\sigma^2_{BFTF} - (1 - r_{BFTF})\,\sigma^2_{BFTF} = \sigma^2_{we}{}'' + \sigma^2_{wh} + 2\sigma^2_{be} + 2\sigma^2_{bh} + 4r_{be.bh}\sigma_{be}\sigma_{bh}$
$$+ 2r_{we.wh}\sigma_{we}{}''\sigma_{wh}$$

This repeats 10 for fraternal twin families. It should be noted that though these formulae distinguish the *we* variance of sibs, identical twins and fraternal twins there seems no reason to multiply unknowns by assuming that the *correlation* of environment and heredity is systematically different in the first and last cases.

It should be noted that the reliabilities in inter-familial variances are the reliabilities for the *mean* score of two sibs or twins.

For completeness we next add four equations, the data for which are obtainable (but not obtained in this research) from families of half-sibs, namely, the children of different fathers born to and reared by one mother, and children of the same father born to and reared by different mothers. Other combinations of birth and rearing are conceivable, but might be far too rare to permit a sufficient sample.

12. $\sigma^2_{HST} - (1 - r_{HST})\,\sigma^2_{HST} = \tfrac{1}{2}\sigma^2_{bh} + \sigma^2_{wh} + \sigma^2_{we} + 2r_{wh.we}\sigma_{wh}\sigma_{we}$

HST equals half-sibs reared together.

CATTELL, BLEWETT AND BELOFF

13. $\sigma^2_{HSA} - (1 - r_{HSA}) \sigma^2_{HSA} = \frac{1}{2}\sigma^2_{bh} + \sigma^2_{wh} + \sigma^2_{we} + \sigma^2_{be} + 2r_{wh.we}\sigma_{wh}\sigma_{we}$
$$+ r_{bh.be}\sigma_{bh}\sigma_{be}$$

This applies to half-sibs apart, typically the same father and different mothers.

14. $\sigma^2_{BHST} - (1 - r_{BHST}) \sigma^2_{BHST} = \frac{3}{2}\sigma^2_{bh} + \sigma^2_{wh} + 2\sigma^2_{be} + \sigma^2_{we} + 3r_{bh.be}\sigma_{bh}\sigma_{be}$
$$+ 2r_{we.wh}\sigma_{we}\sigma_{wh}$$

BHST means among means of pairs of half-sibs reared together, i.e., the supplement of (12).

15. $\sigma^2_{BHSA} - (1 - r_{BHSA}) \sigma^2_{BHSA} = \frac{3}{2}\sigma^2_{bh} + \sigma^2_{wh} + \sigma^2_{be} + \sigma^2_{we} + 3r_{be.bh}\sigma_{be}\sigma_{bh}$
$$+ 2r_{we.wh}\sigma_{we}\sigma_{wh}$$

The assumption in the last four equations is that father and mother contribute equally to the child's heredity, but the existence of the X-chromosome makes this an approximation.

The writers wish to express their great indebtedness to Professor C. R. Rao of the Indian Statistical Institute, Calcutta, for help freely and generously given in searching out errors in the writer's original equations, for improvements, and for proposals for overcoming difficulties in the subsequent solutions.

In principle, the eleven equations offer a complete solution, providing we agree to consider the within-family environmental variance of identical twins to be the same as that of fraternal twins, i.e., $we' = we''$, which is no great assumption, since many parents do not know whether their twins are identical or fraternal. There would then be eleven unknowns: five unknown variances, σ^2_{we}, $\sigma^2_{we'}$, σ^2_{be}, σ^2_{bh} and σ^2_{wh}; and six unknown correlations, as listed in the first article (8).

Unfortunately there is many a slip between the ideal possibility and what can actually be done with a given set of equations. The afore-mentioned linear dependencies, and certain peculiarities of the quadratics, considerably restrict our power of solution. The adaptions made to these restrictions require a section on their own, and are therefore postponed to the computational account in Section 4, while we turn to the psychological measurement data itself.

III. THE Q-DATA PERSONALITY MEASUREMENTS FROM THE J.P.Q. TEST

As indicated above, the only source traits or basic dimensions of personality that have so far received genetic study are those of general mental capacity, rigidity and general neuroticism. The second is not known to be a general *personality* factor, though it was once thought to be, and still apparently remains, a real factor in a certain area of *test* response (6). Although the two true dimensions indicated (intelligence and neuroticism) received prior attention because they were isolated early and assumed to be of greatest practical social and clinical importance, it is now evident that they are no more or less important, in terms of life criteria, than the more recently established personality dimensions. At present, some fifteen or sixteen primary personality factors have been isolated and confirmed, in behavior rating or *L*-data (6) (9), in questionnaire responses or *Q*-data (14) (15), and in objective, behavioral, test responses or *T*-data (9) (10). The matching of factors among the three

INHERITANCE OF PERSONALITY

media is not complete (6) (9) (12) (16) (19), nor do we yet know the significance of some of these factors in various clinical, scholastic, and general life situations. But, we do know that these factors, based on a thorough sampling of behavior, (6), constitute the greater part of the framework upon which a systematic knowledge of personality can be built by further research. Wherever exact measurement and an objective scientific search for laws has proceeded it has encountered these factor structures, and as personality study advances beyond qualitative, philosophical and clinical speculation, it is likely to organize itself increasingly about these factors as functional unities. Accordingly, we have made them the center of our genetic study, in order that the genetic findings may adhere to psychological measurements of permanent value, and also in order that, reciprocally, psychological theory about the nature of the factors may be guided by the first available genetic information.

It is not claimed in principle, nor will it subsequently transpire in fact, that our research clears up the issues as completely as our theoretical approach might suggest. For the geneticist, our contribution is largely methodological, revealing what sizes of sample, reliabilities of measurement, etc., are necessary to give answers of a given accuracy with the multiple variance analysis method. However, although the answers on the specific psychological data do not have the accuracy that the geneticist would require for a "content" contribution, they still offer a real contribution to the psychologist's world, because the latter has been *completely* in the dark regarding the degree of inheritance of personality factors. Even the present conclusions, with their broad margin of standard error, can help the psychologist a lot in choosing directions of valid hypothesis formation for these primary personality factors. For example, it is a waste of experimental effort to explore a physiological, genetic theory of a personality factor if that particular factor proves in our results to be largely environmentally determined. Conversely, much sociological and learning theory "explanation" has already been embarrassingly committed regarding factors which are here shown, whatever the exact figures, to be at least determined substantially by genetic variance.

In short, a proper strategy of investigation of personality source traits requires that the nature-nurture ratios be determined *as soon as measurement of the factors has reached a stage where even a tolerable reliability of measurement exists.* Psychological research of the last fifteen years has succeeded primarily in *demonstrating the factor patterns* as such, i.e., as invariant, replicable, loading constellations from sample to sample. Research has only in the last two or three years turned its attention to developing reliable batteries for measuring these factors (10) (15), to permit the present crucial research.

Admitting, therefore, that the time is not ripe to enter this experiment with expectations of establishing the nature-nurture ratios with *exactness*, we yet assert it is important for the orientation of immediate research that a substantial hint be obtained, as early as possible, as to whether a factor is largely determined by environmental molding influences or by constitution. Accordingly, this research has been undertaken as soon as: (1) it is possible to set up testing batteries; (2) of fair validity and reliability, (3) on an array of factors that have so far been shown to be invariant. A practical difficulty here has been that we can best work with *children*

CATTELL, BLEWETT AND BELOFF

in genetic investigations whereas the advance of factor test measurement has been greatest in the *adult* range and it must be reiterated that we cannot measure these factors in children with the accuracy of, say, intelligence. However, the work of Cattell and Gruen, (14) (16), Beloff (15), Dubin (9), and others in the last few years has provided a reasonably good basis for a child battery, in terms both of question-naire tests and of objective tests.

The present report restricts itself to the results of the questionnaire battery meas-urements. These are of lesser validity but greater convenience than the apparatus tests, and it was felt that to operate first with these would give preliminary results and also smooth out the difficulties of the research design for the ensuing objective test battery. This laboratory had recently finished research on the only existing com-pletely factored questionnaire test for children, *The Junior Personality Quiz*, meas-uring twelve personality factors, one of them being intelligence (15). This test takes less than an hour to administer (¾ of an hour for average subjects) and is only 144 items in length, which means that it proceeds with the maximum validity and re-liability now obtainable from 12 items per factor measurement. It has the advantage that most of its factors can be matched with those of the 16 Personality Factor Questionnaire (13), which is a widely used questionnaire test with adults, and that they are also recognizable in terms of the corresponding behavior rating factors, (16) (19).

The factors measured by the J.P.Q. are those of Cyclothymia vs. Schizothymia (Factor A), Neuroticism vs. Ego-Strength (Factor C), Dominance vs. Submissive-ness (Factor E), Surgency vs. Desurgency (Factor F), General Intelligence (Factor B), Tender-minded vs. Tough-minded (Factor I), Nervous Tension vs. Autonomic Relaxation (Factor Q4), as well as the factors known as D, H, J, K, and Q3. The test is designed in the reading vocabulary of an eleven to fifteen year old child. With the indicated brevity of 12 items for each factor the reliabilities of factor measures range from .25 to .83 with a median at .51. Since the construction of the test (15) is such as to avoid any common factors, other than the primary factor concerned, in the halves of the factor measure, the internal validities of the tests, in terms of the extent to which they measure the factor back of the actual questions, are the square roots of these values, and accordingly range from .50 to .91 with a median value of .71. The Junior Personality Quiz is a new test which has been widely used in the first year of its existence, but because of its newness the results of such use have not yet appeared in terms of publication of *specific* criterion validities. Such data is expected to become available during the time of our present publication.

IV. ADMINISTRATION OF THE J.P.Q. AND CALCULATION OF VARIANCE VALUES

Our aim was to test a sufficient population of identical twins, fraternal twins, sibs together, sibs apart, unrelated pairs reared together and the general population—all in the 11–15 age range. What restrictions we could afford to keep, as to sex, social range, etc., depended on the relation between the population size we considered adequate, and the available population.

Prior to experiment there is no way of knowing what population sizes will give variances of adequate stability. We aimed ideally at 100 pairs in each category, and

INHERITANCE OF PERSONALITY

reached this essentially in two categories: sibs together, and general population. But in spite of search in three major cities we finished, in the case of fraternal twins, with only some thirty-two pairs; in sibs apart, thirty-one pairs; and in unrelated children together, thirty-six pairs. Even in these short categories, however, we have about the same order of population size as the chief previous studies. (Newman, Freeman and Holzinger had 50 identicals and 50 fraternals. Eysenck and Prell had 25 identical pairs and 25 fraternal pairs.)

For the guidance of other researchers in this area it may be helpful to indicate that the number of cases obtained, even with the best school and press campaign, and the assistance of the principal social welfare and placement agencies falls short by perhaps 75% of the theoretically available cases in the area (calculated, for twins, for example, on the basis of one child in forty being born a twin). For this reason we found the Chicago area did not provide sufficient cases, and we were compelled to add Boston and New York. The *most* difficult cases to obtain were siblings reared apart from birth, and the next most difficult the unrelated children reared together.

Our deficiency of fraternal twins was due to our own error, of apparently asking in the press campaign for identical twins, whereupon we got a group which proved later to be largely identicals. More fraternals would otherwise have come in, and are coming in, in a supplementary study now in progress. As the data gathering proceeded it became evident that we could not get enough cases within the strictest form of homogeneity—same sex and male—so our goal was changed to same sex pairs, male *or* female. It is relatively unimportant whether ratios first be obtained for more or for less homogeneous families, providing we know which the obtained variance ratios apply to, and providing we do not employ the within-family identical twin variance term for families of *un*like sex pairs. (In other words, the *we* and *wh* terms in the above equations need a multiplication of primes if we take pairs of differing sex composition. The former is necessary because of the culture pattern difference of treatment of boys and girls and the latter because of the X chromosome.)

We wish to express our great indebtedness to a wide range of people who assisted in this location of cases—the most difficult part of the research. In particular we are glad to record our thanks to Dr. Kenneth Lund and his assistants in the Chicago Schools' Psychological Clinic; to Dr. S. Cook of New York University; to the school superintendents and principals in Chicago, Evanston, Winnetka, and Champaign, Illinois; the Catholic Home Bureau and the City Department of Welfare in Chicago; the Massachusetts Division of Child Guardianship; the Catholic Home Bureau in New York City and the Angel's Guardian Home in Brooklyn, New York. Especially we express our indebtedness to Dr. Benjamin Burack and the authorities of Roosevelt College for generously providing central research rooms for the Chicago testing and to Dr. Norton Kristy for organizing case work. The children to be tested were brought to a central clinic or testing center, and responded to the J.P.Q. questionnaire under the immediate supervision of the psychologist. This was done in a quiet session after the objective tests, physical measurements and photographs had been taken. The results were obtained as raw scores, by the keys provided with the handbook, and the following computational procedures ensued.

1. *Correction for Age.* In those factors—B, I, J, K and Q_3—in which a significant

age trend has been found, all scores were corrected, by the table in the handbook (13), to the 11 year level. Thus all statements, e.g., about inter-sibling variance, must be considered to be independent of trend differences due to age. The reader should be alerted that this possible source of contamination of variance has not been eliminated in some studies with which ours may need to be compared.

2. *Calculation of Variances.* Wherever the pattern was that of two cases per family the within variance was most readily calculated by summing the squares of the differences of the two pair members; while the basis for the between variances was obtained by summing the squares of the corresponding sums. (These sums of raw scores, in the latter case are then converted by the usual $\Sigma X^2 = \Sigma X^2 - (\Sigma X)^2/N$). Both of the variance values thus obtained need to be halved because they are calculated on a doubled scale. Indeed, the *between* variance total would need to be divided by four if one were not already needing doubled values to fit the "mean square" equations 7 through 11, as explained above.

A check on the within variance may be obtained by working out the intra-class correlation coefficient, as is commonly used in correlating twins.

The degrees of freedom for these variances are (1) $km - k$ for the within variances, m being the number in each family, i.e., 2, and k the number of families. (The d.f. are thus equal to the number of families) and (2) $k - 1$ for the between variances. In a few instances, in unrelated reared together, we had data for three in a family, and here it is necessary to calculate means throughout, allowing two degrees of freedom for the within variance in such a family.

3. *Correction for Experimental Error of Measurement.* As indicated in the above equations, the variance as obtained in (2) consists of true variance inflated by error variance, and our nature-nurture relations are required only for the estimated true factor variances. Since the error is $\sigma^2(1 - r)$ the true values on the left are computationally obtained by multiplying the obtained values by the consistency coefficient.

At this point two alternative procedures become possible. We can either take the best estimate of the consistency coefficient for the "population", from which twins, sibs, etc., are samples; or we can accept the value for each sample as an indication of the error in that sample. Some statisticians have recommended the former, but it must be recognized that we are in fact dealing with both sampling error and experimental error. The latter may indeed vary from sample to sample through other than sampling errors and this *should* be reflected in the correction. Retaining a constant population figure for consistency on one factor throughout all equations would not give a different solution from using uncorrected variances (for the left side of every equation would be reduced in exactly the same proportion), and the first alternative would therefore make sense only if the consistency coefficient were modified in each sample according to the variance, which is naturally systematically different for twins, sibs, etc. This is done by

$$\sigma_x(1 - r_x) = \sigma_p(1 - r_p)$$

where we know (by estimate) r_p, the consistency in the general population, σ_p for the population, and σ_x for the special sub-group.

INHERITANCE OF PERSONALITY

In another analysis we shall recompute the solutions on the basis of variances uncorrected for error, to see how much difference results. But here we have followed what seems to us the best course, namely, to correct. And we have compromised between the two extremes of such correction, taking the mean of the r_z obtained as above and the consistency r obtained for the actual sample. For using the latter alone, empirically obtained on small samples, and for factors of lower reliability, produces gross variations in the estimated error-free variance, whereas the former cannot strictly be accepted because it ignores real differences in reliability of testing from sub-group to sub-group.

V. THE EXPERIMENTAL DATA AND ITS TREATMENT IN THE SIMULTANEOUS QUADRATIC SOLUTIONS

Table I(a) sets out the actually obtained variances as derived from raw scores (possible range 0–12) for each of the 12 factors in the J.P.Q., corrected to 11 years of age as indicated above. Table I(b) contains the corresponding consistency coefficients (reliabilities) calculated as the mean of the standard-deviation-corrected general population value and the value empirically obtained in the sub-group concerned.

As indicated earlier, a complete solution for eleven unknowns—six variances and five of the six correlations—by the eleven equations above was found to be impossible because five of the equations turn out to be linearly dependent upon the remainder. This arises largely from the supplementary relation of within family variances in the first five equations and between family in the last five, with respect to equation six.

TABLE I

(a) EXPERIMENTALLY OBTAINED, OBSERVED VARIANCES

Group	Factor											
	1	2	3	4	5	6	7	8	9	10	11	12
Identical Twins.......	2.27	3.05	2.55	2.51	2.70	2.21	2.43	3.47	4.30	2.21	1.89	1.40
Fraternal Twins.......	3.33	4.75	4.09	2.71	3.64	2.39	3.27	4.83	3.86	3.48	2.78	2.68
Sibs Together.........	3.44	4.66	3.57	3.52	2.79	2.40	2.99	4.78	3.87	3.24	2.65	3.18
Sibs Apart...........	4.09	6.16	4.29	4.21	2.77	3.80	4.16	5.38	4.88	3.29	3.00	3.29
Unrelated Together....	3.53	5.72	4.05	3.88	2.94	3.96	6.42	4.63	5.29	5.81	4.05	3.41
General Population....	5.04	5,55	4.00	4.83	3.72	3.31	5.87	4.65	5.49	3.47	4.10	3.73

(b) RELIABILITIES OF MEASUREMENT
(Mean of two estimates)

Group	Factor											
	1	2	3	4	5	6	7	8	9	10	11	12
Identical Twins.......	.60	.55	.47	.35	.27	.19	.30	.47	.31	.24	.44	.65
Fraternal Twins.......	.51	.59	.38	.40	.23	.18	.30	.45	.35	.22	.48	.58
Sibs Together.........	.68	.61	.44	.49	.30	.20	.37	.53	.38	.33	.56	.55
Sibs Apart...........	.54	.56	.47	.44	.26	.24	.48	.59	.44	.42	.40	.69
Unrelated Together....	.68	.53	.42	.49	.31	.25	.26	.53	.38	.20	.37	.58
General Population....	.67	.55	.52	.47	.25	.32	.31	.54	.37	.34	.41	.63

But even if we had not encountered this, some indeterminacy would remain because of the quadratics and the spreading ambiguity of equally possible solutions.

Accordingly, and since four of the six r's are almost certainly zero, we decided to take five equations and solve for five variances, fixing the two r values in ways to be explained. At this point we had a choice of which of two linearly dependent equations to drop, and we decided on the following bases:

(1) The relative importance of the unknowns involved. The variances, as indicated, were considered more important than r's.

(2) The size of samples on which we had data at the time of this decision. On this basis we decided to drop either sibs reared apart or fraternal twins as too few.

(3) The desirability of dropping equations involving r's that could not so confidently be considered zero. Actually $r_{we,wh}$ and $r_{be,bh}$ had to be retained for it is these alone that cannot be considered zero.

Although our choice was a careful one, it is still possible that a better combination of five equations than ours can be found, and certainly others exist. In this compromise we are forced to two assumptions we had wished to avoid, namely, (1) we assumed there are only two kinds of within family environmental variance—that of sibs and identical twins and that of fraternal twins. (2) we assumed only the correlations of *environment and heredity* to be significant, and only in the same realm (within family or between family). These are therefore *not* eliminated, as stated above. They can only be handled, however, either by ulterior empirical evidence as to what they should be, or as here, by assigning a reasonable range of values to them, which permits (a) seeing how much the variances are affected by such a range and (b) obtaining a *range* of variance solutions each conditional on an explicitly assumed correlation.

Although our results are reported on the second basis we have also explored the first, by taking examples where an appreciable hereditary variance exists and is tolerably known, and here we tended to find $r_{we,wh}$ with low negative values. This would agree with expectations from *the law of overt and covert trait deviation* (5), though this applies to traits where deviations are socially undesirable. It implies a general tendency of society, within and without the family, to bring environmental pressure to bear on *deviant* hereditary tendencies, i.e., to press all individuals toward the social norm presented by the existing mean for any trait. This is unlikely to apply to such desirable traits as intelligence, ego-strength and super ego-strength, and, indeed, our final results suggest there are more positive than negative (8 to 4) relations of heredity to environmental influences. However, *a priori*, either might arise, for even in intelligence it may be pointed out that society allows the bright to mark time while it concentrates special education on raising the less bright.[1] Our final results

[1] We find it widely assumed in the literature that the parable of the talents applies, and that the more intelligent get the more intelligence-provoking environment (see 1, 24, 31 and 46 in (8)). This, as we have argued elsewhere (4) is surely a naive and question-begging assumption. For example, both among school teachers and among the parents whom we questioned, even the consciously accepted "obvious thing to do" was more frequently to concentrate intellectual stimulation around the less bright. However, since the converse view was also met we have entered the intelligence equations, just like those for other factors, with both positive and negative correlations, in alternative solutions.

suggest culture tends to be negatively related to heredity where heredity is powerful, but otherwise positive relations predominate.

In general, through lack of space for specific discussion we have assumed within and between family heredity-environment relations have the same sign; though differences could sometimes be justified.

Although the available evidence thus suggests both positive and negative values according to social circumstances, the only acceptable procedure in handling this r, which cannot be assumed zero and yet which cannot be determined, would seem to be to take a spread of values through the most likely range and see how much the resulting variances are affected by this range of assumptions. Accordingly we have systematically, in all factors, tried four values: $\pm$ .10 and $\pm$ .50, while in intelligence we have also tried $\pm$ .30 and $\pm$.60.

The equations finally used from Section 2 above were 1, 2, 3, 5, and 6—the equations for sibs raised apart and for the "between variances" being dropped. However, another solution, using all available data and equations, by the method of least squares, has also been made and will later be reported.

For purposes of easy computation the five equations used—1, 2, 3, 5 and 6 above—were solved for the standard deviations, whereby the latter could be calculated by putting in the empirical values directly. The solutions are:

$$(1) \quad \sigma_{we} = \sqrt{\sigma_{ITT'}^2}$$

$$(2) \quad \sigma_{be} = -r_{be \cdot bh}\sqrt{\sigma_{UT'}^2 - \sigma_{ST'}^2} \pm \sqrt{\sigma_{UA'}^2 - r_{be,bh}^2 \sigma_{ST'}^2 - (1 - r_{be,bh}^2)\sigma_{UT'}^2}$$

$$(3) \quad \sigma_{wh} = -r_{we.wh}\sqrt{\sigma_{ITT'}^2} \pm \sqrt{\sigma_{ST'}^2 - (1 - r_{we.wh}^2)\sigma_{ITT'}^2}$$

$$(4) \quad \sigma_{bh} = \sqrt{\sigma_{UT'}^2 - \sigma_{ST'}^2}$$

$$(5) \quad \sigma_{we''} = -r_{we.wh} \pm \sqrt{\sigma_{FTT'}^2 - \sigma_{wh}^2(1 - r_{we,wh}^2)}$$

For uniformity, all solutions are kept as standard deviations and need squaring to give variances. They are best solved in this order, since earlier values are needed to insert in later equations. These equations represent only the positive solutions, since a negative standard deviation is meaningless. Even so there are potentially two solutions for σ_{wh} and $\sigma_{we''}$, though in all cases it happens that one vanishes, being negative. The question of the particular correlation values to be inserted is taken up in the next section on particular factors. Where four different r's are tried there are of course, typically four solutions for σ_{wh}, σ_{be} and $\sigma_{we''}$, as shown for each factor below.

The actual empirical variances on which these equations are worked are those set out in Table II, representing corrected values, though, as stated, a separate study will also report the use of uncorrected variances. Since these variances (for any one factor, in different sib, twin, etc., samples) should not behave as samples from a single population we have applied the F test to a random 100 pairings and obtained

CATTELL, BLEWETT AND BELOFF

TABLE II.—CORRECTED, "TRUE" VARIANCES FROM THE FIVE KINDS OF GROUPS USED

Group	1	2	3	4	5	6	7	8	9	10	11	12
Id. Twins Together	1.36	1.68	1.21	.88	.73	.42	.73	1.63	1.33	.53	.83	.91
Frat. Twins Together	1.70	2.80	1.52	1.08	.84	.43	.98	2.17	1.35	.77	1.34	1.55
Sibs Together	2.34	2.84	1.57	1.73	.84	.48	1.11	2.27	1.47	1.07	1.48	1.75
Unrelated Together	2.40	3.03	1.70	1.90	.91	.99	1.67	2.45	2.01	1.16	1.50	1.98
General Population	3.38	3.05	2.08	2.27	.93	1.06	1.82	2.51	2.03	1.18	1.68	2.35

TABLE III.—SIZES OF SAMPLES AND DEGREES OF FREEDOM

Identical Twins	Fraternal Twins	Sibs Together	(Sibs Apart)[1]	Unrelated Together	Unrelated Apart[2]
104	64	182	(62)	72	540
d.f. = 52	d.f. = 32	d.f. = 91	(Not used)	d.f. = 36	d.f. = 539

[1] Not used in this analysis.

[2] General Population. In this case d.f. = 539 since they are not taken in pairs but from a common mean.

69% of differences significant at the 1% level and 26% at the 5% level, while 5% did not break the null hypothesis.

The general population variance used here (originally in Table I) is the mean of two estimates: (1) from taking one child from each pair, i.e., a random representative from each of our 210 families, and (2) from a second and larger sample of 330, 11–15 year old boys and girls from towns in Illinois. The general population variance is thus understood, by our age correction of scores, to be the variance of a *one year (11 year old) cross section of the population*, including no two members of the same family (except for the one case in forty which is a twin). The numbers in the other groups, and resulting degrees of freedom, are shown in Table III.

VI. THE CONTRIBUTORY VARIANCE RATIOS DISCOVERED FOR PERSONALITY FACTORS

It is proposed now to set out the obtained variances and ratios, factor by factor. These give four values (set out in corresponding order) for σ_{b_e} and σ_{b_h} (theoretically eight, but four are always negative), and possibly up to eight for $\sigma_{w_e''}$, but actually never more than five.

Although, in general, the alternative r's rarely carry the resulting ratio from a predominantly hereditary to a predominantly environmental one, or vice versa, it is desirable to indicate in each case an r value preferable on some grounds to the others, and to accept consistently the other values which go with this. In this, our considerations, apart from specific ones, brought in below, are: (1) Decided correlations (say .50 or more) between personality and sociological influences are rare. Other things being equal, we should prefer the 0 or ± .10 values. (2) A negative or positive r is to be preferred according to whether or not the trait is one which society seeks to hold in check at its extremes. (3) The r associated with the more central value among the alternatives is to be preferred, rather than a more extreme estimate.

INHERITANCE OF PERSONALITY

(4) In general we may expect rather smaller relations of heredity and environment within society ($r_{be.bh}$) than in the family, ($r_{we.wh}$), since the person's qualities are more constantly understood in the family. However, in one case, intelligence, we know of some appreciable $r_{be.bh}$ values, notably of $+0.3$ between intelligence and social status (4)(35). (5) Most guidance can perhaps be gained from the assumption that the relation of σ^2_{bh} and σ^2_{wh} is likely to stay in fairly narrow limits. This is because we are dealing with a relation common to most hereditary mechanisms and little affected by specific social conditions. In many cases this at once rules out all but one of the four alternative algebraic solutions for σ_{wh}, and at the same time indicates the preferred $r_{we,wh}$ correlation. Two possibilities[1] have to be considered in this last, but they indicate ratios of σ^2_{bh} to σ^2_{wh} probably only ranging from 2 to 1 to 1 to 2.

Factor I. Commonly called "I": Tender-minded vs. Tough-minded
(Also Sensitive, Anxious, Emotionality vs. Tough Poise)

Computed values:

$\sigma^2_{we} = 1.36$ ($\sigma^2_{we''} = .77$ or .64 ($r = \pm 10$); .86 ($r = +50$)

$\sigma^2_{wh} = .77$ and 1.23 ($r = \pm 10$); .32 and 2.99 ($r = \pm 50$)

$\sigma^2_{be} = .93$ and 1.03 ($r = \pm 10$); .74 and 1.26 ($r = \pm 50$)

$\sigma^2_{bh} = .06$

The above form will be followed in setting out all factor values. The four values correspond to the four possible correlations, in the order indicated. A total consistency will decide the preferred solution, and in this the *wh/bh* ratio will be given prime consideration, but also the psychologically preferred *r* and the central tendency of the estimates, as well as the closeness of *we″* to *we*. In this case the $+50$ (or, less well, the $+10$) gives the best agreement of *we* and *we″* (choice of latter underlined) and also gives the only value, .32, for *wh* that brings it nearest the expected order of relation to *bh*. Accepting this system we find that between families, environmental differences are of the order of twelve to fifteen times as effective as hereditary differences in accounting for individual differences in *I*. Correspondingly, within the

---

[1] They are: (1) with random, unassortative mating and (2) with some degree of positive correlation of husband and wife. In the latter the between family hereditary variance is likely to climb relative to within variance. Parenthetically, no such guidance can be sought from an inherent law of relationship of "within" and "between" *environmental* variance. For the relationships there are not beyond the control of man and are subject to all sorts of specific and culturally fluctuant manipulations. But the hereditary ratio of σ^2_{wh} and σ^2_{bh} should be constant within limits useful enough to guide our choice among the four mathematically alternative answers for σ^2_{wh}, (for, in our calculations at least, σ^2_{bh} is free of ambiguity). For an estimate of this ratio we can turn (a) to general evidence from other genetic fields, which points to something of order of 1:2 in non-assortative mating for the ratio of σ^2_{wh} to σ^2_{bh}, and (b) to a calculation from the variance of the mid-parent relative to the total society, which as pointed out below, would make σ^2_{bh} greater than σ^2_{wh}. The mean value for all our factors on all estimates, of σ^2_{wh} and σ^2_{bh}, actually gives a ratio of 3.6 to 1. Since there is no reason to suppose the hereditary mechanism is other than polygenic, for all these personality dimensions the preferred σ^2_{wh} value should be the one approximating a ratio of between 1 to 1 and 1 to 2 to the fixed σ^2_{bh}.

CATTELL, BLEWETT AND BELOFF

family, environment predominates, being about four (two to five) times as important as heredity. The values finally chosen are italicized.

In short this pattern is largely environmentally determined, and on more accurate analysis might prove to be wholly an environmental mold trait (6). The larger ratio for *between* family environment suggests that this resides in some sort of family atmosphere—almost certainly an over-protective, gentler tradition as opposed to a Spartan roughness. The size of positive correlation suggests some selection of gentler temperaments to the gentler environment.

Factor 2. Commonly called Q_4. Nervous Tension vs. Autonomic Relaxation
(Also called "Somatic Anxiety" (12))

$\sigma^2_{we} = 1.69\ (\sigma^2_{we''} = 1.64\ (r = \pm 10);\ 1.64\ (r = +50)\ 1.52$ and $.52\ (r = -.50)$

$\sigma^2_{wh} = .92$ and $1.49\ (r = \pm 10);\ .37$ and $3.63\ (r = \pm 50)$

$\sigma^2_{be} = .01$ and $.03\ (r = \pm 10);\ .01$ and $.23\ (r = \pm 50)$

$\sigma^2_{bh} = .19$

Again the correlation which makes for most consistency is one of about +50. In such consistency, it should be pointed out, we do not assume that the ratio of *bh/be* should equal that of *wh/we*, nor that the correlation should be the same in the two cases. However, one might reasonably expect them to be in the same direction, in general, and of the same sign, in the case of *r*, with $r_{be,bh}$ lower.

The bulk of the variance in this factor is within families. Taking the σ^2_{bh} value, .37, which alone stands in any acceptable ratio to σ^2_{bh}, we find environment predominating, standing four times as influential as heredity *within* families, and about twice as important *between*.

This is perhaps not unexpected, clinically, in that we are dealing with one of the major forms of neurotic anxiety. Presumably the intra-family events are those early experiences so emphasized by psychoanalysts and others. Incidentally, in general, it is probable that large emphasis on *within family* environment generally means emphasis on early life effects, since the effects of the family status within society—the interactions of family with society—are not usually operative until later.

Factor 3. Commonly called "C" (or "O"): General Neuroticism vs. Ego Strength

$\sigma^2_{we} = 1.21\ (\sigma^2_{we''} = 1.21$ and $1.21\ (r = \pm 10);\ 1.21\ (r = +50),\ 1.23$ and $.05$
$(r = -50)$

$\sigma^2_{wh} = .25$ and $.52\ (r = \pm .10):\ .06$ and $1.86\ (r = \pm .50)$

$\sigma^2_{be} = .34$ and $.40\ (r = \pm .10);\ .20$ and $.69\ (r = \pm 50)$

$\sigma^2_{bh} = .13$

In this case the most central tendencies and those best in keeping with the within family hereditary variation being of the same order as the "between," are those de-

INHERITANCE OF PERSONALITY

rived from an r between hereditary proneness and environmental provocation of about $+.40$.

Whatever r is adopted, the predominant influence is to environment, in within and between family situations together. The preferred r would give a 10 to 1 relation within the family and about 2 to 1 as between families.

This result, to our surprise, favors the standard clinical and psychoanalytic viewpoint and possibly the degree of hereditary determination found by Scott in animals (29) rather than the recent major emphasis on heredity in neurosis by Eysenck and Prell (18). Within environment the weight of causation is partly on the total family atmosphere but more on the specific happenings to individuals within the family. Briefly, the following reconciliations may be suggested. (1) We believe Eysenck and Prell's factor of neuroticism is different from our C, being based on (a) less complete factor extraction and (b) on determination by criterion rotation rather than simple structure. Criterion rotation could lump together parts of several distinct factors distinguishing neurotics from normals. Our Q_4, for example, is probably included in such a composite. (2) Eysenck's samples were smaller and, as has been usual in twin studies, no correction was made for difference between the test measurement and the factor measurement. (3) Correlation of variances was not allowed for in that study. Accordingly, we feel entitled to conclude that the greater environmental variance found here is likely to be nearer the truth.

Factor 4. Commonly called Q_3: Will Control (13)

$$\sigma^2_{we} = .88 \ (\sigma^2_{we''} = .29 \text{ and } .10 \ (r = \pm 10), .40 \ (r = +50))$$

$$\sigma^2_{wh} = .13 \text{ and } .30 \ (r = \pm 10); .03 \text{ and } 1.25 \ (r = \pm .50)$$

$$\sigma^2_{be} = .33 \text{ and } .42 \ (r = \pm 10); .18 \text{ and } .72 \ (r = \pm 50)$$

$$\sigma^2_{bh} = .17$$

A moderate positive correlation, about .20, of within environment and within heredity, gives the most consistent relation here. This, or even fairly wide variations from it, will give environment a predominance over heredity reaching about 8 to 1 within the family. Although superficially the pattern of Q_3 looks like one of acquired precision, moral standards and self discipline, it must evidently be founded appreciably also on an hereditary pre-disposition which decides how far this self concept will "take" as between one family and another. A rather unusual discrepancy of twin and sib environmental variance here requires psychological explanation.

Factor 5. Commonly called "D": Impatient Dominance, Immaturity or Sthenic
Emotionality (6) (15)

$$\sigma^2_{we} = .73 \ (\sigma^2_{we''} = .72 \ (r \pm 10) .72 \ (r = +50) .72 \text{ and } .02 \ (r = -50))$$

$$\sigma^2_{wh} = .07 \text{ or } .19 \ (r = \pm 10), .01 \text{ or } .95 \ (r = \pm 50)$$

$$\sigma^2_{be} = .01 \text{ or } .03 \ (r = \pm 10); .004 \text{ or } .11 \ (r = \pm 50)$$

$$\sigma^2_{bh} = .07$$

CATTELL, BLEWETT AND BELOFF

A zero or slightly negative r is all that is indicated here. Practically all solutions make most of the variance in this factor depend upon within-family environment.

This finding agrees with some as yet unpublished evidence, that the level of the Impatient Dominance factor is related to degree of spoiling and favoritism encountered. It suggests that some particular family position influences could profitably be investigated as major determiners of this pattern.

Factor 6. Commonly called "A": Cyclothymia vs. Schizothymia (6) (13)

$\sigma^2_{we} = .42$ ($\sigma^2_{we''} = .37$ ($r = \pm 10$), .37 ($r = +50$), .29 or .04 ($r = -50$)

$\sigma^2_{wh} = .04$ and .10. ($r = \pm 10$); .01 and .53 ($r = \pm 50$)

$\sigma^2_{be} = .04$ and .12 ($r = \pm 10$); 01 and .66 ($r = \pm 50$)

$\sigma^2_{bh} = .51$

These figures suggest that mating may be less assortative on this trait than others (perhaps the non-easy-going seeks the easy-going) and/or that environment acts *against* hereditary deviations, with a negative r of perhaps $-.50$. For the first time we encounter a factor in which heredity is *more* important than environment within the family, and about equally important between families.

The higher emphasis on genetic influences here agrees with the findings of Kretschmer (21), Sheldon (30) and Stockard (32) of strong body build associations with cyclothymia vs. schizothyme tenseness, and the psychiatric findings of Kallmann (20), Rosanoff (27), Slater (31) and others, of appreciable hereditary determination of whether mental disorder shall take manic-depressive or schizophrenic forms. The environment of twins is indicated to be more alike than that of sibs in influence on this factor.

Factor 7. Commonly symbolized "H": Adventurous Cyclothymia vs.
Withdrawn Schizothymia

$\sigma^2_{we} = 73$ ($\sigma^2_{we} = .62$ and .58 ($r = \pm 10$), .62 ($r = + .50$))

$\sigma^2_{wh} = .28$ and .51 ($r = \pm .10$), .10 and 1.39 ($r = \pm .50$)

$\sigma^2_{be} = .10$ and .22 ($r = \pm .10$), .03 and .83 ($r = \pm 50$)

$\sigma^2_{bh} = .56$

In this case an r of about $-.50$ to $-.60$ would seem to give the best fit and to agree also with psychological expectations. For education, both within and between families, aims to "bring out" the shy and to repress the unduly boisterous. Nevertheless the strongest hereditary determination yet encountered is found here, showing roughly equal action between families and a two to one predominance regarding within family variations.

The theory propounded elsewhere (6), that A and H represent hereditary and environmental factors in the schizothyme pattern must be modified, for unless later research alters the values *both* components have substantial hereditary roots.

INHERITANCE OF PERSONALITY

Factor 8. Commonly called "K": Socialized Morale vs. Boorishness (6) (13) (14)
(Also called Trained Mind vs. Rejection of Education)

$\sigma^2_{we} = 1.63$ ($\sigma^2_{we''} = 1.54$ and 1.52 ($r = \pm .10$), 1.54 ($r = +50$), 1.31 or $.27$ ($r = -50$)

$\sigma^2_{wh} = .46$ and $.88$ ($r = \pm 10$); $.15$ and 2.76 ($r = \pm .50$)

$\sigma^2_{be} = .04$ and $.09$ ($r = \pm 10$); $.01$ and $.29$ ($r = \pm 50$)

$\sigma^2_{bh} = .18$

Absence of correlation between the two influences gives the best internal consistency. Hereditary influence then predominates more than two to one between families, while the reverse holds within families. By the apparent psychological nature of the factor, a larger environmental influence might be expected, though an interpretation as "temperamental susceptibility" to culture has also been previously hypothesized (6).

Factor 9. Commonly symbolized by "E": Dominance or Independence vs.
Submissiveness

$\sigma^2_{we} = 1.33$ ($\sigma^2_{we''} = 1.21$ and 1.20 ($r = \pm 10$), 1.21 ($r = +50$), 1.04 or $.08$ ($r = -50$))

$\sigma^2_{wh} = .08$ and $.26$ ($r = \pm .10$), $.01$ and 1.60 ($r = \pm .50$)

$\sigma^2_{be} = .01$ and $.06$ ($r = \pm .10$), $.001$ and $.58$ ($r = \pm .50$)

$\sigma^2_{bh} = .54$

One would almost certainly have to accept a negative correlation here, from the psychological evidence that our culture encourages the meek and frustrates the dominant; and indeed the $-.10$ correlations gives the best *wh/bh* relationship. Heredity would then be about ten times as important as environment *between* families, but one fourth as important within families. The latter suggests that the juxtaposition of highly dominant persons in one family results inevitably in some modification of dominance, to a greater extent than in the outside world.

These conclusions—hereditary emphasis and within family modification—fit the animal experimentation results (23) as well as, say, Sheldon's concept of mesomorphy, and the endocrine evidence.

Factor 10. Commonly called "J": Energetic Conformity vs. Quiet Eccentricity (6) (15)

$\sigma^2_{we} = .53$ ($\sigma^2_{we''} = .25$ and $.18$ ($r = \pm .10$), $.30$ ($r = +.50$)

$\sigma^2_{wh} = .44$ and $.66$ ($r = \pm 10$), $.21$ and 1.40 ($r = \pm .50$)

$\sigma^2_{be} = .01$ and $.03$ ($r = \pm .10$), $.003$ and $.12$ ($r = \pm .50$)

$\sigma^2_{bh} = .09$

CATTELL, BLEWETT AND BELOFF

The emphatic feature here is the predominance of within family variance. An r of about $+.40$ is probably indicated, and this would give a roughly 10 to 1 predominance to heredity between family and an environmental predominance within family of about $2:1$. The large within variance and relatively small twin environment variance suggests a possible family position effect and a lack of relation to cultural and status variables.

Factor 11. Symbolized "F": Surgency vs. Desurgency (6) (13) (14)

$\sigma^2_{we} = .83$ $(\sigma^2_{we''} = .70$ or $.69$ $(r = \pm .10)$, $.72$ $(r = + .50)$

$\sigma^2_{wh} = .52$ and 81 $(r = \pm 10)$, $.22$ and 1.90 $(r = \pm .50)$

$\sigma^2_{be} = .17$ and $.19$ $(r = \pm .10)$; $.13$ and 24 $(r = \pm .50)$

$\sigma^2_{bh} = .02$

Small bh values are, by the nature of the equations, unstable, and one suspects this might be nearer, say, 0.6, corresponding more to the lowest wh. The interesting fact to those who have studied the surgency factor in various contexts is the predominance of environmental determination. "Between" families environment would be three to ten times as influential, and, if the above positive r is accepted, it could possibly reach four times the intra-familiar variance (though twice may be more likely). Family climate is evidently very important, as one would expect with a dimension which has been hypothesized to be general inhibition level.

This environmental emphasis should help in the conceptual distinction from the H factor, with which it is often phenotypically confused.

Factor 12. Symbolized by "B" (or "g"): General Intelligence (6) (13)

$\sigma^2_{we} = .91$ $(\sigma^2_{we''} = .74$ and $.67$ $(r = \pm .10)$, $.76$ $(r = + .50))$

$\sigma^2_{wh} = .68$ and 1.03 $(r = \pm .10)$, $.31$ and 2.27 $(r = \pm .50)$

$\sigma^2_{be} = .32$ and $.43$ $(r = \pm 10)$, $.17$ and $.79$ $(r = \pm .50)$

$\sigma^2_{bh} = .23$

Since correlation of husbands and wives on intelligence is of the order $+0.40$ to $+0.50$, the ratio of bh to wh can be assumed to be on the high side. This would, in spite of our theory of intelligence and environmental stimulation, compel us to accept a positive r, at least within the family, if not in school. Accepting an r of $+.50$ would make heredity more important than environment between families but less important within families. A negative r might even make sense *within* the family, and one of $-.10$ is tentatively taken, at which heredity predominates.

This substantial environmental influence is at first very surprising, for despite lapse of years, there is no reason to doubt the massive evidence summarized by such investigators as Schwesinger (28), Thorndike (33) and Woodworth (35) for a decidedly higher hereditary contribution than this. The present result might therefore reflect either a systematic bias in the new method or a peculiarity of the intelligence test. If we consider the way in which the method has dealt with the whole range of factors we see that it has made some largely hereditary and others largely environmental, though there *does* seem to be some systematic tendency for the environmental ratios to run higher; but there is no independent evidence that this is definitely wrong.

Accordingly we do well to examine the test, which is typical of verbal intelligence tests. The senior author has proposed elsewhere that nature-nurture ratios should not be determined on verbal tests, which can be demonstrated to have considerable cultural association, but on Culture-Free, Perceptual tests (7). It happened that for the general purposes for which the J.P.Q. is intended (15) the verbal form was alone appropriate, but in the experiment reported later it was supplemented by the Culture Free Tests. The use of the same method on the new data may help decide whether our present assumption is correct; that the anomalous intelligence factor findings here are due to rather heavy educational content in the test itself.

SUMMARY OF CONCLUSIONS

1. A multiple variance analysis method (8) has been applied for the first time to psychological, heredity-environment analysis, attempting from five linearly independent equations (survivors of eleven possible equations) to determine five variances. The sample consisted of 104 identical twins, 64 fraternal twins, 182 siblings reared together, 72 unrelated children reared together and 540 children in the general population. The measures were for twelve personality factors (including intelligence as one) on the Junior Personality Questionnaire Test.

2. A critical evaluation of the findings requires more extended discussion of the confidence limits of the variance ratios than is possible here. Debate ranges overestimates that the $2\frac{1}{2}\%$ limits of a 1 to 10 ratio are approximately 1 to 8 and 1 to 12 to estimates which give a standard error as large as the ratios obtained, in certain cases. The matter will be handled systematically in the pending publication applying exactly the same equations to objective test measures on the same sámples.

Meanwhile, this presentation may be taken as a demonstration of the method and as providing estimates, admittedly not sufficiently reliable to stand by themselves, but capable of giving cumulative evidence when compared with future estimates by ourselves and others, as to the true values. Both this unreliability (as shown in the instability of some values such as σ^2_{bh}, which arise as fine differences between two observed variances), and the failure of some sample differences to refute the null hypothesis (section V above) now show that for good solutions the experiment must be carried out on a scale *at least two or three times as large* as ours. And, as our experience shows, this will require thorough case research in three or four large cities, and a generous endowment.

3. In each factor we have presented not so much a solution as a series of solutions, depending on various assumptions of correlation. In some cases variation of r proves to affect the solution relatively little, but in a few it would invert the relative importance of heredity and environment. To lessen the range we have attempted to

CATTELL, BLEWETT AND BELOFF

choose a preferred value on the basis of an expected $\sigma^2_{wh}/\sigma^2_{bh}$ ratio of roughly unity[1]; on psychological considerations; and on internal consistency of the results (predominance, in one factor, of heredity or environment, in both within and between relations). More attention could advantageously be given to determining the wh/bh ratio, from known highly inherited traits and in relation to known assortativeness of mating, for it frequently permitted an instant rejection of one of the superfluous algebraic solutions. Frequently, alternative algebraic solutions are negative or absurd, so that in fact the method gives more unambiguous answers than might be theoretically expected. It is proposed to check elsewhere on the present solutions by using a least squares method that will permit more of our equations to be used. A solution is also being based on variances uncorrected for test unreliability, to compare with the present.

4. In spite of uncertainties on individual values, there is in general considerable internal consistency, and consistency with psychological understanding of the nature of the factor.

Some factors are predominantly environmentally determined, consistently in both "between" and "within" estimates. These are I, Tender-Mindedness; C, General Neuroticism; F, Surgency-Desurgency; Q_3 Will Control, and Q_4, Somatic Anxiety. However, in the neuroticism and anxiety factors heredity has an appreciable role as *between* families.

Four factors show about an equal role of heredity and environment but with heredity predominating *between* families; J, Energetic Conformity, E, Dominance, K, Socialized Morale, and D, Impatient Dominance.

Some three factors have larger roles for heredity than environment. These are: A, Cyclothymia vs. Schizothymia; H, Adventurous Cyclothymia vs. Submissiveness, and, B or General Intelligence.

The inferred correlations of hereditary and environmental influences range from $-.60$ to $+.50$, but most are positive. The strong negatives occur with A, H and E, which could be considered socially undesirable at either extreme, but the same might be said of F, where the indicators were of a positive r. In general the negative correlations are found with more highly inherited traits.

Some observations of interest to psychologists have been made at appropriate points regarding the relation of these conclusions to other psychological evidence, e.g. the twin studies on neuroticism and intelligence, body-build data, animal experiment. In the main there is convergence, but the present findings give a somewhat larger role to environment, and particularly to within family environment, in neuroticism, anxiety and verbal ability than do the twin studies. A number of provocative indications arise for psychological research *per se*, in terms of the direction to look for origins of particular source trait patterns e.g. family position.

The writers wish to thank those who have given help in the statistical discussion (but who are not responsible for our particular conclusions). In addition to our specific indebtedness to Dr. C. R. Rao, mentioned above, we had invaluable help

---

[1] The actual ratio of the mean *wh* variance to the mean *bh* variance accepted for these twelve factors is 1.6. With random mating and simple averaging of parental values, one would expect the *bh* value to be larger than this implies. A problem remains to be solved here.

INHERITANCE OF PERSONALITY

from Dr. W. G. Madow and Dr. C. R. Blythe of the University of Illinois, Dr. D. R. Saunders of the Educational Test Service, and from an unknown member of the editorial board of this journal.

This research was supported in major part by a research grant from the Institutes of Mental Health, of the National Institutes of Health, United States Public Health Service.

REFERENCES

1. BLEWETT, D. B. 1953. An experimental study of the inheritance of neuroticism and intelligence. Unpublished thesis, University of London.
2. BURKS, B. S. 1928. The relative influence of nature and nurture upon mental development. 27th Yearbook. *Nat. Soc. Stud. Educ.* 219–316.
3. BYWATERS, J. H. 1937. The hereditary and environmental portions of the variance in weaning weights of Poland China pigs. *Genetics* 22, 457–468.
4. CATTELL, R. B. 1940. Effects of human fertility trends upon the distribution of intelligence and culture. *39th Yearbook (I). Nat. Soc. Stud. Educ.* 221–233.
5. — 1951. "Principles of Design in 'Projective' or Misperceptive Tests of Personality". Chap. 3 in Anderson, H. H. and Anderson, G. H. (ed.). *Projective Techniques.* New York: Prentice Hall.
6. — 1950. *Personality: A Systematic, Theoretical and Factual Study.* New York: McGraw-Hill.
7. — 1950. A Culture Free Intelligence Test: Scales 1, 2, and 3. Institute for Personality and Ability Testing, 1608 Coronado Drive, Champaign, Illinois.
8. — 1953. Research design in psychological genetics with special reference to the multiple variance method. *Amer. J. Hum. Genet.* 5, 76–93.
9. — 1953. A universal index for psychological factors. Adv. Public. No. 3, Lab. of Person. Assess., Univ. of Illinois, December.
10. — 1954. The Objective Analytic Personality Test Battery. Institute for Personality and Ability Testing, 1602 Coronado Drive, Champaign, Illinois.
11. — & MALTENO, E. V. 1940. Contributions concerning mental inheritance. V. Temperament. *J. Genet. Psychol.* 57, 31–47.
12. — & SAUNDERS, D. R. 1950. Inter-relation and matching of personality factors from behavior rating questionnaire and objective test data. *J. Soc. Psychol.* 31, 243–260.
13. —, SAUNDERS, D. R., AND STICE, G. F. 1950. The 16 Personality Factor Questionnaire. Institute for Personality and Ability Testing, 1602 Coronado Drive, Champaign, Illinois.
14. —, & GRUEN, WALTER G. 1954. Primary personality factors in the questionnaire medium for children eleven to fourteen years old. *Educ. and Psychol. Meas.* 14, 50–76.
15. — & BELOFF, H. 1953. Research origins and construction of the IPAT Junior Personality Quiz. *J. Consult. Psychol.* 17, 436–442.
16. — & BELOFF, J. R. 1955. Personality factor structure in three media for 11 year old children (in press).
17. CHAPMAN, ARTHUR B. 1946. Genetic and Non-Genetic Sources of Variation in the Weight Response of the Immature Rat Ovary to a Gonadotrophic Hormone. *Genetics* 31, 494–507.
18. EYSENCK, H. J. AND PRELL, D. B. 1951. The inheritance of neuroticism: an experimental study. *J. Ment. Sci.* 97, 441–465.
19. FRENCH, J. W. 1953. *The Description of Personality Measurement in Terms of Rotated Factors.* Princeton: Educ. Test. Service.
20. KALLMANN, F. J. 1946. The genetic theory of schizophrenia. *Amer. J. Psychiat.* 103, 309–322.
21. KRETSCHMER, E. 1929. *Körperbau und Charakter.* Berlin: Julius Springer.
22. LUSH, J. L., HETZER, H. O., AND CULBERTSON, C. C. 1934. Factors affecting birth weights in swine. *Genetics* 19, 329.
23. MOWRER, O. H. 1941. Animal studies in the genesis of Personality. *Tr. N. Y. Acad. Sc.* Series 2, Vol. 3, No. 1.

CATTELL, BLEWETT AND BELOFF

24. NEWMAN, H. H., FREEMAN, F. N., AND HOLZINGER, K. J. 1937. *Twins: A Study of Heredity and Environment*. Chicago: Univ. Chicago Press.
25. PRICE, B. 1950. Primary biases in twin studies. *Amer. J. Hum. Genet.* 2, 243–253.
26. ROBINSON, H. F., COMSTOCK, R. E., AND HARVEY, P. H. 1949. Estimates of Heritability and the Degree of Dominance in Corn. *Agronomy J.* 41, 353–359.
27. ROSANOFF, A. J., HANDY, L. M., PLESSET, I. R., BRUSH, S. 1934. The etiology of so-called schizophrenic psychoses with special reference to their occurrence in twins. *Amer. J. Psychiat.* 91, 247–286.
28. SCHWESINGER, G. C. 1933. *Heredity and Environment*. New York: Macmillan.
29. SCOTT, J. P. 1950. The relative importance of social and hereditary factors in producing disturbances in life adjustments during periods of stress in laboratory animals. Chap. 4, *Res. Publ. Ass. Nerv. Disease* 29, 61–71.
30. SHELDON, W., STEVENS, S. S. AND TUCKER, W. B. 1940. The Varieties of Human Physique. New York: Harper Bros.
31. SLATER, E. AND SHIELDS, J. 1953. Psychotic and neurotic illness in Twins. M.R.C. Special Report. Series 278. London: HMSO.
32. STOCKARD, C. R. 1931. *The Physical Basis of Personality*. New York: Norton.
33. THORNDIKE, E. L. 1944. The resemblance of siblings in intelligence test scores. *J. Genet. Psychol.* 64, 265–267.
34. THURSTONE, L. L. & THURSTONE, T. G. 1941. Factorial Studies of Intelligence. Psychom. Monog. No. 2. Chicago: Univ. Chicago Press.
35. WOODWORTH, R. S. 1941. Heredity and Environment: a critical survey of recently published material on twins and foster children. *Soc. Sci. Res. Co. Bull.* 47, 1–95.
36. YULE, F. G. 1935. The resemblance of twins with regard to perseveration. *J. Ment. Sci.* 81, 489–501.

From I. I. Gottesman (1963). Psychological Monographs, *77,* 1-21, *by kind permission of the author and the American Psychological Association*

HERITABILITY OF PERSONALITY
A DEMONSTRATION [1]

IRVING I. GOTTESMAN [2]

Harvard University

Ss were 68 pairs of adolescent twins from the public schools of an urban area. They comprised 60% of the same-sexed twin population. Zygosity diagnosis was determined by blood grouping for 9 groups; half of the sample was identical (MZ) and half was fraternal (DZ). Personality was assessed by the MMPI and Cattell's HSPQ. 24 standard scales were analyzed by intraclass correlations (R) and heritability indexes (H). Holistic analyses of MMPI profile similarity were done clinically and statistically. 6 personality scales had significant genetic components as revealed by higher MZ Rs. 11 scales had appreciable hereditary variance. Pooled accuracy of profile similarity judgments matching zygosity was 68% (p = .005). The general idea that psychopathology in man has a substantial genetic component, especially the psychoses, was supported. A dimension of introversion was the most heavily influenced by genetic factors.

MANKIND in general and life scientists in particular have long been curious about the basic nature of man. In recent years curiosity and speculation have given way to experimentation and controlled observation. One of the eventual outcomes of such research will be a knowledge of the sources of the individual differences in human behavior so that the variation may be explained, predicted, or controlled. The genetic source of variation in human personality is the focal concern of the present research. *Genetic* is used in the strict sense to refer to that science launched by Mendel's work with peas and not, as is common in psychology, as an abbreviation for *ontogenetic*. Although it is axiomatic that the phenotypic expression of a trait is dependent upon the resultant of interaction between genotype and environment, much heat and little light has been generated by attempts to answer the question, "How much of Trait X is due to heredity and how much to environment?" Since neither agent alone can produce the observed behavior, the question as stated is meaningless. The question has precise meaning only when framed in terms of the variation between individuals. Two answerable questions should be posed in the nature-nurture issue: (*a*) How much of the *variability* observed within a group of individuals in a specified environment on a specific measure of a specific trait is attributable to genetic factors? (*b*) How modifiable by systematic environ-

[1] This paper is based upon a doctoral dissertation submitted in partial fulfillment of the requirements for the PhD degree at the University of Minnesota, 1960.

I wish to express my appreciation to my adviser and mentor, R. D. Wirt. I was fortunate to have also had the encouragement and friendship of S. C. Reed, Director of the Dight Institute for Human Genetics, University of Minnesota, Minneapolis.

The cooperation of the Minneapolis, Saint Paul, and Robbinsdale, Minnesota, public school systems through the efforts of H. Cooper, N. C. Kearney, and F. C. Gamelin, Assistant Superintendents, is gratefully acknowledged. A number of other persons contributed their skills and support to this study. Among them are Marianne Briggs, Joan Drues, A. C. Wahl, and Jane Swanson. Conversations with D. Freedman, R. Rosenthal, and D. S. Jones helped me to clarify a number of my thoughts. I benefited from the comments of S. G. Vandenberg and W. R. Thompson on this revised manuscript. Other individuals are given credit in later pages for their specific contributions.

Funds in support of this research were provided by the Tozer Foundation of Stillwater, Minnesota, and the Dight Institute for Human Genetics. The large expense of blood typing was borne by the Minneapolis War Memorial Blood Bank through the interest of G. A. Matson. Subsequent analyses of the data for sex differences were financed by a grant from the Laboratory of Social Relations, Harvard University. Preparation of this monograph was aided in part by Grant M-5384 from the National Institutes of Mental Health.

[2] Formerly at the University of Minnesota.

mental manipulation is the phenotypic expression of each genotype? The answers to these questions will vary according to age, sex, culture, trait, and method of assessment. The importance of genetic factors will range from almost none to overwhelming for those individuals who have been found to have either more or less than 46 chromosomes (Lejeune & Turpin, 1961).

The genes exert their influence on behavior through their effects at the molecular level of organization. Enzymes, hormones, and neurons may be considered as the sequence of complex path markers between the genes and the aspects of behavior termed personality. The inability of behavioral genetics to demonstrate this·type of reduction at the present time need be no more embarrassing than the lack of information concerning the biochemical changes associated with habit formation is to the psychology of learning. It may be that measures of behavior qua behavior are the only reliable indicators of certain kinds of genetic differences (Fuller, 1957; Fuller & Thompson, 1960). For our purposes the best way to conceptualize the contribution of heredity to a personality trait is in terms of heredity's determining a norm of reaction (Dobzhansky, 1955) or of fixing a reaction range (Gottesman, 1963). Within this framework a genotype determines an indefinite but circumscribed assortment of phenotypes, each of which corresponds to one of the possible environments to which the genotype may be exposed. Allen (1961) pointed out that the most probable phenotype of some genotypes may be such a deviant one that even the most favorable of currently known environments would not suffice to bring it within the normal range.

Within the broad context of evolution the demonstration of heritable components for personality traits involves more than an academic exercise. The one nonrandom genetic process which accounts for the adaptive orientation of evolution is differential success in reproduction. If there are heritable aspects to some personality traits and if there is assortative mating for these traits, the frequencies of the associated genes will increase in the gene pool of the population. Tryon (1957) has proposed a behavior genetics model of society

which suggests that relative reproductive isolation between social strata plus social mobility could account for some of the class differences observed in achievement and personality.

In the brief history of contemporary psychology the search for genetic aspects of personality has been dominated by an understandable emphasis on mental illness and mental deficiency (Allen, 1958; Kallmann, 1959). Almost all of such research has occurred within a context of classical Mendelian major gene mechanisms. The inappropriateness of this model ›for the observed quantitative variation in normal personality traits has been one of the inhibitors to investigations by psychologists. Although the classical study by Newman, Freeman, and Holzinger (1937) focused on intelligence and achievement, a number of the personality tests then available were included in the battery administered to their large sample of twins. From their results the authors concluded,

The only group of traits in which identical twins are not much more alike consists of those commonly classed under the head of personality [p. 352].

With very few exceptions (Cattell, Blewett, & Beloff, 1955; Vandenberg, 1962) this conclusion appears to have been accepted as a valid statement of the relationship of genetics to normal personality. Improvements ̀in personality measurement (Cronbach, 1960) and a new era of sophistication about the construction and application of psychometric devices (Cronbach & Meehl, 1955; Loevinger, 1957) make it possible for us to re-examine the relationship in question. This study is an effort in this direction.

The present research attempted to improve upon the methodology of previous twin studies by incorporating a number of refinements. The sample was selected after the entire population of same-sex twins had been enumerated in a large area; the representativeness of the sample to the population was then ascertained. Accuracy and objectivity of zygosity diagnosis were ensured by means of serological tests for 46 different phenotypes in nine different blood group systems and by the use of fingerprints, height, and photographs. Two types of objectively scored personality inventories were used, each purporting to be comprehensive but parsimonious in its characterization of the personality domain. Unlike the tests which historically have been used in an effort to elucidate the "nature and nurture" of personality, both types of tests in the present research have a recognized claim on construct validity (Cronbach, 1960, p. 122). One test depends upon the process of factor analysis for the derivation of "pure" trait measures while the other stems from item analyses which separate criterion groups on various empirical dimensions.

A primary goal of the present research is to answer the first question posed above about *how much* of the variability on various traits for a specified sample reared in a particular environment is attributable to genetic factors and how much to environmental. Earlier criticisms of this strategy (Anastasi, 1958; Loevinger, 1943) are well taken but do not render it obsolete. Fuller (1960) has noted that, while the question has no significance for an individual, the contribution of heredity to total variance in a population

is still a useful object of inquiry, though with increased sophistication we have come to see that the answer to "How much?" is not a universal constant [p. 43].

PROCEDURE

This section gives the details of twin selection as well as a description of the first application in psychological research of the Smith and Penrose (1955) method for the determination of zygosity by extended blood grouping. The efficiency of this method is compared with the methods of the past. Only questionnaire measures of personality were used so as to facilitate the handling of scale scores within the context of quantitative genetics; the tests and their validity and reliability are described. A brief rationale of the twin method is presented followed by a description of the scheme of data analysis.

Selection of the Twin Sample

In sound twin methodology, it is essential that the sample be a miniature of the population of twins. This ensures proportional representation of the two kinds of twins (identical or MZ and fraternal or DZ) and allows accurate genetic analysis with the computed heritability indexes or concordance rates. It is also essential that the two groups of twins in the sample be matched on as many variables as possible so that differences in variance cannot be attributed to differences in age, sex, intelligence, socioeconomic

status, or other factors which may influence personality other than the independent variable, genotype.

All class cards for the over 31,000 children in public school Grades 9 through 12 in the cities of Minneapolis, Saint Paul, and Robbinsdale, Minnesota, were examined. All pairs of children with the same last name, same sex, same address, and same birthdate were recognized as the twin population available. Opposite-sexed fraternal twins were not included in the study in order to eliminate the questionable procedure of comparing a boy with a girl on the same personality traits.

The best data available to date about the incidence of twin births in the United States "white" population are those of Strandskov and Edelen (1946) who reported that 1.129% of all births are twin births. Of these, one third are opposite-sexed fraternals, one third are same-sexed fraternals, and one third are identicals. The best known twin studies (Kallmann, 1946; Newman et al., 1937) assumed that only one fourth of all twins are identical.

A total of 163 pairs of same-sex twins were located in the schools' files of 31,307 children. Based on the incidence of twin *births,* 1.129%, the expected incidence of same-sex twins would have been 237 pairs. After calculating neonatal mortality, however, Allen (1955) found that the incidence of twins at 1 month of age had already been lowered to .87 pairs per 100 children (.87%). Based upon this incidence, the expected number of same-sex twin pairs in the entire population would have been 182. After 1 month of age, the mortality of twins is the same as that of single born survivors. By subtracting the known mortality rate in the general population for children reaching the age of 15 (5%), the final expected number of same-sex twin pairs was 173.[3] At the time the present study was conducted, there were no adolescent twins in either the correctional or mental institutions (not counting the two housing mental defective and brain damaged cases) of the state. It would appear that virtually the entire population of same-sex adolescent twins in the public high schools of the three communities was enumerated.

The parents of all pairs in Minneapolis and Robbinsdale and of those in the largest high school in Saint Paul were sent a letter describing the project and a return postcard on which was printed a medical release authorizing blood typing. After 10 days, telephone calls were made to those who had not returned the card indicating the voluntary participation of their children. After another 10 days, a second and last, hopefully persuasive, telephone call was made. These efforts secured the initial cooperation of 26 pairs of boys and 48 pairs of girls. By the end of the study 6 pairs of twins had defaulted for various reasons: 1 pair was lost as a result of fear of the intravenous removal of the blood specimen, one member of another pair had cerebral palsy and could not take the personality tests in the stand-

---

[3] Evaluation of the sampling adequacy was suggested by and facilitated by E. Anderson.

ard manner, and 4 pairs were unavailable at the times provided for the tests which were Saturday afternoons and mornings.

The final study sample, then, consisted of 23 pairs of boys and 45 pairs of girls. These 68 pairs, disregarding sex, represented 60.2% of the total possible 113 pairs in the schools sampled. The sample contained, respectively, 43.4% and 75.0% of the male and female twin pairs. The sample of the present study compares favorably in size with the majority of twin studies reported in the psychological literature. In representativeness, it is superior to the majority. The simplest explanation for the preponderance of girls over boys is the reluctance of adolescent boys to volunteer their spare time for taking paper-and-pencil tests, especially on Saturdays. The children came from 13 different high schools (all that were sampled), some of which included a ninth grade, and 5 different junior high schools. Participation ranged from 8 out of 8 pairs to 3 out of 8 in the high schools. There was a tendency toward better participation as the economic level of the neighborhood increased.

After the parents of a twin pair had returned the signed authorization for participation and blood typing, an appointment was made to drive the pair to the Minneapolis War Memorial Blood Bank. An appointment was then made for the personality tests. The children were tested in small groups ranging up to 12 pairs. At the time of testing, the children filled out a personal history data sheet, the Minnesota Multiphasic Personality Inventory (MMPI), and the High School Personality Questionnaire (HSPQ; Cattell, Beloff, & Coan, 1958); they were weighed, measured for height, fingerprinted, and photographed. The entire procedure usually took between 3 and 4 hours for each group.

John D. Douthit, Identification Officer with the Minnesota Bureau of Criminal Apprehension, fingerprinted about half of the twins and, after being tutored in the technique, the author fingerprinted the rest. The Faurot inkless method was used with acceptable results and a considerable saving of time. It makes use of a colorless fluid and chemically sensitive paper. An ordinary bathroom scale was used for weighing. Height measurement is estimated to be correct within 5 millimeters. Photography was done by the author with a 35 mm. camera; both a front view and a profile were shot of the head and shoulders.

Some descriptive characteristics of the sample are presented in Table 1. By a serological procedure described in the next section, the 68 pairs of twins were classified into 34 pairs of MZ and 34 pairs of DZ. That this split corresponds to genetic theory is a stroke of luck and an illustration of the representativeness of the sample. About 90% of the twins reported they were of Scandinavian or Western European extraction. In addition to obtaining Otis IQs on the sample, the same data were obtained for 30 more pairs of twins who had not volunteered in Minneapolis and Robbinsdale so that any selection for intelligence might be revealed. It should be noted

that the total of 98 pairs accounts for information about the IQs of 86.7% of the *population* of same-sex twins in the schools used. A sampling bias was revealed by the fact that the mean IQ of the non-sample twins was 97, while those of the MZ and DZ samples were 105 and 108, respectively. A *t* test for the significance of these differences showed that both study samples were significantly different from the nonvolunteers ($t = 2.66$, $p < .01$; $t = 3.66$, $p < .001$).

Criteria for the Diagnosis of Zygosity and an Evaluation of their Relative Efficiencies

One of the most serious criticisms of much twin research is the inaccuracy of zygosity diagnosis. In reaching a judgment in the past, reliance has been placed on an evaluation of the type of birth membrane or the degree of physical resemblance between the twins. Diagnoses based upon the birth membranes are unreliable because while monochorionic (i.e., a single membrane surrounding both fetuses) twins are always MZ, the presence of two chorjons is known to occur with both MZ and DZ twins (Stern, 1960, p. 536). In addition, when studying adult or adolescent twins, it is difficult to obtain accurate information about the birth membrane. Diagnosis by means of the placenta is even more unreliable. In evaluating the extent of physical resemblance, geneticists have used such traits as sex, height, weight,

TABLE 1

DESCRIPTIVE CHARACTERISTICS OF THE SAMPLE

Character	MZ	DZ	Combined
Pairs of boys	12	11	23
Pairs of girls	22	23	45
Age			
14	0	2	2
15	15	4	19
16	9	13	22
17	7	10	17
18	3	5	8
Grade			
9	7	5	12
10	15	11	26
11	7	11	18
12	5	7	12
Level of paternal occupation [a]			
I and II	15	9	24
III	7	13	20
V and VI	12	12	24
M Otis IQ	105	108	107
IQ *SD*	12	12	12

[a] The Minnesota Scale for Paternal Occupations, Institute of Child Welfare, University of Minnesota.

eye color, hair color and form, familial appearance, and various types of fingerprint or palmprint analyses. Although there is an unavoidable subjective element in evaluating many of these characteristics, one expert has estimated the error to be no greater that 1 in 10 (Newman, 1940). That this estimate may be in error is demonstrated below.

If twins differ in sex or any other known inherited characteristic, they cannot be MZ twins. However, if the characteristics are alike, the possibility still remains that the twins are DZ. Given a number of simply inherited and widely distributed traits, it is possible to state the probability of monozygosity or dizygosity for a given pair of twins. It is to be noted, however, that all such diagnoses of monozygosity, no matter how many characteristics are identical, will always be statements of probability; that is, the probability of sharing the given number of traits in common.

Numerous criteria were examined in this study with the hope that the various suggestions in the literature for the diagnosis of zygosity might be objectively evaluated against the recognized best method of extensive blood typing recently quantified by Smith and Penrose (1955). Thus blood type alone was compared with blood type combined first with height, second with a difference in total fingerprint ridge count, and then with both height and ridge count. The accuracy of fingerprints alone and height alone was ascertained. In addition, three groups of judges, geneticists, psychologists, and artists, looked at photographs of the twins and made another form of judgment.

All blood specimens were drawn and typed by the Minneapolis War Memorial Blood Bank, Incorporated. The following blood group systems (Race & Sanger, 1958) were used: ABO, MNSs, Rh, P, Lutheran (Lu), Kell (K), Duffy (Fy), Kidd (Jk), and Lewis (Le).

Smith and Penrose (1955) tabulated the probabilities used for an objective determination of the likelihood of dizygosity based on the incidence of phenotypic sib-sib concordance for the above blood groups. A specific example will illustrate the basic principle underlying the origin of the tabulated probabilities. Blood typing of a large Caucasian population in Great Britain shows that the frequency of Type B blood is .084509 and the frequency of two sibs being B is .040062. The probability that if one of two sibs is B the other is also becomes .040062/ .084509 or .4741. Since DZ same-sex twins are genetically as similar as ordinary sibs, the probability of DZ twins both being Type B is equally .4741. Probabilities derived in this manner are listed in the upper part of Table 2 together with the initial probability that Caucasian, United States twins are DZ and that of a DZ pair being the same sex. Multiplication of all these independent probabilities results in the probability of finding twins who are DZ and alike in all the gene loci involved. A more extensive discussion of the Smith and Penrose method together with the rationale for the derivation of probabilities for the morphological traits used can be found elsewhere (Gottesman, 1960).

TABLE 2

EXAMPLE OF THE SMITH AND PENROSE METHOD FOR ZYGOSITY DETERMINATION

Character	Independent relative chance
Initial odds	1.9246
Likeness in sex	.5000
Likeness in ABO	.6891
Likeness in MNSs	.4556
Likeness in Rh	.5021
Likeness in Le	.8681
Likeness in K	.9485
Likeness in Fy	.8036
Likeness in Jk	.8531
Likeness in Lu	.9614
Likeness in P	.5699
Total relative chance p_{DZ} (blood)	.0470
Total chance $p_{DZ}/(1+p_{DZ})$	.0448
Difference in ridge count	.2288
Total relative chance (blood + ridges)	.0107
Total chance	.0106
Difference in stature	.4671
Total relative chance (blood + stature)	.0219
Total chance	.0214
Total relative chance (all of above)	.0050
Total chance	.0050

As a result of the blood typing, 34 pairs of twins were diagnosed as definitely DZ, that is, they differed on at least one of the independently inherited blood groups. Using only blood, the remaining 34 pairs were diagnosed as MZ with the probability of accuracy no less than 95 times in 100. Table 3 summarizes the results of the accuracy for the various combinations of blood and physical characteristics. It seems paradoxical that while additional information increased the accuracy of some of the diagnoses, it was at the expense of serious errors, e.g., using all the characters resulted in calling 22 pairs MZ at the .01 level or better, but at the expense of 6 pairs failing to meet the criterion of the .05 level. The primary reasons for this are the lack of cross validation and the small samples upon which the fingerprint and height probabilities are calculated, 52 and 50 pairs of MZ, respectively. This resulted in a range of within-pair differences too narrow to allow for those found in the present sample of MZ twins. The probability figure given was too much in the DZ direction to be overcome by any amount of additional information. Eight pairs of MZ twins had differences of ridge count which were tabulated at probabilities greater than 1.0 in favor of the DZ contingency. Similarly, five pairs were "penalized" for differences in height larger than the tabulated ones for the 50 criterion pairs of MZ twins on which they were based. Differential growth rates during adolescence may have been another attenuating factor in the use of the probabilities attached to differences in height.

Let us turn now to two different analyses of the fingerprints: one clinical and the other statistical. Given the 68 pairs of fingerprints and no information as to the base rates, i.e., incidence of DZ and MZ twins in the sample, how accurately can an expert diagnose the two kinds of twins? Douthit undertook this task and was able to correctly identify 30 MZ pairs and 23 DZ pairs. Most important in his clinical decisions were three components (Cummins & Midlo, 1943): differences in pattern slope for the same finger in a twin pair, similarities in slope but different patterns, and differences in the range of dermal ridges for paired fingers. His decisions were not purely clinical in the Meehl (1954) sense of the word in that he subjectively assigned different weights to these components, and used the scores a pair of prints obtained. The statistical method used was for the author to· assign what appeared to be the optimum cutting score (Meehl & Rosen, 1955) to the distribution of differences between total ridge count. This cutting score was then cross validated by applying it to the original distribution (Smith & Penrose, 1955) from which the aforementioned probabilities were determined. A cutting score of 30 classified 33 of 34 MZ pairs and 20 DZ pairs correctly. This score correctly classified 51 of the original 52 MZ pairs at the expense of misclassifying 39 of 101 (38.6%) like-sex siblings. The clinical and statistical methods tied in their accuracy for diagnosing the entire present sample with both hitting 78%. Both Newman, Freeman, and Holzinger (1937) and Slater (1953) make use of some aspects of fingerprints in their diagnosis of zygosity.

Judgments of photographs constituted the final method of zygosity determination evaluated in this section. A summary of all the methods attempted is then presented. Three groups of judges were utilized; three geneticists, three child psychologists, and three artists.[4] Although the front and profile pictures of the head were black and white 35 mm. contact prints, expressions of dissatisfaction with their quality were minimal.

It is obvious that previous estimates (e.g., Newman, 1940) of a 10% error in the diagnosis of zygosity by general appearance are subject to doubt. Jackson's (1960) contention that he observed a "striking difference" between photographs of MZ and DZ twins in the literature needs to be re-evaluated. Even allowing for the quality of photographs and the absence of the cues from the twins' physical presence, the median accuracy of 72% for all nine judges was significantly less than an expected 90% ($\chi^2 = 24.33$, $p < .001$). Poor reliability of judgments may be inferred from the fact that for only 13 MZ pairs and 14 DZ pairs were there one or no inaccurate judgments. There was a total of 84 errors in judging

the MZ twins and 70 errors in judging the DZ twins. Judging the MZ girls seemed to be the most difficult. To the extent that the data in Table 3 were stable, only the geneticists made sufficient allowance for the variability that existed between MZ twins.

Summary

For the sake of clarity, the accuracy of zygosity determination for all the methods described thus far is presented in Table 3.

It should be noted that the three columns cannot be evaluated independently of one another. A judge of the photographs or fingerprints could maximize his accuracy in one category at the expense of the other. It is the final column which conveys the most meaning. The blanks in the table derive from the fact that the DZ twins were absolutely removed from further consideration by the blood typing methodology in the Smith and Penrose scheme.

Psychometric Devices

Both instruments used to measure personality in this study come under the category of objective as contrasted with projective tests. Within the former group there are two major types of questionnaires: one is derived empirically from its ability to discriminate among behavioral phenotypes and the scales may be said to have functional unity, and another type is derived by factor analysis and the scales may be said to have statistical unity. The MMPI was selected as an example of the first type and the HSPQ of the second.

Widespread usage of the MMPI precludes the necessity for a detailed description (Dahlstrom & Welsh, 1960). The test was constructed to provide,

---

[4] I am grateful for the assistance of Vivian Phillips, Elizabeth Reed, S. C. Reed, J. E. Anderson, Mildred C. Templin, R. D. Wirt, Carol Safer, L. Safer, and Ane Wolfe Graubard.

TABLE 3

ACCURACY SUMMARY FOR METHODS OF ZYGOSITY DETERMINATION

Method	MZ %	DZ %	Total %
Blood ($p \leq .05$)	100	100	100
Blood + Height	85	—	—
Blood + Ridge count	88	—	—
Blood + Height + Ridge count	82	—	—
Height + Ridge count	0	—	—
Fingerprints			
Clinical	88	68	78
Statistical	97	59	78
Photos			
Best geneticist	97	74	85
Best psychologist	59	82	71
Best artist	79	91	85
Pooled judges (6/9 agreement)	68	88	78

in a single instrument, measures of all the more important phases of personality of interest to the psychiatrist. Items were selected from 26 subject-matter categories, e.g., general health, sensory disturbances, family problems, sexual and social attitudes, masculine and feminine interest patterns, and schizophrenic thinking disturbances. The 550 items were answered *true* or *false*. Use of the MMPI with normal adolescents may be questioned, but this practice is becoming more popular as experience accumulates with this age group (Hathaway & Monachesi, 1961; Wirt & Briggs, 1959). A basic assumption of the present research was that personality scales represent dimensions or continua of behavior, not categories. Such scales thus lend themselves to the assumptions of quantitative inheritance and permit the use of nonpsychiatric subjects. Numbers have been assigned to the MMPI scales instead of their Kraepelinian based names by the developers of the test so as to facilitate fresh associations to the meaning of the scales as personality constructs. There is no simple translation from MMPI data into descriptive terms for normal populations, but adjectives associated with the behavior of subjects with different scale patterns are easily obtained (e.g., Black, 1953).

The group form of the test was used and scored in the usual fashion for the four validity indicators and 10 clinical scales, 1 through 0 (or Hypochondriasis —Hs—through Social Introversion—Si). In addition, 6 experimental scales (Hathaway & Briggs, 1957), Ego Strength (*Es*), Anxiety (*A*), Repression (*R*), Dominance (*Do*), Dependency (*Dy*), and Social Status (*St*) were scored and analyzed. The 5 scales requiring a *K* correction were analyzed after the correction had been made.

Test-retest reliability coefficients on the 10 standard MMPI scales for a sample of 100 male and female college students after a 1-week interval (Dahlstrom & Welsh, 1960, p. 472) range from .56 to .90. These particular coefficients were chosen because they are most comparable to the circumstances under which the HSPQ reliabilities were computed.

The HSPQ is new to the literature on personality tests and requires more exposition than the MMPI. Cattell, Beloff, and Coan (1958) constructed this instrument by factor analysis especially for adolescents 12 through 17 years in the tradition of the Cattell (1946, 1950) laboratory. It is said to cover all the major dimensions involved in any comprehensive view of individual differences in personality (Cattell et al., 1958).

It consists of 280 forced-choice items, all of which are scores, which form 14 independent, equal length, scales. Although printed in two forms of 140 items each, the authors [5] recommend the use of both to obtain sufficient reliability. It is also suggested that raw scores rather than standard scores be used for research purposes and this suggestion was followed. The scale designations and their titles are given in

[5] R. B. Cattell, personal communication, February 1959.

Table 4. Test-retest correlations based on 112 children aged 13 through 15 tested 2 weeks apart with the full test range from .68 to .80.

In the opinion of the constructors, validity for the 14 scales is satisfactorily established. The main technique used to demonstrate this is the computation of a multiple correlation from factor-item correlations. This gives a median *r* of .81. Although no correction for Test-Taking Attitude is used, there are equal numbers of "yes" and "no" keyed answers on each scale.

It should be obvious that the reliabilities of the MMPI and the HSPQ are on much firmer ground than the validities. Unfortunately, the magnitude of the test-retest correlations has no direct bearing on the construct validity of a scale (Loevinger, 1957). An inherent difficulty in measuring personality traits is the observation that they change with the passage of time and with intervention. After the data of the present study are analyzed, there should be more evidence for the validity, or lack thereof, of the various scales. At the least one might expect significant correlations between MZ twin siblings. Another speculation would be the absence of negative correlations between either class of twins unless there were some parsimonious explanation of a within-pair interaction on a trait.

Twin Method

Bacteria, fruit flies, and mice have contributed greatly to the body of genetic knowledge, but the application of this knowledge to the causes of variation in human behavior raises difficulties. Moreover, relatively few direct methods are available to the

TABLE 4
HSPQ Symbols and Titles [a] for Test Dimensions

Symbol	Low score	High score
A	Stiff, Aloof	Warm, Sociable
B	Mental Defect	General Intelligence
C	General Neuroticism	Ego Strength
D	Phlegmatic Temperament	Excitability
E	Submissiveness	Dominance
F	Sober, Serious	Enthusiastic
G	Casual, Undependable	Super Ego Strength
H	Shy, Sensitive	Adventurous, Thick-Skinned
I	Tough, Realistic	Esthetically Sensitive
J	Liking Group Action	Fastidiously Individualistic
O	Confident Adequacy	Guilt Proneness
Q_2	Group Dependency	Self-Sufficiency
Q_3	Uncontrolled, Lax	Controlled, Showing Will Power
Q_4	Relaxed Composure	Tense, Excitable

[a] A mixture of technical and popular terms was used here.

researcher in human behavior genetics because of such problems as those introduced by uncontrolled mating, small numbers of offspring, heterogeneous environments, and the uniqueness of one individual's heredity. Of the available methods, the twin method approaches the ideal experimental design. Galton (1875) first called attention to the possible usefulness of twins for casting light on the nature-nurture problem. The underlying principle is simple and sound: since MZ twins have identical genotypes, any dissimilarity between pairs must be due to the action of agents in the environment, either postnatally or intrauterine; DZ twins, while differing genetically, have certain environmental similarities in common such as birth rank and maternal age, thereby providing a measure of environmental control not otherwise possible. When both types of twins are studied, a method of evaluating either the effect of different environments on the same genotype or the expression of different genotypes under the same environment is provided. This means, with respect to any given genetically determined trait, that there should be a greater similarity between MZ than between DZ twins. If both members of a twin pair develop the same phenotype in a given environment, they are called *concordant* for the trait under study; *discordant* is the designation for differing phenotypes. When dealing with a single gene difference, such as Huntington's chorea, MZ twins should always be concordant; DZ twins may be either concordant or discordant. The expected difference in concordance can then be used to give a measure of heritability (H) of the trait if the traits are amenable to discrete classification.

Inasmuch as few traits in the normal range of human personality are dichotomous, another approach is needed to estimate H when traits are continuous and the genetic component is of the polygenic variety. In the present research, H will be defined as the proportion of total trait variance associated with genetic factors. Holzinger (1929) suggested that the best comparison to make in evaluating the nature-nurture interaction for a quantitative characteristic is that between the intraclass correlation coefficients (R) for MZ and like-sexed DZ twins. Holzinger's H gives the proportion of variance produced by genetic differences *within families*. The method underestimates the effects of heredity in the general population by a factor of approximately 2 since the genetic variance is estimated from the genetic overlap between DZ twins which is .5. The index of heritability, h^2, computed in animal behavior genetics (e.g., Falconer, 1960; McClearn, 1961) is different from H in that it is an estimate of the proportion of trait variance in a population determined by genotypic variation in that population. Both between- and within-families variance components are used to compute h^2.

Holzinger gave two formulas for his estimate of heritability, one based on R and another, statistically equivalent, based on the within-pair variances.

$$H = \frac{R_{MZ} - R_{DZ}}{1 - R_{DZ}}$$

$$H = \frac{V_{DZ} - V_{MZ}}{V_{DZ}}$$

where,

$R_{MZ} = $ intraclass correlation between MZ twins
$R_{DZ} = $ intraclass correlation between DZ twins
$V_{MZ} = $ within-MZ pairs variance estimate (mean square)
$V_{DZ} = $ within-DZ pairs variance estimate (mean square)

Falconer has suggested that the difference between the MZ and DZ Rs could be taken as an estimate of half the heritability if there were no nonadditive genetic variance; since the latter assumption is probably not warranted, the difference can only be regarded as setting an upper limit to half the heritability.

Limitations and Criticisms of the Twin Method

After reviewing probable natal and prenatal influences on twin development, Price (1950) was willing to conclude,

In all probability the net effect of most twin studies has been underestimation of the significance of heredity in the medical and behavior sciences [p. 293].

This appears to be the result of biases of two sorts. Inferences drawn from data on twins are subject to both statistical and biological biases. In the first category, it is basic to the kinds of analyses discussed above that the samples be proportional and therefore representative of the population of MZ and like-sexed DZ twins before *the* concordance or *the* variance used in the formulas can be assumed to be valid enough to support the inferences. This assumption is difficult to meet. Use of the twin method also assumes that the within-pair environmental variance is the same for the two types of twins. This is not necessarily true for the personality traits as measured by the tests, since one can proceed only on the assumption that such variance is not too different for the two types of twins. Loevinger (1943) mentioned some additional difficulties underlying the use of the variance method, chief among which were the assumption that influences combine additively and the assumption that estimates of the error variance are eliminated from the computation of H. Again the extent to which these conditions are met is hard to assess. Cattell (1953) concluded that approximations of a solution to the nature-nurture issue, with an awareness of methodological shortcomings, were better than postponing all research in the area. The author is inclined to agree.

Biological biases have been reviewed by Price (1950) who divided them into natal factors (e.g., position in utero), lateral inversions, and effects of mutual circulation. No attempt to evaluate these factors will be made since data are not available. Postnatal biological biases are often overlooked on the apparent assumption that the general environment for a pair of twins is the same. Once more the assumption is questionable. Should one of a pair, for example, contract some form of encephalitis with its well-known sequelae, the results on personality measurement would be obvious.

The main limitations of twin studies were viewed in somewhat different terms by Kallmann and Baroff (1955) as the following:

(a) twins cannot be separated before they are born, nor can they be provided with two mothers of different age, personality, or health status; (b) two-egg twins are no more dissimilar genotypically than brothers and sisters and like them, are rarely raised in different cultures; therefore, even fraternal twins are unlikely to fall into the extremes of theoretically possible genetic and cultural differences; and (c) the average difference between one-egg twin partners is no precise measure of environmentally produced variation, nor does an increase over the average difference between two-egg twins represent the exact contribution of genetic influences even in relatively comparable environments [p. 303].

Intraclass Correlation Analysis of Personality Traits

Following the diagnosis of zygosity and the collection of the personality test data, each scale of the two tests and the IQ from the school records were analyzed by means of the intraclass correlation coefficient, first for the two classes of twins and then for the two sexes within each class. A total of 186 coefficients was obtained from 186 simple one-way analyses of variance using T scores for the MMPI, raw scores for the HSPQ, and Otis IQs.

Haggard's (1958) book on the intraclass correlation gives a detailed exposition of the method used here. Although the *intraclass* correlation was formerly computed by calculating the *interclass* correlation after constructing a symmetrical table with double entries for a pair of scores and then dividing by 2, it now is recognized as a simple function of variances. Haggard (1958, p. 11) gives this formula for the computation:

$$R = \frac{BCMS - WMS}{BCMS + WMS}$$

where,

$BCMS$ = between-classes (twin pairs) mean square
WMS = within-classes (twin pairs) mean square

This means that the unbiased estimate of R may be obtained in terms of the mean squares (i.e., variance estimates) of the analysis of variance table. This formula is the specific one to use for pairs of scores. The relationship of F, the variance ratio, to R is given by:

$$F = \frac{1 + R}{1 - R}$$

The level of statistical significance of R is identical with that of the corresponding F (i.e., $BCMS/WMS$). In other words, the hypothesis that an observed R could have come from a population with a true correlation of zero can be tested by the F ratio computed from the same mean squares, with the appropriate degrees of freedom, as were used to obtain R.

In order to test the significance of the differences between two independently obtained Rs, they were converted into Fisher's z (Fisher & Yates, 1949) which has an approximately normal distribution with variance:

$$V = \frac{k}{2(c - 2)(k - 1)}$$

where,

k is the number of individuals within a class, i.e., 2 (MZ or DZ twins), and c is the number of classes, i.e., 34 (pairs).

The distribution of the difference between the corresponding z values is approximately normal with variance:

$$V_d = \frac{k_1}{2(c_1 - 2)(k_1 - 1)} + \frac{k_2}{2(c_2 - 2)(k_2 - 1)}$$

Dividing the difference between z's by the square root of the above gives a normal deviate, the p value of which is found in the usual manner. A one-tailed test of significance was appropriate and was used.

Recapitulating, the objectives of this intraclass correlation analysis of traits are (a) to demonstrate that the traits are significantly and positively correlated in MZ twins and may or may not be in DZ twins and (b) to demonstrate that for any genetically influenced trait the correlation within MZ pairs will be significantly greater than that within DZ pairs.

Subsequent to this analysis, the heritability indexes were computed as described in the previous section using the independently obtained WMS or within variances. It should be noted that the two procedures, intraclass correlation analysis and computation of heritability indexes, involve simple and complex assumptions, respectively. The correlation analysis is sufficient to show that heredity has something to do with individual differences. Estimates of the relative importance of nature and nurture as indicated by H must be considered as suggestive rather than definitive in human behavior genetics.

Configural (Holistic) Analyses of Personality Similarity

Following a scale-by-scale analysis, one of the two personality tests was selected for holistic profile analyses. The MMPI was chosen because MMPI configurations have been treated extensively in the literature. Recent emphasis on the study of profiles has resulted from the realization that interpretation of an individual's set of scores must frequently be based on the pattern of scores rather than examination of one scale at a time or the use of a linear sum of the scale deviations. General and specific methodological difficulties arise which weaken any confidence that may be attached to the quantification of profile similarity. Only a few of the difficulties

362

noted by students of the problem (Cronbach & Gleser, 1953; Osgood & Suci, 1952) will be discussed.

Similarity as a general quality of personality is nebulous but necessary for communication. Cronbach and Gleser (1953) say:

> *similarity is not a general quality. It is possible to discuss similarity only with respect to specified dimensions (or complex characteristics).* This means that the investigator who finds that people are similar in some set of scores cannot assume that they are similar in general. He could begin to discuss general similarity only if his original measurement covered all or a large proportion of the significant dimensions of personality [p. 457].

Other general methodological difficulties involve the loss of information by reducing the relationship between two configurations to a single index; lack of comparability between indexes of similarity; and violations of assumptions about ratio scales, uncorrelated measures, and equal reliability among subtests.

There are two aspects of profiles which matching may involve: the shape or configuration of scores and the general elevation from the mean of the norm group. It is logical to distinguish between matching for absolute agreement, in which both shape and elevation are considered, and relative agreement, in which only shape is considered. Three statistical and one clinical indexes of similarity were computed for the two classes of twins. In addition, the profile of each twin was coded according to the methods of both Hathaway and Welsh (Dahlstrom & Welsh, 1960) to facilitate further clinical assessment (Gottesman, 1960).

Statistical Indexes

Rank-Difference Correlation. This well-known measure, Spearman's rho, was the first index computed. It yielded a nonarbitrary number which reflected similarity of shape but disregarded elevation. One of its disadvantages was that a rho of 1.00 did not necessarily indicate perfect similarity and another was that two pairs of profiles with the same coefficient need not be equally similar. Rho's were calculated from the Welsh codes; ties were resolved by using the scales in numerical order.

D Coefficient. This index, sometimes known as the generalized distance function, was then computed. Cronbach and Gleser (1953) devote considerable attention to this index which is designed to reflect both shape and elevation. The D coefficient is based on the geometric principle that in a space of N mutually orthogonal dimensions, the distance between two points is equal to the square root of the sum of the squared differences between the coordinates of the points on each dimension. Since profiles may be considered as points in N space, where N equals the number of scales (i.e., 10), the distance between them serves as a measure of similarity. Note that orthogonality does not obtain for the MMPI. The D coefficient results in an arbitrary number whose value depends on the number of scales.

Concordance of Test Behavior (TT'). In the context of discovery it was decided to compute the absolute percentage of MMPI items answered in the same direction by a pair of twins, i.e., one twin's answer sheet was used to score the other's. Of course the MMPI was not designed to be used this way and in this instance serves primarily as an item pool. The percentage of agreement for the 566 items has been termed TT', to signify the comparison of one twin with his sibling. No provision was made for the few items which are repeated, but any question omitted by either twin was subtracted from 566 before the percentage was calculated. This process was then repeated using only those items appearing on the 10 clinical scales (337 items).[6]

Clinical Index

Visual Judgment. The only quantifiable clinical index of similarity used was the accuracy of visual judgment in sorting the profiles into four categories: Very Similar, Similar, Dissimilar, and Very Dissimilar. By *accuracy* was meant the number of MZ pair profiles placed in the first two categories and the number of DZ in the last two. Three psychologists[7] skilled in the use of the MMPI were the judges. Another indication of similarity was provided by comparison of the accuracy of visual judgments in the extreme categories with the overall accuracy.

Recapitulating, the objective of each of the above four procedures was to search for a greater similarity of personality, as measured by the configural aspects of the MMPI, for the MZ twins than for the DZ twins.

RESULTS

The presentation of the findings is organized around the two instruments of assessment; first the MMPI with its 10 clinical scales, 6 experimental scales, and K (a validity scale thought to have personality referents); and second the HSPQ with its 14 factored scales. Indexes of H are presented separately after each correlational analysis. Results are displayed for the total sample of 34 pairs each of MZ and DZ twins, then for the female subsample (22 MZ and 23 DZ pairs) and then for the male subsample (12 MZ and 11 DZ pairs). The results by sex are provocative but any extensive discussion of

---

[6] Hathaway's linear statistic CC' was also calculated with no improvement over any of the statistical methods reported here. Data are available upon request.

[7] Thanks are due Jan Duker, H. Gilberstadt, and R. D. Wirt.

TABLE 5

MMPI INTRACLASS CORRELATIONS FOR MZ AND DZ TWINS FOR TOTAL GROUP, FEMALES, AND MALES

Scales	Total Groups' R		Females' R		Males' R	
	MZ	DZ	MZ	DZ	MZ	DZ
1 Hs	39**	21	14	19	44	25
2 D	47**	07	44*	25	48*	−19
3 Hy	47**	41**	36*	51**	65**	30
4 Pd	57***	18	45*	25	66**	−07
5 Mf	52***	32*	52**	35*	55*	28
6 Pa	44**	18	44*	31	43	−10
7 Pt	55***	20	62***	11	40	31
8 Sc	59***	19	50**	12	65**	19
9 Ma	24	−07	29	−28	11	42
0 Si	55***	.08	37*	18	73**	−04
K	32*	−02	30	03	40	−26
Es	25	47**	17	49**	48*	30
A	45**	04	46*	12	42	−35
R	29*	.22	20	15	50*	42
Do	46**	21	22	40*	72**	−44
Dy	52***	25	59**	47**	28	−37
St	47**	53***	28	63***	72**	24

* $p \le .05$.
** $p \le .01$.
*** $p \le .001$.

them is vitiated by the size of the samples. This section concludes with the results of the configural and holistic MMPI profile analyses. Thorough discussion of the results is deferred to the next section.

Minnesota Multiphasic Personality Inventory

The excellent matching of the two classes of twins and their representativeness of adolescents in general were observed on the mean scores and standard deviations of the 3 validity scales and the 10 clinical scales. Intraclass correlation coefficients for the twins are given in Table 5. Nine of the 10 standard MMPI scales were significantly different from zero at the .01 level for the MZ twins. Fifteen of the 17 MMPI MZ scale correlations were larger than the corresponding correlations for DZ twins. It should be noted that for 6 of the 8 total MZ scale correlations for which test-retest reliability data on adolescents were available, the magnitudes are about the same.

Rozeboom (1960) has reminded us that the primary aim of a scientific experiment is not to precipitate decisions, but to make an appropriate adjustment in the degree to which one accepts, or

believes, the hypothesis or hypotheses being tested [p. 420].

Since the traditional null hypothesis tests in psychological research pay no attention to the utilities of various outcomes, he suggested that the basic statistical report should be in the form of a *confidence interval* whenever possible. It is obvious, in the case of correlation coefficients, for example, that the researcher is concerned with more than the fact that a particular coefficient is not zero—he hopes he is in a position to account for more than a trivial amount of variation. In sympathy with the Rozeboom position, a few of the 90% confidence limits for the data in Table 5 will be mentioned. For the largest nonzero R in the total sample of MZ twins, .59 for Schizophrenia (Sc), the limits are .35 and .74; for the smallest nonzero R, .39 for Hs, the limits are .13 and .61. For the corresponding Rs, in the sample of DZ twins, .19 for Sc, the limits are −.10 and .44; for Hs, .21, the limits are −.08 and .46.

The results of testing whether or not the correlation between MZ pairs is significantly greater than that between DZ are presented in Table 6. All Rs were first converted to

TABLE 6

ONE-TAILED TEST OF THE DIFFERENCE BETWEEN MZ AND DZ MMPI SCALE INTRACLASS CORRELATIONS FOR TOTAL GROUP, FEMALES, AND MALES

Scale	Total group		Females		Males	
	Normal deviate	p	Normal deviate	p	Normal deviate	p
1 Hs	.79	.21	−.16		.47	.32
2 D	1.76	.04	.69	.24	1.56	.06
3 Hy	.30	.38	−.59		1.01	.16
4 Pd	1.86	.03	.73	.23	1.88	.03
5 Mf	.98	.16	.68	.25	.72	.24
6 Pa	1.16	.12	.48	.31	1.22	.11
7 Pt	1.66	.05	1.97	.02	.22	.41
8 Sc	1.94	.03	1.37	.08	1.27	.10
9 Ma	1.26	.10	1.88	.03	−.73	
0 Si	2.15	.02	.66	.25	2.11	.02
K	1.40	.08	.89	.19	1.50	.07
Es	−1.02		−1.17		.46	.32
A	1.78	.04	1.20	.11	1.77	.04
R	.30	.38	.16	.43	.22	.41
Do	1.14	.13	−.64		3.00	.001
Dy	1.28	.10	.54	.30	1.47	.07
St	−.32		−1.45		1.44	.08

Fisher's z's. The MZ twins appeared to be significantly higher than DZ on 5 of the 10 standard MMPI scales (p less than or equal to the 5% level). The results from the correlational analyses then left 5 of the 10 standard scales, 2—Depression (D), 4—Psychopathic deviate (Pd), 7—Psychasthenia (Pt), 8—Schizophrenia, and 0—Social Introversion, which appeared to have significant genetic (i.e., gene determined) components for the combined group.

The heritability estimates for the MMPI scales, which only utilize within-pair variances, are presented in Table 7. While there is no method yet for the computation of confidence limits for H, the suggested way for testing its significance is a function of the significance of the F ratio formed by the within-DZ pair variance divided by the within-MZ pair variance. Even when the computation of H in the present study showed that 42% of the observed within-family variance for the total group could be accounted for by genetic factors, the associated F was not statistically significant at the .05 level. The infrequent reporting of the significance of H in the literature together with the paucity

of positive results for even intellectual and psychomotor tasks (Vandenberg, 1962) suggests a need for mathematical clarification of H. Within the limits of the assumptions for this kind of analysis, this attempt at quantification of the proportion of scale variance accounted for by heredity gave positive results for the same five scales identified by the correlational analysis. Scales Pt and Sc showed appreciable variance accounted for by heredity but with environment predominating. Scales D and Pd showed about equal contributions of heredity and environment. Scale 0, Social Introversion, showed a predominance of variance (.71) accounted for by heredity. The value of H for the Si scale is of the same magnitude as that found in this study and others for intelligence as measured by standard IQ tests.

Cattell's Factored Test

Once again the excellent matching of the two classes of twins and their representativeness of adolescents in general may be inferred from the comparison of mean scores on the 14 scales with the normative data. Intraclass correlation coefficients for the MZ and DZ twins are given in Table 8. Eight of the 14 scales had correlations between MZ twins greater than zero. Two scales, A and J, were not significantly different from zero for both MZ and DZ twins.

Six of the 14 factors resulted in correlation coefficients which were not significantly different from zero for the MZ twins. That DZ should obtain significant correlations on 4 of these 6 was paradoxical. It is difficult to reconcile claims of construct validity for these 6 scales with these results. Unless there were some logical a priori grounds for identical twins to be opposed on some trait, their identical heredity and/or their very similar environment would lead us to expect other than a zero correlation between them for a personality trait. The factor derivation of all the scales and their low intercorrelations permitted acceptance and interpretation of the remaining eight scales on their own merit. Factors B, F, G, H, I, O, Q_2 and Q_3 at this point in the analysis have the potential for showing a predominance of genetic variance.

For the largest nonzero R in the total sample of MZ twins (other than the intelligence

TABLE 7

MMPI Scale Heritability Indexes for Total Group, Females, and Males

Scale	Total group H	Total group F[a]	Females H	Females F[a]	Males H	Males F[a]
1 Hs	.16	1.19	.25	1.33	.01	1.01
2 D	.45	1.81	.22	1.28	.65	2.83
3 Hy	.00	.86	.00	.56	.43	1.74
4 Pd	.50	2.01	.37	1.60	.77	4.35
5 Mf	.15	1.18	.00	.99	.45	1.83
6 Pa	.05	1.05	.00	.70	.52	2.09
7 Pt	.37	1.58	.47	1.89	.24	1.31
8 Sc	.42	1.71	.36	1.56	.50	2.00
9 Ma	.24	1.32	.33	1.50	.00	.81
0 Si	.71	3.42	.60	2.49	.84	6.14
K	.06	1.06	.00	.95	.26	1.35
Es	.00	.73	.00	.69	.00	.84
A	.21	1.26	.22	1.28	.18	1.22
R	.00	.82	.00	.79	.00	.86
Do	.00	.95	.00	.76	.33	1.50
Dy	.24	1.32	.03	1.03	.45	1.82
St	.34	1.52	.14	1.16	.63	2.69

[a] The three values of F required for significance at the .05 level are 1.78, 2.04, and 2.72.

factor), .60 for Q_2, the 90% confidence limits are .38 and .75; for the smallest nonzero R, .30 for Q_3, the limits are .02 and .54. For the corresponding Rs in the sample of DZ twins, .15 for Q_2, the limits are $-.13$ and .42; for Q_3, .12, the limits are $-.16$ and .39.

In Table 9 are presented the results of testing whether or not the correlation between MZ pairs is significantly greater than that between DZ. All Rs were first converted to Fisher's z's.

The MZ twins were significantly higher than DZ on only one HSPQ factor, Q_2. For 8 of the 14 factors the differences were in the predicted direction. The results from both the correlation analyses then left only 1 factor, Q_2—Group Dependency versus Self-Sufficiency, which appeared to have significant genetic (i.e., gene determined) components.

The heritability indexes for the HSPQ scales, computed only from the within-pair variances, are presented in Table 10. Within the limits of the assumptions for this analysis, this attempt at quantification of the proportion of scale variance accounted for by heredity gives positive results for 6 of the 14 factors. Factors E, Submissiveness versus Dominance; H, Shy, Sensitive versus Adventurous; and J, Liking Group Action versus Fastidiously Individualistic showed apprecia-

TABLE 9

ONE-TAILED TEST OF THE DIFFERENCE BETWEEN MZ AND DZ HSPQ SCALE INTRACLASS CORRELATIONS FOR TOTAL GROUP, FEMALES, AND MALES

Factor	Total group Normal deviate	p	Females Normal deviate	p	Males Normal deviate	p
A	$-.34$		$-.50$		$-.32$	
B	$-.03$		$-.05$		$-.02$	
C	$-.46$		$-.23$		-1.45	
D	-1.21		-1.56		$-.07$	
E	-1.10		-2.07		1.13	.13
F	1.56	.06	$.44$	.33	1.56	.06
G	$.36$	.36	$-.33$		$.77$	.22
H	$.78$	.22	$.33$	.37	1.09	.14
I	$.40$	.34	$.86$	.19	$.54$	.29
J	1.20	.11	1.23	.11	$.56$	.29
O	$.40$	.34	$-.04$		$.53$	.30
Q_2	2.13	.02	2.00	.02	$.24$	.41
Q_3	$.74$	.23	$.88$	.19	$.46$	.32
Q_4	$-.25$		$.63$	.26	-1.78	

ble variance accounted for by heredity but with environment predominating. Factors F, Sober, Serious versus Happy-Go-Lucky; Q_2; and O, Confident Adequacy versus Guilt Proneness showed about equal contributions of hereditary and environmental variance (.56, .56, and .46).

Results of the Otis IQ analysis

The results of the school administered intelligence test are given at this point because Factor B of the HSPQ is a brief 20-item measure of intelligence. Intraclass correlations for the MZ and DZ twins were .83 and .59, respectively, both significant at the .001 level with the first significantly greater than the second at the .02 level. The H value computed from the Otis within variances was .62. This means that 62% of the within-family intelligence variance measured by the Otis is accounted for by hereditary factors in this sample.

Configural and Holistic Analyses

Rank-Difference Correlations for the Coded MMPI Profiles

Table 11 shows the distribution of the Spearman rho's for the 68 pairs of profiles by twin type. It is obvious that the overlap is too great to permit other than chance discrimi-

TABLE 8

HSPQ INTRACLASS CORRELATIONS FOR MZ AND DZ TWINS FOR TOTAL GROUP, FEMALES, AND MALES

Factor	Total groups' R MZ	DZ	Females' R MZ	DZ	Males' R MZ	DZ
A	19	27	26	40*	-10	05
B	60**	61***	65***	66***	56*	57*
C	28	38*	05	12	33	76**
D	21	47**	23	62***	19	23
E	16	41**	-06	53**	33	-18
F	47**	12	29	16	64**	04
G	49**	42**	23	33	76***	56*
H	38*	20	42*	34	34	-15
I	55***	47**	26	00	37	14
J	26	-04	29	-08	24	-01
O	45**	37*	50**	51**	20	-04
Q_2	60***	15	54**	-02	51*	42
Q_3	30*	12	56**	34	-01	-22
Q_4	27	32*	35*	16	12	73**

* $p \leqq .05$.
** $p \leqq .01$.
*** $p \leqq .001$.

Irving I. Gottesman

TABLE 10
HSPQ Factor Heritability Indexes for Total Group, Females, and Males

Factor	Total group		Females		Males	
	H	F[a]	H	F[a]	H	F[a]
A	.10	1.11	.00	.97	.24	1.32
B	.05	1.05	.00	.96	.18	1.22
C	.03	1.03	.25	1.34	.00	.43
D	.00	.62	.00	.37	.42	1.72
E	.31	1.44	.00	.80	.74	3.84
F	.56	2.29	.45	1.81	.74	3.83
G	.00	.97	.01	1.01	.00	.79
H	.38	1.62	.42	1.73	.34	1.52
I	.06	1.07	.05	1.05	.10	1.11
J	.29	1.41	.27	1.37	.34	1.51
O	.46	1.85	.22	1.29	.69	3.18
Q_2	.56	2.28	.60	2.52	.47	1.89
Q_3	.12	1.13	.31	1.44	.00	.99
Q_4	.00	.53	.18	1.22	.00	.09

[a] The three values of F required for significance at the .05 level are 1.78, 2.04, and 2.72.

nation ($\chi^2 = .47$, $p > .25$) between the two kinds of twins on the basis of their MMPI profile rank-difference correlation coefficients. A cutting score for a rho of .40 and above would correctly classify 53% of all the twin pairs.

D Coefficient

Table 12 shows the distribution of the generalized distance function computed from the 68 pairs of profiles. This index abstracts information about the shape and elevation of the profile. There was a tendency for the identical twins to have a lower D, i.e., be less dissimilar; 19 of the MZ pairs were below the

TABLE 11
Distribution of MZ and DZ MMPI Profile Code Rho's

Rho	MZ	DZ
.80–.89	2	1
.70–.79	2	1
.60–.69	3	3
.50–.59	6	6
.40–.49	4	4
.30–.39	3	2
.20–.29	3	2
.10–.19	3	5
0–.09	2	1
− .50 to − .01	6	9

TABLE 12
Distribution of MZ and DZ MMPI Profile D Coefficients

D	MZ	DZ
15–19	1	0
20–24	4	3
25–29	10	8
30–34	8	5
35–39	5	4
40–44	3	4
45–49	1	2
50–54	1	3
55–59	0	3
60–64	1	0
65–69	0	1
70–74	0	1

median of the combined group as contrasted with 15 of the DZ pairs ($\chi^2 = .94$, $p < .17$). Using the median D as a cutting score resulted in correct classification of 56% of the profiles.

Concordance of Test Behavior (TT')

The percentage of all MMPI test items (566) answered in the same direction for a pair of twins is given in Table 13. There was a tendency for the identical twins to have a greater overlap in their responses to all the items; 21 of the MZ pairs were above the median of the combined group as contrasted with 15 of the DZ pairs ($\chi^2 = 2.35$, p < .06). Using the median TT' of 72% as a cutting score resulted in correct classification of 59% of the profiles. There was some improvement in the use of this index when only the items in the 10 clinical scales were used as the denominator (337); 21 of the MZ pairs ex-

TABLE 13
Distribution of MZ and DZ Total MMPI Item Agreement Percentages (TT')

TT'	MZ	DZ
85–89	1	1
80–84	6	4
75–79	4	3
70–74	13	11
65–69	7	10
60–64	2	2
55–59	0	2
50–54	1	1

ceeded the median compared to 14 DZ pairs ($\chi^2 = 2.94$, $p < .05$). The cutting score was the same and correctly classified 60% of the profiles.

Clinical Judgment of Profile Similarity

The extent to which the judges' clinical assessment of personality similarity agreed with the zygosity of the twin pairs is given in Table 14. Computing the combined p levels (Mosteller & Bush, 1954, p. 329) for the accuracy of the three judges on their sorting of all profiles resulted in a p equal to .003. The comparable figure for accuracy of judging the two extreme groups of Very Similar and Very Dissimilar was .004. By pooling the ratings for each pair (i.e., 2 of 3, or 3 of 3 votes) in an effort to correct for the various sources of attenuation in the "configural powers" of the clinician, the accuracy of the total sort increased to 67.6% ($z = 2.90$, $p = .005$).

DISCUSSION

In the introduction the purpose of the present research was said to be to answer this question—How much of the variability observed within a group of individuals in a specified environment on a specific measure of a specific personality trait is attributable to genetic factors? Implicit in the posing of this question was the assumption, subsequently confirmed by the data, that there were measurable genetic influences for at least some of the aspects of human personality tapped by the selected personality tests. Since the quantification of genetic variability derived from the computation of heritabilities by the classi-

cal twin method, and since this method rests upon some unproved assumptions, the results are recognized as suggestive and heuristic rather than definitive. While the data language for this research consists of scores on scales of personality tests, the discussion which follows is in terms of the underlying biophysical traits which the scales (read constructs) reflect.

The first section of the discussion deals with the specific traits and their configurations demonstrated to have been influenced by hereditary factors together with some of the implications of these data for personality theory and the etiology of mental illness. This is followed by an attempt to explain the apparent failure of some of the holistic analyses of personality to support strongly the findings of the trait analyses.

To what extent can the results of the present study be applied to human behavior in general? The representativeness of the twin sample to Minnesota adolescents in general suggests that this kind of extrapolation is fairly safe. There is the possibility that the twins, preponderantly of Scandinavian extraction, sample a unique gene pool. Whether the further extrapolation to adults can be safely made is dubious and difficult to assess. When *rate* of development enters the picture, biological influences on a trait might be emphasized compared to a final adult stage. The present results could be very different if derived from adult twins as suggested by studies of morphology (Osborne & DeGeorge, 1959). Another important question is the extent to which these data from normal nonhospitalized individuals can be applied to identifiable psychiatrically ill. A basic assumption throughout this project was that the measured aspects of personality varied continuously, and that any underlying genetic mechanisms were polygenic in nature. The possibility that the extremes of distributions for some personality characteristics constitute discrete series exists, but this phenomenon would be masked by the strategy used. The net effect would be the underestimation of the importance of heredity since concordances in MZ twins for low incidence Mendelian or polygenic characteristics would pass unnoticed in the analysis of quantitative variability.

TABLE 14

AGREEMENT OF CLINICAL JUDGMENTS OF MMPI
PROFILE SIMILARITY WITH TWIN ZYGOSITY

Judge	Total sort	z	p	Extreme pile sort	z	p
A	64.7%	2.43	.01	67.6%	2.06	.03
B	61.8%	1.95	.03	73.5%	2.74	.006
C	58.8%	1.45	.08	58.8%	1.03	.16
Combined p			.003			.004

Genetic Aspects of Personality

A total of 6 traits out of the standard 24 in the two tests met a criterion which classified them as significantly influenced by genetic factors; that is, correlations between the scores of indentical twins were significantly higher than those between the scores of fraternal twins. Beyond this, for 23 of the total 31 scales analyzed in the two personality tests, the differences were in the predicted direction. Trait Q_2, Self-Sufficiency, was the only survivor of the 14 HSPQ measures. Although Factor Q_2 is not thought to be clearly established, the item content suggests that a person who is resolute and accustomed to making his own decisions will obtain a high score, while low scorers would be described as followers and conformists. A synthesis of this trait and F, Surgency (significant at the .06 level), is provided by Cattell's large second-order factor, Extraversion versus Introversion, which is composed of four factors. Two of the four are F and Q_2. Tying in neatly with the MMPI findings which are discussed next is a study on the construct validity of the adult form of the HSPQ by Karson and Pool (1957). These authors found the highest MMPI scale correlate of Factor F to be Scale Si, Social Introversion, and the highest correlate of Q_2 to be Si also with correlations of − .48 and .32, respectively. Together such results appear to identify a general dimension closely related to introversion-extraversion as one which is heavily influenced by genetic factors. Such a conclusion has also been reached by Eysenck (1947, 1956) who isolated introversion-extraversion as one of the two (now three) dimensions of personality by a factor analysis of ratings and personal data on 700 neurotic soldiers. He considers his findings to represent a confirmation of the theoretical ideas of Jung (1933). Genetic factors are given a prominent place in Eysenck's typology; his twin study (Eysenck, 1956) using statistics similar to those in the present study, yielded a tentative value for H on a factored measure of introversion-extraversion of .62.

The trait of introversion as measured by the MMPI may also have implications for one of the genetic theories of schizophrenia. Patients with very high scores on Scale Si are clinically described as "schizoid" and Kallmann (1953) and others have suggested that the schizoid individual may represent the genetic "carrier state" of the recessive schizophrenic gene. In other words, the schizoid individual may represent the heterozygote and the schizophrenic may represent the homozygote. If the schizoid carrier can be identified, Kallmann's hypothesis about recessivity is no longer tenable. The mode of inheritance must then be that of incomplete *dominance* or polygenic, thus better accounting for the high familial incidence of schizophrenia (cf. Gregory, 1960). The magnitude of the heritability for Scale Si was the largest found in the present study. The belief in the genetic contribution to intelligence has come to have a fairly secure status in contemporary psychology (Gottesman, 1963); the results of this investigation indicate that a similar status is appropriate for the more pure personality trait of introversion.

The results concerning the four remaining MMPI scales, D, Pd, Pt, and Sc, lend support to the general idea that in human beings psychopathology, especially psychosis, has a substantial genetic component. The scoring keys for these scales were developed for the purpose of locating patients with respect to psychiatrically diagnosed states of depression, psychopathic personality, psychasthenia, and schizophrenia. Patients of each type were compared, item by item, with a normal group. Those items which statistically differentiated a diagnostic group from normals were then included in the appropriate scale. Taken *singly*, these MMPI scales are able to discriminate about 60% of the patients corresponding to their label at a cost of 5% false positives among the normals; however, the single scale approach has been largely supplanted by the interpretation of the entire profile with particular attention to the two or three highest scores. The use of the pattern types formed by the various combinations of high scores has led to their establishment as constructs which can be used in lieu of diagnostic classes. Many correlations have been observed between other variables and the personality construct patterns. For the D-Sc pattern, for example, a majority of the diagnoses among psychiatric patients obtaining such a configuration were psychotic ones, either depression or schizophrenia.

Heredity, defined here rather crudely simply as psychosis in siblings or parents, tended to be unfavorable in these individuals [Hathaway & Meehl, 1956, p. 143].

Recent research on the *D-Pt* type (Gilberstadt & Duker, 1960) showed that it could be analyzed into three subtypes. Among other important findings, the authors observed that the *D-Pt-Sc* type of MMPI profile was characterized by a diagnosis of chronic undifferentiated schizophrenia and that such patients had much in common with descriptions in the literature of pseudoneurotic schizophrenia (Peterson, 1954). Surveys of the significance of major configural patterns are available in Hathaway and Meehl (1951) as well as in Dahlstrom and Welsh (1960).

A discussion of the results of the attempted quantification of hereditary influence adds some new information but it is not on the same firm footing as the correlational results. Eleven of the 24 traits measured by the two tests showed at least an appreciable genetic component. By *appreciable* is meant one third or more of the trait variance accounted for relative to the contribution of environmental factors (this required an *H* of .25 or more so that *H* divided by one minus *H* equalled one third). HSPQ factors, F, Q_2, and O showed about equal roles for heredity and environment. Factor O in the Karson and Pool (1957) study correlated most highly, .77, with MMPI Scale 7 (Psychasthenia) and .54 with Scale 0 (Social Introversion). Scale 7 was also found to have an appreciable genetic component in the present study. Three more HSPQ factors survived the criterion, E, H, and J. H along with F and Q_2 formed three of the four factors in Cattell's second-order factor Extraversion versus Introversion. In a study using an early form of the HSPQ (Cattell et al., 1955) both E and J were found to have appreciable genetic components. All five of the MMPI scales surviving the correlation criterion appeared in the quantitative analysis as having an appreciable genetic component. Only Scale *Si*, as noted above, was predominantly genetically determined.

Heritability values given in Tables 7 and 10 as well as those in other twin studies give the proportion of variance produced by genetic differences *within* families and underestimate the effects of heredity in the general population. *If* we could assume random mating for the traits measured, the values in Tables 7 and 10 would have to be multiplied by a factor of approximately two to indicate the true degree of genetic determination. The values thus obtained are remarkable even when compared with the results from animal behavior genetics. McClearn (1961) reported a value of .69 for activity in strains of mice. Fuller and Thompson (1960) reported a heritability of .59 for exploratory behavior in two strains of mice. In animal breeding intense selection pressure permits the value of heritability to become large for such characters as egg weight and wool length (Falconer, 1960). An overview of the relative contributions of heredity and environment to within-family variance on the personality traits measured leads to the observation that environment is the preponderant influence in a majority of the traits. Cattell, Stice, and Kristy (1957) reached a similar conclusion for both within- and between-family variances.

Sex Differences

It is difficult to evaluate the meaning to be attached to the observed sex differences in heritability of the various traits since the sample sizes are reduced. It is tempting to speculate about the possible evolutionary origin of sex differences. Confidence in, and extension of, the interpretations which follow must await the completion of an ongoing study using 180 pairs of twins. To suggest that variation in a personality trait is more under genetic control in one sex than the other, it is only necessary to be reminded of the range of secondary sex differences already observed in physical and behavioral characters in both man and animal. The differentiation of such traits is brought about by hormones; the latter are one of the links in the gene to behavior pathway.

Changing from an expressive environment to a suppressive one will lower the heritability of a trait. Suppose, for example, that early experience in fighting is essential for inducing aggressive behavior. Genetic differences in variability on the *Pd* scale will not be detected in boys reared without this experience. The process of sex typing in our culture restricts certain types of behavior in the two sexes. Fighting is not tolerated and is suppressed in little girls so that we might expect the value of *H* for females on the *Pd* scale to be less than that for males. The results for Factor E, Submissiveness versus Dominance, and for Surgency reveal the same pattern of greater heritability for males than females. This attempt at an environmental explanation for the sex difference observed in trait heritability should not be thought of as appropriate for all the patterns observed.

Factorially Derived Scales versus Empirically Derived Scales

The positive correlational results for the 1 of 14 HSPQ factors could have been attributed to chance. In comparison with the positive results for 5 of the 10 MMPI scales, the harvest from the factorially derived personality test looks poor. The validity of 6 of the 14 HSPQ scales was cast into doubt by finding a zero correlation between identical twins. Many psychologists (e.g., Hall & Lindzey, 1957) have noted that factors derived by factor analysis are often not psychologically meaningful and do not agree with reality. Perhaps the empirical derivation of the MMPI scales was such as to allow Nature to be carved, albeit imperfectly, at the joints. The ease with which MMPI scales can be factored into subscales may mean that the original scales and those derived in similar fashion are equivalent to the large second-order factors of the factor analysts. The *Si* scale, for example, correlates with 10 of Cattell's factors (Karson, 1958). Demonstration of behavioral correlates for factors, such as Eysenck's (1950) criterion analysis, could result in a formidable merger of the ideas of Cattell, Eysenck, Hathaway, and Meehl.

Fate of Attempts at a Holistic View of Personality

Although all three statistical measures of MMPI profile similarity, rho, *D,* and *TT',* tended to support the hypothesis of greater personality similarity between isogenic individuals, only the clinical judgments of similarity gave substantial support. Inasmuch as the statistical method usually surpasses the clinical in psychology (Meehl, 1954), these findings require close attention. Factors favoring successful clinical prediction in a profile sorting task have been suggested by Meehl (1959). Perhaps the most directly relevant factor he mentioned was the clinician's ability to analyze a configural relationship existing between predictor variables and a criterion, when the function is not derivable on rational grounds.

Even casual inspection of the results of the clinical judgments of personality similarity are conducive to accepting the general hypothesis of this research—the greater the gene similarity, the greater the overall personality similarity. The judging task required a discrimination between sisters, for example, of the same age, with the same parents, sharing more or less the same environment for their entire lives, but who differed in the amount of genetic overlap by a factor of only two. We might speculate that the task would have been easier had the pairs consisted of unrelated individuals or first cousins of the same age, sex, and social class background contrasted with identical twins. Misjudgments from the pooled ratings of the judges afford some insight to the range of heredity-environment interactions. The amount of variability available to the same genotypes is shown by the fact that 10 of the 34 pairs of identical twins' profiles were classified as dissimilar. Conversely, the lack of variability in personality available to genotypes with only half their genes in common is shown by the fact that 12 of the 34 fraternal twins' profiles were classified as similar.

Summary and Conclusions

The present study was carried out in the context of behavior genetics, the interdisciplinary science combining the knowledge and procedures of modern genetics with those of psychology. By means of the classical twin method, as it has been recently improved, and objective personality tests, the purpose of the research was to answer the question, how much of the variability observed within a group of individuals in a specified environment on specific measures of specific personality traits is attributable to genetic factors? It was recognized that the genetic variance, heritability (*H*), could vary according to such things as age, sex, culture, trait, and method of trait assessment.

Among the key constructs from genetics, *reaction range* and *polygenic inheritance* are central to the methodology used and interpretation of results. Heredity fixes a reaction range; within this framework a genotype determines an indefinite but circumscribed assortment of phenotypes, each of which corresponds to one of the possible environments to which the genotype may be exposed. The classical Mendelian model of dominant and recessive gene inheritance will not handle the data on continuous variation, the kind observed with human behavior. Polygenic systems are posited to account for quantitative inheritance, the phenotypic effects being simply a function of the number of genes present. Both the twin method and its limitations were discussed.

Thirty-four pairs each of identical (MZ) and fraternal (DZ) same-sex adolescent twins from the public high schools of Minneapolis, St. Paul, and Robbinsdale, Minnesota, served as the sample. The entire population of same-sex twins among the 31,000 children in the schools was first enumerated. Forty-five pairs of girls and 23 pairs of boys volunteered which represented 75% and 43%, respectively, of the total possible twin pairs available in the selected sample of schools. Disregarding sex, the twins comprised 60% of the possible 113 pairs.

At the time of testing, the twins filled out a personal history data sheet, the Minnesota Multiphasic Personality Inventory (MMPI), and Cattell's High School Personality Questionnaire (HSPQ); they were weighed, measured for height, fingerprinted, and photographed. The diagnosis of zygosity was based upon extensive blood grouping with respect to nine blood groups. This resulted in 100% accuracy in the diagnosis of DZ twins and at least 95% for MZ twins. A methodological contribution to twin diagnosis was made by the comparison of the accuracies of various methods and their combinations. Blood typing

is necessary and sufficient for the accuracy required in human behavior genetics research.

Each scale of the two personality tests and the school recorded Otis IQ were first analyzed by means of the intraclass correlation coefficient for the two classes of twins and for sex differences. Subsequent to this analysis, the heritability indexes were computed; *H* is defined as the proportion of personality scale variance attributable to genetic factors. The correlation analysis of the 14 HSPQ scales suggested that two factors (F, Sober, Serious versus Enthusiastic, Happy-Go-Lucky, and Q_2, Group Dependency versus Self-Sufficiency) had significant genetic (i.e., gene determined) components. The correlation analysis of the 10 MMPI scales resulted in five, Scale 2 (Depression), Scale 4 (Psychopathic Deviate), Scale 7 (Psychasthenia), Scale 8 (Schizophrenia), and Scale 0 (Social Introversion), which appeared to have significant genetic components.

Within the limits of the assumptions, the attempt at quantification of the proportion of scale variance accounted for by heredity gave positive results for six of the HSPQ factors. Factors E, Submissiveness versus Dominance; H, Shy, Sensitive versus Adventurous; and J, Liking Group Action versus Fastidiously Individualistic showed appreciable variance accounted for by heredity but with environment predominating. Factors F, Q_2, and O, Confident Adequacy versus Guilt Proneness, showed about equal contributions of heredity and environment. The same kind of analysis of the MMPI gave positive results for 5 of the 10 scales. Scales 7 (Psychasthenia) and 8 (Schizophrenia) showed appreciable variance accounted for by heredity but with environment predominating. Scales 2 (Depression) and 4 (Psychopathic Deviate) showed about equal contributions of heredity and environment. Scale 0 (Social Introversion) showed a predominance of variance ($H = .71$) accounted for by heredity. The value of *H* for the Otis IQ in this study was .62.

Following the scale-by-scale analysis, three holistic statistical analyses and one clinical holistic analysis of the MMPI profiles were done. The rank-difference correlations (rho) for the coded MMPI profiles, the generalized distance function (D), and a measure of test item verbal behavior concordance (TT') all showed a tendency for the MZ profile pairs to be more similar. The tendency was not strong enough to discriminate between the two classes of twins on the basis of any of the three measures. Clinical judgments of profile similarity by three experts supported the general hypothesis that the greater the gene similarity, the greater the personality similarity. The pooled accuracy of the agreement of clinical judgments of MMPI profile similarity with twin zygosity was 68% ($p=$ .005).

Elaboration of the various biochemical or structural differences in the gene to behavior pathway which correspond to the results reported here might be intellectually satisfying, but progress in personality genetics need not await this step. A useful taxonomy of the aspects of behavior termed personality can be facilitated by the use of relatively invariant psychometric configurations to describe behavioral phenotypes. An important by-product of the study of twins and a concern with human behavior genetics is the emphasis given to the need for a multidisciplinary analysis of behavior ranging from biochemistry through evolution. Granting that the difficulties in accurately assessing the contribution of heredity to variation in socially important behavior are great, such efforts will not have been in vain if they contribute to a greater understanding of the sources of individual differences. The provision of an optimum environment for the optimum development of the various aspects of human behavior should follow such increased understanding.

REFERENCES

ALLEN, G. Comments on the analysis of twin samples. *Acta genet. med. Gemellolog.*, 1955, 4, 143–160.

ALLEN, G. Patterns of discovery in the genetics of mental deficiency. *Amer. J. ment. Defic.*, 1958, 62, 840–849.

ALLEN, G. Intellectual potential and heredity. *Science*, 1961, 133, 378–379.

ANASTASI, ANNE. Heredity, environment, and the question "How?" *Psychol. Rev.*, 1958, 65, 197–208.

BLACK, J. D. The interpretation of MMPI profiles of college women. Unpublished doctoral dissertation, University of Minnesota, 1953.

CATTELL, R. B. *The description and measurement of personality*. New York: World Book, 1946.

CATTELL, R. B. *Personality*. New York: McGraw-Hill, 1950.

CATTELL, R. B. Research designs in psychological genetics with special reference to the multiple variance method. *Amer. J. hum. Genet.*, 1953, 5, 76–91.

CATTELL, R. B., BELOFF, H., & COAN, R. W. *Handbook for the IPAT High School Personality Questionnaire*. Champaign, Ill.: Institute of Personality Ability Testing, 1958.

CATTELL, R. B., BLEWETT, D. B., & BELOFF, J. R. The inheritance of personality. *Amer. J. hum. Genet.*, 1955, 7, 122–146.

CATTELL, R. B., STICE, G. F., & KRISTY, N. F. A first approximation to nature-nurture ratios for eleven primary personality factors in objective tests. *J. abnorm. soc. Psychol.*, 1957, 54, 143–160.

CRONBACH, L. J. *Essentials of psychological testing*. New York: Harper, 1960.

CRONBACH, L. J., & GLESER, GOLDINE. Assessing similarity between profiles. *Psychol. Bull.*, 1953, 50, 456–473.

CRONBACH, L. J., & MEEHL, P. E. Construct validity in psychological tests. *Psychol. Bull.*, 1955, 52, 281–302.

CUMMINS, H., & MIDLO, C. *Fingerprints, palms, and soles*. Philadelphia: Blackiston, 1943.

DAHLSTROM, W. G., & WELSH, G. S. (Eds.) *An MMPI handbook*. Minneapolis: Univer. Minnesota Press, 1960.

DOBZHANSKY, T. *Evolution, genetics, and man*. New York: Wiley, 1955.

EYSENCK, H. J. *Dimensions of personality*. London: Paul Kegan, 1947.

EYSENCK, H. J. Criterion analysis. *Psychol. Rev.*, 1950, 57, 38–53.

EYSENCK, H. J. The inheritance of extroversion-introversion. *Acta psychol.*, Amsterdam, 1956, 12, 95–110.

FALCONER, D. S. *An introduction to quantitative genetics*. New York: Ronald, 1960.

FISHER, R. A., & YATES, F. *Statistical tables for biological, agricultural and medical research*. (3rd ed.) New York: Hafner, 1949.

FULLER, J. L. The genetic base: Pathways between genes and behavioral characteristics. In, *The nature and transmission of the genetic and cultural characteristics of human populations*. New York: Milbank Foundation, 1957. Pp. 101–111.

FULLER, J. L. Behavior genetics. *Annu. Rev. Psychol.*, 1960, 11, 41–70.

FULLER, J. L., & THOMPSON, W. R. *Behavior genetics*. New York: Wiley, 1960.

GALTON, F. The history of twins as a criterion of the relative powers of nature and nurture. *Fraser's Mag.*, 1875, 12, 566–576.

GILBERSTADT, H. G., & DUKER, JAN. Case history correlates of three MMPI profile types. *J. consult. Psychol.*, 1960, 24, 361–369.

HERITABILITY OF PERSONALITY

GOTTESMAN, I. I. The psychogenetics of personality. Unpublished doctoral dissertation, University of Minnesota, 1960.

GOTTESMAN, I. I. Genetic aspects of intelligent behavior. In N. Ellis (Ed.), *The handbook in mental deficiency*. New York: McGraw-Hill, 1963. Ch. 7.

GREGORY, I. Genetic factors in schizophrenia. *Amer. J. Psychiat.*, 1960, **116**, 961–972.

HAGGARD, E. A. *The intraclass correlation coefficient*. New York: Dryden, 1958.

HALL, C. S., & LINDZEY, G. *Theories of personality*. New York: Wiley, 1957.

HATHAWAY, S. R., & BRIGGS, P. F. Some normative data on new MMPI scales. *J. clin. Psychol.*, 1957, **13**, 364–369.

HATHAWAY, S. R., & MEEHL, P. E. *An atlas for the clinical use of the MMPI*. Minneapolis: Univer. Minnesota Press, 1951.

HATHAWAY, S. R., & MEEHL, P. E. Psychiatric implications of code types. In G. S. Welsh & W. G. Dahlstrom (Eds.), *Basic readings on the MMPI*. Minneapolis: Univer. Minnesota Press, 1956. Pp. 136–144.

HATHAWAY, S. R., & MONACHESI, E. D. *An atlas of juvenile MMPI profiles*. Minneapolis: Univer. Minnesota Press, 1961.

HOLZINGER, K. J. The relative effect of nature and nurture influences on twin differences. *J. educ. Psychol.*, 1929, **20**, 241–248.

JACKSON, D. D. A critique of the literature on the genetics of schizophrenia. In D. D. Jackson (Ed.), *The etiology of schizophrenia*. New York: Basic Books, 1960. Pp. 37–87.

JUNG, C. G. *Psychological types*. New York: Harcourt, 1933.

KALLMANN, F. J. The genetic theory of schizophrenia. *Amer. J. Psychiat.*, 1946, **103**, 309–322.

KALLMANN, F. J. *Heredity in health and mental disorder*. New York: Norton, 1953.

KALLMANN, F. J. Psychogenetic studies of twins. In S. Koch (Ed.), *Psychology: A study of a science*. Vol. 3. *Formulations of the person and the social context*. New York: McGraw-Hill, 1959. Pp. 328–362.

KALLMANN, F. J., & BAROFF, G. S. Abnormalities of behavior (in the light of psychogenetic studies). *Annu. Rev. Psychol.*, 1955, **6**, 297–326.

KARSON, S. Second order personality factors and the MMPI. *J. clin. Psychol.*, 1958, **14**, 313–315.

KARSON, S., & POOL, K. B. The construct validity of the Sixteen Personality Factors Test. *J. clin. Psychol.*, 1957, **13**, 245–252.

LEJEUNE, J., & TURPIN, R. Chromosomal aberrations in man. *Amer. J. hum. Genet.*, 1961, **13**, 175–184.

LOEVINGER, JANE. On the proportional contribution of differences in nature and in nurture to differences in intelligence. *Psychol. Bull.*, 1943, **40**, 725–756.

LOEVINGER, JANE. Objective tests as instruments of psychological theory. *Psychol. Rep.*, 1957, **3**, 635–694.

McCLEARN, G. E. Genotype and mouse activity. *J. comp. physiol. Psychol.*, 1961, **54**, 674–676.

MEEHL, P. E. *Clinical versus statistical prediction*. Minneapolis: Univer. Minnesota Press, 1954.

MEEHL, P. E. A comparison of clinicians with five statistical methods of identifying psychotic MMPI profiles. *J. counsel. Psychol.*, 6, 1959, 102–109.

MEEHL, P. E., & ROSEN, A. Antecedent probability and the efficiency of psychometric signs, patterns, or cutting scores. *Psychol. Bull.*, 1955, **52**, 194–216.

MOSTELLER, F., & BUSH, R. R. Selected quantitative techniques. In G. Lindzey (Ed.), *Handbook of social psychology*. Boston: Addison-Wesley, 1954. Pp. 289–334.

NEWMAN, H. H. *Multiple human births*. New York: Doubleday, 1940.

NEWMAN, H. H., FREEMAN, F. N., & HOLZINGER, K. J. *Twins: A study of heredity and environment*. Chicago: Univer. Chicago Press, 1937.

OSBORNE, R. H., & DEGEORGE, F. V. *Genetic basis of morphological variation*. Cambridge: Harvard Univer. Press, 1959.

OSGOOD, C. E., & SUCI, G. J. A measure of relation determined by both mean difference and profile information. *Psychol. Bull.*, 1952, **49**, 251–262.

PETERSON, D. R. The diagnosis of subclinical schizophrenia. *J. consult. Psychol.*, 1954, **18**, 198–200.

PRICE, B. Primary biases in twin studies. *Amer. J. hum. Genet.*, 1950, **2**, 293–352.

RACE, R. R., & SANGER, R. *Blood groups in man*. (3rd. ed.) Springfield: Charles C Thomas, 1958.

ROZEBOOM, W. W. The fallacy of the null-hypothesis significance test. *Psychol. Bull.*, 1960, **57**, 416–428.

SLATER, E. *Psychotic and neurotic illnesses in twins*. London: Her Majesty's Stationery Office, 1953.

SMITH, SHELIA M., & PENROSE, L. S. Monozygotic and dizygotic twin diagnosis. *Ann. hum. Genet.*, 1955, **19**, 273–289.

STERN, C. *Principles of human genetics*. (2nd ed.) San Francisco: Freeman, 1960.

STRANDSKOV, H. H., & EDELEN, E. W. Monozygotic and dizygotic birth frequencies in the total, in the "white" and the "colored" U. S. populations. *Genetics*, 1946, **31**, 438–446.

TRYON, R. C. Behavior genetics in social psychology. *Amer. Psychologist*, 1957, **12**, 453. (Abstract)

VANDENBERG, S. G. The hereditary abilities study: Hereditary components in a psychological test battery. *Amer. J. hum. Genet.*, 1962, **14**, 220–237.

WIRT, R. D., & BRIGGS, P. F. Personality and environmental factors in the development of delinquency. *Psychol. Monogr.*, 1959, **73** (15, Whole No. 485).

(Received February 7, 1963)

From L. Eaves and H. J. Eysenck (1975). Journal of Personality and Social Psychology, *32*, 102-112, *by kind permission of the authors and the American Psychological Association*

The Nature of Extraversion: A Genetical Analysis

Lindon Eaves
Department of Genetics,
University of Birmingham,
Birmingham, England

Hans Eysenck
Institute of Psychiatry,
University of London,
London, England

A biometrical–genetical analysis of twin data to elucidate the determinants of variation in extraversion and its components, sociability and impulsiveness, revealed that both genetical and environmental factors contributed to variation in extraversion, to the variation and covariation of its component scales, and to the interaction between subjects and scales. A large environmental correlation between the scales suggested that environmental factors may predominate in determining the unitary nature of extraversion. The interaction between subjects and scales depended more on genetical factors, which suggests that the dual nature of extraversion has a strong genetical basis. A model assuming random mating, additive gene action, and specific environmental effects adequately describes the observed variation and covariation of sociability and impulsiveness. Possible evolutionary implications are discussed.

One of the central problems in personality research has been the question of whether such higher order factors as extraversion can be regarded in any meaningful sense as *unitary* or whether there are several independent factors, such as "sociability" and "impulsiveness," which should not be thrown together artificially. Carrigan (1960) concluded her survey of the literature by saying that "the unidimensionality of extraversion/introversion has not been conclusively demonstrated" (p. 355); she further pointed out that several joint analyses of the Guildford and Cattell questionnaires show that at least *two* independent factors are required to account for the intercorrelations between the extraversion–impulsiveness variables. These two factors, she suggested, may correspond to the European conception of extraversion, with its emphasis on impulsiveness and weak superego controls, and the American conception, with its emphasis on sociability and ease in interpersonal relations. Eysenck and Eysenck (1963) have reported quite sizable correlations between sociability and impulsiveness, a conclusion replicated by

Sparrow and Ross (1964); this would suggest that there is a close connection between the two conceptions (Eysenck & Eysenck, 1969). Furthermore, Eysenck and Eysenck (1967) have shown that the correlations of extraversion items (whether sociability or impulsiveness) with subjects' reactions on a physiological test devised on theoretical grounds were proportional to their loadings on the extraversion factor. The recognition that extraversion is a unitary factor in behavior is thus vindicated by prediction from a psychological theory as much as by a correlation between primary factors (Eysenck, 1967).

We now develop a model for the genetical and environmental determinants of extraversion and of its primary components, sociability and impulsiveness. Our intention is to analyze the phenotypic variation and covariation of sociability and impulsiveness into their genetical and environmental components in order to determine, as far as our data permit: (a) the simplest model for the genetical and environmental variation of extraversion considered as a unitary trait and (b) the simplest model for the genetical and environmental determination of the interaction between subjects and the component tests of extraversion, sociability and impulsiveness.

In fulfilling these aims, we are led to compare the unitary and dual models of extraversion with regard to their relative contri-

We are indebted to the Colonial Research Fund and the British Medical Research Council for their support of the investigation. We are grateful to J. Kasriel for the collection of data and to the twins for their continued cooperation.

Requests for reprints should be sent to Lindon Eaves, Department of Genetics, University of Birmingham, Birmingham, B15 2TT, England.

LINDON EAVES AND HANS EYSENCK

butions to the representation of both genotypic and environmental determinants of variation among the responses of subjects to a personality inventory.

Earlier research from the standpoint of the psychological theory underlying this work has mainly been concerned with the analysis of extraversion as a unitary trait (Shields, 1962). Claridge, Canter and Hume (1973) reported analyses of extraversion, sociability, and impulsiveness, but these authors themselves admitted that their samples were too small to justify the kind of analysis we attempt here. Our model will be derived from an analysis of twin data and will, therefore, inevitably reflect the limitations of twin studies as sources of genetical information (Jinks & Fulker, 1970). Even twin studies, however, have seldom been used to best advantage. We hope that our particular analysis will have the additional virtue of demonstrating how twin data in general may be manipulated to test simple hypotheses about the causes of variation. We have adopted the methods and notation of biometrical genetics (Mather & Jinks, 1971) because we believe them to be the most precise and general, while embodying a defined procedure for the analysis of continuous variation which may be extended readily to the analysis of human behavior (Jinks and Fulker, 1970).

DATA

The analysis is based on the responses of 837 pairs of adult volunteer twins to an 80-item personality inventory. Of these items, 13 formed a scale of sociability, and 9 items were scored to provide a measure of impulsiveness. The relevant items are given in Table 1. On the basis of a short questionnaire concerning similarity during childhood, the twins were classified as monozygotic or dizygotic.[1] Such a procedure is surprisingly reliable (Cederlöf, Friberg, Jonsonn, & Kaij, 1961). A sample of

[1] The twins were asked: (a) "Do you differ markedly in physical appearance and coloring?" and (b) "In childhood were you frequently mistaken by people who knew you?" If consistent replies were not given, reference was made to previous questionnaires, twins' letters, and additional information in an attempt to assess zygosity. Many of the twins have been blood-typed subsequently, and the original diagnoses have generally been confirmed (Kasriel, J., personal communication, December 1974).

TABLE 1

PERSONALITY INVENTORY ITEMS INCLUDED IN THE ANALYSIS

Item	Key
18. Do you suddenly feel shy when you want to talk to an attractive stranger?	−S
23. Generally, do you prefer reading to meeting people?	−S
27. Do you like going out a lot?	+S
30. Do you prefer to have few but special friends?	−S
36. Can you usually let yourself go and enjoy yourself a lot at a gay party?	+S
40. Do other people think of you as being very lively?	+S
44. Are you mostly quiet when you are with other people?	−S
48. If there is something you want to know about, would you rather look it up in a book than talk to someone about it?	−S
56. Do you hate being with a crowd who play jokes on one another?	−S
66. Do you like talking to people so much that you never miss a chance of talking to a stranger?	+S
69. Would you be unhappy if you could not see lots of people most of the time?	+S
75. Do you find it hard to really enjoy yourself at a lively party?	−S
77. Can you easily get some life into a rather dull party?	+S
1. Do you often long for excitement?	+I
4. Are you usually carefree?	+I
8. Do you stop and think things over before doing anything?	−I
12. Do you generally say things quickly without stopping to think?	+I
16. Would you do almost anything for a dare?	+I
20. Do you often do things on the spur of the moment?	+I
33. When people shout at you, do you shout back?	+I
59. Do you like doing things in which you have to act quickly?	+I
62. Are you slow and unhurried in the way you move?	−I

Note. S denotes an item scored for sociability, I for impulsiveness; + indicates that "yes" scored 1, and − indicates that "no" scored 1 for scale under consideration.

digzygotic twins of unlike sex has been included in our study because these provide a critical diagnostic test of sex limitation. The composition of the sample by sex and zygosity is given in Table 2.

The mean sociability and impulsiveness scores of the five groups are given in Table 3. An analysis of the variation between and within groups revealed highly significant (but substantively fairly small) differences between groups with respect to the sociability scores. The groups did not differ with respect to their mean impulsiveness scores. We shall regard

TABLE 2
Structure of Twin Sample

Twin type	No. pairs
Monozygotic female	331
Monozygotic male	120
Dizygotic female	198
Dizygotic male	59
Unlike-sex dizygotic	129

the groups as representative of the same population as far as their means are concerned. The groups are homogeneous with respect to their dispersion, as will become clear from the subsequent genetical analysis. The pooled standard deviations within groups were 3.0015 and 1.7586 for sociability and impulsivenses, respectively.

Since we wished to minimize the possibility of spurious interaction between subjects and tests, we standardized the raw scores of the twins on both sociability and impulsiveness by dividing the scores by the corresponding average within-groups standard errors. For each group of twins separately, the mean squares within pairs and between pairs were calculated for each of the standardized scales. The analogous within-pairs and between-pairs mean products were also calculated. The mean squares and mean products form the basic statistical summary for the analysis to follow (see Table 4).

We studied the inheritance of extraversion by analyzing the mean squares derived from the subjects' total scores of the two standardized tests. The mean squares for the twins on the measure of extraversion (E) may be

TABLE 3
Mean Sociability and Impulsiveness Scores of Twin Groups

Twin type	N	M	
		Sociability	Impulsiveness
MZf	662	6.5045	3.7039
MZm	240	5.7875	3.8125
DZf	396	6.6869	3.7525
DZm	118	6.6441	4.0678
DZos	258	6.4884	3.7054

Note. Abbreviations are as follows: MZf = monozygotic female, MZm = monozygotic male, DZf = dizygotic female, DZm = dizygotic male, and DZos = unlike-sex dizygotic.

TABLE 4
Mean Squares and Mean Products Within and Between Twin Pairs for Standardized Sociability and Impulsiveness Scores

Item	df	MS (S)	MS (Imp)	MP (S-I)
Between MZf pairs	330	1.5339	1.3777	.6517
Within MZf pairs	331	.5394	.6403	.1762
Between MZm pairs	119	1.5595	1.2904	.3126
Within MZm pairs	120	.4817	.6630	.1497
Between DZf pairs	197	1.0855	1.1804	.3069
Within DZf pairs	198	.8380	.8408	.2918
Between DZm pairs	58	1.3919	.9799	.6309
Within DZm pairs	59	.6693	.8441	.1516
Between DZos pairs	128	.9457	1.2839	.3638
Within DZos pairs	129	.9290	.7697	.3581

Note. Abbreviations are as follows: MZf = monozygotic female, MZm = monozygotic males, DZf = dizygotic female, DZm = dizygotic male, and DZos = unlike-sex dizygotic. MS = mean square. MP = mean product; S = Sociability and I = impulsiveness. No correction for the main effect of sex was necessary for the DZos.

derived directly from the mean squares and mean products (MP) of Table 4, since MS_E = $MS_{(S+I)} = MS_S + MS_I + 2MP_{S,I}$, where S and I refer to sociability and impulsiveness.

Just as we obtained an E score for each subject by summing over tests, so we may obtain a difference (D) score for each subject by taking the difference between his scores on the standardized tests. The MS derived from these differences summarizes the variation arising because subjects do not perform consistently on the two tests. We may obtain the MS for the D scores directly from the raw MS and mean products of Table 4, since

$$MS_D = MS_{(S-I)} = MS_S + MS_I - 2MP_{(S,I)}.$$

The mean squares for E and D are found in Table 5. Clearly, since the mean products are all positive, the MS_E's are larger than the corresponding MS_D's. Since we are only concerned with these particular tests, the mean squares between subjects for E contain none of the interaction variation. Thus the fact that the MS_E's are approximately twice as large as the MS_D's is an indication that E accounts for more of the total variation of the two tests than D.

We analyze the MS_E to provide a genetical model for variation in extraversion, and we analyze the MS_D to determine the extent to which genetical or environmental factors contribute to the resolution of E into sociability and impulsiveness. Finally, we show that the covariation of sociability and impulsiveness reflects both genetical and environmental factors by an analysis of the raw mean squares and mean products of Table 5.

METHODS

Formulation of the Model

Most analyses of classical twin studies have merely demonstrated the existence of a genetical component of variation by showing that monozygotic twins are more alike than are dizygotic twins. Such an intuitive approach is imprecise and does not lead to any exact predictions about the similarity between other degrees of relatives. For this reason the classical approach is not very helpful in guiding the design of future research. In adopting the methods of biometrical genetics we are able to specify, for a given set of assumptions about the kinds of gene action and environmental effects, precise expectations for the components of variance (and consequently for the mean squares) derived from the analysis of variance of any group of relatives. Furthermore, having specified our assumptions and the consequent expectations of mean squares, we are able to provide a statistical test of the agreement between observations and expectations and, consequently, to test the validity of the assumptions we made at the outset.

Clearly, twin data of the kind we have summarized in this article do not allow us to test any but the simplest set of assumptions about the causes of variation. We also recognize that failure of particular assumptions in principle may not lead to failure of the model in practice, either because sample sizes are too small for the test to be sufficiently powerful (see, e.g., Eaves & Jinks, 1972) or because failure of certain assumptions may contribute more to a bias in estimation than to departures of what is observed from what is expected.

We now consider individually the assumptions we make in the analyses which follow. Some of these are an undesirable necessity of the limited data we have available and may not be tested very powerfully by our analysis. Other assumptions are quite likely to be disproved in practice, even with the data available, if they are unjustified. We emphasize that these limitations apply not to the method, which is the most explicit and flexible available, but to the particular data upon which we seek to build our model. Other experimental designs would enable us to test with greater conviction the assumptions which we now make tentatively, (Eaves, 1972; Jinks & Fulker; 1970).

1: *Alleles and loci act additively and independently.* We assume that there is no dominance, epistasis, or linkage for the loci contributing to variation of the traits under consideration. If our other assumptions are justified, nonadditive variation may be detected in principle with our data, but in practice the necessary sample sizes are likely to be too large (Eaves, 1972). Failure of either of the two following assumptions may make the de-

TABLE 5

MEAN SQUARES FOR EXTRAVERSION AND INTERACTION OF SUBJECTS AND COMPONENT TESTS

Item	df	MS	
		E = S + I	D = S − I
Between MZf pairs	330	4.2150	1.6082
Within MZf pairs	331	1.5321	.8273
Between MZm pairs	119	3.4751	2.2247
Within MZm pairs	120	1.4441	.8453
Between DZf pairs	197	2.8797	1.6521
Within DZf pairs	198	2.2624	1.0952
Between DZm pairs	58	3.6336	1.1100
Within DZm pairs	59	1.8166	1.2102
Between DZos pairs	128	2.9572	1.5020
Within DZos pairs	129	2.4749	.9825

Note. Abbreviations are as follows: MZf = monozygotic female, MZm = monozygotic male, DZf = dizygotic female, DZm = dizygotic male, and DZos = unlike-sex dizygotic. E refers to extraversion, and D refers to the interaction of subjects and component tests. S and I refer to sociability and impulsiveness, respectively.

tection of nonadditive variation virtually impossible with the data of our study.

2: *Mating is random.* There is little evidence of assortative mating for extraversion. We might expect to detect the genetical consequences of assortative mating provided there is substantial genetical variation and a fairly high correlation between spouses (Eaves, 1973a). The design of the present study, however, since it involves twins reared together, makes it impossible to distinguish the effects of assortative mating from those of environmental influences shared by members of the same twin pair. Eysenck (1974) reports a nonsignificant correlation for the extraversion scores of husbands and wives. This suggests that assortative mating can safely be discounted as a factor contributing to the genetical variability of extraversion.

3: *All environmental effects are specific to individuals within families.* Most of the twins in our study lived together, especially when they were young. The fact that both individuals in a pair have the same biological mother and grew up in the same family may make both monozygotic and dizygotic twins more alike than we would expect on the basis of our simple genetical and environmental model. For twins reared together, such effects are formally indistinguishable from those of assortative mating and, if they are substantial, may contribute to failure of our simple model, which assumes that assortative mating and common environmental influences make a negligible contribution to the observed variation. We have some independent test of the contribution of postnatal shared environmental influences for extraversion because we would expect the intrapair differences of twins to increase with the period of separation. Although age and duration of separation are, of course, highly correlated, we can detect no relationship between the intrapair difference for extraversion scores

THE NATURE OF EXTRAVERSION

TABLE 6

A GENETICAL AND ENVIRONMENTAL MODEL FOR A SET OF OBSERVED MEAN SQUARES

MS	Coefficient of parameter	
	D_R	E_1
Between MZf pairs	1	1
Within MZf pairs	.	1
Between MZm pairs	1	1
Within MZm pairs	.	1
Between DZf pairs	$\frac{3}{4}$	1
Within DZf pairs	$\frac{1}{4}$	1
Between DZm pairs	$\frac{3}{4}$	1
Within DZm pairs	$\frac{1}{4}$	1
Between DZos pairs	$\frac{3}{4}$	1
Within DZos pairs	$\frac{1}{4}$	1

Note. Abbreviations are as follows: MZf = monozygotic female, MZm = monozygotic male, DZf = dizygotic female, DZm = dizygotic male, and DZos = unlike-sex dizygotic. D_R refers to an additive genetical component, and E_1 refers to a within-family environmental component.

and the age or duration of adult and juvenile separation of these twins. We hope to make a detailed consideration of this issue the subject of a future publication. We assume, until we have evidence to the contrary, that any environmental variation for the traits in question is the result of influences which are unique to particular individuals rather than shared by members of the same family. If such an assumption were clearly unjustified, then we would find our observations quite obviously did not coincide with our expectations and we would be forced to reject our simple model.

Jinks and Fulker (1970) showed in their biometrical genetical reanalysis of Shields's (1962) extraversion data that common environmental influences must be fairly unimportant. This adds some weight to our assumption that common environmental influences can be ignored, but we should first indicate the likely sensitivity of our experiment for detecting such effects if they still contribute to the variation between pairs.

Power calculations, familiar in the context of biometrical genetics, (e.g., Eaves, 1972; Eaves & Jinks, 1972; Kearsey, 1970) reveal that a sample of approximately 220 pairs of monozygotic and the same number of dizygotic pairs would allow us to be roughly 50% certain of detecting common environmental influences which accounted for 20% of the total variation against the background of an additive genetical component which accounted for about 40% of the total variation. This gives some indication of the power of the present study to detect common environmental influences (and the confounded consequences of assortative mating), provided there is no nonadditive genetical variation. To be 95% certain of detecting a common environmental component of this magnitude, sample sizes would have to be about four times as great.

4. *Sex linkage and sex limitation are absent.* If we were to adopt the usual practice of analyzing correlations

rather than mean squares, we would have only poor tests of sex linkage and sex limitation. We would, however, expect the numerical values of comparable mean squares to vary significantly between sexes in the presence of sex linkage or sex limitation except under very restrictive assumptions about the magnitudes and types of gene effects (see Mather & Jinks, 1971). In applying our model to the mean squares rather than to the correlations, we may expect any gross distortion due to either of these causes to result in significant failure of the model.

5. *Genotypic and environmental deviations are uncorrelated.* Under some circumstances we might expect genotype–environmental covariation to contribute to failure of our simple genetical model for monozygotic and dizygotic twins. These circumstances, however, are rather restricting for a study of this type, and we should be cautious about assuming that the adequacy of the model for twin data means that we can ignore this source of variation. As a consequence of the covariation of genotype and environmental effects we could, in principle, find that the environmental components for dizygotic and monozygotic twins are no longer comparable. In practice we are unlikely to detect such differences with these data.

6. *Any variation due to the interaction of genotype and environment is confounded with the environmental variation within families.* It is inevitable that any interaction between genotypic effects and those environmental influences specific to individuals will be confounded with variation due to specific environmental factors in human studies (Jinks & Fulker 1970). We hope that an analysis of such interactions for personality variables will be the subject of a future article. If we are justified in our assumption that there are no common environmental influences, then we are also justified in our assumption that these do not interact with the genotype. Should our model fail because of common environments, we would find that our estimate of the additive genetical component was biased by the variation due to any interaction of these influences with genotypic factors.

We represent the six assumptions by writing a model for the *mean squares* for pairs of monozygotic and dizygotic twins in terms of an additive genetical component (D_R) and a within-family environmental component (E_1). Mather and Jinks (1971) showed how D_R may be defined in terms of the frequencies and effects of many loci. The coefficient chosen for D_R will depend on the mating system. Since we are assuming mating to be random, the coefficients involve no further unknown parameter and may be written for monozygotic and dizygotic twins as they are shown in Table 6. The expectation for a *within-pair mean square* is simply the expectation for the corresponding *within-family component of variance*, σ_w^2, and the expectation for a *between-pair mean square* is σ_w^2 plus twice the expectation for the corresponding *between-families component of variance*, σ_b^2. Full tables of expectations of mean squares and variance components for different kinds of relatives may be found elsewhere (e.g., Eaves, 1973a; Jinks & Fulker, 1970; Mather & Jinks, 1971).

Estimating Parameters and Testing the Model

If we consider only one trait we have, in this study, 10 observed mean squares. Let these be written as the column vector x. Our model (see Table 6) involves two parameters whose coefficients in the expectations of x may be represented by the 10×2 design matrix A. We may obtain our estimates of the two parameters, denoted by the two-element vector $\hat{\theta}$, by solving the simultaneous equations:

$$\hat{\theta} = (A'WA)^{-1}A'Wx,$$

where W is the (10×10) matrix of information about the observed statistics. When the x are mean squares, the amount of information about mean square x_i is $n_i/2(\varepsilon x_i)^2$, where n_i is the degrees of freedom corresponding to x_i. Clearly we do not know εx until the model has been fitted so we have to use the observed x to provide trial values for the amounts of information and proceed iteratively until our εx are stable. In practice, however, it is often unnecessary to go beyond the first cycle provided the model is adequate, since x will then be a close approximation to εx. For the case in which we are considering a single trait and our mean-squares are all independent, W is diagonal and the computations for simple models are not tedious. Providing that our observed statistics are normally distributed, our estimates of θ are the maximum-likelihood estimates and the scalar

$$S = (x - \varepsilon x)'W(x - \varepsilon x)$$

is distributed as a chi-square with degrees of freedom equal to the number of statistics less the number of parameters estimated from the data. The assumption of normality is probably not far from the truth with the sample sizes available. Should this chi-square be significant, we would be compelled to reject our model as inappropriate for the description of the variation for the trait under consideration.

Although the preceding statistical considerations are not new, they have not been generally applied to the genetical analysis of human behavior, with the result that data have been used inefficiently, standard errors of estimates have rarely been quoted, and assumptions rarely tested. The usual analyses of twin data either concentrate on the variation within pairs or on a comparison of monozygotic and dizygotic correlations. The method we employ combines both approaches in a single test of a simple model. In effect, our test of the D_R, E_1 model is not merely testing whether the within-pair variances differ for the two types of twins but whether the estimates derived from within-pair comparisons can be used to predict the variation between pairs. We expect the prediction to be poor if certain of our assumptions fail. These and other considerations, such as that of sex limitation, are all combined in our weighted least-squares analysis of the full set of raw mean squares.

RESULTS

Genetical Analysis of Extraversion

The estimates of the parameters and the elements of their covariance matrix, $(A'WA)^{-1}$,

TABLE 7
GENETICAL ANALYSIS OF EXTRAVERSION

Parameter	Estimate	χ^2	df	P
D_R	2.2487	98.50	1	< .001
E_1	1.5280	276.04	1	< .001
Residual		7.05	8	.50
V D_R	.051336	—	—	
V E_1	.008458	—	—	
Cov $D_R E_1$	−.011814	—	—	

Note. D_R refers to an additive genetical component, and E_1 refer to a within-family environmental component. V and Cov refer to variance and covariance, respectively.

are given for extraversion in Table 7. We see from the nonsignificant residual χ^2 that our model is clearly adequate so that the data give no reason to suppose that our assumptions are unjustified. We divide the square of each estimate by the corresponding variance term to give, for each estimate, a $\chi^2(1)$ which tests the significance of that parameter. Clearly both D_R and E_1 are highly significant components of the variation in extraversion.

On the basis of our tests of the model we tentatively adopt the view that most of the genetical variation is additive and most of the environmental variation can be attributed to E_1. We may use our estimates to estimate the proportion of the population variance for extraversion which can be attributed to genetical causes. Since all of the variation is additive, we have no need of the distinction between "broad" and "narrow" heritability in the present context; we just estimate:

$$\hat{h}^2 = \tfrac{1}{2}\hat{D}_R/(\tfrac{1}{2}\hat{D}_R + \hat{E}_1)$$
$$= .424 \text{ for extraversion.}$$

This means that 42% of the variation in extraversion may be attributed to genetical causes. In the present case E_1 includes variation due both to "unreliability" and "real" specific environmental influences. There seems little point in correcting for unreliability if all predictions are to be made on the basis of one administration of a test such as that analyzed here. If our genetical model is in fact appropriate, we may predict the correlations between other degrees of relatives for extraversion as measured by this test. For parents and offspring, for example, we would expect a correlation of $\tfrac{1}{2}h^2 = .21$. Such data as we have suggest that the observed correlation is

TABLE 8

GENETICAL ANALYSIS OF INTERACTION BETWEEN SUBJECTS AND TESTS OF SOCIABILITY AND IMPULSIVENESS

Parameter	Estimate	x^2	df	P
D_R	.8591	62.94	1	<.001
E_1	.8359	288.95	1	<.001
Residual	—	8.76	8	>.30
V D_R	.011727	—	—	—
V E_1	.002418	—	—	—
Cov $D_R E_1$	−.003277	—	—	—

Note. D_R refers to an additive genetical component. and E_1 refers to a within-family environmental component. V and Cov refer to variance and covariance, respectively.

somewhat lower but not significantly so. Such a difference, if it turned out to be significant, might be attributed to the interaction of the genotypic difference between individuals with an overall differences between the environments of parents and offspring or to the fact that our estimate of the heritability is somewhat biased by undetected common environmental effects. A common environmental effect which accounted for about 10%–15% of the total variance might explain the disparity and is more likely than not be to undetected in our study.

We obtained estimates of the internal consistency of the scales. For sociability the reliability was about .75 and for impulsiveness, .60. We may correct our heritability estimate for unreliability provided we can assume the Subjects × Items interactions estimate experimental error only. Using the estimates of genetical and environmental variance and covariance obtained below, we found the heritability of extraversion, after correction, to be .57. By correcting for unreliability, we have attempted to partition the environmental variation for extraversion into that part which may reflect stable environmental influences on the development of the trait and that part due to experimental error. If subjects and items interact, the contribution of experimental error to E_1 will be overestimated. Such interactions may have a genetical component which we could analyze using the methods adopted in this article. Confounded with our "true" environmental variation will remain variation reflecting day-to-day changes in behavior whose contribution can only be assessed by repeated measurement.

Genetical Analysis of Subject × Tests Interaction

The results of the analysis of the mean squares for the D scores appear in Table 8. Broadly speaking the results for the interaction are very similar to those for E. The main difference is the reduction by half, in this case, of the estimates of D_R and E_1. This reflects the greater discriminating power of E resulting from the positive covariation of sociability and impulsiveness. However, the simple model is again adequate, since the residual $x^2(8)$ is not significant. D_R and E_1 are, once more, highly significant. This means that the discrimination between sociability and impulsiveness is justified in genetical terms. We have to conclude that not all the genetical factors contributing to variation in sociability and impulsiveness contribute equally and consistently to both. We estimate the heritability of the interaction to be .339. Although this value is somewhat lower than that for E, the difference is not large and we must notice that the *relative* contribution of unreliability variation will be greater for the interaction than for E. Using the reliabilities given above, and the estimates of the genetical and environmental variance and covariance components from a later analysis (see below), we estimate the heritability of the interaction of subjects and tests to be .72. The marked change reflects the relatively large positive environmental correlation between sociability and impulsiveness, particularly when the environmental variances are corrected for unreliability.

Table 9 summarizes the results of both analyses in terms of the proportions of the total variation of sociability and impulsiveness

TABLE 9

THE RELATIVE CONTRIBUTIONS OF GENOTYPIC AND ENVIRONMENTAL FACTORS OF EXTRAVERSION AND SUBJECTS × TESTS INTERACTION TO THE VARIATION BETWEEN SUBJECTS FOR SOCIABILITY AND IMPULSIVENESS

Causal factor	Psychological factor		Total
	Extra-version	Inter-action	
Genetical	.2870(.3402)	.1096(.2631)	.3966(.6035)
Environmental	.3900(.2156)	.2134(.1807)	.6034(.3963)
Total	.6770(.5558)	.3230(.4440)	1.0000(.9998)

Note. Proportions of estimated reliable variation are given in parenthesis.

LINDON EAVES AND HANS EYSENCK

TABLE 10
RESULT OF FITTING SIMPLE MODEL TO VARIATION AND COVARIATION
OF SOCIABILITY AND IMPULSIVENESS

Parameter	Estimate	Covariance ($\times 10^4$) of estimate with estimate of						$\chi^2(1)$
		D_{RS}	D_{RI}	D_{RSI}	E_{1S}	E_{1I}	E_{1SI}	
D_{RS}	.9214	67.05	8.54	23.89	−14.80	−1.61	−4.92	126.63*
D_{RI}	.7132		68.38	24.01	− 1.62	−19.34	−1.93	74.33*
D_{RSI}	.3419			38.08	− 4.92	− 5.64	−9.30	30.70*
E_{1S}	.5410				10.42	1.11	3.41	280.77*
E_{1I}	.6441					14.32	9.92	290.45*
E_{1SI}	.1758						6.68	46.27*

Note. The parameters D_{RS}, D_{RI}, D_{RSI}, E_{1S}, E_{1I}, and E_{1SI} correspond to the components of the mean squares of sociability, impulsiveness, and the mean products of the two traits, respectively.
* $P < .001$.

scores which may be attributed to the genetical and environmental components of extraversion and the interaction of subjects and tests. Approximately three fifths of the total variation is environmental (from the row totals of Table 9) and two thirds of the total variation is attributable to the extraversion factor (from the column totals of Table 9). The proportion of environmental variation is fairly consistent over columns, and the proportion of variation accounted for by extraversion is fairly consistent over rows. In Table 9 we also present a summary for the scales after the environmental components have been corrected for unreliability. So far we have sl own that genetical factors probably contribute to individual differences in both E and D scores. A qualitative consideration of the conclusion suggests that E is more discriminating than D genetically and environmentally and leads us to the view that the positive covariation of sociability and impulsiveness has a basis which is both genetical and environmental. We could verify this directly by a statistical comparison of our estimates to test whether the estimates of D_R and E_1 are significantly greater than the corresponding estimates for D. We prefer, however, to estimate separately the genetical and environmental components of the variation and covariation of sociability and impulsiveness scores, since this will allow us to estimate the genetical and environmental correlations between the traits.

Analysis of Variation and Covariation of Sociability and Impulsiveness

The weighted least-squares procedure described above may be extended with ut undue complication to the simultaneous analysis of the variances and covariances of multiple variables (Eaves & Gale, 1974). In this case, however, separate D_R's and E_1's are fitted for the variance and covariance terms. The information matrix, **W**, is no longer diagonal, since the model is fitted to mean squares and mean products which are no longer independent because each subject yields measurements on every trait.

In this instance the model is fitted to the 30 statistics of Table 5. Now six parameters are specified, D_{RS}, D_{RI}, $D_{RS,I}$, E_{1S}, E_{1I}, and $E_{1S,I}$. These correspond to the components of the mean squares of sociability, impulsiveness, and the mean products of the two traits, respectively. The method and the definition of the parameters is discussed in more detail by Eaves and Gale (1974).

There are thus 30 statistics. Six parameters are estimated from the data, so the residual chi-square for testing the goodness of fit of the model has 24 degrees of freedom. This chi-square changed by less than .2% between the first and second cycle of the weighted least-squares analysis, when $\chi^2(24) = 29.41$, $p \simeq .20$. Thus the adequacy of the D_R, E_1 model for the variation and covariation of sociability and impulsiveness was confirmed.

The estimates of the six parameters and their covariance matrix are given in Table 10. Clearly all the estimates differ significantly from zero. We estimate the heritability of sociability to be .460 and that of impulsiveness to be .356. Using, once more, our estimates of reliability, we infer that about 54% of the environmental variation for sociability is "reliable" variation, assuming that we have accounted for all the unreliability. For impulsiveness the comparable figure is 38%. We may now obtain estimates of the proportion of *reliable* variance which is due to genetical causes. Our estimates are .61 for sociability and .60 for impulsiveness. There is, therefore, convincing evidence that both traits are under some degree of genetical control. This finding is not new. Claridge, Canter, and Hume (1973) reported an apparent genetical component of variation for both scales. Our model-fitting approach, however, leads us to suggest that there is no evidence of nonadditive genetical variation and no evidence of common environmental effects. Furthermore, we have demonstrated that the covariance of sociability and impulsiveness probably has a genetical basis but that environmental factors also contribute significantly to the covariation of the two scales. The extent to which the two traits may be regarded as sharing common genetical and environmental factors is represented by the genetic and environmental correlations r_{D_R} and r_{E_1}, respectively:

$$r_{D_a} = D_{RS,I}/(D_{RS} \cdot D_{RI})^{\frac{1}{2}}$$
$$= .42$$
$$r_{E_1} = E_{1S,I}/(E_{1S} \cdot E_{1I})^{\frac{1}{2}}$$
$$= .32.$$

Variation due to unreliability contributes to E_1 but not to D_R so we might expect the observed environmental correlation to be less than the genetic correlation. These correlations are a little less, though not considerably less, than the phenotypic correlation of .468 reported for sociability and impulsiveness by Eysenck and Eysenck (1969).

Providing we are justified in assuming the unreliability components of sociability and impulsiveness to be uncorrelated, we may correct our estimate of r_{E_1} for unreliability using the estimates of reliability given above. We now find that r_{E_1} is .66. This indicates that the unitary nature of extraversion is clearly evident in the environmental determinants of the trait, even though the genetical correlation between sociability and impulsiveness is rather less. Eaves (1973b) suggested, on the basis of a multivariate genetical analysis of monozygotic twins, that "the apparently unitary nature of extraversion at the phenotypic level could be due to environmental rather than to genetical

influences." The different analysis we have presented here confirms this conclusion.

We should perhaps clarify what this finding means. It does not necessarily support the view that extraversion is an "environmental mold" trait, to use the conception of Cattell, that is, a trait which reflects the structure of environmental influences inherent in the environment itself. We may obtain exactly the same picture because the organism, by virtue of the integration of its nervous system, *imposes* a unitary structure on externally unstructured environmental influences contributing to the development of behavior.

CONCLUSIONS

The analyses presented above suggest the following principal conclusions.

1. Genetical factors contribute both to the variation and covariation of sociability and impulsiveness.

2. Environmental factors also contribute to the covariation of sociability and impulsiveness.

3. The genetical correlation between the two factors is estimated to be .42, the environmental correlation to be .66 after correction for unreliability.

4. Combining sociability and impulsiveness scores by addition to provide a measure of extraversion provides the most powerful single means of discriminating between individuals with respect to the genetical and environmental determinants of their responses to the sociability and impulsiveness items of the questionnaire.

5. The interaction between subjects and tests has a significant genetical component, so there is some justification for regarding sociability and impulsiveness as distinguishable genetically.

Furthermore we conclude:

6. About 40% of the variation in sociability, impulsiveness, and their combinations, as measured by this questionnaire, can be attributed to genetical factors.

7. Our data are consistent with the view that the genetical variation is mainly additive.

8. We find no evidence for a large effect of the family environment on any of the traits studied, but the environmental influences

specific to individuals (including unreliability of measurement) account for about 60% of the variation.

9. Mating is effectively random for the traits in question.

10. The genetical and environmental determinants of variation are homogeneous over sexes, suggesting that the effects of sex linkage and sex limitation are negligible.

DISCUSSION

Our analysis is necessarily tentative because it is based only on monozygotic and dizygotic twins. We would be particularly cautious about discounting genotype–environment correlations as an additional source of variation. It must also be emphasized that genotype–environment interaction may well be confounded with E_1 so that variation which we have ascribed to environmental factors may itself have a genetical component. We hope to clarify this matter in the future.

Between 30% and 40% of the variation in components of extraversion may be due to environmental factors that cannot be attributed to the inconsistency of the test. All of the detectable environmental variation is specific to individuals rather than common to families. This suggests that attempts to relate extraversion to aspects of the individual's "family background" are unlikely to be productive unless the family background has a direct genetical association with extraversion. Even though we might be able to measure social and domestic factors shared by members of the same sibship, we would not expect these to be very highly correlated (say, not more than $r = .2$) with the mean extraversion score of the sibship. Consistently larger correlations between such shared environmental factors and the mean raw E scores of sibship would lead us to suspect our simple model.

Since a considerable proportion of the variation in extraversion and its components is clearly due to environmental influences specific to individuals, we could expect, in principle, to relate the intrapair differences of monozygotic twins to differences in their environmental experiences. That this is feasible in principle, however, does not aid our efforts to specify or detect such likely influences. Attempts to predict the variation in extraversion for a

random sample of individuals by measuring concomitant social or other variables, however, may be misleading, because any association we find could reflect either genetical or environmental communality of the traits in question. Merely attaching the label "social" to a trait does not constitute a prior case for environmental causation. Analyses of the kind we have conducted for the covariation of components of extraversion would have to be employed for the other variables if we were to discriminate between environmental and genetical association between extraversion and other variables in the social "environment."

The fact that between 60% and 70% of the "reliable" variation is genetically determined does not, of course, suggest which genes are involved nor what may or may not be done to modify the trait. It does, however, suggest that the segregation and recombination of alleles may be a primary cause of variation in the dimension of personality we have studied here. At the level of population biology it means that extraversion, like most other traits, reflects genetical polymorphism and as such is exposed to the directional, stabilizing or disruptive influence of natural selection. As far as we can judge from studies on other organisms (Kearsey & Kojima, 1967; Mather, 1966; 1967), we find that directional selection has been characteristically associated with the evolution of a genetical system demonstrating a large amount of directional dominance and duplicate gene interactions. When natural selection has favored intermediate phenotypes, the genetical system involves predominately additive effects, and dominance, if any, is ambidirectional. It would be too early to say whether our failure to detect nonadditive variation merely reflects the design of our study, the (relatively) low heritability, or the small amount of dominance relative to the additive variation. It may be difficult to obtain a definite answer to such questions for this trait because of the large samples required and because of the formal inability to disentangle completely the additive, dominance, and epistatic components of gene action for natural populations even when these can be raised in strictly experimenal situations (Mather, 1974). We suggest very tentatively that the polymorphism we detect for extraversion and its components may be subject to stabilizing selection because, as far as we can tell at-the-moment, the genetical variation is additive. That is, we should conclude that neither extreme introversion nor extraversion has_been favored systematically during human evolution. It is possible that without either extreme the fitness of a human population would have suffered at sometime or other. We can at least conceive of situations in which individuals of more impulsive or sociable temperament may well have promoted the survival of themselves and their close relatives. Similarly, we can imagine that there are times or situations in which it would be advantageous to have the persistent, attentive behavior characteristic of introverts. In contrast to this, we may consider a trait such as high intelligence for which there is as uggestion of directional dominance (Jinks & Eaves, 1974; Jinks & Fulker, 1970) and for which, therefore, we suspect a history of directional selection. In the case of intelligence, it is difficult to conceive of as many plausible situations in which relatively high intelligence could not confer upon an individual greater reproductive fitness than average. Such speculations about the evolutionary significance of personality are less well founded at this stage because we cannot infer the genetical system with any great degree of confidence. We believe, however, that such speculations are legitimate if they engender a more systematic and thoughtful approach to the collection and analysis of data on human behavioral traits.

REFERENCES

Carrigan, P. M. Extraversion-introversion as a dimension of personality: A reappraisal. *Psychological Bulletin*, 1960, *57*, 329–360.

Cattell, R. B. The description and measurement of personality. New York: World Book, 1946.

Cederlöf, R., Friberg, L., Jonsonn, E., & Kaij, L. Studies in similarity of diagnosis in twins with the aid of mailed questionnaires. *Acta Genetica (Basel)*, 1961, *11*, 338–362.

Claridge, G., Canter, S., & Hume, W. I. *Personality differences and biological variations: A study of twins.* New York: Pergamon Press, 1973.

Eaves, L. J. Computer simulation of sample size and experimental design in human psychogenetics. *Psychological Bulletin*, 1972, 77, 144–152.

Eaves, L. J. Assortative mating and intelligence: An analysis of pedigree data. *Heredity*, 1973, *30*, 199–210. (a)

Eaves, L. J. The structure of genotypic and environmental covariation of personality measurements: An analysis of the PEN. *British Journal of Social and Clinical Psychology*, 1973, *12*, 275–282. (b)

Eaves, L. J., & Gale, J. S. A method for analysing the genetical basis of covariation. *Behavior Genetics*, 1974, *4*, 253–267.

Eaves, L. J., & Jinks, J. L. Insignificance of evidence for differences in heritability of I.Q. between races and social classes. *Nature*, 1972, *240*, 84–88.

Eysenck, H. J. *The biological basis of personality.* Springfield, Ill.: Charles C Thomas, 1967.

Eysenck, H. J. Personality, premarital sexual permissiveness and assortative mating. *Journal of Sex Research*, 1974, *10*, 47–51.

Eysenck, H. J., & Eysenck, S. B. G. On the unitary nature of extraversion. *Acta Psychologica*, 1967, *26*, 383–390.

Eysenck, H. J., & Eysenck, S. B. G. *Personality structure and measurement.* London: Routledge & Kegan Paul, 1969.

Eysenck, S. B. G., & Eysenck, H. J. On the dual nature of extraversion. *British Journal of Social and Clinical Psychology.* 1963, *2*, 46–55.

Jinks, J. L., & Eaves, L. J. I.Q. and inequality. *Nature*, 1974, *248*, 287–289.

Jinks, J. L., & Fulker, D. W. A comparison of the biometrical genetical, MAVA and cassical approaches to the analysis of human behavior. *Psychological Bulletin*, 1970, *73*, 311–349.

Kearsey, M. J. Experimental sizes for detecting dominance variation. *Heredity*, 1970, *25*, 529–542.

Kearsey, M. J., & Kojima, K. The genetic architecture of body weight and egg hatchability in *Drosophila melangaster. Genetics*, 1967, *56*, 23–37.

Mather, K. Variability and selection. *Proceedings of the Royal Society of London, Series B*, 1966, *164*, 328–340.

Mather, K. Complementary and duplicate gene interactions in biometrical genetics. *Heredity*, 1967, *22*, 97–103.

Mather, K. Non-allelic interaction in continuous variation of randomly breeding populations. *Heredity*, 1974, *32*, 414–419.

Mather, K., & Jinks, J. L. *Biometrical Genetics.* London: Chapman Hall, 1971.

Shields, J. *Monozygotic twins.* Oxford: University Press, 1962.

Sparrow, N. H., & Ross, J. The dual nature of extraversion: A replication. *Australian Journal of Psychology*, 1964, *16*, 214–218.

(Received March 11, 1974)

From R. H. Dworkin, B. W. Burke, B. A. Maher and I. I. Gottesman (1976). Journal of Personality and Social Psychology, *34*, 510-518, *by kind permission of the authors and the American Psychological Association*

A Longitudinal Study of the Genetics of Personality

Robert H. Dworkin, Barbara W. Burke, and Brendan A. Maher
Harvard University

Irving I. Gottesman
University of Minnesota

A longitudinal twin study was conducted to determine whether personality traits with significant heritability in adolescence remain so in adulthood. A subsample of a group of twins who had been administered the Minnesota Multiphasic Personality Inventory and the California Psychological Inventory in adolescence was readministered the same two inventories 12 years later. The subsample was found to be representative of the sample from which it was drawn. Different patterns of significant heritability were found for the two ages studied: Several personality traits demonstrated evidence of significant heritability in either adolescence or adulthood, while others demonstrated evidence of significant heritability at both ages. In addition, genetic influences on the change from adolescence to adulthood were found for several personality traits. The results raise important questions for the interpretation of twin research and the understanding of genetic influences on personality development.

There has been renewed interest in the biological bases of personality (e.g., Buss & Plomin, 1975; Claridge, Canter, & Hume, 1973; Eysenck, 1967). One consequence of this is an increased reliance on the twin method in determining the importance of genetic influences on personality traits (for reviews of twin studies of personality, see Mittler, 1971, and Vandenberg, 1967). Most twin studies of personality have used adolescent twins, because of the relative ease with which such samples can be collected. An assumption of many of these studies has been that results from one age would be comparable with results from other ages. Although often implicit, this assumption has been clearly stated by Buss and Plomin (1975) and Vandenberg (1967). These authors have argued that personality traits that are under substantial genetic control at one age should remain so at other ages and should show longitudinal stability. Although not incompatible with this position, others have emphasized that the extent to which traits are under genetic control (heritability estimates) may be expected to differ from one age to another (Cavalli-Sforza & Bodmer, 1971; Gottesman, 1963, 1974; Thompson, 1967).[1] For example, Morton (1975; Rao, Morton, & Yee, 1974) has recently presented evidence suggesting that the heritability of IQ is very much lower in adults than in children; he argued that questions about heritability are meaningless without specifying the age group studied.

The issue is an important one. If twin studies at one age are inconclusive regarding genetic influences at other ages, then studies of personality using adolescent twin samples, although of interest in their own right, may yield little or no information with regard to

This research was supported in part by grants from the Milton Fund to the third author and from the Department of Psychology and Social Relations of Harvard University, and by a National Institute of Mental Health Graduate Traineeship to the first author and a Scottish Rite Fellowship for Research in Schizophrenia to the second author.

We thank Andrea L. Megela and Sarah W. Bartlett for valuable assistance at several stages of the research, Ronald S. Wilson for advice regarding data analysis, and John C. Loehlin for a critical reading of the manuscript.

Requests for reprints should be sent to Robert H. Dworkin, Department of Psychology and Social Relations, Harvard University, 33 Kirkland Street, Cambridge, Massachusetts 02138.

[1] The terms *heritability* and *genetic variance* will be used interchangeably in this article. Strictly speaking, the terms are not equivalent; the twin study method as it is typically used estimates genetic variance (Cavalli-Sforza & Bodmer, 1971).

the importance of genetic influences on adult personality. Indeed, even when personality traits are examined in an adult twin sample (e.g., Eaves & Eysenck, 1975), the age range studied should perhaps be as narrow as feasible, since it might be the case that the degree of heritability varies at different ages within the span of adulthood. It is also possible that whether a trait is under genetic control at all varies as a function of the age at which it is studied. If the latter possibility proved to be true, reviews of twin studies that investigate, without regard to age, whether a given personality trait shows a significant degree of heritability in several different samples would have to be reexamined, taking into account the ages of the twins studied.

The question of the comparability of estimates of the heritability of personality traits obtained at different ages has been examined by several authors who have divided their twin samples into older and younger groups (Buss, Plomin, & Willerman, 1973; Claridge et al., 1973; Partanen, Bruun, & Markkanen, 1966; Willerman, 1973). Results from this type of investigation have been equivocal, often because of the small sample sizes resulting when twin pairs are divided into two groups. Because these investigations were not initially designed to examine the question of age effects in the heritability of personality, the age analyses typically involved dividing the sample at the mean age and hence did not usually compare meaningful age groups. Another strategy has been to administer, to one age twin sample, a personality measure for which twin data already exist for a different age twin sample. In only two instances has this type of comparison been made. Reznikoff and Honeyman (1967) administered the Minnesota Multiphasic Personality Inventory (MMPI) to a small sample of adult twins and compared their findings with Gottesman's (1963) results for adolescent twins. They concluded that the comparison substantiated Gottesman's conjecture that the extrapolation of his findings on adolescents to adults would probably not be appropriate. Horn, Plomin, and Rosenman (1976) compared their results on the heritability of the California Psycho-

logical Inventory (CPI) scales in an adult male sample with those obtained by Nichols (1966) for high school boys. They concluded that the average differences between the intraclass correlations for monozygotic (MZ) and dizygotic (DZ) twins were approximately the same in both samples. We calculated the Spearman rank-order correlation coefficient of the heritabilities obtained in the two studies, a more sensitive index of the extent to which the results of the studies are similar, and found it to be nonsignificant ($r_s = .29$).

Given the sensitivity of estimates of heritability to sampling considerations and numerous genetic and environmental factors (Fuller & Thompson, 1960), conclusions about the comparability of such estimates obtained from these types of cross-sectional investigations are understandably inconclusive. In order to determine whether the personality traits that show evidence of significant heritability at one age are also under significant genetic control at another, a longitudinal investigation was conducted. A subsample of a group of twins who had been administered two personality inventories in adolescence was readministered the same two inventories approximately 12 years later. There has not been a previous longitudinal investigation of the heritability of personality traits using personality inventories, and it was hoped that the results of this study would speak to the questions raised above regarding the nature of genetic influences on personality at different points in the life cycle and the extrapolation of the results of twin studies from one age group to another.

METHOD

Subjects

In 1961 and 1962 Gottesman administered the MMPI and CPI to a sample of 178 high school age same-sex twin pairs in the Boston area (Gottesman, 1965, 1966). Of the 147 pairs for which both twins had valid MMPIs in adolescence (see Gottesman, 1966, for the criteria used in determining validity), 43 pairs were located at follow-up and readministered the two inventories. One of these pairs was dropped from further analysis because of an invalid MMPI for one of the twins at follow-up. Of the 42 remaining pairs of twins with valid MMPIs at both initial and follow-up testing, 25 pairs were MZ (16 female, 9 male) and 17 pairs were DZ (8 female, 9 male).

The original twin sample was collected through cooperating school systems, advertisements in neighborhood newspapers, and Mothers of Twins Clubs. Additional sampling and demographic data are reported by Gottesman (1966). The zygosity of most of the pairs in the original sample was established by extensive blood grouping. For reasons of economy, some pairs who were clearly MZ or DZ were not blood typed. The average age of the 42 retested pairs when seen in adolescence was 15.9 years and when seen at follow-up was 27.9 years.

Procedure

At both the initial and follow-up contacts, most twins were administered the MMPI and CPI in groups of varying size. At follow-up several twins were individually tested. Both inventories were completed in a single session, the CPI always being administered first. A few twins were mailed the two inventories with instructions on how to complete them in their homes. Biographical information was collected at both ages. Twins were paid for their participation at both contacts.

Data Analysis

Evidence of significant heritability in the MMPI and CPI scales was assessed by two complementary techniques (Gottesman, 1963). For each personality scale, the intraclass correlation coefficients for the MZ pairs and the DZ pairs were calculated with the formula suggested by Haggard (1958). The MZ intraclass correlation coefficients (R_{MZ}) and the DZ intraclass correlation coefficients (R_{DZ}) for each scale were then transformed into z scores. Whether R_{MZ} is significantly greater than R_{DZ}, as the genetic hypothesis predicts, was tested with a one-tailed test. In addition, the F ratio consisting of the DZ within-pair mean square divided by the MZ within-pair mean square, which has been widely used as a significance test for the presence of genetic variance in twin data, is also reported for each scale. Because there is some dispute in the literature regarding the relative merits of these two approaches (e.g., compare Christian, Kang, & Norton, 1974, with Jinks & Fulker, 1970), both are presented here.

Quantitative estimates of heritability are not reported. Loehlin, Lindzey, and Spuhler (1975) and Eaves (1972) have shown that the confidence limits around estimates of heritability are very wide with samples of the size typically used in twin studies. Given the small sample size on which our data are based, we have limited our analyses to determining the presence of significant genetic variance for the personality traits studied and have not attempted a numerical estimate of the extent of genetic variance present. However, both Holzinger's (1929) and Falconer's (1960) estimates of heritability can be easily calculated from the data we present. Another consequence of the small sample size is the impossibility of analyzing the data for sex differences, although we realize that they are important for some traits (Gottesman, 1963, 1966).

RESULTS

Representativeness of the Retested Subsample

Since the sample of retested pairs is only 29% of the sample of pairs with valid MMPIs at the initial testing, the demonstration that this subsample is a representative one is essential for interpreting subsequent findings. In Figure 1 the mean MMPI profiles for males and females for the entire sample of 178 pairs and for the retested subsample at adolescence are presented. The norms used are those given by Dahlstrom, Welsh, and Dahlstrom (1972) for 16-year-olds, without K correction. As can be seen from the figure, in adolescence the subsample that was retested in adulthood was very similar to the entire adolescent sample. The slight but consistently greater elevation of the entire sample when compared with the subsample is a result of the fact that the subsample was drawn from only those pairs in the sample having valid MMPIs. This is made especially clear by the differences between the subsample and entire sample on the L and F scales, since these were the scales used in establishing validity. Figure 1 also demonstrates what many twin studies have neglected to examine: that the sample of twins studied is representative of the population in general, in this case, the population of 16-year-old adolescents. This is true for both the entire sample of twins and for the subsample.

Although the comparison of the mean MMPI profile of the subsample at adolescence with the mean MMPI profile of the entire sample has demonstrated substantial similarity, another method exists for assessing the representativeness of the subsample. This is to determine whether the personality scales that showed significant evidence of genetic variance in the subsample at adolescence are the same as those that showed significant evidence of genetic variance in the entire sample. For the original sample of pairs with valid MMPIs at adolescence, six of the MMPI clinical scales and six CPI scales demonstrated statistically significant evidence of genetic variance (see Gottesman, 1965, 1966, and revised values in Table 1). For the retested subsample's adolescent data, four of these six MMPI scales and three of

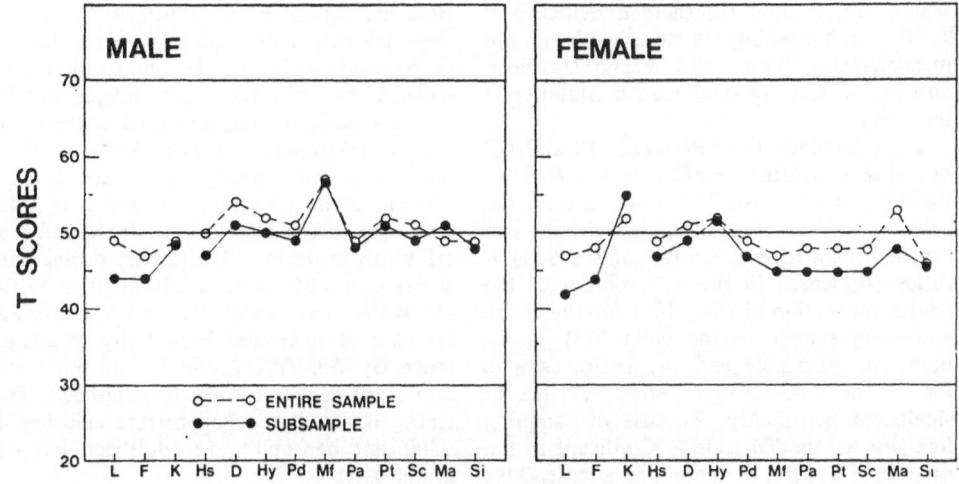

FIGURE 1. Mean Minnesota Multiphasic Personality Inventory profiles for retested subsample at adolescence and entire sample at adolescence. (T scores, with a mean of 50 and a standard deviation of 10, are based on norms for 16-year-olds, without K correction.)

these six CPI scales were also significant. Given the small size of the retested sample, these results provide further evidence of its representativeness.

Homogeneity of Variance

Inasmuch as heterogeneity of the total variances of the MZ and DZ pairs invalidates the model on which twin study data analysis is based (Kempthorne & Osborne, 1961), the F ratio of these variances for each scale at each age was calculated (the method suggested by Haseman and Elston, 1970, was used). Of the 66 two-tailed tests calculated, 5 were significant at the .05 level. Only 2 of these, the tests for MMPI scales Pa and A at adolescence, were for scales that demonstrated evidence of significant genetic variance.

Comparison of Adolescent and Adult Twin Data

With respect to the adolescent subsample that was retested in adulthood, Table 1 shows MZ and DZ intraclass correlation coefficients and F ratios for the 10 MMPI clinical scales, the K scale, and four research scales. These data can be compared with the F ratios (presented in the last column of the

adolescent section of the table) for the entire adolescent sample having valid MMPIs (cf. Gottesman, 1965, for preliminary analysis). In both the subsample and the entire sample, the D, Pd, Pa, and Sc scales show evidence of significant heritability. Because of sampling fluctuations, the Mf scale is significant in the subsample but not in the entire sample, while the Hy and Si scales are significant in the entire sample but not in the subsample.

The adolescent data for the subsample demonstrate that the significance of the F ratio and the significance of the difference between R_{MZ} and R_{DZ} do not always correspond. This is a function of both the small sample size and, presumably, some nonsignificant heterogeneity of variance. Another consequence of the small sample size is that several of the R_{DZ}s are zero or negative when there is evidence of significant heritability, a finding that with a larger sample would be considered counter to the genetic expectation.

When the adult MMPI results presented in Table 1 are examined, a different pattern of heritabilities emerges. The clinical scales for which there was evidence of significant heritability in adolescence are not under significant genetic control in adulthood. For three

A LONGITUDINAL STUDY OF THE GENETICS OF PERSONALITY

scales, *Ma, K,* and *Es,* there is evidence of significant heritability in adulthood but not in adolescence. Two scales, *A* and *Dy,* demonstrate evidence of significant heritability at both ages.

Table 2 reports the adolescent MZ and DZ intraclass correlation coefficients and *F* ratios for the 18 CPI scales. These data are for the subsample that was retested in adulthood and can be compared with Gottesman's (1966) *F* ratios (presented in the last column of the adolescent section of the table) for the entire adolescent sample having valid MMPIs. In both the subsample and the entire sample, the *Do, Sy,* and *Sa* scales show evidence of significant heritability. Because of sampling fluctuations, the *To* scale is significant in the subsample but not in the entire sample. This is also the case for *Ai* and *Ie,* although there was evidence of significant heritability for these scales in the female subset of the original sample. Three scales, *Sp, So,* and *Gi,* were significant in the entire adolescent sample but not in the subsample.

As was true for the MMPI, when the adult CPI results presented in Table 2 are compared with the adolescent data, different patterns of heritability emerge. The only CPI scale with significant genetic variance in both adolescence and adulthood is *Do.* The results for the *Sc* and *Gi* scales are not clear-cut:

Both are significant in adulthood but not in the adolescent subsample; however, there is evidence of significant heritability for the *Gi* scale in the entire adolescent sample and for the *Sc* scale in the female subset of the entire sample (Gottesman, 1966). Both of these findings are most simply interpreted as a result of sampling fluctuations, and it is probably best to consider both of these scales as exhibiting evidence of heritability during both adolescence and adulthood, in addition to the *Do* scale. Five scales for which there was evidence of significant heritability in adolescence, *Sy, Sa, To, Ai,* and *Ie,* are not under significant genetic control in adulthood. Two scales, *Wb* and *Py,* demonstrate evidence of significant heritability in adulthood but not in adolescence.

The results of the preceding analyses are summarized in Table 3. The different patterns of significant heritability that were found in adolescence and adulthood are a function of changes in both MZ and DZ similarity. As shown by the intraclass correlations and within-pair mean squares in Tables 1 and 2, MZ similarity tends to increase with age, while DZ similarity tends to decrease for the MMPI and CPI scales that are significant in adulthood but not in adolescence. For the MMPI scales that are significant in adolescence but not in adulthood, DZ similarity

TABLE 1

ADOLESCENT AND ADULT MINNESOTA MULTIPHASIC PERSONALITY INVENTORY INTRACLASS
CORRELATION COEFFICIENTS AND *F* RATIOS

	Adolescent						Adult				
Scale	R_{MZ}[a]	R_{DZ}	MZ within-pair MS	DZ within-pair MS	F (17, 25)	F[b] (68, 79)	R_{MZ}[a]	R_{DZ}	MZ within-pair MS	DZ within-pair MS	F (17, 25)
Hypochondriasis (*Hs*)	.07	.47	36.48	39.09	1.07	1.00	.42	.30	30.20	55.65	1.84
Depression (*D*)	.43	.15	34.10	92.27	2.71*	1.80**	.49	.56	42.50	37.29	.88
Hysteria (*Hy*)	.23	.20	35.08	69.62	1.98	1.51*	.16	.40	53.36	46.68	.87
Psychopathic Deviate (*Pd*)	.49	.30	32.62	75.44	2.31*	1.64*	.44	.34	58.66	68.21	1.16
Masculinity–Femininity (*Mf*)	.64*	.17	37.82	106.97	2.83**	1.36	.79	.81	34.34	42.97	1.25
Paranoia (*Pa*)	.19	−.19	52.56	161.21	3.07**	1.69*	.21	−.27	91.20	68.09	.75
Psychasthenia (*Pt*)	.41	.14	51.30	77.15	1.50	1.46	.28	.19	71.54	75.32	1.05
Schizophrenia (*Sc*)	.47	.24	47.08	100.44	2.13*	1.48*	−.15	.55	76.04	50.32	.66
Hypomania (*Ma*)	.46	.31	57.76	91.32	1.58	1.17	.72**	.08	37.44	76.79	2.05*
Social Introversion (*Si*)	.45	.26	33.04	50.56	1.53	1.69*	.50	.25	44.14	67.35	1.53
K	.45	.29	53.62	47.32	.88	1.13	.47**	−.27	47.42	73.82	1.56
Anxiety (*A*)	.58*	−.04	49.20	54.06	1.10	1.12	.71**	.00	25.42	69.88	2.75*
Repression (*R*)	.37	−.04	81.22	92.03	1.13	1.24	.40	.12	50.58	74.88	1.48
Ego Strength (*Es*)	.35	.14	43.24	72.50	1.68	1.35	.53*	−.06	30.12	63.82	2.12*
Dependency (*Dy*)	.53**	−.21	53.92	72.85	1.35	.85	.76**	−.05	26.26	86.18	3.28**

Note. MZ = monozygotic; DZ = dizygotic.
[a] Significance levels given in R_{MZ} column are for $R_{MZ} > R_{DZ}$.
[b] Revised values for entire adolescent sample (cf. Gottesman, 1963, for preliminary analysis).
* *p* < .05.
** *p* < .01.

DWORKIN, BURKE, MAHER, AND GOTTESMAN

TABLE 2

ADOLESCENT AND ADULT CALIFORNIA PSYCHOLOGICAL INVENTORY INTRACLASS CORRELATION
COEFFICIENTS AND F RATIOS

	Adolescent						Adult				
Scale	R_{MZ}[a]	R_{DZ}	MZ within-pair MS	DZ within-pair MS	F (17, 25)	F[b] (68, 79)	R_{MZ}[a]	R_{DZ}	MZ within-pair MS	DZ within-pair MS	F (17, 25)
Dominance (Do)	.62	.45	34.62	76.41	2.21*	1.95**	.70**	.09	46.06	125.03	2.71*
Capacity for Status (Cs)	.64	.64	49.74	67.74	1.36	1.34	.40	.45	53.94	53.94	.68
Sociability (Sy)	.61	.24	30.08	84.85	2.82**	1.97**	.29	.21	64.40	68.24	1.06
Social Presence (Sp)	.39	.52	60.82	42.53	.70	1.55*	.47	.43	51.44	57.09	1.11
Self-Acceptance (Sa)	.66	.44	38.78	83.32	2.12*	1.85**	.48	.33	74.90	78.09	1.04
Sense of Well-Being (Wb)	.56	.35	84.20	87.29	1.04	1.11	.65**	−.01	35.92	91.59	2.55*
Responsibility (Re)	.77	.61	25.94	48.74	1.88	1.35	.43	−.03	48.64	66.59	1.37
Socialization (So)	.51	.31	41.84	83.35	1.99	1.48*	.69	.46	31.86	46.06	1.45
Self-Control (Sc)	.57	.26	49.04	68.03	1.39	1.38	.62**	−.16	40.98	106.50	2.60*
Tolerance (To)	.75*	.29	45.32	98.91	2.18*	1.37	.42	−.06	70.18	50.44	.72
Good Impression (Gi)	.40	.33	51.82	55.85	1.08	1.60*	.46*	−.14	57.38	108.00	1.88
Communality (Cm)	−.05	−.07	56.44	56.44	1.00	1.23	.22	.29	48.66	21.18	.44
Achievement via Conformance (Ac)	.49	.57	77.38	48.82	.63	.87	.43	.05	57.76	83.41	1.47
Achievement via Independence (Ai)	.70*	.16	48.24	144.77	3.00**	1.31	.41	−.02	67.80	84.35	1.24
Intellectual Efficiency (Ie)	.78*	.33	36.42	87.71	2.41*	1.22	.54	.15	49.62	49.24	.99
Psychological Mindedness (Py)	.37	.04	77.72	72.15	.93	1.46	.45*	−.10	48.52	79.59	1.64
Flexibility (Fx)	.40	.46	60.48	71.15	1.18	1.17	.56	.31	76.80	95.56	1.24
Femininity (Fe)	.42	.55	55.84	57.29	1.03	1.36	.32	.18	59.32	36.74	.62

Note. MZ = monozygotic; DZ = dizygotic.
[a] Significance levels given in R_{MZ} column are for $R_{MZ} > R_{DZ}$.
[b] Values for entire adolescent sample (Gottesman, 1966).
* $p < .05$.
** $p < .01$.

tends to increase with age, while there is no consistent trend in MZ similarity. For the CPI scales that are significant in adolescence but not in adulthood, MZ similarity tends to decrease with age, while there is no consistent trend in DZ similarity. The relationship between changes in twin similarity with repeated measurements and heritability has been discussed by Thompson and Wilde (1973).

Twin Similarity in Personality Change

Wilson (1968, 1974) has developed an analysis of variance for longitudinal twin data that yields values for R_{MZ} and R_{DZ} reflecting twin similarity in the pattern of change over age. With data for two ages, as in the present study, this analysis is equivalent to an analysis of variance of difference scores between the two ages (Winer, 1971). The 15 MMPI scales and the 18 CPI scales were each analyzed for adolescence-to-adulthood change by this method, and whether R_{MZ} was significantly greater than R_{DZ} was tested for each scale. For five MMPI scales, Hs, A, R, Es, and Dy, and two CPI scales, Wb and To, MZ similarity was significantly greater than DZ similarity at the .05 level, one-tailed test. This indicates that for these scales, the change in

score from adolescence to adulthood is under significant genetic control. That the A and Dy scales show significant heritability in the retested subsample in both adolescence and adulthood as well as significant heritability for adolescence-to-adulthood personality change supports the importance of genetic influences on these scales. Data for the Hs, R, Es, Wb, and To scales suggest that the development

TABLE 3

SCALES WITH SIGNIFICANT F RATIOS OR $R_{MZ} > R_{DZ}$
IN ADOLESCENCE AND/OR ADULTHOOD

	Scales with significant Fs or $R_{MZ} > R_{DZ}$		
Inventory	Adolescence only	Adulthood only	Adolescence and adulthood
MMPI	D, Pd, Pa, Sc, Mf,[a] Hy,[b] Si[b]	Ma, K, Es	A,[a] Dy[a]
CPI	Sy, Sa, To,[a] Sp,[b] So,[b] Ai,[d] Ie[d]	Wb, Py	Do, Sc,[c] Gi[b]

Note. For first and third columns, scales had significant F ratios or $R_{MZ} > R_{DZ}$ in both the entire adolescent sample and the adolescent subsample, unless otherwise noted. MMPI = Minnesota Multiphasic Personality Inventory; CPI = California Psychological Inventory.
[a] Significant in subsample only.
[b] Significant in entire adolescent sample only.
[c] Significant in female subset of entire adolescent sample only.
[d] Significant in subsample and female subset of entire adolescent sample only.

A LONGITUDINAL STUDY OF THE GENETICS OF PERSONALITY

of some traits may have a significant genetic component even though cross-sectional assessments of the heritability of these personality traits are not significant at both ages.

DISCUSSION

The most important result of this study is that different patterns of significant heritability were found in adolescence and adulthood. Three meaningful clusters of scales were found to be under significant genetic control in adolescence but not in adulthood: MMPI clinical scales originally constructed to assess psychopathology, CPI scales that are related to sociability, and CPI scales associated with achievement and intelligence. Exceptions to these generalizations were the MMPI *Ma* scale, significant in adulthood only, and the CPI *Do* scale, significant at both ages. A fourth group of scales was found to be under significant genetic control in adulthood but not in adolescence: several MMPI and CPI scales commonly thought to reflect emotional stability, self-confidence, and insightfulness. The characterization of the scales that demonstrated significant heritability in both adolescence and adulthood is less clear-cut. The three scales best representing the first factors of the MMPI and CPI (scale *A* for the MMPI and *Sc* and *Gi* for the CPI; Dahlstrom, Welsh, & Dahlstrom, 1975; Megargee, 1972) are included in the group of five scales for which there was evidence of significant heritability at both ages. This suggests that the major sources of variance in these two inventories correspond to traits that have a significant degree of genetic variance in both adolescence and adulthood.

In general, these patterns of significant heritability are supported by other investigations. In a cross-sectional twin study of the MMPI using a Minneapolis adolescent twin sample, Gottesman (1963) found evidence of significant heritability for the *D, Pd, Pt, Sc, Si,* and *A* scales. With the exception of *Pt,* these scales were also under significant genetic control in the Boston adolescent sample. As with our adult sample, Reznikoff and Honeyman (1967) failed to find significant heritability in their adult sample for the MMPI scales that are significant in the Minneapolis and Boston adolescent samples.

Nichols (1966) reported substantial heritability for the group of CPI scales related to sociability and, to a lesser extent, for the scales related to achievement and intelligence in a large sample of adolescent twins. Although Horn et al. (1976) have studied the CPI in 45- to 55-year-old twins, the substantially younger age of our adult twins makes any comparison inconclusive.

It is important to point out that while we have discussed the results in terms of the presence or absence of significant heritability at one or both ages, the small sample size involved makes it impossible to distinguish between the presence of genetic variance that is not statistically significant and the absence of any genetic variance at all. In other words, we have not shown that personality traits that are under genetic control at one age may be under no genetic control at another. However, we have demonstrated that there are substantial changes with age in which personality traits show evidence of significant heritability.[2]

How can such age effects in genetic variance in personality traits be explained? Since a change in any of the components of the total phenotypic variance will affect the value of the genetic variance, several explanations of the results are possible. Perhaps most appealing, but also most difficult to prove, is that the changes in genetic variance with age are a function of gene regulation (see Gottesman, 1974), genotype–environment interaction and correlation, and/or epistasis (interactions between genes at two or more loci). It is also possible that when compared with either initial or final levels, development is associated with an increase in genetic influences on a trait (Gottesman, 1963; Vandenberg & Falkner, 1965). If this were the case, it would be expected that a greater number

---

[2] Because the adult sample is considerably smaller than the original adolescent sample, certain scales (*Hs, Si,* and *Ac*) have *F* ratios that while not significant in the adult sample, would have been significant in a sample the size of the larger adolescent sample. However, even if we consider these scales as exhibiting significant genetic variance in adulthood, the patterns of significant heritability described above are not substantially altered.

of traits are under genetic control in adolescence, as was found in this study, since this is a period when rate of development is accelerated.

Changes in other components of the phenotypic variance could also account for the results. Fuller and Thompson (1960) pointed out that heritability will decline both as a function of increases in the environmental variance, which can be brought about by relaxing environmental controls, and as a result of changing from an expressive environment to a suppressive one. Heritability can be increased by corresponding reductions in the environmental variance and by changing from a suppressive environment to an expressive one. It can also be argued that MZ twins are more similar in personality than DZ twins because their shared environment is more similar. As adolescent twins become adults this similarity is less likely to occur; thus there appears to be a reduction in the heritability of personality traits. This explanation fails to account for the finding of significant heritability for several MMPI and CPI scales in adulthood but not in adolescence and for the meaningful patterns that emerged.

One final interpretation of the results should be mentioned. That a given MMPI or CPI scale exhibits significant heritability at one age but not at another might be the result of the scale measuring two different traits at the two ages (or conceivably, one trait at one age but nothing reliable at the other). Correlational and multivariate longitudinal analyses that can be expected to shed light on this question are in progress.

It is not possible from the data collected in this study to determine which of the explanations offered above account for the results. However, this research has furnished the first set of data suggesting that age is a variable that must be considered in future research on the genetics of personality. It is no longer possible to assume that studies of the heritability of personality traits in one age group yield valid information with regard to other age groups, and it is no longer meaningful to review twin studies of personality without taking into account the ages of the different

samples studied (Scarr, 1969; Vandenberg, 1967). Prospective longitudinal twin studies with large samples and longitudinal adoption studies have the potential to specify in greater detail the nature of the changes in the heritability of personality with age and thereby answer the many questions that this research has raised.

REFERENCES

Buss, A. H., & Plomin, R. *A temperament theory of personality development.* New York: Wiley, 1975.

Buss, A. H., Plomin, R., & Willerman, L. The inheritance of temperaments. *Journal of Personality,* 1973, *41,* 513–524.

Cavalli-Sforza, L. L., & Bodmer, W. F. *The genetics of human populations.* San Francisco: W. H. Freeman, 1971.

Christian, J. C., Kang, K. W., & Norton, J. A., Jr. Choice of an estimate of genetic variance from twin data. *American Journal of Human Genetics,* 1974, *26,* 154–161.

Claridge, G., Canter, S., & Hume, W. I. *Personality differences and biological variations: A study of twins.* Oxford, England: Pergamon Press, 1973.

Dahlstrom, W. G., Welsh, G. S., & Dahlstrom, L. E. *An MMPI handbook* (Vol. 1: Clinical interpretation). Minneapolis: University of Minnesota Press, 1972.

Dahlstrom, W. G., Welsh, G. S., & Dahlstrom, L. E. *An MMPI handbook* (Vol 2: Research applications). Minneapolis: University of Minnesota Press, 1975.

Eaves, L. J. Computer simulation of sample size and experimental design in human psychogenetics. *Psychological Bulletin,* 1972, 77, 144–152.

Eaves, L., & Eysenck, H. The nature of extraversion: A genetical analysis. *Journal of Personality and Social Psychology,* 1975, *32,* 102–112.

Eysenck, H. J. *The biological basis of personality.* Springfield, Ill.: Charles C Thomas, 1967.

Falconer, D. S. *Introduction to quantitative genetics.* New York: Ronald Press, 1960.

Fuller, J. L., & Thompson, W. R. *Behavior genetics.* New York: Wiley, 1960.

Gottesman, I. I. Heritability of personality: A demonstration. *Psychological Monographs,* 1963, 77(9, Whole No. 572).

Gottesman, I. I. Personality and natural selection. In S. G. Vandenberg (Ed.), *Methods and goals in human behavior genetics.* New York: Academic Press, 1965.

Gottesman, I. I. Genetic variance in adaptive personality traits. *Journal of Child Psychology and Psychiatry,* 1966, 7, 199–208.

Gottesman, I. I. Developmental genetics and ontogenetic psychology: Overdue détente and propositions from a matchmaker. In A. D. Pick (Ed.), *Minnesota Symposia on Child Psychology* (Vol. 8). Minneapolis: University of Minnesota Press, 1974.

A LONGITUDINAL STUDY OF THE GENETICS OF PERSONALITY

Haggard, E. A. *Intraclass correlation and the analysis of variance.* New York: Dryden, 1958.

Haseman, J. K., & Elston, R. C. The estimation of genetic variance from twin data. *Behavior Genetics,* 1970, *1*, 11–19.

Holzinger, K. J. The relative effect of nature and nurture influences on twin differences. *Journal of Educational Psychology,* 1929, *20*, 241–248.

Horn, J. M., Plomin, R., & Rosenman, R. Heritability of personality traits in adult male twins. *Behavior Genetics,* 1976, *6*, 17–30.

Jinks, J. L., & Fulker, D. W. Comparison of the biometrical genetical, MAVA, and classical approaches to the analysis of human behavior. *Psychological Bulletin,* 1970, *73*, 311–349.

Kempthorne, O., & Osborne, R. H. The interpretation of twin data. *American Journal of Human Genetics,* 1961, *13*, 320–339.

Loehlin, J. C., Lindzey, G., & Spuhler, J. N. *Race differences in intelligence.* San Francisco: W. H. Freeman, 1975.

Megargee, E. I. *The California Psychological Inventory handbook.* San Francisco: Jossey-Bass, 1972.

Mittler, P. *The study of twins.* Baltimore, Md.: Penguin, 1971.

Morton, N. E. Analysis of family resemblance and group differences. *Social Biology,* 1975, *22*, 111–116.

Nichols, R. C. The resemblance of twins in personality and interests. *National Merit Scholarship Corporation Research Reports,* 1966, *2*, 1–23.

Partanen, J., Bruun, K., & Markkanen, T. *Inheritance of drinking behavior.* Helsinki: Finnish Foundation for Alcohol Studies. 1966.

Rao, D. C., Morton, N. E., & Yee, S. Analysis of family resemblance. II: A linear model for familial correlation. *American Journal of Human Genetics,* 1974, *26*, 311–359.

Reznikoff, M., & Honeyman, M. S. MMPI profiles of monozygotic and dizygotic twin pairs. *Journal of Consulting Psychology,* 1967, *31*, 100.

Scarr, S. Social introversion-extraversion as a heritable response. *Child Development,* 1969, *40*, 823–832.

Thompson, W. R. Development and the biophysical bases of personality. In E. F. Borgatta & W. W. Lambert (Eds.), *Handbook of personality theory and research.* Chicago: Rand-McNally, 1967.

Thompson, W. R., & Wilde, G. J. S. Behavior genetics. In B. B. Wolman (Ed.), *Handbook of general psychology.* Englewood Cliffs, N.J.: Prentice-Hall, 1973.

Vandenberg, S. G. Hereditary factors in normal personality traits (as measured by inventories). In J. Wortis (Ed.), *Recent advances in biological psychiatry* (Vol. 9). New York: Plenum Press, 1967.

Vandenberg, S. G., & Falkner, F. Hereditary factors in human growth. *Human Biology,* 1965, *37*, 357–365.

Willerman, L. Activity level and hyperactivity in twins. *Child Development,* 1973, *44*, 288–293.

Wilson, R. S. Autonomic research with twins: Methods of analysis. In S. G. Vandenberg (Ed.), *Progress in human behavior genetics.* Baltimore, Md.: The Johns Hopkins Press, 1968.

Wilson, R. S. Twins: Mental development in the preschool years. *Developmental Psychology,* 1974, *10*, 580–588.

Winer, B. J. *Statistical principles in experimental design* (2nd ed.). New York: McGraw-Hill, 1971.

(Received January 15, 1976)